The Etruscans and the History of Dentistry

"This study is vitally important for our knowledge of the history of dentistry, especially for the Etruscan period. It is extensively researched and combines the subjects of biological anthropology, medical history and material cultural studies to provide a rounded approach to the history of dentistry. This book is a valuable contribution to scholarship on ancient perceptions of dental health and conceptions of beauty and is highly recommended for anyone interested in the medical humanities."

Dr. Patty Baker, *University of Kent, UK*

The Etruscans and the History of Dentistry offers a study of the construction and use of gold dental appliances in ancient Etruscan culture, and their place within the framework of a general history of dentistry, with special emphasis on appliances, from Bronze Age Mesopotamia and Egypt to modern Europe and the Americas. Included are many of the ancient literary sources that refer to dentistry—or the lack thereof—in Greece and Rome, as well as the archaeological evidence of ancient dental health. The book challenges many past works in exposing modern scholars' fallacies about ancient dentistry, while presenting the incontrovertible evidence of the Etruscans' seemingly modern attitudes to cosmetic dentistry.

Marshall Joseph Becker is Emeritus Professor of Anthropology at West Chester University, USA, and is a Distinguished Member of the American Anthropological Association.

Jean MacIntosh Turfa is Lecturer in Classical Studies at the University of Pennsylvania, USA, where she is also a Consulting Scholar in the Mediterranean Section of the University Museum.

Routledge Monographs in Classical Studies

Rome and Provincial Resistance
Gil Gambash

The Origins of Ancient Greek Science
Michael Boylan

Athens Transformed, 404–262 BC: From Popular Sovereignty to the Dominion of the Elite
Phillip Harding

Translating Classical Plays: The Collected Papers
J. Michael Walton

Athens: The City as University
Niall Livingstone

Forthcoming:

Resemblance and Reality in Greek Thought
Arum Park

Attic Oratory and Performance
Andreas Serafim

Childhood in Antiquity
Lesley Beaumont, Nicola Harrington, and Matthew Dillon

TransAntiquity: Cross-Dressing and Transgender Dynamics in the Ancient World
Domitilla Campanile, Filippo Carlà-Uhink, and Margherita Facella

Aeschylus and War: Comparative Perspectives on Seven Against Thebes
Isabelle Torrance

The Etruscans and the History of Dentistry

The Golden Smile through the Ages

Marshall Joseph Becker and Jean MacIntosh Turfa

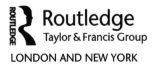
Routledge
Taylor & Francis Group

LONDON AND NEW YORK

First published 2017 by Routledge

2 Park Square, Milton Park, Abingdon, Oxfordshire OX14 4RN

52 Vanderbilt Avenue, New York, NY 10017

Routledge is an imprint of the Taylor & Francis Group, an informa business

First issued in paperback 2020

British Library Cataloguing-in-Publication Data
A catalogue record for this book is available from the British Library

Library of Congress Cataloging-in-Publication Data
Names: Becker, Marshall Joseph, author. | Turfa, Jean MacIntosh, 1947– author.
Title: The Etruscans and the history of dentistry: the golden smile through the ages/by Marshall Joseph Becker and Jean MacIntosh Turfa.
Other titles: Routledge monographs in classical studies.
Description: Abingdon, Oxon; New York, NY: Routledge, 2017. |
Series: Routledge monographs in classical studies | Includes bibliographical references and index.
Identifiers: LCCN 2016031094| ISBN 9781138677913 (hardback: alk. paper) | ISBN 9781315559254 (ebook)
Subjects: | MESH: Dental Prosthesis—history | Gold Alloys—history | Esthetics, Dental—history | Prosthesis Design—history | History, Ancient | Western World—history | Italy
Classification: LCC RK651 | NLM WU 11 GI8 | DDC 617.6/9—dc23
LC record available at https://lccn.loc.gov/2016031094

ISBN: 978-1-138-67791-3 (hbk)
ISBN: 978-0-367-59532-6 (pbk)

Typeset in Times New Roman
by Swales & Willis Ltd, Exeter, Devon, UK

In memory of our parents,
and of
Tamara Launags, DDS,
and Arthur R. Marsilio, DDS

Contents

Illustrations

Figures

Tables

Preface

The intensive study of what many would consider a marginal aspect, a curiosity, of Etruscan civilization—ancient "false teeth"—has resulted in some major reversals of past opinions on ancient life.

Our research into the unusual finds of Etruscan gold-band dental appliances, both bridges and braces, has led to our own discoveries of some startling aspects of the ancient world and insights into modern dentistry. We have formed a new respect for the significance of Etruscan culture for the history of society and technology, in spite of the fact that we cannot link the Etruscans (or any pre-Roman culture) to any formal practice of dentistry or oral medicine (that is one surprise). Other shocks: the ancient Egyptians never made or used "false teeth" and certainly never practiced any sort of dentistry—this is confirmed by respected Egyptologists, in spite of the glib comments of popular or ill-informed writers. The Etruscans, a first-millennium BCE Italian culture different in language, wealth and customs from all their neighbors, were the first and nearly the only people to attempt the replacement of lost teeth or the permanent securing of loose teeth, and they seem to have applied the most advanced technology of their day to this procedure. The experts who produced appliances were Etruscan and Italic goldsmiths—there were no dentists or dental surgeons. (The earliest *known* "practitioner" was an unnamed barber–surgeon, not a doctor or dentist, who operated out of a shop-front on the Roman Forum in the early days of the Empire.)

In terms of dentistry and medicine, this exposes a perplexing situation: in the history of dentistry there were no serious attempts at tooth replacement until essentially the modern era, except for the brief flourishing of Etruscan civilization, when, over a period of perhaps five centuries, a few scores of women of the ruling classes of society wore golden appliances to replace their front teeth. The first and the most useful (and showy) appliances began in central Italy in the seventh century BC. These women were the only ones flashing golden bling. No wonder Etruria's women got racy reputations among the Greek and Roman writers! By the first centuries BCE–CE, some of the Roman satirists were criticizing their own socialites for pathetic attempts to cover up age with false teeth—yet only a single burial has ever been found of a Roman woman wearing such things. Likewise, Late Antique Jewish texts mention women inserting false teeth, although no such actual bridges have ever been found. Greek medical writers mentioned shoring up loosened teeth with gold wire, but, besides the Roman example, only six such wire appliances (plus one in silver wire) have been found—in Phoenicia, Egypt and Greece. All came centuries later than the development of the more substantial Etruscan gold-band appliances.

The Etruscan appliances were made, and presumably installed, by goldsmiths who for just this purpose perfected techniques of purifying gold that greatly exceeded the standards applied to the gold jewelry for which they were justly famous. Again, we did not know this until our research led to the application of new analytical techniques in 2015 in the laboratory of the University of Liverpool's Department of Archaeology, Classics and Egyptology. (We hope this will encourage other museums to submit their specimens for non-invasive testing.)

Anthropologist Marshall Becker has spent several decades studying Etruscan human remains, developing the identification of cremated individuals from urn burials in central Italy; with the late Loretana Salvadei, he conducted a groundbreaking double-blind study of the burials from pre- and proto-historic Osteria dell'Osa (the Latin region of ancient Gabii). He has assisted Italian teams in identifying inhumation and cremation burials at Tarquinia and elsewhere in Italy, and with Jean MacIntosh Turfa and Bridget Algee-Hewitt, has published a study of the human remains found in Etruscan and Italic burials in the collection of the University of Pennsylvania Museum. In 2015 Becker was invited to study the human remains found in the "Tomb of the Hanging Aryballos" (Tarquinia Tomb 6423, *c.*600–575 BCE), where the undisturbed skeleton of a 40-year-old woman was accompanied by a box holding a sewing kit and a molar—apparently hers! (the tomb will be published by the Italian excavators). Becker has concentrated in recent years especially on ancient dental appliances, including the recent discovery in the Roman Collatina necropolis, and also the find of a drain full of human teeth extracted by a barber surgeon at a shop in the Roman Forum (*c.*50–110 CE).

Jean MacIntosh Turfa worked with Becker on the human remains from Italy in the University of Pennsylvania Museum, and has studied at length the Liverpool appliances, as part of her project to publish a complete catalogue of the splendid Etruscan collection in the Liverpool World Museum; she has viewed several of the appliances displayed in Italy. Her research as an Etruscologist has delved into Etruscan medicine, as reconstructed from anatomical models given as votive offerings, and from practices of divination. The unusual bits of evidence show that Etruscans were aware (though not through modern-type, empirical studies) of the effects of industrial pollution from metal-working and parasitic contamination in agriculture and husbandry, and that they were even, on rare occasions, attempting post-mortem C-sections for fetal salvage. Etruscan metallurgy was highly developed, their metal vessels sought even by discerning Greeks, but it was still a surprise to find that their goldsmiths were ahead of their rivals in refining gold for the false teeth.

Marshall Becker has supplied the material on the history of dentistry as well as all the first-hand measurements and descriptions of actual appliances, including an explanation of his attempts at sleuthing the whereabouts of some lost pieces. A small number of appliances or burials had to be described from published sources and illustrations where specimens were not available when a museum or collector was approached for permission (these are noted in the catalogue). Jean MacIntosh Turfa has supplied archaeological background on Etruscan civilization and Greek and Roman literature, including translations of ancient texts where not otherwise noted. The history of the golden smile goes on today, with rock and rap stars (and those who would emulate them) acquiring gold caps, bridges or inlays for purely aesthetic or social purposes—we comment on this at the end of the book, but you will undoubtedly find more examples in your daily news!

Acknowledgments

Marshall Joseph Becker

My research with Etruscan dental appliances and the history of dentistry began in 1985 as an ancillary aspect of studies of human skeletons from archaeological sites in Italy. Subsequently, this specific research program focused on the examination and detailed study of those examples of ancient dental prostheses that today can be identified. The intent of this research was to provide the necessary evidence to understand the origins and development of the technology involved as well as to understand the social processes related to the use of these artifacts. A great number of colleagues at more than two dozen institutions in seven countries graciously helped me to gather and verify the data presented in this work. My many thanks are due to each of them as well as to the following individuals who offered notable aid.

Very special thanks are due Professor L. Bliquez for his generous sharing of data, constant encouragement and advice, and for his considerable aid in correcting and editing one of the final drafts of this manuscript, as well as generously sharing illustrations with us. His help and particularly his encouragement has been critical to the development of this study.

My sincere thanks are due Dr. Penelope M. Allison, Professor Avis Allman, Dr. Kurt W. Alt (Univ. Düsseldorf), Professor George Bass, Professor Graeme Barker, Dr. Anna Maria Bietti Sestieri, Malcomb Browne, Dr. Ester Console (Vatican Museums), Dr. T. Biro Katalin (Hungarian National Museum), Professor Larissa Bonfante, Dr. Niels Bruun, Professor George Claghorn and his staff, Mrs. Eve Cockburn, Professor Robert S. Corruccini, Dr. Alessia Donadio, Professor Arthur Einhorn, Professor F. Emptoz, Professor Gioacchino Falsone, Professor Dr. Klaus-Dietrich Fischer, Dr. L. Gorelick, Jack W. Gottschalk, DDS (John Harris Dental Museum), Professor Thomas Grynaeus, M.D. (Budapest), Dr. A. M. Haeussler, Xia Haibin (Wuhan, China), Professor Birthe Højby-Nielsen, Dr. Ralph Jackson (The British Museum), Professor Jean-Louis Jannot, Professor Francis Johnston, Dr. Ernst Künzl, Professor Jodi Magness, Professor Charles S. Mandel, Professor Alan Mann, Dr. Ilona Marz, Martha McCartney, Dr. Timothy McNiven, Dr. Jacopo Moggi-Cecchi (Firenze), Dr. Theya Molleson (British Museum, ret.), Professor Sergio Musitelli, Dr. Thomas Nickol,

Dr. Inge Nielsen, Dr. Elsa Pacciani, Dr. Paola Pelagatti, Professor Joanne Phillips, Professor Michael Pietrusewsky, Professor Adele Ré, Mrs. Dina L. Rudman, Professor John Scarborough, Dr. and Mrs. John Shedd, Dr. Rolf Sinclair, Mag. Karen Slej, Professor Jocelyn Penny Small, Dr. Deborah Anne Smith (GlaxoSmithKline), John Spellman, DDS (West Chester, PA), Dr. Nigel Spivey, Dr. Tamara Stech, Dr. Wolf-Rudolf Teegen, Molly Unger (CBC Radio), Professor Jean-Claude Verger-Pratoucy, Professor Dianne Wayman, and Dr. Joseph Zias, for sharing important information or otherwise supporting this project.

For research relating to gold metallurgy our sincere thanks are due again to Professor Gioacchino Falsone as well as to Dr. Georges Tsoucaris (Louvre Museum) and Professor Guy Demortier (Université de Notre-Dame, Bruxelles), for their generous aid in various aspects of this research. Thanks also are due to Professor Ludovico Riva di Sanseverino (Erice, 2001), and for his continuing contributions to important scientific meetings. For specialist advice our thanks are due to Dr. Eli Kaufman and Professor Fred Monson.

At the *Museo Nazionale di Archeologia, Firenze*, the study of their materials was conducted through the gracious aid of Dr. Anna Maria Esposito, with the kind permission of the then Director of the Museum, Dr. Francesco Nicosia. Their aid, plus that of Bruno Michelucci and many other helpful members of the staff, is gratefully acknowledged. Special thanks are due to Professor Lucos Cozza for pointing out important archaeological data relating to the discovery of the Valsiarosa appliance, and to Professor Luigi Capasso for his aid in locating references and his generous sharing of data relating to this project. Thanks also to Professor J. -F. Roulet (Freie Universität Berlin), and Professor Zuhrt, for information relating to the Teano example, and to Dr. Ernst Stirnad for information about copies now in Germany. Thanks in particular are due to Dr. Demetrius Waarsenburg for kindly sharing data that he gathered in his important program of related research. The extensive computer and art work of Professor Fred Danziger is most gratefully acknowledged.

Thanks also are due the staff of the Danish Academy in Rome and to the former director Dr. Th. J. Meijer, and to the entire staff of the Istituto Olandese di Roma, as well as to Amanda Claridge (Oxford University) and Maria-Pia Malvezzi (British School in Rome) for their assistance in various aspects this research. Christopher Moss (Princeton University) graciously provided an IBYCUS search of the Classical literature. Professor Krishna Kumar's 1993 attempts to locate examples of Near Eastern appliances in Cairo also are very much appreciated.

Sincere thanks are due Søren Dietz, Keeper of the Department of Near Eastern and Classical Antiquities (National Museum, Copenhagen), for permission to publish the example in Copenhagen (Becker 1992a, 1994b). Thanks also are due to Dr. Helle Salskov Roberts, the late Dr. Pia Guldager Bilde, and Dr. John Lund for considerable aid in various aspects of this research in Copenhagen.

The aid of the late Dr. Christopher Mee (School of Archaeology and Oriental Studies, University of Liverpool) in arranging for Becker to study the ancient dental appliances in Liverpool, plus his hospitality and many kindnesses are gratefully acknowledged. At the Liverpool Museum Mr. Edmund Southworth (then Keeper of Antiquities) graciously gave permission to study their material. His assistant, Ms F. A. Paton, and Ms Philpot provided considerable assistance with this project. Thanks also are due the Librarian and entire staff at the offices of the British Dental Association (London), who most graciously provided support in the final stages of this research.

Special thanks are due Stewart Emmens (Assistant Curator, Public Health, The Science Museum, London) for his extensive aid in identifying the copies of these dental appliances originally held in the collections of the Wellcome Museum of the Wellcome Institute, and for his continuing interest in this research. Thanks also are due Julia Shepherd, at the Wellcome Institute in London, and her assistant for their aid in tracing the Wellcome copies. Thanks also are due Dr. Claude Rousseau, DSO, DDS, conservator of the *Musée Pierre Fauchard* in Paris, for providing data on the Guerini copies in that collection, and to Armelle Debru for aid with various French sources. The aid of Patricia Heller and the many helpful members of her staff at the Library of the Dental School at the University of Pennsylvania also is most gratefully acknowledged.

Dr. Giovanni Scichilone (former Director of the Museo Nazionale di Villa Giulia and Superintendent for Etruscan Archaeology) very kindly gave permission for me to study these materials in their collections. My thanks also are due Sig. Marino and the entire staff of the Villa Giulia Museum for their constant support in various projects, and to Dr. Rita Cosentino (*Soprintendenza Archeologica per l'Etruria Meridionale*) for arranging (through Dr. Anna Maria Moretti Sgubini, Il Primo Dirigente, Soprintendente Vicario) for a permit (Prot. no. 8322) for me to study the Valsiarosa appliance, which is displayed at the Museo di Forte Sangallo in Civita Castellano. Thanks also are due Dr. Pettinelli of that museum for his generous assistance in that study, and to Dr. Gabriella Barbieri (Museo Archeologico, Viterbo) and Dr. Mariolina Cataldi Dini for their considerable help in facilitating the research in Civita Castellana.

The aid of Professor *emerita* Ingrid Edlund-Berry (University of Texas, Austin) as well as that of Professor William Feagans (Dean of the Dental School, State University of New York at Buffalo) and many kind people in Buffalo, New York was of great value in attempting to locate the appliances brought to America by Dr. Barrett. Although this search has yet to bear fruit, the efforts of these scholars have provided the basic direction for future work. The observations of Professor Eli Kaufman, DMD (University of Buffalo) on the cold working and welding of gold, based on his observations of his father's skills, were extremely helpful.

Fresh thanks are due to Joel Irish, and to Patricia Baker for her publications on medical instruments and to Sergio Musitelli for sharing offprints. Dr. Simona Minozzi and Dr. Gino Fornaciari shared news and publications of the Collatina (Rome) dental appliance, and generously shared their publications. It was a great honor for Turfa to discuss ancient health with Dr. Fornaciari during his visit to Penn (May 2016).

Funding for this research has come from many sources. Most of my initial research was conducted while I was working on other projects that brought me close to the artifacts reviewed here. Preliminary arrangements for the Copenhagen portion of this study were made while the author was there conducting research on Native American objects in the National Museum of Denmark, a project funded by the American Philosophical Society (1987). Comparative research at the Villa Giulia Museum in Rome was funded entirely by a grant from the Italian Studies Center of the University of Pennsylvania joint program with L'Aquila University (1988). Several other trips to Italy were aided by a series of small awards from Dean Jennie Skerl (College of Arts and Sciences, West Chester University of Pennsylvania (1989–1994), plus a small grant for research awarded by the State System of Higher Education (Pennsylvania) and from the Jacqueline and Daniel Colyer Foundation (1993). Re-examination of the appliances in Tarquinia was made possible through a generous research grant from the National Geographic Society (Grant no. 5326-94) to study Etruscan skeletal remains in 1994.

Jean MacIntosh Turfa

In addition to very many of the scholars, also my friends, named above I owe a great debt of gratitude to several friends who have helped me with the study of certain appliances, and with the editing of this manuscript:

Dr. Margarita Gleba (Director, PROCON Ancient Textile project, Macdonald Laboratory, Cambridge), for generous hospitality, ongoing assistance and specialized photography, especially in the Liverpool World Museum. Cynthia Reed, goldsmith, archaeologist and former dental hygienist, for advice and sanity during study tours in Italy, the UK and USA, study photography and ongoing technical advice on many topics. Roger Thomson, goldsmith and husband of Cindy, in addition to patiently supporting our travels, has often shared sage advice on technological matters as well. Professor *emerita* Ingrid Edlund-Berry has helped inestimably and well beyond the call of scholarly duty, in the USA and abroad, and had even studied years ahead of me, the Barrett Collection of New York State.

Dr. Georgina Muskett, Curator (retired), Classical Antiquities, Liverpool World Museum, for hospitality, assistance with collections study and photography, and continuing advice. Dr. Chrissy Partheni, Curator, Classical Antiquities, Liverpool World Museum, for recent photography and kind assistance with study of the collection. They and the Liverpool staff made it possible to have the Etruscan gold tested. The late Drs. Margaret Warhurst and Glenys Lloyd-Morgan made it possible for me to study the Liverpool appliances—and much more—during my residence in the UK (1979–1981). Their efforts on behalf of collections of Etruscan and Italic antiquities in the United Kingdom are recalled fondly by many of us.

Elena Yandola, Esq., for irreplaceable assistance in editing the manuscript through multiple variations, and for help in examining materials in the UK and Philadelphia. Dr. Jacopo Tabolli, Director, MAVNA (Museo Archeologico

Virtuale di Narce Antica), for ongoing discussions, advice, and rare bibliography. Professor David George, St. Anselm College, New Hampshire, who, with Professor Mary Kate Donais, kindly shared the results of his research in XRF techniques. Professor Claudio Bizzarri, Director, Orvieto Archaeological Park, Dr. Rosalie David, *emerita*, Manchester Mummy Project, Dr. Judith Swaddling, Greek and Roman Department, British Museum, Dr. Laura Orsi (Florence), in addition to friendship have assisted with rare information and more. Virginia Greene (Tikal Excavations), Francine Sarin and Jennifer Chiappardi (Penn Museum Photo Studio) provided special help and encouragement. Stephanie Budin likewise provided needed advice and encouragement.

In 2015 Dr. Matthew J. Ponting and Dr. Pablo Fernández-Reyes of the Department of Archaeology, Classics and Egyptology, University of Liverpool kindly performed technical analysis of the Liverpool gold prostheses: it was a very special day when I arrived at the Garstang Museum, Liverpool and he informed me of the new findings on the purity of the Etruscan gold.

Thanks to the Royal Collection Trust and the Wellcome Collection, for generous provision of photographs; also, through the kind permission of the Wellcome Collection and Team Votives I was able to examine anatomical votives and related materials from the Wellcome study collection, administered by the Science Museum, London, then (2015) in Blythe House. My research was not funded by grants, but was undertaken in part during other travel supported by St. Joseph's University (Philadelphia), the Lorant Memorial Lecture Program (British Museum), and the Haynes Lecture Program (Oxford). My study of the human remains, and Etruscan collection, at Penn would not have been possible without the kindness of my colleagues in the Mediterranean Section of the University of Pennsylvania Museum, Lynn Makowsky, Ann Blair Brownlee, Brian Rose and Don White. Nor would my participation have been possible without the constant support and encouragement and scientific advice of my exceptional husband, Alex Turfa.

We are indebted to the Routledge staff for kind and patient support, especially Amy Davis-Poynter and Lizzi Thomasson. Naturally, the ideas and opinions expressed in this study, as well as any errors of presentation or interpretation, are the responsibility of the authors alone.

Background
The main ancient cultures associated with dental appliances listed in alphabetic order

Egypt, "late period" (Persian domination, Ptolemaic kingdom)

Three of the seven extant wire appliances were found in tombs in Lower Egypt (the region of the Nile Delta, Cairo, and the Pyramids). One was found at El-Qatta as part of a secondary deposit within a *mastaba*-tomb (a low, bench-shaped tomb) built in the time of the pharaohs (probably Old Kingdom, the third millennium BCE). It was deposited (with its wearer) when the tomb was re-used during Roman times, the first or second century CE. The silver-wire appliance from Tura el-Asment was in a necropolis of the Ptolemaic period (331–330 BCE), when Egypt was ruled by the Macedonian (Greek) dynasty that followed Alexander the Great and ended with the death of Cleopatra VII and the Roman conquest of Egypt by Octavian/Augustus. The third, from the Ibrahimieh necropolis of Alexandria, comes from the first-century CE Roman occupation of Egypt.

Background

Becker, M. J., 1997. "Early dental appliances in the Eastern Mediterranean," *Berytus* 42 (1995/1996): 71–102.

Morkot, R. G., 2005. *The Egyptians.* New York: Routledge.

Myśliwiec, Kurt, 1998. *The Twilight of Ancient Egypt: First Millennium B.C.E.*, trans. D. Lorton, Ithaca, NY: Cornell University Press.

Etruscans (Etruria)

The Etruscans controlled large portions of Central Italy during much of the first millennium BCE, especially the region today known as Tuscany, extending from the Arno that flows through Pisa and Florence to the Tiber that separated Rome from Etruria. Etruscan material culture and language also spread south, from Capua through the Bay of Naples and also east, across the Apennines into the Upper Adriatic. In the northeastern part of this territory, the Etruscan city of Felsina became modern Bologna. Excavating beneath the floors of buildings at Pompeii destroyed by Vesuvius in 79 CE, archaeologists found Etruscan artifacts and inscriptions, an indication of how wide-reaching Etruscan civilization once was.

The Etruscan language is not Indo-European like the Latin spoken by their Roman neighbors, nor is it Semitic like Phoenician or Hebrew. As one of the last surviving non-Indo-European languages, it marked them as proudly different from the surrounding Italic tribes and Greek colonies in Italy. Etruscan society allowed women much greater freedom and authority than their counterparts in Greece or Rome, another factor that fueled jealous commentary. Etruscan art, often in terracotta or bronze, was more colorful and energetic than much comparable Greek art, producing masterworks such as the Apollo of Veii and the bronze Chimaera of Arezzo. Etruscan material culture, with its advanced metallurgy, surveying and construction specialties, formed the basis for the art and technology of the Italic tribes, such as Latins and Faliscans, who occupied the rest of the Italian peninsula. Trading in Etruria's iron ore and other natural resources during the seventh–sixth centuries BCE, the great cities such as Populonia, Chiusi, Vulci, Tarquinia, Caere (modern Cerveteri) and Veii grew to rival their Greek and Levantine competitors and to dominate the seas of the central Mediterranean. Etruscan kings ruled Rome for most of the sixth century, but the Roman revolution of 510 BCE resulted in the Republic and initiated political decline and gradual loss of Etruscan autonomy to Rome. By the era of Cicero and Caesar (first century BCE), Etruria had been incorporated into the Roman political and economic system, and its distinctive language faded from written records.

Although some Romans (including the Emperor Claudius) appreciated Etruria's culture and history, Etruscan literature was allowed to fall into oblivion, so that we have only the words of their Greek and Roman enemies to describe Etruscan society. The Greek historian Herodotus, writing in the fifth century, told a tale of Etruscan origins in ancient Lydia (in Asia Minor), but more academic scholars such as Dionysius of Halicarnassus offered evidence that they belonged in Italy. In spite of some hasty modern studies of their DNA, early Etruscans seem more closely linked to prehistoric Europe, their language a rare survival of the many pre-Indo-European languages that once existed.

Etruscan-style gold-band dental appliances have been associated with several affluent Etruscan cities: Bisenzio, Orvieto (and perhaps its successor Bolsena), Chiusi, Populonia and Tarquinia, the source of the greatest number (five) of appliances. Two appliances in Liverpool probably came from the great necropoleis of Vulci, although this has not been substantiated; another is said to be from a tomb found near Lake Bracciano, also in the southern Etruscan region.

Background

Haynes, Sybille, 2000. *Etruscan Civilization: A Cultural History*. Los Angeles, CA: J. Paul Getty Museum.

Smith, Christopher, 2014. *The Etruscans: A Very Short Introduction*. Oxford: Oxford University Press.

Turfa, Jean MacIntosh, ed., 2013. *The Etruscan World*. London: Routledge.

Faliscans (the *Ager Faliscus*—"Faliscan territory")

Indo-European languages such as Latin, brought to the Italian peninsula by Italic tribes, were firmly embedded by the first millennium BCE, to judge from material culture. (As with Etruscan, we must await the arrival of the alphabet and the recording of inscriptions, during the eighth century BCE, to verify specific languages.) Oscans settled around the Bay of Naples, Umbrians to the east around modern Perugia, and Picenes on the Adriatic shore. The Italic tribe known as Faliscans was based near Rome, to the east and south of Etruria at the sites of Narce (modern Mazzano Romano) and *Falerii* (modern Civita Castellana). The Faliscans were allies of Etruscan states such as Veii, and shared much Etruscan technology such as metallurgy; they also borrowed their alphabet and numerals from Etruria. Faliscans intermarried with Etruscans and the two cultures shared religious cults and sanctuaries. Faliscan temples were decorated with Etruscan-inspired sculpture, and Faliscan political fortunes waned in tandem with Etruscan loss of autonomy during the fifth–first centuries BCE.

An important gold-band appliance was excavated in a tomb at Valsiarosa, the site of a necropolis of the Faliscan city of *Falerii Veteres* ("Old Falerii," modern Civita Castellana). It was probably made during the fourth century when Falerii experienced a renaissance of building and artistic production. The city was terminated in 241 BCE when it was defeated by Rome and survivors relocated to *Falerii Novi* ("New Falerii").

Background

De Lucia Brolli, M. A. and J. Tabolli, 2013. "The Etruscans and the Faliscans" in J. M. Turfa, ed., *The Etruscan World*, 259–280. London: Routledge.

Greeks (Greece: cities of Tanagra and Eretria)

One distinctly Etruscan-style gold-band appliance was found in a tomb at Tanagra in the region known as Boeotia, Greece. This territory, to the east of Attica and Athens, despite the pejorative view of other Greeks who knew it for pork production, supported a rich agricultural society that already during the Archaic period (seventh–sixth centuries BCE) produced fine architecture and works of art. Boeotia had become a military powerhouse during the fourth century. Its economy revived during the Hellenistic period following the Macedonian conquests, fostering rich offerings found in burials, especially the elegant terracotta "Tanagra figurines." The Tanagra dental appliance is said to be from a tomb of the Early Hellenistic era, the end of the fourth through the third century BCE, and attests to the affluence of this age of world travel and commerce.

A single gold-wire appliance was found buried in a tomb at Eretria, one of the cities on the large island of Euboea, on the eastern shore of mainland Greece. Euboea had been one of the richest regions during the Geometric and

Archaic periods (the first half of the first millennium BCE), and continued to support religious sanctuaries and artistic schools. During the eighth century BCE, the Euboean cities of Chalkis and Eretria founded colonies such as Pithekoussai, on the island of Ischia off the Bay of Naples, where artisans of many nationalities (Greek, Phoenician/Syrian, Etruscan, Italic) produced iron, metal goods and painted pottery and traded across the entire Mediterranean. The Eretria appliance came from a necropolis of the fourth–third century BCE, when the city was still known for a famous shrine of Apollo.

Background

Bugh, Glenn R., ed., 2006. *The Cambridge Companion to the Hellenistic world*. Cambridge: Cambridge University Press.
Ridgway, David, 2002. *The First Western Greeks*. Cambridge: Cambridge University Press.

Phoenicians (Phoenicia)

The Phoenicians were the Iron Age descendants of the Bronze Age Canaanites who inhabited much of the coastal Levant, including what is now North Syria, Lebanon and Israel. From *c.*1000 to 500 BCE Phoenician culture spread through the Mediterranean, and parts of the Red Sea/Indian Ocean, Atlantic Iberia and North Africa, with commercial routes and bustling colonies. (Carthage in Tunisia and Cadiz and Cartagena in Spain, Cagliari in Sardinia and Palermo in Sicily are examples of their rich colonial cities.) Phoenicians were famous for their purple-dyed textiles, ivory carvings and furniture, glassmaking, and goldworking technology, which they taught to Etruscans and other cultures in the Mediterranean. The two cities of Tyre and Sidon on the southern coast of Lebanon are mentioned in the Bible; they dominated eastern Mediterranean trade and shipbuilding. Other homeland cities include Berytus (Beirut), Byblos, Tripolis and Arwad. The city of Sidon had been a monarchy since before 1,000 BCE, and supported numerous Phoenician industries and commercial ventures; the great aristocratic families participated in colonization initiatives and maintained tombs similar to those of royalty. Phoenician craftsmen were loaned by King Hiram of Tyre to King Solomon to decorate the Temple in Jerusalem, and precious Phoenician metal goods, ivory furniture and gold jewelry have been identified in the ruins of Assyrian royal palaces (as booty and tribute), Greek sanctuaries (as votives), and Etruscan tombs (as gifts to rulers). Located on a pathway between Egypt, Mesopotamia and Anatolia, Phoenicia was conquered or at times survived as a tributary of the Egyptians, Hittites, Assyrians, Babylonians, and Persians. Alexander the Great restored the King of Sidon deposed by the Persians, but material culture after the fourth century resembles the Hellenistic *koine* of the eastern Mediterranean. Phoenicia has given us our alphabet (handed down via Greece, Etruria and Rome) and many technological and economic developments, including even businessmen's white shirts (from the white linen tunic, called *chiton*, of Phoenician traders).

Several seventh-century Etruscan and Latin tombs at Caere, Tarquinia, and Praeneste hold fine specimens of Phoenician vessels and ornaments in gold, silver and bronze, but the two gold-wire appliances found in different aristocratic necropoleis of Sidon are dated to the fourth century, when Phoenicia was restive under Persian control. It appears that gold-band technology was created by Etruscan goldsmiths whose forebears may have once trained as apprentices of Phoenician masters.

Background

Grainger, John D., 1991. *Hellenistic Phoenicia*. Oxford: Clarendon Press.
Markoe, Glenn E., 2005. *Phoenicians.* London: British Museum.

Romans/Latins (Rome, Latium, and other Italic tribes)

The Romans were part of the Latin-speaking ethnic group, distinguished in their early days by distinctive pottery and metal types and by inhumation burial rather than the cremation practiced in Etruria. The region they inhabited included other tribes, under the historical name *Latium Vetus* ("Old Latium"). Early in the first millennium BCE Rome was a tiny enclave of Latin hut villages, which coalesced into a growing city during the eighth century (a development attributed by later historians to Romulus and Remus). Following 250 years of monarchy, and ending a century of flourishing under Etruscan rulers, the city of Rome became a Republic, and began a methodical takeover of the peninsula and the Mediterranean world. This long process was punctuated by slave revolts and wars with Carthage, Iberia, Gaul and Britain, and the eastern dynasties that succeeded Alexander in Greece, Asia Minor, Mesopotamia and Egypt. Civil wars of the first century BCE led to the Empire, begun by Octavian/Augustus when he conquered Cleopatra VII of Egypt, ending the last of the Hellenistic kingdoms and launching an era of relative prosperity throughout the Mediterranean and much of Europe, until the barbarian conquest of Rome in 410 CE. The great era of Roman literature, which has provided authors' comments on false teeth, and a single example of a dental appliance, was the first century BCE and first–second centuries CE.

Gold-band appliances have been found in burials at the Latin-speaking towns of Satricum and Praeneste (modern Palestrina). The Satricum appliance has been dated to the seventh century, the so-called "era of the princely tombs," when the ruling classes of cities were buried with lavish tokens of wealth and power. The Praeneste example was a chance find, and the necropolis it came from, while famous for extravagant seventh-century tombs, was also used into the Hellenistic period, so the date of the appliance remains obscure. Another gold-band appliance came from Teano, ancient *Teanum Sidicinum* ("Teanum of the Sidicini," an Oscan/Italic tribe) situated in Campania, north of modern Caserta and Capua, about halfway between Naples and Rome. The tomb in which it was found was dated to the fourth–third centuries BCE, by which time the region was under Roman domination.

Literature on Greece and Rome is massive: for a quick lookup of names, dates, facts, maps, see Adkins, Lesley and Roy A. Adkins, 1994. *Handbook to Life in Ancient Rome*. Oxford: Oxford University Press.

Introduction

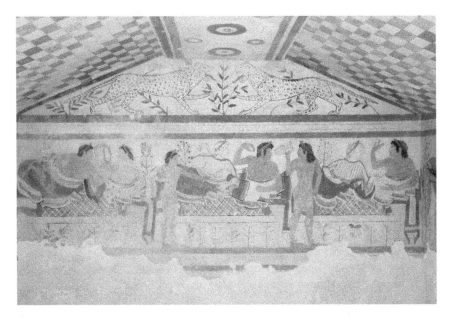

Figure I.1 Women's public presence in Etruria: banquet scene with aristocratic women reclining beside their husbands. Tarquinia, *Tomb of the Leopards*, fresco on back wall, *c*.480–470 BCE.

Source: Odyssey-images/Alamy.

Humans are the only creatures with special facial muscles that allow them to smile, independent of other functions. Our ability to succeed socially is due in part to such non-verbal communication, expressing approval or aloofness, or mastery of a situation. The golden smile of ancient Etruscan women is one rare development of this ability, and one that resonates with our own civilization's embracing modern dentistry.

Picture a large, aristocratic family gathering with several women arriving to join their menfolk for a banquet, children and slaves in tow. More than one of them flaunts lovely, but probably artificial, blonde hair, and all wear brightly colored garments, calf-length to facilitate walking, and to show off their red and black boots with upturned toes. They recline on tall couches, each beside her husband, and drink from gold and silver cups. Someone tells a joke, and everyone laughs—Larthia and Velia flash smiles and we catch the gleam of gold—their perfect, white teeth are decorated with thin bands of pure gold! And perhaps those teeth are not quite as perfect as they seem: they are replacements for lost front teeth, skillfully (and probably painfully) inserted thanks to Etruria's advanced technology.

The Etruscans were often slandered by their enemies/neighbors, both Greek and Roman, who felt disadvantaged politically and economically in their dealings with them. It is true that the Etruscans grew rich—ostentatiously so—well ahead of their competitors, and although their literature is lost, artistic representations such as murals in their tombs give a picture of the society that Greek observers and others could only envy. The Greek author Theopompus, writing in the fourth century BCE, said some extravagant things about Etruscan women, comments that betray a certain ignorance of his subject, as well as envy. Many such criticisms are known today only because they were quoted by later writers. Greeks called the Etruscans "Tyrrhenians," naming the sea west of Tuscany after them; Romans called them *Tusci* or *Etrusci*, but these too probably began as ethnic slurs; the Etruscans called themselves *Rasna* or *Rasenna*.

Athenaeus, a Greek from Naukratis in Egypt writing during the Roman Empire (second century CE), quotes from the lost work by Aristotle *On the Customs of the Etruscans*: "But the Tyrrhenians banquet with their own wives, reclining both of them under the same cloak." (*Deipnosophistae* 1.23d, JMT's translation). The Greek appears below:

Ἀριστοτέλης ἐν Τυρρηνῶν Νομίμοις· « Οἱ δὲ Τυρρηνοὶ δειπνοῦσι μετὰ τῶν γυναικῶν ἀνακείμενοι ὑπὸ τῷ αὐτῷ ἱματίῳ. »

Greeks seem to have been scandalized to think that wives—as opposed to call girls—would be seen in public at banquets alongside their husbands. (In this regard it is easier for us Westerners to empathize with the Etruscans—what American wife would stay hidden at home when other women will be attending the banquet?) Athenaeus also preserves more of the prejudiced comments by Greek authors about the Etruscans; these likely began as misunderstandings of images, like the Underworld Banquet scenes painted in Etruscan tombs, or of social events where women were included in contrast to Greek segregation of the sexes. Such differences in social traditions are magnified when only the literature of one side survives. From Athenaeus again:

Theopompus in the 43rd book of his *Histories* says it is customary among the Tyrrhenians to share their women in common. These women take special care of their bodies and often exercise naked, among themselves and even with men: for it is no shame for them to appear naked. [He says] they dine not with their own husbands but alongside whatever men happen to be present, and they propose toasts to any of those they care to. Further, their faces are exceptionally beautiful and they are also skillful at drinking. [He says that] the Tyrrhenians raise all the offspring that are born without knowing whose father is whose.

Θεόπομπος δὲ ἐν τῇ τεσσαρακοστῇ τρίτῃ τῶν Ἱστοριων καὶ νόμον εἶναί φησιν παρὰ τοῖς Τυρρηνοῖς κοινὰς ὑπάρχειν τὰς γυναῖκας· ταύτας δ' ἐπιμελεῖσθαι σφόδρα τῶν σωμάτων καὶ γυμνάζεσθαι πολλάκις καὶ μετ' ἀνδρῶν, ἐνίοτε δὲ καὶ πρὸς ἑαυτάς· οὐ γὰρ αἰσχρὸν εἶναι αὐταῖς φαίνεσθαι γυμναῖς. Δειπνεῖν δὲ αὐτὰς οὐ παρὰ τοῖς ἀνδράσι τοῖς ἑαυτῶν, ἀλλὰ παρ' οἷς ἂν τύχωσι τῶν παρόντων, καὶ προπίνουσιν οἷς ἂν (517e) βουληθῶσιν. Εἶναι δὲ καὶ πιεῖν δεινὰς καὶ τὰς ὄψεις πάνυ καλάς. Τρέφειν δὲ τοὺς Τυρρηνοὺς πάντα τὰ γινόμενα παιδία οὐκ εἰδότας ὅτου πατρός ἐστιν ἕκαστον.

(*Deipnosophistae* 12.517d–e)

In point of fact, there are murals on the walls of noble tombs, especially at Tarquinia, one of Etruria's premiere cities, that depict women reclining at banquet with men—but inscriptions and other evidence show that the couples depicted are married to each other, that children's genealogies were carefully recorded often for many generations, and that there are logical, often religious, explanations for whatever details of the paintings seem shocking to us (or to ancient Greeks). An outsider, perhaps even a tomb robber, however, would not have the background to interpret the scenes correctly. . . Etruscan women in public in showy robes, with dyed hair and gold jewels would have seemed alien, no doubt threatening, to Greek or early Roman observers—certainly Athenian women did not sport golden dentures, for this technology was a purely Etruscan phenomenon in the first millennium BCE, shared, but just barely, with their Latin in-laws in nearby *Ruma* (Rome), Praeneste and Satricum.

The focus of this book is on the unique phenomenon of Etruscan dental appliances, or bridges in modern terminology, that were made to be worn by a few elite women in central Italy, Etruria and its environs, from the seventh century down to the end of the first millennium BCE. We find only a very few of them preserved in the burials of such women (thanks to the efforts of tomb robbers), and they were probably never very common—they represent too much wealth (gold), skill (of a goldsmith, not a dentist in the modern sense), and pain (for the wearer in having them fitted and maintained). Nonetheless, the tradition seems to have been carried on by Roman women of the Late Republic and Empire, still in very small numbers, although such women were indeed remarked upon.

Like Catullus before him, the poet Martial (*c.*40–103/4 CE) at times turned his sharp tongue, in pithy epigrams, on such women who he encountered in society. Various women and men are mocked for their attempts to disguise their age, and are said to have few teeth or discolored teeth (*Epigrams* 1.19, 2.41, 6.74, 8.57).

Galla, one of his society targets, is said to put away her teeth at night just like she does her silk gowns (*Epigram* 9.37.1–6), Aegle has teeth of bone and Indian horn (1.72), and Laelia can use her "bought teeth" but cannot so easily replace her failing eye (12.23). A famous quip from the poet's acid tongue says that Thais (a popular name for a courtesan) has black teeth, but that's because they are genuine; Laecania's white teeth are bought (*Epigram* 5.43). There is mention, too, of cosmetic services, including dentistry apparently, for up on the Aventine, "Cascellius extracts or repairs an ailing tooth" (*Epigram* 10.56). (For more on these poems, see Chapter 1; likewise for some recent information on Roman extractions!)

Roman men, too, could be self-conscious about their teeth: for most men this would have meant hiding discolored or decayed dentition, keeping their mouths closed when smiling or speaking cautiously. But a few (thankfully) rare individuals did the opposite, for they were proud of a perfect set of teeth (presumably the results of good dental hygiene). The *louche* Republican poet Catullus (*c*.84–54 BCE) criticized a man for ostentatiously showing off his nice, clean teeth, in a poem full of what may have been mild ethnic slurs (on the *obesus etruscus*, see Turfa 2016):

> Catullus, *Carmen (Ode)* 39.11
> Si urbanus esses aut Sabinus aut Tiburs
> aut pinguis Vmber aut obesus Etruscus
> aut Lanuvinus ater atque dentatus
> aut Transpadanus, ut meos quoque attingam,
> aut quilubet, qui puriter lavit dentes,
> tamen renidere usque quaque te nollem:
> nam risu inepto res ineptior nulla est.

> Even if you were a refined person or a Sabine, or a man from Tivoli,
> or a portly Umbrian or a fat Etruscan,
> or a swarthy or toothy Lanuvian
> or a man from beyond the Po, to touch upon my own people,
> or whoever you like, who cleans his teeth with pure water,
> I still don't want you to be grinning all the time:
> because nothing is dopier than a silly smile.

What the Roman works show is a self-conscious society noticing physical traits like teeth and reading value judgments or status symbols into them. Etruscan society may have behaved in similar fashion, but for them, the addition of a golden bridge was a rare status symbol.

The technology and skilled labor represented in the golden appliances is just as interesting to analyze. Ancient Etruscan goldsmithing skills are well known to archaeologists and art collectors (see, for instance, De Puma 1987, Cristofani 1983; Formigli 1985; Formigli and Nestler 1994; Formigli *et al.* 1995.) The skills of these Etruscan crafters formed the basis for the Roman gold-working tradition, which, according to many scholars, peaked in the Imperial Period (second–third centuries CE; Pirzio 1992). The Etruscan origins of numerous and complex techniques that were employed in gold-working long before the development of the Roman state have been discussed by many scholars (Cristofani 1983; Formigli 1979; Strøm 1990; Mauro and Martelli 1983; Buchner 1979: 129–138). Etruscan primacy in applying their varied gold-working abilities beyond the manufacture of elaborately decorated jewelry, however, is less well known. The ancient application of decorative design to functional devices in central Italy will not surprise students of art history or of technology. More than 2,600 years ago, Etruscan goldsmiths were constructing the earliest true dental appliances in the Mediterranean and Europe, and creating complex dental bridges (pontics), which had cosmetic as well as therapeutic value.

This phenomenon, treated as a curiosity prior to the 1880s, coincidentally came to the attention of medical historians about the same time that modern dentistry became professionalized, and some professionals of that era were involved in both movements. Since then a steady flow of publications have made reference to these ancient appliances, but a complete and accurate corpus had never been assembled, and many inaccuracies were inadvertently propagated. These appliances have over the last century received sporadic attention from dentists and archaeologists, with some publications far better than others.

Documentation of the existence of these gold dental prostheses can be traced through ancient literary sources to one of the most archaic of Roman documents, the *Laws of the Twelve Tables (XII Tabulae)*. The surviving text was published as early as the fifth century BCE but the law was probably developed even earlier, perhaps in the era of the Etruscan kings of Rome, the sixth century BCE. Additional references are dated to the second century BCE. Various references to dental gold continued to appear in medical texts through the medieval period (see Reinach 1918, and others). Rarely, however, has the archaeological evidence been carefully matched with the anthropological data for ancient dental disease (e.g. Geist-Jacoby 1896, Emery 1963) and for extant dental appliances. An in-depth analysis of these ancient dental appliances will help us to understand their origins and functions.

The principal contributions of this book to our understanding of early dental prostheses are the detailed, first-hand descriptions of existing Etruscan dental appliances. These data, plus records from the close examination of the teeth now associated with the appliances provide the basis for reconstructing an important part of Etruscan culture. Several additional bridges that are no longer preserved, or the whereabouts of which are no longer known, have been studied through publications and images, to complete the catalogue of known gold-band or wire prostheses. A complete bibliography of the literature that relates to this subject supports a comprehensive view of this unprecedented social as well as medical phenomenon, a phenomenon that, with few exceptions, would not reappear for almost 2,000 years.

In addition, we list certain famous items formerly described as "dental appliances" but clearly found to be spurious (Appendix III). There has been a long history of efforts to replace missing teeth, dating back to the 1700s. This history, culminating in the very recent success in developing dental implants, has led several archaeologists to make claims to the discovery of early "examples" of dental implants (see Becker 1998b, 1999c). All can be explained by other, more likely phenomena. Despite efforts to enlighten our scholarly colleagues, the market for popular mythology on this subject seems infinite.

Perhaps the single most interesting finding of our research program derives from the study of the teeth of the people who wore the gold-band appliances made in central Italy. Based on the findings of Garn and his colleagues (1967) regarding sex differentiation in tooth size within a population, a test of this method was directed toward an Iron Age population ($N = 650$) in central Italy. The results of the study of dentition at Osteria dell'Osa (Becker and Salvadei 1992) confirm the results of previous studies and indicate that even for ancient central Italy sex can be predicted from odontometric data (size measurements of teeth) with great reliability. The metric data from teeth associated with these ancient dental appliances, previously ignored, provide evidence that the Italian examples of these prostheses all were worn by women.

This observation regarding the gender of the people wearing the appliances calls to mind the heightened public identity of Etruscan women, so often cited by ancient as well as modern historians. Etruscan women normally dined together with men, as clearly contradistinguished from contemporary Greek and Republican Roman dining customs (see Loraux 1993). Among the Greeks, a common avoidance taboo was associated with eating, as it remains among Turkish and most Middle Eastern peoples to this day. Without going into the anthropology of gender specific avoidance taboos, which many Europeans still maintain in the area of bathroom use, for instance, it is clear that Etruscan women dined in public with males, as was depicted in several famous tombs at Tarquinia (cf. Spivey 1991: 64). The fact that only women appear to have worn these ancient dental prostheses, and the fact that the technology appears at an early date only within the Etruscan sphere, suggests that a public presentation was an important part of the use of the devices. The decline in use of these appliances may correlate with the decline of Etruscan cultural traditions as the Roman state, and Roman habits, came to dominate all of Italy.

The catalogue of 28 ancient examples presented here is intended to provide a complete listing of these interesting devices. We also include an identification of all those spurious examples that have been generated by some published commentaries. The spurious "examples" generally seem to have been created when authors failed to make direct observations of the actual dental appliances, the originals of which were widely distributed throughout Europe and America, and in several cases are now lost (cf. Torino *et al.* 1996). The literature on the subject has become bewildering in its multiplication (especially where one author merely repeated another's comments, never having seen the real objects—see Becker 1994b). However, in at least two cases where the original dental appliances no longer exist (no. 6—Populonia, and one of the Tarquinia series), we may still unwittingly be repeating errors found in the literature, and possibly compounding them (this is noted in the catalogue under nos. 6 and 9, 11, 12).

The recent discovery of a gold-band appliance in the tomb of a noble family at Lucca is fresh evidence of an interest in this technology in Italy before 1600; before the writings of Ambroise Paré (1564, 1585) describing various pontics. (See S. Minozzi, D. Panetta, M. DeSanctis and V. Giuffra in Clinical Implant Dent. and Related Res. (2016) DOI 10.1111/cid.12460.) Sixteenth-century practitioners reveal a continuity in aspects of the ancient Etruscan traditions.

"Modern" interest in things Etruscan, leading to the decision in 1726 to form a "*biblioteca comune,*" is considered by Barocchi and Gallo (1985: 33) to be the basis for the ultimate formation of *L'Accademia etrusca*. Levi (1985a: 109–110) discusses the beginnings of both academic and private collections of Etruscan artifacts during the period 1724–1750 (see also Levi 1985b: 120–121). In particular, Levi (1985a) reviews the work of the Scottish antiquarian Thomas Dempster, and illustrates a "chest" depicted by this early investigator (Dempster 1726: pl. LXXXIII; see de Angelis 2013). Yet we have no idea when the first dental prosthesis entered any local collection of Etruscan artifacts.

We do not know when the first Etruscan dental appliance was discovered, but systematic searches for "treasures" from the past were well under way by the beginning of the eighteenth century (Dempster 1724–1726; see Pannozzo 1986). The first archaeological evidence for the presence of ancient gold dental appliances, in the form of an excavated example, has been available since the late eighteenth century (Böttiger 1797: 63). The discovery of a dental bridge from excavations somewhere in central Italy confirmed the validity of those ancient texts that made mention of dental appliances. Where this appliance had been found, as well as its present disposition, remains unknown—its existence is known only from Böttiger's description recorded in 1797. It once belonged to Sir William Hamilton, but was apparently lost (see Appendix 1A).

By the late nineteenth century more than a half dozen ancient prostheses had been identified from archaeological contexts in Etruria and environs. These examples led the German archaeologist Wolfgang Helbig (1886: 26) to suggest that sufficient numbers of gold dental appliances had been recovered from "dated" contexts to permit a chronology to be established. No archaeological evidence ever was presented for these suppositions, and the assignment of dates by various authors appears to have been based on inferences regarding "types" of dental appliances, rather than exact chronologies or archaeological contexts. A chronology is certainly desirable, but the findings of our study suggest that no dates can be assigned with confidence to any specific *types* of appliances. Today we can identify more than a score of dental appliances, in an amazing variety of shapes and sizes, but few of them can be reliably dated—they came from antiquities dealers or were found so long ago that no one preserved details of the bodies or tombs in which they were found. The one condition of which we can be sure is the Etruscan primacy in this field. No other Mediterranean culture produced this particular type of artifact using gold bands, and, with one or two exceptions, the rare finds outside of Italy date from the Hellenistic or Roman periods (and use wire rather than bands, a very different technique). This information also implies that the manufacture and use of gold dental appliances was related specifically to the high status of Etruscan women, and that the absorption of Etruscan culture by the Romans led to the demise of this aspect of ancient dentistry.

The goal of our research has been to provide a synthesis of various perspectives that have been published concerning these appliances, and to clarify some of the problems that have arisen in the literature through incomplete or naive descriptions of these ancient dental bridges, and the contexts in which they were found or now appear. While they are frequently cited by archaeologists, dental prostheses tend to be a subject more frequently discussed by dental or medical historians, yet their immense value for social documentation is outstanding.

More than 100 years ago Alfred Jones (1884) offered a brief commentary on dentistry in the classical world as gleaned from ancient texts, with barely a brief note on the use of gold dental prostheses. Another complicating factor is the reliance of most past (and too many recent) scholars on literary as opposed to archaeological sources. This puts Etruscan culture at a great disadvantage for, as we know from their Greek and Roman rivals' historians, the Etruscans' own rich literature, written on perishable media of papyrus, linen, and wax, has not survived. Jones's study appeared just before the flurry of discoveries generated by the developing interest in Etruscan dental appliances (see Waite 1885b). These newly discovered ancient dental appliances have formed the basis for important sections in various histories of dentistry that have emerged. Unfortunately, most of these summaries provide only superficial and popularized reviews of the secondary literature (cf. Ramos Calvo 1986).

Guerini's (1909) work, announced with enthusiasm by M'Manus (1905), remains one of the better texts relating to this specialized portion of dental history. However, none of the many scholars directing their attentions to dental appliances worked out the problems that began to develop quite early through the lack of direct (primary) observations by these authors, as well as the absence of a detailed catalogue.

Deneffe (1899) was the first to attempt to provide a catalogue of ancient gold dental appliances, but since then, we have seen a considerable number of inventories emerge (Sudhoff 1926, Casotti 1947, Bobbio 1958). Tabanelli (1963) attempted a true catalogue, with 14 potential examples of dental appliances. Dental as well as other ancient prosthetic devises are reviewed by Bliquez (1983, cf. 1996), whose study of specific information regarding various dental prostheses and their history remains one of the most complete inventories. The Bliquez inventory also includes many of the best photographs of these items available before 1990, thereby providing an important contribution to the clarification of this problematical literature. The attempt by Emptoz (1987) to update Deneffe's (1899) compendium includes some valuable information, but does not bring order to the subject. To the best of our knowledge, the following study includes every major reference that has been made to these ancient dental appliances, as well as a number of the minor notes. Excluded from this study are general surveys of dental or medical history that offer little more than brief reference to the existence of ancient dental appliances. The bibliography notes every work consulted for this study.

With one notable exception, most of the previous descriptions of these ancient prostheses have been somewhat superficial, rendering indistinguishable many of the individual examples. This problem, in turn, led to individual examples "multiplying" in the literature as the same object was described in more than one entry (as Waarsenburg 1991a has warned). In an insightful study Bliquez (1996) resolved the interesting problem of these "created" examples that had been generated by poor or inadequate scholarship. Bliquez demonstrates that multiple "examples" sometimes were created accidentally from the same piece through printing the original photographic negatives upside down or backwards. A single negative can be printed in four positions, and some authors have confused the reversed or inverted images of the same appliance as being separate examples. In addition, spurious prostheses also are "created" through poor or erroneous observations, especially when an author has not examined ("autopsied") an appliance in person. Professor Bliquez courageously offers corrections to the many published works that erroneously "created" supposedly new examples of these ancient appliances.

Another situation of poor scholarship leading to the "creation" of false examples may be found in those reports that treat modern *copies* of these appliances (see Appendix II) as if they were originals. During the early part of the twentieth century a number of copies were fashioned in order to depict examples of early "dentistry." In no case does this appear to be forgery—a deliberate attempt to create a modern replica in order to sell or represent it as an original. The list of spurious dental appliances (see Appendix III) reflects the ease with which such appliances became listed among the "examples" of some authors.

A third source of error involves mistaken inferences about the Egyptian origin of ancient dental appliances. Some imagined Egyptian "prostheses," as well as false "examples" from Italy, appear even in recent lists (e.g. Emptoz 1987, signaled by Bliquez 1996). New "examples" continue to be generated (as detected by Waarsenburg 1991a). In order to clarify some of these problems we have included in Appendix III lists of the better known spurious examples, along with a list of known copies (Appendix II) and a list of votives and amulets (Appendix IV) that often have been confused with, or interpreted as being, dental appliances. This specific problem of spurious Egyptian prostheses is reviewed as a special topic, in Chapter 2. The difficulties created by these poor evaluations of "pseudo-prostheses" are compounded by several superficial reviews of the subject, which rarely help to clarify these issues (cf. Cali 1901; Micheloni 1976; Eriksson 1988; also Puech, Cianfarani and Puech 1990: 2006). However, incorrect or garbled accounts purporting to describe these dental appliances continue to be published (e.g. Capasso and Di Tota 1993), and others can be expected to appear *ad infinitum*.

Adding to this problem is the general lack of data concerning the archaeological contexts from which most of these pieces were recovered. Not only is basic contextual data for most appliances wanting, but often the human remains were discarded (!) and only the gold portion was saved. Even the human and false teeth that were associated with these prostheses are largely absent, not to mention other parts of the skeletons. Only rarely is the entire skull present, and only one prosthesis can be associated with what today would be considered a basic archaeological record.

These various difficulties can be remedied only by detailed studies of each of the appliances, such as Clawson's outstanding contribution (1934), and also by including careful study of the dental and skeletal materials found in association with these prostheses. Some of the archaeological evidence, recovered from unpublished notes, journals, and reports, is the focus of a paper on the Valsiarosa appliance (no. 15, Waarsenberg 1991a). This specimen had been one of the most problematical examples, despite Waarsenburg's attempts to clarify the literature, because no first hand description had been made prior to 1993. As noted earlier, our book now offers a series of accurate descriptions of nine of these pieces, in addition to an inventory of the other known appliances.

Also important for understanding the social system within which these dental appliances were made and used is the related evidence provided by the literary sources for ancient dentistry, including literary evidence of the relationship of practitioners of medicine to those persons who performed dental extractions in ancient societies. This study, which appears in Chapter 1, provides clear evidence of how available this type of prosthetic adjustment was among the Etruscans and Romans. The literary evidence reflects the long history of dental appliances, which now can be documented archaeologically.

The manufacture of these ancient dental appliances was a skilled activity apparently in the hands of goldsmiths rather than the work of barbers or physicians, as appears to have been the case in recent centuries. The rediscovery of processes of making dental bridges (also called pontics, from the Latin word for "bridge") as an aspect of dentistry has had a varied history, but one that may be researched with great success from written records. Sissman (1968: 10) notes that jewelers, barbers, and blacksmiths all participated in fashioning dentures in the post-Renaissance period. Sissman also points out that the famous American silversmith, Paul Revere, also created dentures for his clients, using ivory, gold and silver.

Three approaches to the question of the Etruscan origins of dental pontics are incorporated within this volume. The first to be discussed is the "literary" approach. This is not the point of departure that sheds the most light on the subject, but it has been the traditional approach to these objects. As such, it reveals much regarding the confusion about the origins of this technology. The inference that the written sources document the origins of this technology is clearly refuted by the archaeological evidence—the oldest appliance (Satricum, no. 18) has been dated by context to the seventh century BCE, while the literary sources only begin with the fifth century, and are fullest in the first centuries BCE and CE. Thus the second approach, here embedded in the catalogue of our corpus of ancient prostheses, is a review of the archaeological evidence. The core of this study, involving the third approach to the subject, is the direct analysis of as many of these dental prosthetics as are now available for detailed study.

This book is intended as a fresh look at these exceptional artifacts and their archaeological and social contexts, which have much yet to tell us about the development of technology and medicine in ancient Italy. They also attest to the special character of the Etruscan society and ideology, which became the foundation (via its absorption by Rome, credited or not) of our own culture.

Becker has autopsied most of the items in the Etruscan catalogue (see Table 5.1 for those no longer available), and has attempted to track down or verify the disappearance of the lost pieces. During this research it became apparent that much of the published information was disparate at best and often woefully inaccurate: ancient false teeth (like George Washington's) are strange, inter-esting items, and reporters recognize their draw, whether they are correctly analyzed or not. All previous bibliography known to us has been cited in the catalogue, but all descriptions and interpretations are our own and will often be seen to contrast with familiar, older references. Turfa has studied the Liverpool appliances firsthand (1980–1981, 2011, 2015), both before and after their theft in 1989 and later return (unscathed), and has seen some others on display in Italian museums (Tarquinia, Villa Giulia, Orvieto, 2009). We are grateful for the additional advice and help of Margarita Gleba and of Cynthia Reed (goldsmith) in the study of the pieces in Liverpool and Italian museums.

The Corpus and this study of dental appliances

One of the major advantages of conducting a direct study of the known examples of Etruscan dental appliances has been the ability to describe the exact methods of manufacture, and to use that information to provide a general understanding of the ways in which these appliances actually were fitted into the mouths of the owners. During the detailed examination of the nine available appliances, it became evident that they were primarily fitted to the anterior teeth of Etruscan and Italic women and for cosmetic purposes. By deriving conclusions from the direct study of these appliances, we have avoided at least some of the errors generated by earlier authors. The common use of earlier and equally limited publications, rather than making detailed examinations of the actual appliances, has created a plethora of fanciful commentary.

Perhaps a more important contribution to this study has been the identifica-tion of the wearers of the prostheses, through examination of the actual teeth and bone associated with the appliances. Gender can be evaluated by relative tooth size (see Becker and Salvadei 1992), and so even where the skeleton is lacking, measurements of the spaces in gold prostheses can indicate the sex of the original wearer. The degree of confidence in gender evaluation is indicated by the numbers of question marks after the evaluation (0 to 3). Thus an evalu-ation as "Male," or "M" would indicate high confidence, while "M???" would indicate only that this "might" be a male, but with a low degree of confidence in this gender evaluation. This study also provides an entirely new dimension to our understanding of these appliances, based on Becker's 30 years of experi-ence in the excavation and analysis of human skeletons. However, it appears that none of the bone now with the available appliances, and possibly only some

Table I.1 Correlation between the Becker direct tooth referencing system and the International Standard for Adults

Becker:	Left																Right
Maxilla	^{3}M	^{2}M	^{1}M	^{2}PM	^{1}PM	C	^{2}I	^{1}I	I^1	I^2	C	PM^1	PM^2	M^1	M^2	M^3
Mandible	$_3$M	$_2$M	$_1$M	$_2$PM	$_1$PM	C	$_2$I	$_1$I	I$_1$	I$_2$	C	PM$_1$	PM$_2$	M$_1$	M$_2$	M$_3$

International Standard for Adults (See Robetti 1983)

Maxilla	18	17	16	15	14	13	12	11	21	22	23	24	25	26	27	28
Mandible	38	37	36	35	34	33	32	31	41	42	43	44	45	46	47	48

Alt 1997: 26 Left | | | | | | | | | *Right*

Maxilla	18	17	16	15	14	13	12	11	21	22	23	24	25	26	27	28
Mandible	48	47	46	45	44	43	42	41	31	32	33	34	35	36	37	38
Deciduous maxilla				55	54	53	52	51	61	62	63	64	65			
Deciduous mandible				85	84	83	82	81	71	72	73	74	75			

of the teeth, can be confirmed as being original. For the teeth now associated with these appliances, or bound by or replaced by these bridges, we have used a reference system that specifies the tooth's position, the side (quadrant) of the jaw, and possible placement in upper or lower jaw (maxilla, mandible). Other systems of notation exist, and Table I.1 is offered to reduce possible confusion.

1 Dentistry in medical history

Classical roots

The main purpose of this book is to present to a variety of readers, experts and laymen, yet another invention or innovation that in a way we owe to the Etruscans: the dental appliance. Those found in the burials of ancient Etruscan women were the first such devices known; they were cosmetic in purpose, and not strong enough for heavy-duty everyday biting and chewing. They represent the main elements of dental prostheses: the insertion of replacement teeth, anchored to living teeth in the mouth, and the use of gold, which enabled them to be fitted, and happens to make them safe (non-toxic) in the mouth. Other cultures have given the modern world such inventions as amalgam fillings (China), but the Western world follows Etruscan design and goldsmiths' innovations in the use of bridges and braces.

First, for full background, and an indication of how many centuries elapsed between the Etruscan appliances and the next time such prostheses (somewhat improved) appeared in Western society, we offer here a brief history of dental science and(/or) artistry, including the latest finds from archaeological sites across Europe and the Mediterranean world. The technological advances illustrated by ancient dental appliances, such as the "parting" (purification) of gold, will also be considered, for valuable new evidence has come from the excavations of Sardis, capital of the Lydian kingdom of the famous Croesus, and from new techniques of materials analysis such as XRF (X-ray fluorescence).

Ancient texts provide a considerable range of information regarding activities in the Classical world that today fall under the umbrella of dentistry. The most important of these are presented through direct quotes. These include oral hygiene, dental extractions, and the manufacture and use of dental prosthetics and/or braces. Claims of ancient Mesopotamian dentistry merit a separate line of research inasmuch as few modern scholars have provided more than a note concerning this subject (see Musitelli 1996: 213–217, notes 12–21). The Babylonian cuneiform texts contain no "indication that would suggest any form of replacement of teeth" (Hoffmann-Axthelm 1970: 81). Certainly there was never anything like the dental appliances, especially the bridges ("pontics" to use the Latin-derived term) that elite Etruscan and Italic women used during the seventh to first centuries BCE.

Egypt, that source of so much technological development, seems never to have engaged in actual dentistry. Apart from magical or pharmaceutical treatments for toothache or sore gums, neither the Egyptian papyri nor the Egyptians' mummies furnish any evidence of dental intervention. The first Egyptian examples of gold wiring for loose teeth were found in burials of Ptolemaic and Roman date from the region of Alexandria and Giza (see Catalogue nos. W-3 to W-5), thus many centuries after the Etruscan phenomenon of gold-band appliances had flourished in Italy. Still, the mystique of Egypt in the popular press has caused many people to believe that false teeth were known in Pharaonic Egypt—so we discuss that situation at length in Chapter 2.

In the Classical world of Greece, Rome and Etruria from about 700 BCE to 500 CE, oral hygiene, dental extraction and dental appliances appear to have been quite distinct areas of activity (Musitelli 1996: 217). At that time hygiene and extractions were more closely linked to each other than either was to the use of dental appliances. For each of these three areas of interest we now have more written resources than archaeological evidence such as actual appliances or skeletons with evidence of dentistry. The archaeological record continues to grow in quality and quantity, providing us with better means by which the ancient texts may be interpreted and distinctions among these medical specialties may be recognized.

An impressive inventory of gold dental appliances from the ancient Mediterranean world has been known for some time (Bliquez 1996; Becker 1994c).[1] These provide direct evidence for the Etruscan practice of cosmetic dentistry as early as the seventh century BCE (see also Johnstone 1932b, Tabanelli 1963, Scarborough 1969)—we use the term "dentistry" for the technical process without implying that it was identical to the modern, medical profession of dentistry. The archaeological evidence for Etruscan dentistry, however, is nowhere directly documented by the Etruscan written record, despite the claims of some authors (Corruccini and Pacciani 1989, 1991). We have lost virtually all of the rich literature that Etruria once produced. Somewhere in the dramas and histories that Romans knew as Etruscan, there were probably references to the repair of lost teeth, but we may never know since works in Etruscan failed to survive the takeover by Roman culture in the course of the first millennium BCE.[2] Etruscan books were written on linen and papyrus, and have not survived in the soils of Italy.

One rich resource is the body of medical literature attributed to the fifth-century BCE Greek physician and teacher, Hippocrates, although much of this was actually recorded or created well after his lifetime. The treatise *On Joints* (32–34), one of the works possibly written in Hippocrates' own era (many others under his name are later additions), noted that teeth displaced or loosened through an injury to the jaw could be braced with gold (almost certainly wire) or thread (fiber) until they were firmly fixed in place (Hippocrates 1928: 258–265).[3] The few examples of dental appliances now known from the Eastern Mediterranean (Becker 1997) confirm the use of tooth conservation techniques mentioned in this early literature— they originated at the end of the fifth century, however, and continued in the Hellenistic or Roman periods, and do not predate the corpus of Etruscan examples. In contrast, however, the Etruscan production of dental appliances appears to be a profession associated with goldsmiths, and quite distinct from dentistry as it was then practiced (and that involved only the removal of teeth). Skilled, or at least regularly active, dental technicians may have been practicing (extracting teeth presumably) considerably earlier, but no evidence for this has been detected anywhere. Direct evidence for the practice of tooth extraction in antiquity is extremely rare, until recently limited to references to dentists on tombstones with an occasional depiction of what some scholars believe may be a dental forceps (Lanciani 1892: 353, see below). Collections of medical curiosities often include such instruments, but cannot demonstrate their exact application (and usually lack context as well: cf. for example, Thompson 1921: 580–581). The following consideration of those aspects of dentistry that involve oral hygiene and extraction as they existed in the Classical world will serve as a useful point of departure from which we may examine the origins and development of dental appliances.

The recent discovery of direct *archaeological* evidence for the practice of dentistry—tooth pulling—in a *taberna* (shop) within the podium of the Temple of Castor and Pollux in the Roman Forum provides evidence for the early history of this profession—but it was not early in human history, dating only to the first century CE (see Appendix VI). Associated artifacts suggest that a barbershop (or beauty salon?) and pharmacy were the principal trades plied at this location (Nielsen and Zahle 1987, Nielsen 1992: 109–111). The evidence from the human teeth in the shop's drain shows clearly that one form of dentistry was an important adjunct to these other activities, and that the practitioners were rather successful at this aspect of their trade (Becker, 2000a).

The interpretation of the new archaeological data can be enhanced if we review critically the ancient literary evidence from authors who made reference to teeth and activities related to oral hygiene. Some texts are medical in nature, but many of the most useful ones are satirical or otherwise circumstantial in character. A few sources appear to refer to the use of dental appliances, which obviously were related to the preservation of loose teeth or the replacement of missing teeth. While these generally are the consequences of failed dental hygiene, or dental disease, some appliances in the form of simple bands may have been meant to stabilize teeth loosened by a blow rather than by periodontal disease. And we cannot discount the possibility that some such simple bands may have been purely ornamental.

Development of dentistry

Two basic histories of dental surgery and oral medicine in general (Guerini 1909, Hoffmann-Axthelm 1973) provide useful reviews of the earlier literature. The following information is intended to re-examine and expand upon these sources from the perspective of the period during which the shop in the Temple of Castor and Pollux was functioning, the early years of the Roman Empire. These data will be reviewed in the cultural context of Roman history, and compared with related developments in the care and preservation of teeth. This will enable us to scrutinize the origins and development of the technology of dental prosthetics.

The first Western evidence for practitioners comes from Greece and Rome; other commentaries from Egypt or Mesopotamia are older but do not even encompass extractions, let alone other dental procedures.

We might have expected a discussion of such matters in the early Greek medical texts, attributed to the great healer of Kos, Hippocrates—but in vain. The almost complete absence of data concerning diseases of the gums or teeth in the original Hippocratic works, assembled between 425 and 300 BCE,[4] reflects ancient Greek attitudes towards oral health as a category distinct from other aspects of medicine. Ancient Greeks saw tooth loss as a minor problem associated with the normal process of aging, a view held by many people in the modern world. This ancient conceptual separation of dentistry from internal medicine appears to have continued until modern times. Nevertheless, medical observers did recognize quite early that periodontal disorders were a principal cause of tooth loss, and devised numerous treatments for diseased gums. Treatments for dental decay, as indicated by the compilations of Pliny (first century CE, see Appendix V), also were numerous, but probably few if any of them were efficacious.

The dominant theory of dental decay in the ancient world seems to have been the "tooth worm" theory (see Gorelick and Gwinnett 1987b; Ghalioungui 1973: 117, fn. 181). Dental practitioners as well as the ancient public believed that small worms eating the teeth caused decay and pain, and assumed that killing these worms would stop the pain. Leek (1967b: 51) documents the presence of the tooth worm theory in Egypt as early as the nineteenth century BCE. While drilling techniques similar to those used in modern dentistry were well known throughout the ancient world for making artifacts (Gorelick and Gwinnett 1987a; Bennike and Fredebo 1986; also Gwinnett and Gorelick 1979), they were never applied to the physical removal of these theoretical worms. The use of gold foil techniques of considerable complexity also existed in antiquity (for constructing jewelry), but the merger of drilling and foil use within the realm of dentistry is a very recent phenomenon. In fact, except for extractions there were no remedies for dental decay before the relatively modern procedure of drilling and filling of carious teeth emerged in the 1870s (see Künzl and Weber 1991).[5]

Since the removal of teeth could, in theory, be effected by almost anyone with a pair of pliers and the inclination to attempt the procedure, extractions may have been performed quite frequently by people who were not trained in any particular aspect of the medical arts. The procedures developed in ancient Greece for the extraction of teeth were quite basic and probably extremely effective. Only advances in tools (see Bliquez 1994, 1996, 2015), and possibly in the related use of anesthetics, have improved upon knowledge that must have been common to the more skilled of these ancient practitioners. The use by early dental specialists of ancillary and effective surgical procedures, together with the application of ointments such as were part of the pharmacists' trade, created a natural affinity, which must have emerged quite early. Pharmacy, barbering, and what is now called cosmetology in America (hair, face, and general care of the skin), may all have been part of the same trade, just as it was conducted in the shop excavated in the Temple of Castor and Pollux in Rome.

Dental extractions in antiquity

For obvious practical reasons basic dental anatomy has been known by all skilled practitioners of dental extractions since at least the fifth century BCE. These skills probably developed hundreds of years before the appearance of the written records that note observations relating to this part of dentistry. On the other hand, recorded information about shape variations, numbers, and other features associated with the teeth was slow to develop as a *scholarly* pursuit (see Lindsay 1953). We do not know at what date specialized instruments were developed for dental work, but the earliest dental texts, Hellenistic Greek and later Roman works, note that any kind of extracting instrument, whether a dental forceps or simple pincers, should be used only in the final phases of an extraction. Any attempt to extract decayed teeth using ordinary pliers can result in the shattering of the fragile crowns. Aristotle (*Mechanics* 854a 16–32) uses the term *odontagra* for "tooth forceps" and other Greek writers seem to have called it *odontagogon*, with the meaning of grasping or pulling a tooth (see Bliquez 2015: 239–240 for the texts and references to over 20 Roman examples of simple iron forceps).

Information concerning proper extraction methods was known to the Roman author Celsus who lived during the reign of emperor Tiberius (14–37 CE). He cited it in the surviving medical arts portion (*Artes*) of his encyclopedia; the knowledge has continued to be disseminated as a basic rule in dental extractions. The proper removal of a tooth is a very skilled operation, since any bit of roots remaining within the jaw after an unsuccessful extraction will prevent proper healing. Even the earliest professional dentists were aware that the intact tooth had to be removed for the operation to be successful. The use of scaling instruments, or specialized blades for cutting the gum to expose the root, must have a long history. Simple tools can be fashioned to give the dentist a better grip on the instrument used to cut away the bone surrounding the roots of the tooth to be extracted. Specific tools of this type were quite common in Roman culture by the first century BCE (see Jackson 1990), but they began centuries earlier.

The use of dental forceps appears to be depicted in one of the four scenes worked in repoussé in the surface of an electrum vase from the Kul Oba kurgan-tomb (of a royal Scythian woman) in the Kerch Peninsula on the Black Sea, dating from the fourth century BCE (Alexeyev 2012: 190–191, color fig. p. 190; Weinberger 1948: 106–107, fig. 35). Long-haired, trouser-clad Scythians draw a bow or treat a foot-injury, while another has a tooth pulled, perhaps scenes from a myth or epic. This frequently illustrated vessel, and others like it, may have been made and ornamented by Greeks upon the commission of some important personage from the Scythian world (Siberia and the northern Black Sea shore).

The legend of the physician Erasistratus of Keos, during the same period (*c.*300–245 BCE), has him seeing among the votive offerings in the Temple of Apollo at Delphi a forceps made of lead: in the words of Larry Bliquez, this is "a reminder that only those teeth loose enough to be removed with an instrument as malleable as lead should be pulled" (Bliquez 2015: 240; ancient source: Caelius Aurelianus 1950, *Chronic Diseases* 2.4.84). But forceps also were used for many other medical purposes. Nikol (1991: 24) provides a useful summarization of data on dental forceps (*odontagra*) as distinct from bone forceps, and notes why Milne (1907: 137) concluded that probably the same instrument was used in both situations. The most up-to-date discussion on surgical/dental forceps, with reference to actual instruments, is that of Bliquez 2015: chapter 4.

The fabrication of specialized tools for extraction, and perhaps dental surgery, has been inferred from archaeological finds at Roman sites (e.g. Künzl 1982; Eschebach 1984; Künzl and Weber 1991). These finds, including a tombstone engraved with a forceps and tooth (Laviosa, Capasso and Baggieri 1993: 132, fig. V6), suggest that by Roman times the profession of dentistry was well established in urban areas. Not surprising, therefore, are the rich finds within shops and houses at Herculaneum, buried beneath masses of volcanic mud and ash, which include artifacts which may relate to pharmacy appropriate to dentistry (Scatozza Höricht 1986: 72, 115). Glass containers and instruments used in the pharmaceutical trades may indicate the presence of physicians and/or pharmacists, but no clear evidence for dentistry has been recovered from either Pompeii or Herculaneum. Estelle Lazer's survey of the Pompeian dead (2009: 168–179) shows rather poor oral hygiene, tooth wear from mineral particles in food, some tooth loss, periodontal disease, caries and abscesses, including many instances where tooth extraction would have alleviated suffering, but none where actual extraction could be demonstrated. She noted (2009: 176) "No unequivocal evidence of dental intervention was observed in the available Pompeian sample," nor were any dental forceps identified among the Pompeian instruments (cf. Bliquez 1994: 78). Forceps were found in the excavation of the Roman army fort at Vindonissa (Switzerland), although their uses and meanings could have been varied, not necessarily for dentistry (see Baker 2004: 13, fig. 2a.). (For the congenital and pathological conditions identified among burials of ancient Italy, including Magna Graecian settlers, Italic ethnics and Romans, see Gourevitch's (2007) illustrated synopsis of Baggieri 2005. Pontecagnano in Campania was carefully studied by Fornaciari *et al.* 1985, for the seventh- to sixth-century Etruscan cultural period contrasted with the fifth- to fourth-century Oscan occupation. For Roman-era dental health in Italy, see Minozzi *et al.* 2012.)

Given the rich variety of cultures represented within Rome itself one could expect that a variety of practitioners were at that time using several approaches to dental extractions, just as many different forms of religious rituals were being followed (cf. Becker 1988, 1995c). We remain uncertain as to *who* performed tooth extractions in Rome. What is today a medical art may have been performed by specialists or may have been a minor part of some more generalized profession, such as pharmacy or barbering, as in the shop at the Temple of Castor. Still, the basic archaeological and documentary evidence for ancient dentistry remains remarkably limited. The skill of tooth extraction could have been practiced by tooth-drawers unassociated with other medical activities, but the need to employ specialized tools must have helped to establish the extractive aspect of dentistry firmly within one or another of the allied medical professions at an early date. The relationship between the shaving razor and the surgeon's scalpel, plus the skill in dealing with cuts and wounds renders obvious the reason for dentistry to have become associated with barbering, so that by the Middle Ages the barber-surgeon commonly extracted teeth.

One piece of archaeological evidence, less clearly documented than the shop in the Roman Forum, has been interpreted to suggest that Roman medicine included dentistry as a subspecialty. Excavations at a Roman camp at Novaesium on the lower Rhine (Koenen 1904: 180–183, pl. XIII) revealed a complete military hospital complex within the large encampment. Evidence from this hospital has been interpreted to indicate that both dentistry and pharmacy were recognized aspects of medical treatment at that time (see Allbutt 1921: 468, n. 2; also Davies 1970, 1972). However, the Novaesium hospital represents an all-purpose frontier situation that is quite different from medicine as practiced in urbanized Roman Italy. In contrast, Eschebach (1984) was able to describe 18 buildings at Pompeii believed to be associated with the practice of medicine or pharmacy, but found no establishments yielding any evidence for the practice of dentistry, nor any barbershops (Pagano 1996, 1997; see Bliquez 1986).

This could be an effect of conditions, both ancient and modern, in the cities of Vesuvius. See Estelle Lazer's (2009: 284–288) chapters 5 and 10 for conditions of research with the human remains there. Bliquez (1994) provides a detailed list of 21 sites at Pompeii that may have had medical associations, but only the shop in the Forum of Rome appears to hold direct evidence for dentistry in the form of the actual teeth that were extracted.

Dental extractions in antiquity: archaeological evidence

The Taberna in the Roman Forum

Only one archaeological site furnishes unequivocal evidence for the practice of tooth extraction as part of a specific profession. Excavations in the 1980s by a team of Scandinavian and Italian archaeologists focused on the area of the Temple of Castor and Pollux, a ruin in the heart of ancient Rome whose three surviving columns are a familiar landmark in the southeast corner of the *Forum Romanum*. The temple's location, between the *Vicus Tuscus ("Etruscan Street")* and the Fountain of Juturna, marks the spot where the twins Castor and Pollux were seen watering their steeds after the fledgling state of Rome won the Battle of Lake Regillus in 496 BCE. The temple was an important focal point in ancient Rome, often used for meetings of the Senate. The area behind heavy metal doors in the temple's podium was the repository of the state weights and standards, and its strong-rooms protected state and private wealth.

The excavations confirmed the presence of "*taberna*-like recesses between the pilasters of the marble facade" (Strong and Ward-Perkins 1962: 25), revealing an extensive series of 29 separate commercial facilities built into the temple's massive podium. Most of these small shops, or *tabernae*, measure about 2.0 by 4.3 meters. Many had been used by moneychangers, the currency traders essential to conducting business in the diverse coinages of antiquity. Other *tabernae* were occupied by people engaged in the banking trades. One shop, however, appears to have belonged to a barber or beautician (Guldager and Slej 1986: 33; Ginge *et al.* 1989; Guldager 1990; Nielsen 1992: 109–111; Poulsen 1992: 56; Becker 2014). These cosmetological trades are indicated by the discovery of large numbers of small glass bottles, tiny bowls and ointment jars, delicate ivory tools such as spatulas and picks, and other such pharmaceutical or cosmetic gear. Such items were part of the equipment of ancient "barbers" and continued to be part of medieval and even some modern barbershops. Large numbers of human teeth were discovered in a drain associated with this *taberna:* it appears that dental extractions were one aspect of the trade conducted there, shortly before the temple burned down around the end of the first century CE. The excavators have dated the context with the teeth *c.*50–*c.*110 CE. As such, this well-documented setting provides the best evidence for this aspect of dentistry from any context in the ancient world.

The 86 human teeth (almost all molars) indicate that this shop must have served as the operating room of a practitioner of dental extractions.

Most of the teeth were found within the opening and pipes of the drainage system beneath the floor, along with fragments of pharmaceutical jars and many tools (see Appendix VI; also Becker 2014). Although the artifacts alone are indicative of the trades of pharmacy and possibly cosmetology, the effectively extracted diseased teeth indicate that dentistry was associated with at least the pharmaceutical aspect of these trades.

The number of people who had a tooth pulled by a professional here may have equaled the number of teeth found, thus close to 86; Becker has estimated

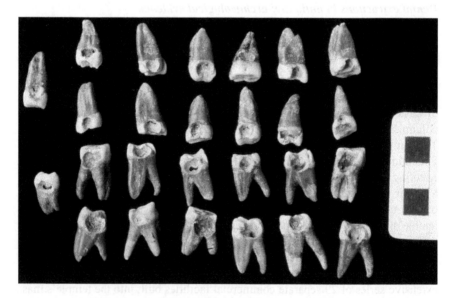

Figure 1.1 A selection of the extracted teeth found in the drain at the *taverna* (shop) in the Roman Forum (*c.*50–110 CE), as in *Archaeology* 42: 35.

Source: photo M. J. Becker.

(2014: 214) that *at least* 50 individuals are represented by the teeth here, and we cannot know how many more teeth were swept up or otherwise lost in antiquity. Most of the molars came from adult men, relatively few are the smaller size that we would expect from women. Perhaps Roman women went elsewhere to have decayed teeth treated, or simply suffered at home. A very few of the teeth that appear healthy have come from women (as estimated by their size), but X-ray studies might reveal additional problems. Dental wear patterns on the teeth suggest that most patients were from 30 to 60 years of age; very few came from elderly persons, who probably suffered more from periodontal disease and loose teeth than caries. While age can only be loosely estimated, it appears that most of the terribly decayed teeth came from men aged between 30 and 40 years, a very different pattern from modern Western populations, where adults suffer less from caries and more from periodontal disease. In modern groups, children have caries that taper off by age 25: a combination of modern factors may be behind this, including fluoridated water supplies, regular dental hygiene and preventive treatments. The pattern seen in the Forum teeth of the incidence of cavities *increasing* with age is similar to that found for the much earlier, Latin population of Osteria dell'Osa (historic *Gabii*) of the early first millennium BCE (Becker and Salvadei 1992). Fornaciari *et al.* (1985–1986) found that in Etruscan Pontecagnano males had more and more severe dental problems, and suggested that this was related to men's longevity compared to that of women, many of whom did not live long enough to develop certain problems.

The teeth themselves attest to the skill of the practitioner. Many have decayed so extensively that only thin, fragile shells remain, yet these were not broken by the extraction process. The ancient texts accurately describe the process of grasping and rocking the tooth gently until it could be removed by hand. Molars with complex roots might have required cutting the gum and even the surrounding bone in order to achieve a complete extraction. Even more drastic measures were required when the carious lesion was more advanced. One example of the very badly decayed molars, which was in danger of breaking and leaving an infected portion in the jaw, was found with a small portion of alveolar bone from the jaw that had been pinched against the tooth and extracted along with it. While seemingly a crude extraction, this deliberate effort guaranteed that the entire fragile

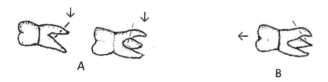

Figure 1.2 Root fractures on extracted teeth found in the Roman Forum (*c.*50–110 CE):
(a) fracture resulting from forced extraction, without preliminary loosening;
(b) post-extraction fracture, resulting from trampling.

Source: sketch by M. J. Becker.

crown and roots of the tooth were cleanly removed, thus reducing the danger of breakage and infection. Extracting a bit of adjacent bone was the procedure recommended by Celsus (early first century CE), who also urged practitioners not to extract children's teeth unless they were hampering the growth of adult teeth, and only 2 of the 86 teeth from the shop's drain are from children.

All but one tooth from the *taberna* were molars, many showing advanced decay and damage; the only other one was a premolar, indication that front teeth were not normally lost or extracted in this population. Most of those relieved of a bad tooth would have been suffering constant pain, as the cavities were deep, penetrating and often occupying the entire pulp chamber. A study of the carious teeth by Feyerskov *et al.* (2012: 210) found that most of the carious "lesions had a hypermineralized zone in the dentin at the advancing front of the carious cavities," a situation interpreted by Becker as indicating the use of strong analgesics while they suffered with the bad tooth or teeth. The many little ointment or drug pots found in the shop lead us to assume that many of these cases received treatment to control their pain and heal their infections. Full data on the teeth and bibliographic references on the Temple of Castor and Pollux *taberna* appear in Becker 2014.

Extractions, additional and unusual evidence

Dental extractions were a minor facet of medical practice throughout almost all of history. Roman dentists certainly were practicing a trade distinct from that of the physicians of that period, who are frequently represented in various contexts (Hillert 1990, see also Scarborough 1990). The Roman dentists who did extractions used some of the techniques of the surgeon, including cutting back the gum and bone to expose roots, post-operative cauterization (generally with a white-hot iron), and the use of astringent mouthwashes to stop minor bleeding. Crude as these activities may seem, they form the basis for all subsequent treatment of dental pain derived from tooth removal. A brief summary of ancient formulae and treatments for dental and oral diseases has been assembled by Neiburger (1992), but the important subject of pain and its treatment in antiquity warrants some discussion in this context.

One ancient event is surely the work of a pagan mob or professional torturers, but often cited in histories of dentistry: the martyrdom of Saint Apollonia (Sainte Apolline). A deaconess in Alexandria, she was one of a group of Christian virgins murdered by a mob during the reign of the emperor Philip the Arab. Her death in 249 CE is celebrated on February 9 (Benedictine Monks 1989: 56). During her martyrdom her teeth were said to have been broken and extracted with pincers. Thus she is represented as holding a tooth in pincers, and, in the curious logic of hagiography, is invoked as a patron of those with toothaches, and of dentists. A reliquary in the Cathedral of Porto, Portugal displays a tooth said to be hers, held in a small pincers. Her martyrdom is retold in Eusebius' fourth-century CE *Historia Ecclesiae* (1.6.41).

Pain

Ancient Roman dentistry was not oriented toward prevention, although dentifrices and toothbrushes were commonly used. Many of the classical authors did describe means by which dental problems could be reduced (see Porter and Teich 1995; Crawfurd 1914: 22–23). The ability of practitioners to relieve associated pain, using remedies that might leave in place the teeth, or what remained of decayed teeth, was entirely dependent on the use of analgesics. Lufkin (1948: 55) believes that the Greeks Herophilus (335–280 BCE), Erasistratus (304–250 BCE) and Heraclides of Tarentum (c.230 BC) all were aware of dental pathology, and the fact that a badly executed extraction could lead to death.

In any discussion of dentistry the subject of dental pain may arise. In the context of ancient dentistry the nature of available palliatives and anesthetics is almost always noted. Numerous modern authors have focused attention on this particular aspect of medicine (see King 1988; Baumann 1993; Rey 1993), with Indian hemp (hashish) and other plants receiving the most attention. Folk knowledge regarding toxins produced by various frogs' skins is extensive, and derivative analgesics have always been popular. Some painkillers derived from frog skins have the advantage of low toxicity as well as being non-addictive (Bannon *et al.* 1998; also Strauss 1992).

Although many of these narcotic agents were well known and widely employed throughout the classical world, Shapiro and Shapiro (1997) believe that all medicinal treatments until nearly modern times were placebos, at best. Sternberg (1998) refutes this general claim, noting that in addition to the indirect benefits of various painkillers, a number of ancient treatments such as squill (the lily-like plant, *Drimia maritima*, native to the Mediterranean and featured in ancient medications: see Appendix V) have potentially useful applications.[6] Sternberg (1998) notes that a "plant's content of biologically active chemicals can vary with different geographical sources, seasons, years, and plant parts." In addition to these variations, the processes of collecting the plant as well as extracting and storing the active substances all influence potency. In short, control over dosages and the effects of pharmaceutical agents was, until recently, limited but not entirely inefficacious: one can imagine that certain dealers could offer better products, and so earn high reputations.

The landmark work of Theophrastus (born in 370 BCE), *The Enquiry into Plants*, demonstrates the breadth of knowledge of Greek scholars regarding their natural environment and their expertise in identifying narcotic plants that could be used to alleviate pain. Of particular interest in this research is the note that Homer is believed to have indicated Egypt as the source of "*nepenthes*, the famous drug which cures sorrow and passion, so that it causes forgetfulness and indifference to ills" (Theophrastus 1916: 291). Theophrastus also notes the fame of Etruria in this regard, indicating that this was common knowledge among poets such as Aeschylus (*Enquiry into Plants* 9.15.1). (Greek authors referred to the Etruscans as *Tyrrhenians* or *Tyrsenoi*, from whom the name of the Tyrrhenian Sea is derived. For a variety of herbs/drugs gathered in ancient Etruria, in addition to painkillers, see Harrison and Turfa 2010.)

Φαρμακώδεις δὲ δουκοῦσιν εἶναι τόποι μάλιστα τῶν μὲν ἔξω τῆς Ἑλλάδος οἱ περὶ τὴν Τυρρηνίαν καὶ τὴν Λατίνην, ἐν ᾗ καὶ τὴν Κίρκην εἶναι λέγουσιν.

The places outside Hellas [Greece] which especially grow medicinal herbs seem to be parts of Tyrrhenia and Latium (where they say Circe was).

(Enquiry Into Plants 9.15.1)

Καὶ γὰρ Αἰσχύλος ἐν ταῖς ἐλεγείαις ὡς πολυφάρμακον λέγει τὴν Τυρρηνίαν. "Τυρρηνὸν γενεάν, φαρμακοποιὸν ἔθνος."

For Aeschylus too in his elegies calls Tyrrhenia rich in drugs: "The Tyrrhenian tribe, a people skilled in compounding drugs."

(Enquiry Into Plants 9.15.1; see Weiss 1989: 137)

While the Greeks may have been importing pharmaceuticals as well as metals from Etruria, we must note that Theophrastus (1916: 293 (9.15.2)) specifically identifies numerous places in Greece where drugs were produced (see also Theophrastus 1988). In the difficult and disease-ridden ancient world, all agents that could relieve pain must have been in great demand.

The painkillers known to the classical world continued to be in use in medieval Near Eastern pharmacopeias long after the decline of the Roman Empire. Many of the herbs and barks that were the mainstay of Roman pharmacies, such as frankincense SP and myrrh, had Near Eastern origins (see Marin and Cappelletti 1995) and have remained in demand by the medical profession (myrrh, for instance, is still used in some toothpastes). The difficulties in identifying specific plants mentioned in various texts are often noted, but Touwaide (1998) provides an important review of the literature as well as many useful suggestions. With regard to Italy, Wilhelmina Jashemski's *Pompeian Herbal* (1999) offers information on 36 ancient medicinal plants that are known from the region of Pompeii in the Roman period, and several of them continue to be used by the local populace for their pharmaceutical properties. (See also numerous articles in Jashemski's 2002 *Natural History of Pompeii* compendium.)

Heraclides' supposed investigations of the clinical effects of drugs are believed by Lufkin (1948: 55) to have involved the use of opium. (Note that Heraclides, active during the third–second century BCE, was a native of Tarentum in South Italy.) Lufkin, who provides good references, also notes that Pedanius Dioscorides of Anazarbus (Cilicia), *c.*50 CE, discussed the benefits of various drugs. Brunner (1973) even suggests that marijuana was used in the Classical world, probably referring to the various kinds of hemp (hashish) more commonly smoked in the Orient, and certainly known throughout the Roman world. In the Middle East various parts of the hemp plant normally were placed on hot coals to vaporize the active agents. A small tent was erected over the coals and participants placed the nose or face into the tent to inhale the smoke emitted by the burning plant. (Cannabis smoking was described by Herodotus for the Scythians as well—see Herodotus 4.74–75; Emboden 1980: 52–53, fig. 30).[7]

Pliny in the extant books of *Natural History* focuses on agents derived from animal sources for the cure, or amelioration, of dental problems (see Appendix V). This commentary on animal-derived remedies is particularly interesting since plant products clearly formed the majority of those ancient pharmacological agents that would have had any efficacy in treating pain (as in Theophrastus and Dioscorides).

Plants also are listed as the most important ingredients in the earlier, ancient Egyptian treatments for oral disease, but not necessarily dental disorders (see Ebbell 1937; Dawson 1935, 1938; Nunn 1996, also Lucas 1937). A variation on the use of plant products can be seen in the use of alcohol, taken internally, as a method of reducing pain. Thus, wine or beer may have been used to dull pain, but their alcohol content would be too low for the effective treatment of serious dental discomfort unless taken in considerable quantities. Oil derived from the fruits of cloves (*karyophylla: Eugenia caryophyllata* Thunb.) has great efficacy against pain from dental caries, and is still used today. This spice may not have reached the Mediterranean world much before the time of Alexander of Tralles (525–605 AD), since it seems to have been unknown in ancient Rome. Hobbs (1992: 153, from Budge 1913) believes that Assyrian garlic was used both as a food and also as a medicinal agent, being used to fill rotten teeth. What effect, if any, an extract of garlic would have on dental disease is not clear.

More powerful narcotics such as *nepenthe* (purified opium?), for both local and general use, were common to Greek medicine (Allbutt 1921: 61). Some 257 drugs from the Hippocratic corpus are listed by Riddle (1987: 39, see also Riddle 1992, and Moisan 1990), and drug vendors (*pharmakopoloi*) and herbalists (*rhizotomoi*) abounded throughout the ancient world.

Pedanius Dioscorides, one of many physicians writing in the first century CE, often refers to the opium poppy and to hemp. Scarborough (1996) indicates that *opos*, the latex of the opium poppy, was processed by the Romans into a powerful drug. The works of Dioscorides also reflect the incorporation of Indian and Egyptian medical practices into Roman procedures (Scarborough and Nutton 1982; Riddle 1985; Brothwell 1988).[8]

The vast majority of the ancient pain killing prescriptions now known to have been effective involved plant derivatives (see Appendix V, also Ciarella 1993). Many of these plants are known today to contain active agents effective in reducing distress (see Vidal 1983, 1984; Riddle 1985). Many of the less effective remedies were derived from non-venomous animal sources, but most, such as spider, snake or frog venoms, are so powerful, due to high toxicity, that they would have been difficult to handle without extreme danger to the patient (see Myers and Daly 1993; also Bradley 1993; Kreil 1994).

The potentially lethal agents employed in ancient medicine, such as snake venom, were recognized as extremely dangerous. In Homer's epics, the word "*pharmakon*" sometimes translated as "drug" or as "magical spell," may also indicate "poison" depending on the context or qualifying adjectives. The general role of snakes in ancient medicine has been summarized by Angeletti and her colleagues (1993).[9] The relationship between poisons and drugs is quite close, and even today "[m]any of these venoms-toxins are useful pharmacological tools" (Heck *et al.* 1994: 1065).

Many of the painkillers used in antiquity, as today, could easily be taken in fatal quantities. The preparation of suitable doses required the abilities of skilled "pharmacists." Since counters to poisons, or the achievement of immunity to various toxins, were often produced by the use of the same agents, the evolution of pharmacological specifics from these sources can be understood (see Barton 1994; also Appendix V: Note 5).[10]

Experiments known from as early as the second century BCE (Allbutt 1921: 347–388) dealt with the development of appropriate dosages for many pharmaceutical substances that could be lethal if not handled with care. In Rome, retail druggists were marketing these pharmaceutical items on the Via Sacra and presumably on the Vicus Unguentarius, although we do not know the location of the latter. Richardson (1992: 429) suggests further Etruscan associations: "One is inclined to put it in the neighborhood of the Vicus Tuscus, where there is known to have been a concentration of shops dealing in luxuries." Another of the many problems involved with the application of these pharmacological treatments was the problem of addiction. Pliny (*Natural History* 20.200) observes that Erasistratus was opposed to abuse in the use of opium, demonstrating that its addictive effects were well known to the ancients.

The search for medicinal plants continues to this day. The recent identification of the Pacific yew product *taxol* as an agent useful in cancer therapy is part of an ancient tradition, dating from at least the Bronze Age, of focusing trade and exploration on the search for pharmaceuticals. These concerns were important aspects of the discovery of the New World, from which the first great exports were pharmaceutical plants (Griffenhagen 1992). These New World spices (*droghi*, in Italian) included tobacco, which "killeth worms" in the teeth and serves against the "bytings of venomous beasts" (Monardes 1577: 76–91, in Griffenhagen 1992: 136). The arrow poisons of Native American peoples also were sought for the sake of their medicinal potential, but like tobacco, were equally dangerous.

The drugs available in Etruria encompassed healing materials as well as potential painkillers. While it has not been possible to conclusively identify such substances or their raw materials in the archaeological record, there are tantalizing fragments of literary evidence relating to medications for teeth or mouths. Some tiny jars occasionally found in Etruscan sites might have held drugs, but none have yielded proof of their contents as yet: see Becker 2009. For instance, *Millefolium* (water-milfoil) was found in Etruria in antiquity and described by Pliny (*Natural History* 24.152) as good for toothache and wound healing (Harrison and Turfa 2010: 286–287, no. 18).

Personal hygiene and home care

The first tool-using hominids probably availed themselves of the humble toothpick. Toothpick use has been identified as the probable cause of an interproximal groove detected on the lower right molar of the early hominid OH 60 from Olduvai

Gorge in Tanzania (Ungar *et al.* 2001). This early *Homo erectus*, found in 1982, has been dated at 1.7 to 2.1 million years old. Similar grooves have been found on the teeth of Neanderthals. Chewing sticks and/or toothpicks are documented from a number of contemporary tribal societies in Africa (Enwonwu 1974, Oranje *et al.* 1935; see Mays 1998: 152). Thus the concern in ancient Rome with these aspects of oral hygiene is not at all surprising. What is surprising is the lack of direct evidence from their teeth while other sources abundantly indicate the use of tooth-picks and dentifrices by the Romans. Roman use of formal toothpicks, rather than simple sticks of wood fashioned only for immediate needs, had become common by the first century CE. Slips of mastic (*lentiscus* or *lentiscum*) were the preferred variety of wood, but quills also offered "relief" (Martial 3.82, 6.74, 7.53, 14.22, see below under "Martial"). While the wording of the satirical poet Martial makes it seem that toothpicks were for comfort rather than periodontal care, Pliny (*NH* 30.27 = 1963: 294–297) indicates that the use of porcupine quills is conducive to dental firmness, but that using a vulture's feather to pick the teeth would make the mouth sour.

The tooth powder mentioned by Martial (14.56, a gift-tag in verse, to be attached to a container of toothpaste) also seems to have been intended to polish (brighten) the teeth rather than to cleanse them (prophylaxis). Martial implies that tooth powders are for the young and fair and not for the aged who would have false, or purchased, teeth (Lentini 1995). Dioscorides advises the use of *Murex* (shells) for tooth cleaning powder, saying that "being burnt [it] has the property of drying and cleaning the teeth." (Pedani Dioscuridis Anazarbi, 1958: 85–86, from Vol. V: 115). His treatise "On quicklime" (*Peri asbestos*) gives a full review of the many uses for this caustic stuff as made from murex etc. (he also was aware that this was the same material (!) as quicklime made by burning marble, limestone, etc., see Riddle 1985: 134.) The use of the shell of this dye-yielding mollusc is presumably but one of many early applications through which an industrial waste, here the discarded shells, was processed into a saleable byproduct. Dioscorides also (elsewhere) says that the whelk (sea snail) shell filled with salt and burned in the same way also serves to clean the teeth and other things (as cited by Riddle 1985: 135). The extensive lists of dentifrices provided by various ancient authors quite clearly suggest that clean breath and teeth could have been related to a good appearance, and probably to good health.

The connection between dental hygiene and the cleaning or polishing of teeth probably was not understood until centuries later. For instance, as late as about 50 CE, gingivitis and pyorrhea are not described by Celsus (1938; see Musitelli 1996). The lack of descriptions of these common disorders in the ancient medical literature suggests that they were seen as part of the normal aging process and not a disorder that could be cured or prevented. Even Paracelsus's doctrine of *tartarus*, tracing all diseases to the presence of calculi or stones within the body (Schneider 1985) does not appear to include concern with dental tartar. Removal of dental tartar from the teeth appears to be a very modern concern; many ancient skulls contain evidence of unchecked tartar deposits.

Surgical tools and techniques for dental extractions

Numerous sets of ancient surgical instruments, found throughout the Roman world, have been well documented (Milne 1907; Bliquez 2015), and vast numbers of single examples are known. Most of these medical tools date from the first and second centuries CE (see Michaelides 1984). One of the largest sets, consisting of 39 separate instruments from Roman Italy, is in the British Museum (Jackson 1986, also 1987). Interest in this ancient equipment is so great that large numbers of false sets are being created to meet the demands of buyers (Künzl 1986, also Bliquez 1985). The interpretation as dental instruments of various tools found at Roman sites is based on comparisons with modern examples as well as on descriptive passages in classical texts.

Ancient texts listing various types of surgical instruments and attendant paraphernalia are known from as early as the second century CE, in the *Onomasticon* (4.181) of a scholar from Naukratis, Pollux, who wrote *c.*166–176 CE during the reign of Commodus (Pollux 1900: 254–255). These lists are in Greek, which long remained the language of scholars. Latin lists appear by 600 CE; one appears in the writings of the famous etymologist and grammarian, Isidore of Seville (*c.*560–636 CE; Bliquez 1985: 191).

Aside from the Greek terms denoting special instruments, or specific uses for general instruments, there is little information in the texts to distinguish between pliers (as might be used by a jeweler or a blacksmith), a surgeon's forceps, and dental forceps (Anonymous 1987). A number of specialized instruments for dentistry were developed during the medieval period. The specialized tooth gripper called a "pelican," known by this name and its distinctive shape only since about 1500 CE, was designed to grip a decayed tooth, or what was left of it, in order to wiggle it loose in its socket so that it could be drawn without breaking. Since the roots of molars expand into the jaws like the roots of trees, removal of an adult tooth with the root intact depends, to a large degree, upon flexibility. The pelican may have existed earlier, but only one possible example is known from an archaeological context. Künzl (1982: 42 fig.11:1) illustrates an iron tool that looks like a pelican; it came from a kit of 10 instruments excavated in Kallion in Central Greece. Künzl terms this tool a *Zahnzange* ("tooth-forceps"). Two of the other tools appear to be dental chisels, rather than surgical knives; quite possibly the owner had specialized in dentistry. These archaeological finds of medical cases provide the best evidence for the hardware in use during any given period (most seem to be Roman); at least, this is true if the mortuary customs of the times included interment of instruments with the owner.

Two ancient lists of terms for medical tools (Bliquez 1985) provide important evidence relating to ancient dentistry. Both are written in Greek, and Bliquez believes that they originated during the Byzantine period and may have served as checklists for the dozens of instruments that comprised a surgeon's equipment during the ninth to eleventh centuries (see Fischer 1987; also Schöne 1903). Bliquez (personal communication, 1994) indicates that the purpose of these lists remains uncertain, but suggests that they may have been "bookish summaries," an advance on the etymological treatises of Pollux and Isidore.

Among the tools noted in these lists are an *odontoxister* (tooth scaler: Bliquez 1985: 196, from Pollux 1900: 254; Milne 1907: 138) and an *odontagra* (tooth forceps: Bliquez 1985: 201; from Pollux 1900: 254; Cüppers 1981: 40). Many of the other tools listed could have served in various aspects of dental surgery in addition to their principal or originally intended function.

An important observation concerning dental *appliances* is their distribution within a very restricted area, as compared with the very wide distribution of ancient medical tools (e. g. Künzl 1993). While Roman medical and surgical devices are found over nearly the entire width and breadth of the Roman world, actual dental *appliances* have only been recovered from within a remarkably limited zone, mainly central Italy, with a very few Phoenician, Egyptian and Greek outliers.

Status of Roman-era medical and dental practitioners

The status of physicians among the Etruscans remains completely unknown. It is difficult to compare Etruscan medicine with Greek and Roman practices, since none of the Etruscan literature survives. Stray comments in the Greek and Latin authors imply their skill at herbalism, and the wealth of *materia medica* to be harvested in Etruria.[11]

One other field of evidence relating to Etruscan medicine is the corpus of anatomical votive models, which betray some additional anatomical/physiological knowledge during the last centuries of the first millennium BCE. Offerings made in thanks for healing at over 200 sanctuaries across central Italy (both Etruscan and Italic cults) from about 300 BCE into the first century CE, include terracotta models of heads, hands, feet, arms, legs, external and internal genitalia and other internal organs. Plaques with stylized viscera could have been based on what an artist saw in a butcher's shop or sacrificial ritual, resembling beef, pork or fowl, but they were certainly intended as human representations. Sometimes entire statues or torsos display a man or woman's internal organs as if the abdominal cavity or chest were sawed open. The most telling are the model uteri, usually depicted with ridges to indicate the rippling contractions of third-stage labor. These came in a variety of styles, some showing fibroid tumors or a sectioned, multiparate cervix. While extremely stylized, symmetrical and simplified, these can only be primate organs and must have been offered for safe childbirth or the healing of related complications (there is indication that Etruscans attempted post-mortem C-section in special cases) (see Turfa 1994 and 2004; Turfa and Becker 2013: 866–869). While Hellenistic Greek doctors such as Herophilus certainly dealt with surgery, gynecological specialties (and vivisection), the Greek sanctuaries have not yielded this kind of abundant anatomical evidence, and we must acknowledge that Etruscan medicine had a distinctly different character than the philosophical and theoretical brand practiced by Greeks and Greek-trained Romans.

Although the Romans also relied to a great extent on magic (see Önnerfors 1993), surviving literature demonstrates that many Romans placed great emphasis on the quite successful Greek medical tradition and also employed Greek physicians as preferred medical practitioners (also, see Baller 1992; Horstmanshoff 1990). McKechnie (1989: 148, 164–165 n. 61) suggests that Greek physicians enjoyed high status in their communities, and probably among the Italians as well. McKechnie's reliance on Sherwin-White's (1978: 257) data, however, may be unwarranted. H. W. Pleket (1995) believes that the Romans disparaged itinerant Greek physicians, and Latin authors do evince some prejudice for persons who worked with their hands—yet Romans seem to have relied on Greek physicians for medical care over many centuries. The evidence for the status of physicians in Roman Italy is not yet well understood; the type of medicine practiced by individual physicians must have been a factor in the regard in which they were held (see Jackson 1993, Riddle 1993). In general, physicians appear to have been treated as among the more useful hired staff in a Roman household.

The Roman tradition in which doctors are ridiculed for their "kill 'em or cure 'em" treatments is clearly depicted in the satirical epigrams of Martial, a professional poet who wrote for high society in Rome during the second half of the first century CE. His description of the low status of medical practitioners in Imperial Rome is important. Suetonius (*Julius Caesar* 42) writes that civic rights were granted by Julius Caesar to immigrant medical practitioners indicating that their skills were needed and appreciated on some level (see Crawfurd 1914: 16). Also significant are Martial's notes on the presence of medical specialists (Crawfurd 1914: 17). Lucian's comments (see below) on the status of medical practitioners are often the un-cited basis for modern references (e. g. Ring 1986). Pliny's works also furnish references critical of professional physicians. If physicians in ancient Rome generally were Greek in origin or other easterners, and probably freed slaves, they must have been accorded a relatively low status (Hirt 1986; see also Andre 1987).

The status of Roman tooth pullers must have been even lower than that of physicians (see Crawfurd 1914: 20, also 21–22). Lanciani's (1892: 353) note of the discovery in 1864 of the tombstone of the dentist Victorinus (or Celerinus, his inscription preserves only ". . . inus") decorated with an instrument that is probably a forceps and also a chisel or knife (see Figure 1.3a), also provided an early clue as to means by which the status of some of these ancient practitioners could be inferred. These forceps have been interpreted by Northcote as dental forceps.

Lanciani, citing De Rossi the excavator and mirrored by Northcote (1878: 172–173) also noted the name of an "Alexander" whose final resting place (a *loculus* in the cemetery of Calepodius) is decorated with an incised pair of similar forceps (Figure 1.3b). A general surgeon's grave monument in the cemetery of Praetextatus had a small relief of many instruments including the same forceps type (Figure 1.3c). This reference to a general surgeon appears to have led Jackson (1988: 119) to infer that extractions were performed by physicians and surgeons. This certainly would have been the exception rather than the rule.

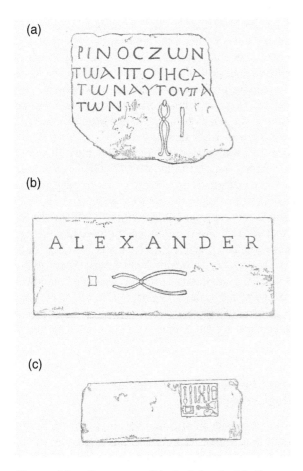

Figures 1.3a-c Images, possibly depicting dental pliers, carved in Roman stone
funerary monuments: (a) tombstone of a dentist (?) incised with
image of forceps for ". . . inus" the damaged inscription probably
named "Victorinus" or "Celerinus," Cyriaca Cemetery on the via
Tiburtina; (b) tomb epitaph of "Alexander," depicting forceps
and tooth, Cemetery of Calepodius, Rome; (c) funerary relief,
uninscribed, possibly of a surgeon, with dental forceps among other
surgical tools, Rome, Catacombs of Praetextatus.

Source: after Northcote 1878: 172–173.

Jackson (1988), in his revision of an earlier paper, suggests that by 100 BCE
Romans were taking over these medical trades from Greek immigrants (or their
descendants?) and that the status of these new professionals had improved (see
also Jackson 1993). However, it is more likely that the eastern physicians and
their descendants simply were known by Roman names, and that the status of
these professionals remained low (see also Joshel 1992).

Treggiari (1978: 162–164) examined the activities and status of laborers in ancient Rome, focusing on jobs described by the upper class as common and sordid. Some 225 specialized jobs can be identified using a variety of sources. Citing Cicero, Treggiari notes that numerous tasks were considered as unsuitable for a free person. These included unskilled manual work, retail trades, workshop employees, and people providing pleasure (entertainers, food sellers, perfume makers), all of whom operated from workshops (*officinae*) or from shops or inns (*tabernae*). Obviously people without even these formal establishments (street venders, street prostitutes) had even lower status.

The labors of skilled crafters were not considered sordid, but still were common. On this level were persons engaged in large-scale commerce, who could be rich, but still had low status. Cicero notes that those whose trades demanded intelligence and provided benefits, such as teachers, architects, and medical practitioners, were honorable for those of suitable station (Treggiari 1979: 48). The implication here is that such jobs were common, but more like the respectable poor of today. These *opifices* practiced manual arts (writing, building, healing) necessary to life. This category probably included physicians, while the still more bloody arts of surgeons and dentists probably occupied the lower end of this already low end of the social scale. Treggiari (1979: 82, n. 11) suggests that some of the Roman goldsmiths may have been women, a factor that might have been an advantage, considering the intimate contact needed for the fitting of dental appliances.

Ancient written evidence for dentistry and dental appliances in chronological order

While Chapter 3 covers the phenomenon of actual dental appliances in the first millennium BCE, we examine here some background in the ancient literary sources (none of them Etruscan) on use of dentures or appliances and on oral hygiene in the Classical world.

Near Eastern sources: Mesopotamia and Egypt

The abundant cuneiform archives from Sumerian and Babylonian Mesopotamia offer a wealth of medical information for the ancient Near East (Biggs 1969, Verderame 1997). Sumerian society had developed full-fledged cities by the third millennium BCE. A thousand years later the people of the Dynastic era were creating impressive monuments and art, with the city of Lagash achieving massive proportions by 2500 BCE. A decline, followed by a brief renaissance about 2050 BCE, is evident from the records that similarly reveal the rise and expansion of the city of Babylon. By 1700 BCE the expanding Babylonian empire dominated the region, with Nippur (southeast of Babylon) a major city. The sack of all Babylonia by Hittites in 1595 led to a long decline until the Assyrian ascendancy in Mesopotamia after 900 BCE. Assyria fell at the end of the seventh century, to be replaced by the Persian Empire, itself conquered by the Macedonian kingdom *c.*331 BCE. The Macedonian, Seleucid and Ptolemaic successors of Alexander were gradually supplanted by Rome, which controlled the entire region from 30 BCE on.

At the beginning of the twentieth century Felix Freiherr von Oefele contributed a landmark study of Babylonian medicine (1902) that includes limited information on teeth and dental history. Oefele's 1905 excavations at Assyrian Nineveh, however, chanced upon the library of Ashurbanipal of Assyria (King Sardanapalus, the first Assyrian king who could read and write: 668–626 BCE; Sudhoff 1922: 11–29, also Thompson 1923). Many of the medical texts recovered during these excavations turned out to be copies of older writings, including those from Sumerian Nippur (*c.*1700 BCE). The continuities in these records over more than 1,000 years parallel, and to some extent duplicate, the records known from contemporary Egypt.

As in ancient Egypt, the texts offer a wide range of information relating to health and disease, with magical (religious) treatments dominating therapies. What have been called Babylonian medical textbooks (see Oefele 1917) are largely discussions of bodily parts affected by disorders that are now difficult to identify; attached to the texts are the applications of rituals and pharmaceuticals to counter them. One of these tablets (K 259, see Oefele 1917: 250) has "a pharmaco-therapeutic list for toothache, shaking tooth, and tooth-decay" that appears to bring together what little was known regarding dental ills (see Stol 1985).

A study by E. J. Neiburger (2000) of the dentition of burials at the Mesopotamian cities of Ur (home of Abraham) and Kish from the period *c.*2000 BCE showed poor dental health, a characteristic of many agrarian people. Neiburger found that 95 percent of the people had experienced dental attrition (tooth loss) in life, but only 42 percent suffered periodontal disease. His suggestion that only 2 percent showed dental caries reveals a faulty methodology, as attrition was certainly a function of dental decay. Total population size for this study was not provided. Mesopotamian urban populations were rather homogeneous, with dental decay probably equally common among the elite as well as common folk. Neiburger's somewhat casual research showed that many individuals lived with congenital or neoplastic (cancerous) lesions in their mouths, and some had TMJ dysfunctions. This would seem to be a fertile field for the practice of dentistry, but effective treatments were, of course, absent.

Apparently the tooth-worm theory of dental decay was generally accepted throughout Egypt and the regions to its east (cf. Dussau 1987, Musitelli 1996; also Febres-Cordero 1966). While widespread dental pathology was recognized among these urban populations, and periodontal diseases were extensive, little effective treatment was available. Ailments such as dental decay and gum disorders are easily recognized in skeletal populations of these periods, but the texts indicate that efforts to deal with them were largely palliative (Powell 1993: 59, see also Neiberger *et al.* 1998). Powell's excellent study (1993) also proposes that Egyptian and Babylonian medicine were equally limited. As throughout the premodern world, pharmaceutical categories were grouped by animal, mineral and vegetable origins, but efficacy was another matter. Anything resembling modern dentistry was absent (Pfeiffer 1978; see also Neiberger 2000). Appliances of any type and for any purpose were absent prior to the arrival of therapeutic wiring techniques (fifth century BCE or later; Becker 1997). Recent references are furnished in a short article by Reid and Wagensonner (2014) in the *Cuneiform Digital Library Bulletin* in presenting tablet texts that refer to "bandages," presumably poultices to treat an aching tooth; the cuneiform sources indicate magic or exorcism more often than science in handling dental problems. The notion of wrapping the jaw for toothache brings to mind the twentieth-century advertisements for remedies with a person in distress wearing a scarf around their face and jaw.

Many general works attribute some expertise in dentistry to the Egyptians, but unfortunately, quite the opposite seems to be the case. Many cases of supposed apicoectomies to relieve abscesses can be shown to be nothing more than natural processes of the abscess eroding through the jawbone: this relieves pressure but can still be a source of systemic infection, and a number of mummies show evidence of this as the cause of death. Likewise reports of false teeth, wooden teeth, etc. found in the mouths of mummies have all proven incorrect. Chapter 2 gives a survey of the Egyptian evidence for—but mainly against—Egyptian professional dentistry, and corrects the false statements on Egyptian dental prostheses.

A recent find taken as evidence for Egyptian filling of cavities is open to various other modes of interpretation: a man's mummy of the Ptolemaic period now in the Redpath Museum of McGill University revealed in a CT-scan a tooth with a lesion that had apparently been packed with linen (Wade *et al.* 2012). It is difficult to envision this sort of fabric filling being durable enough for use in life, but the well-known need for a "whole" mummy, even if missing limbs must be replaced with wooden or papyrus substitutes, makes it likely that this was a part of the mummification process, either for aesthetic purposes or perhaps bandaging impregnated with antiseptic or analgesic substances was being supplied for the eternal comfort of the deceased.

Greek and Roman sources

Loss of teeth as a sign of old age was well known to Classical authors. Aristophanes, in a late play, *Plutus* (*"Wealth"* lines 1056–1060) (probably produced 388 BC rather than 408 BC: see Henderson 2002: 415–420), presents an old woman with her boy-toy who mocks her wrinkles, rouged cheeks and lost teeth, playing a guessing game of how many teeth she has left. One character guesses "three or four," and the gigolo says "she only has one molar" (ἕνα γὰρ γομφίον μόνον φορεῖ—*Plutus* line 1059; also Deneffe 1899: 10). Such comments give us some impression of daily life and social concerns, while the early Greek medical treatises still leave much untold.

Many authors, focusing on the early Greek texts and the Latin versions that followed, underestimate just how much Roman medicine had been influenced by the Etruscan tradition in surgery and dentistry (Tabanelli 1963: 74–89). Greek medical texts tend to focus on lethal disorders (Rolleston 1914: 5), perhaps because of their limited ability to deal with severe medical problems. Minor health problems remained securely in the realm of folk medical traditions. The possible influences on Greek medicine of Egyptian and Phoenician knowledge also have been considered (Saunders 1963), and their combined effects in the development of the Roman medical corpus provide the focus for much speculation. Weiss (1989) is one of the few scholars to provide some indication that Etruscan medicine was the basis for Roman practitioners. We now have clear evidence that gold dental appliances are a distinctive Etruscan invention, confined to a few women of the highest classes of society.

Roman medicine is well known because the Romans developed a complex, and highly literate, society. Roman authors probably incorporated into their texts whatever had been medical verbal tradition among the Etruscans as well as that of the Greeks. Ballér's study (1992) of medical thinking among the educated Roman citizenry is extremely useful in helping us to define what they believed to be health as well as disease. In turn, this information reveals what kinds of treatments would be sought and when. The more specific nature of medical education among the people of ancient Greece and Rome, within the general subject area of ancient medicine, is the focus of a paper by Drabkin (1944; extensively quoted by Weinberger 1948: 109–114). (For basic background, see Nutton 2004 and Scarborough 1969.) Regardless of the sources of influence, medicine in ancient Rome had reached a high degree of sophistication by the second century BCE. Almost all aspects of general dentistry as it is now known, with the exception of tooth filling, seem to have become common medical knowledge by the Early Imperial period. The early development of dental bridgework, although not really a true orthodonture, has a history that can be verified by archaeology to at least the seventh century BCE, and therefore may be presumed to have had its origins at an even earlier date.

As early as 1831 Carabelli had made a basic search of the Classical literature for information relating to ancient dentistry. Heyne (1924) provides a dissertation focusing on dentists and dentistry in the literary sources. A brief review of the literature as it relates to people called dentists also is provided by Brown (1936). Depictions of dentists and dentistry in art (see Pindborg and Marvitz 1960) will not be reviewed here, because no depiction of a dental appliance is known from any work of art. The following summary is not intended to be an exhaustive review, but simply to provide an indication of the course of development, and devolution, in various aspects of dentistry in the ancient world. This summary is intended to serve as a prelude to the direct study of dental appliances, which is the focus of this volume.

The Laws of the Twelve Tables

The famous Roman law codes referred to as the *Twelve Tables* (see Düll 1976: 60–62) were preserved in inscriptions as early as the fifth century BCE, soon after Rome became a republic, but they surely had their origins in the sixth century, as compilations of earlier texts. Giovanni Colonna (1977) proposed revising the date of the origin of *Table X* to *c.*580 BCE (see also Ampolo 1984), a date that

Waarsenburg (1994: 320, n. 982) points out would be contemporary with the great Athenian statesman Solon and with the next-to-last Roman king known as Servius Tullius. Nevertheless, actual dates for the transcriptions of these codes clearly are much later than their putative origins, which must have been monumental, public postings of some sort.

The *Tenth Table* included sumptuary laws, restrictions on the allowable expense or ostentation of funerals, such as the inclusion of gold objects among the funerary offerings, which would have taken gold out of circulation, potentially causing harm to the fragile economy of the young Roman Republic. Similar laws were operating in Athens at the time, and would appear in various states over many centuries. The excerpts were preserved by Cicero when he quoted them: "*neve aurum addito*" ("nor shall anyone add gold") from one law, and "*At cui auro dentes vincti escunt, ast im cum illo sepeliet uretve, se fraude esto.*" ("But whoever has had teeth fastened together with gold, if someone shall bury or cremate him, this shall be with impunity." Thus, "teeth that are joined with gold" are specifically exempted. (Cicero noted this provision for its humane intentions, *De legibus* 2.60, Warmington 1938: xxvi–xxxi, 502–503). As with other early Roman laws, most scholars assume that these have derived from earlier, Etruscan law, although the archaeological evidence for Etruria makes it clear that there were few if any restrictions on the expense of funeral offerings. Certainly, the passage constitutes evidence for familiarity with gold dental appliances in Rome by (and probably before) the fifth century BCE. Only the ruling classes could have afforded gold appliances, and protection of property and the rights of the "haves" are usually the main concerns of early law codes.

Ancient literary sources

The following quotations or summaries from the ancient texts provide an indication of the trajectory of early written scholarship regarding the teeth during the centuries after the initial formulation of the Hippocratic corpus. The course of these writings may be helpful in understanding the history of dental appliances. Although the Hippocratic texts include a treatise on *Dentition* (Hippocrates 1923, II: 322–329; Jones 1946, 1953) no basic information on dentistry appears in this or any of the other available Hippocratic tracts other than the references to wiring of loose teeth. In fact, *Dentition* is not an independent text at all, but quite clearly an early scribal error (Hippocrates 1923: 317–319). The original location of the brief section now commonly called "Dentition" must have been in *Aphorisms* III, between sections XXV (teething) and XXVI (children's tonsils: see Hippocrates 1931, IV: 131). While references by Livy (5.27) and by Herodotus (2.84) may relate to dental concerns, the principal authors whose works closely relate to this study of ancient dentistry appear on the following pages. These citations appear in the chronological order in which they were written, and so can reflect possible developments and changes in the history of dentistry.

In the absence of Etruscan literature we must turn to Greek and Roman authors for written information regarding oral health and medicine. Readers should bear in mind that the Etruscan culture differed considerably from both the Roman and the Greek traditions. Thus these literary findings cannot be taken as exact images of Etruscan behaviors relating to the manufacture and use of dental appliances. When Aeschylus (525/4–456/5 BCE) noted, in his *Elegies* (preserved only in a quote by Theophrastus), that Etruria was rich in medicines he appeared to be speaking about pharmacological plants, the way Europeans in 1500 AD described the New World as being rich in plants with pharmacological value. These data appear in the work of Theophrastus (370–286 BCE), whose *Enquiry into Plants* (9.15.1) notes Etruscan sources of drugs. Both Varro and Virgil appear to cite these ideas of Theophrastus (see Kenney 1980: 288, 322, also 460).

Hippocratic Treatise: On Joints 32

The earliest medical reference to dental appliances of gold appears in the treatise *On Joints*, as part of trauma treatment, and is not presented as dental practice per se. It need not have been dictated by Hippocrates himself, but probably was written close to his lifetime in the fifth century BCE.

> καὶ ἦν μὲν διεστραμμένοι ἔωσιν οἱ ὀδόντες οἱ κατὰ τὸ τρῶμα καὶ κεκινημένοι, ὁπόταν τὸ ὀστέον κατορθωθῇ, ζεῦξαι τοὺς ὀδόντας χρὴ πρὸς ἀλλήλους, μὴ μοῦνον τοὺς δύο, ἀλλὰ καὶ πλέονας, μάλιστα μὲν δὴ χρυσίῳ, ἔστ'ἂν κρατυνθῇ τὸ ὀστέον, εἰ δὲ μή, λίνῳ.

> If the teeth at the point of injury are displaced or loosened, when the bone is adjusted fasten them to one another, not merely the two, but several, preferably with the gold wire, but failing that, with thread, until consolidation takes place.

> (Hippocrates 1928: 258–265)

The term logically translated as "gold wire" (*chrysiō*) is not so precise in the original Greek: it merely means "with gold," with no extra word for "wire." The term for "with thread" (*linō*) can mean "with linen thread" (a term that has carried into English). (It is interesting to note that some dentures found in the eighteenth- to early nineteenth-century burial crypts in Spitalfields, London, were made with thread, albeit silk thread (see Chapter 4).

Cicero: Marcus Tullius Cicero: 106–43 BCE

Writing around 50 BCE, Cicero (*De Legibus* 2.24.60) makes reference to the ancient law proscribing the burial of gold with the dead, from which gold bridgework was specifically exempted. He notes this as a "kind intention" of the lawmakers ("*quam humane excipit altera lex*"). Cicero says of extravagant funeral celebrations, "the law would not have forbidden [such practices] unless they really happened" (*quae et recte toluntur neque tollerentur, nisi fuissent, On the Laws* 2.60). We may certainly assume that gold-band dental appliances were known in archaic Rome, although none have yet been discovered there. Cicero's purpose was to analyze laws rather than discuss medicine, so this passage is especially meaningful in our crediting the Etruscans with this breakthrough in dentistry.

Catullus: Gaius Valerius Catullus: c.84– c.54 BCE

Catullus, a gifted but short-lived young poet among the glitterati of Late Republican Rome (perhaps best known for his presumed obsession with Claudia Pulcher the beautiful sister of an infamous politician), satirized ethnic groups and social players. In his *Carmen (Ode)* 39 (line 11) he criticizes a man who shows off his fine real teeth, which were apparently a rarity among the wealthy, while tossing off an ethnic caricature, the "swarthy or toothy Lanuvian" (*Lanuvinus ater atque dentatus, Ode* 39.11) from a nearby Latin-speaking region outside Rome, as if prominent teeth were a characteristic of this group. (For the text and translation, see the Introduction: this is the famous poem mentioning the *"obesus etruscus."*)

Horace: Quintus Horatius Flaccus: 65–8 BCE

Horace, patronized by the wealthy Etruscan Maecenas (a friend and backer of Octavian-Augustus), published several works of lyric poetry including *Odes, Satires,* letters and pastoral poetry. In his *Satires* (1.8), published between 35 and 30 BCE, Horace notes a courtesan who apparently had false teeth and who he calls Canidia (most poets disguised their victims with such nicknames, knowing that contemporaries would recognize them anyhow). Poor Canidia's bad breath is said to be *peior serpentibus Afris* "more poisonous than African snakes," at *Satire* 2.8.95. She and her friend Sagana are described as practicing witchcraft at night on the Esquiline Hill when a sharp noise frightens them and they run away, dropping their bundles of charms and also, in their haste, Canidia's teeth and Sagana's fancy wig (*Satire* 1.8). For the joke to work, Horace's audience had to already be familiar with women's false teeth.

> Canidiae dentes, altum Saganae caliendrum
> Excidere atque herbas atque incantata lacertis
> Vincula cum magno risuque iocoque videres.

> Canidia's teeth, the tall hairpiece of Sagana
> you will see them with much laughter and fun fall out,
> along with the herbs and charmed love-knots [they carry].
>
> (*Satire* 1.8: 48–50)

Celsus, Aulus (?) Cornelius: c.25 BCE–c.50 CE

Celsus is known today as the author of *De medicina (On Medicine)*, which probably represents only a portion of what was essentially an encyclopedia of this and related topics; only the *Libri Octo (Eight Books)* survive. The extant work provides as complete a statement regarding gold dental appliances as any of those which appeared at any later date, suggesting that his text derives from a well-established literature (see Jones 1953: 103–106). Quite probably, most of the information derives from the Hippocratic corpus, which had developed over the three centuries prior to the birth of Celsus. The archaeological evidence, however, is at odds with literary tradition, which seems to be ignorant of the Etruscan gold appliances.

Celsus is believed to have been born, or lived, in Narbonne (*Gallia Narbonensis*), which had been a part of the Roman state since 121 BCE. He may have been an educated gentleman (member of the landed gentry), rather than a practicing physician (Nickol 1991). His medical works are believed to derive primarily from earlier literature (see Sabbah and Mudry 1995; Nickol 1991: 21), including the Hippocratic corpus, and probably also the works of Asclepiades, Heracleides, and other later Greek physicians.

The enormous range of pharmaceuticals mentioned by Celsus, such as ox-gall, myrrh and rose petals, reflect the important relationship between pharmacy and medicine at that time. Both the ingredients and the prescriptions in *Book* 5.1–25 of Celsus are listed by Spencer in his bilingual Loeb edition of the text (Celsus 1938, II: xv–lxiii, 247–251).

Some 50 years after Cicero had mentioned the law involving gold dental appliances, Celsus (1938, III, 7.12: 370–371), following Hippocrates, indicates that gold (bands or wire?—see translation below, and Chapter 4) could be used to hold teeth in place that had been loosened by a blow, until the surrounding tissue could recover. These also could be used as a permanent means of securing teeth loosened by attrition of the bone. Wiring was obviously a very different procedure from making a bridgework that was meant to be permanent. These Roman sources indicate that such aspects of dentistry probably had become familiar to readers in the Julio-Claudian (Early Imperial) period.

A brief summary of the dental information offered by Celsus appears in his section "On the Mouth" (Book 7.12: see Celsus 1938, III: 368–371; see also Foster 1879: 235–240). This information is best summarized by Nickol (1991), who also offers a useful brief history of the manuscripts in which the text was preserved. Most impressive is Celsus's primary concern with treating the gums first in all cases where oral pain or other symptoms may be a problem. Only if this is unsuccessful should extraction of a tooth be considered. Since there is great danger in extracting a tightly fixed tooth, especially the upper teeth (which have more widely spreading roots), extreme care should be taken.[12]

Celsus recognized that concussions in the delicate boney areas around the temples and eyes might result from poor levering (using the face as a platform on which to rest the tool or the hand) during the extraction of maxillary dentition. The tooth selected for removal should be scraped free of the surrounding gum down to the boney socket. The tooth is then grasped with an instrument and shaken to loosen it. At that point it is removed, preferably with the fingers to ensure a delicate pressure, but with forceps if necessary. When forceps are used, the tooth should be pulled out straight lest the curved roots, particularly in maxillary molars, break off the thin bone within which the tooth is seated (the alveolar portion of the jaw). Celsus points out that there is special danger if the tooth is short (decayed to the stump) in which case the forceps cannot grip the remaining tooth properly. In attempting to grip such a stump the dentist might, in error, grasp and break the bone off under the gum. This bone fragment, just as any piece of the tooth root that may break off, has to be located, by probing or cutting, and removed.

In fact, an example of exactly this problem of breaking off parts of bone surrounding the tooth, where the forceps was applied in such a way as to pinch together the fragile alveolus (bony tissue) as well as the root stump, is found among the teeth discarded at the *taverna* in the Roman Forum (see Figures 1.1 and 1.2). This example is one of the most severely decayed teeth recovered from the excavations at the Temple of Castor and Pollux (Becker, 2014: 210, 214–215; Ginge *et al.* 1989). Nevertheless, this decayed tooth had been removed successfully, with the remains of its decayed crown intact, but with a small segment of the jaw still adhering to it. Quite probably this damage to the maxillary bone was preferable to leaving a small piece of root broken off within the jaw where it would probably have created serious, possibly fatal, problems.

Roots that broke off during an attempt at dental extraction, or stumps of teeth that had decayed extensively, could be removed through the use of a special forceps that the Greeks call *rhizagra* ("root catcher"). Spencer (Celsus 1938, III: 370) believes that examples of this instrument now survive. The name alone is sufficient to indicate that this procedure was known and employed.

In the case of "hollow" (rotted) teeth that had been determined as suitable for removal, Celsus recommended that the decayed cavity should be neatly plugged with lint or lead. This was meant to prevent the crown from breaking under the forceps, presumably in the shaking phase of extraction since he recommends the use of the fingers in the actual removal stage. There does not appear to be any suggestion of the drilling of teeth to prepare them for being plugged. In keeping with the conservative nature of his practice, Celsus says that deciduous teeth only should be pulled if they are impeding the development of the secondary dentition.

Also, teeth that have been loosened by a blow can be fixed in place "by means of gold." As with the Hippocratic reference, it is not clear what shape the gold was in—whether a band or a wire, and most translators actually say "with gold wire."

> At si ex ictu vel alio casu aliquid labant dentes, auro cum iis, qui bene haerent, vinciendi sunt; continendaque ore reprimentia, ut vinum, in quo malicorium decoctum, aut in quo galla candens coniecta sit.
>
> But if teeth are loosened by a blow or any other event, with gold they should be attached [literally chained] together with those teeth that are firmly rooted; in the mouth there should be held repressants, such as wine in which pomegranate rinds have been boiled, or in which burning oak galls have been thrown.
>
> (*De medicina* 7.12(f), see Celsus 1938, III: 371)

Celsus recognized that this would enable the teeth to securely re-establish themselves once the area had recovered from the effects of the injury. Of importance in Celsus' texts is the distinction that he made between oral ulcers, described together with other diseases of the mouth (6.2: 2–6), and ailments of the gums, that were recognized as periodontal problems (4.13: 2–4; see Celsus 1938, II: 261). A series of prescriptions specific to toothache are noted elsewhere in the writings of Celsus (1938, II: 61), within the context of remedies for an assortment of general ills.

For a few centuries after Celsus produced his work we have no evidence of any new information being added to these texts, with practitioners relying on the ancient authors for their accumulated wisdom. In fact, the Western tradition in dental medicine was entering a period of serious decline, from which a recovery only came in the early seventeenth century.

Various unorthodox translations of Celsus, together with specious archaeological confirmations of his writings, are abundant (e.g. Deneffe 1899: 32). Many of these archaeological verifications simply reflect poor excavation techniques and faulty recording and publication of skeletal data.

Scribonius Largus: c.0–c.50 CE

Scribonius, a contemporary of Celsus, was court physician to the emperor Claudius, and *c.*47 CE drew up a list of over 200 of his prescriptions (including some folk remedies, etc.), which were disseminated for hundreds of years (known today by the title *De compositione medicamentorum liber*). The data presented reflect the general information available to physicians at that time and indicate the extent to which medical knowledge had developed and disseminated.[13] Scribonius's extensive data on dentistry (Scribonius 1983: 33–36) begins with remedies for aching teeth, followed by information on dentifrices, and finally on the care of the gums. Scribonius' prescriptions are nicely reviewed by Schonack (1912). The delicate nature of tooth removal, and the need to use an excavator to cut down the gums prior to extraction, are clearly noted by this physician as well.

Pliny the Elder: Gaius Plinius Secundus: 23/24–79 CE.

Pliny was a polymath and author of many works in addition to his famous Natural History; as admiral of the Misenum Fleet, he directed rescue efforts in 79 CE during the Vesuvian eruption, and died observing the event. Perhaps the most significant aspect of Pliny's writings on matters pertaining to dentistry is his massive compilation of folk remedies, as well as medical data, creating a veritable flood of information (Jones 1953: 106–108, also see Appendix V). From this collection we can see how busy the pharmacists of the day may have been. Certainly an aching tooth would have long decayed away before the sufferer could have time to try all the remedies listed, if there were money available to make all of the necessary purchases! (*Natural History* Books 28–32 (see Pliny 1963) furnish data on specific plants, animals and other materials known to provide *materia medica*.)

Lucillius (Greek author, Loukillios): first century CE

Not to be mistaken for any of several Roman authors and statesmen named Lucilius, the Greek satirical author Lucillius lived in Rome under the patronage of Nero, to whom he dedicated some publications (*Palatine Anthology* 9.572). Over 100 of his satirical epigrams were preserved in the *Palatine Anthology*, sometimes known as the *Greek Anthology*. Most mock people for physical deformities or moral/professional inadequacy, in a highly polished style that must have influenced the Latin poet Martial. Lucillius provides an epigram (11.310, see Paton 1956: 212–213) making reference to the purchase of cosmetics, false hair and false teeth:

Ἠγόρασας πλοκάμους, φῦκος, μέλι, κηρόν, ὀδόντας.
τῆς αὐτῆς δαπάνης ὄψιν ἂν ἠγόρασας.

You bought hair-braids, seaweed-rouge, honey, wax, and teeth.
For the same expense you could have bought a face.

Another of his epigrams (11.408, see Paton 1956: 266–267) comments on dyed hair and white lead face powder, among other beauty aids, but does not mention false teeth.

Martial: Marcus Valerius Martialis: c.38/41–c.104 CE

The poet Martial came to Rome from his native Spain and made his living precariously, selling his poetry; many of his short epigrams sound like labels or gift tags intended to accompany presents or monuments. Artifacts and conditions mentioned in the poems must have been familiar to most Romans or they could not have provoked the desired laugh or snicker. Strömgren (1919: 28–30) reviewed some of the related data from Martial's well-known epigrams (see also Deneffe 1899: 43–45) for information on dentistry. A compendium of data relating to physicians and medicine in general from the works of Martial was published some 70 years ago by Spallicci (1934), and the *Epigrams* were authoritatively translated for the Loeb Classical Library editions by W. C. A. Ker in 1925 (see Ker 1968, 1978) and then in an updated translation in three volumes by D. R. Shackleton Bailey (Bailey 1993). (Translations below are by JMT.)

The loss of teeth was a frequent target for Martial, as for other satirists.

Si memini, fuerunt tibi quattuor, Aelia, dentes:
Expulit una duos tussis et una duos.
Iam secura potes totis tussire diebus:
Nil istic quod agat tertia tussis habet.

If I recall, there were four teeth you had, Aelia.
One cough expelled two, another two more.
Now you can safely cough for days on end.
There is nothing there for a third cough to disturb.

(1.19)

The fear of losing remaining teeth is like other people's worries that wind will blow off a wig or sun and rain will melt copious makeup:

> tu puella non es,
> et tres sunt tibi, Maximina, dentes,
> sed plane piceique buxeique.
> quare si speculo mihique credis,
> debes non aliter timere risum
> quam ventum Spanius manumque Priscus,
> quam cretata timet Fabulla nimbum,
> cerussata timet Sabella solem
> [. . .]
> You are not a girl,
> and you have only three teeth, Maximina,
> but they are clearly pitch-black and like boxwood.
> So if you believe me and your mirror,
> you have got to be afraid to laugh,
> just like Spanius fears the wind and Priscus fears a touch,
> like powdered Fabulla fears a raincloud,
> like made-up Sabella fears the sun.

(2.41.5–12)

Men too could suffer rather harsh mockery for lost teeth:

> Medio recumbit imus ille qui lecto,
> calvam trifilem semitatus unguento,
> foditque tonsis ora laxa lentiscis,
> mentitur, Aefulane: non habet dentes.

> That man reclining at the foot of the middle couch [the place of honor],
> the one whose bald head has three hairs slicked down with oil,
> and who digs out his loose mouth with mastic toothpicks,
> he lies, Aefulanus: he doesn't have any teeth.

(6.74)

> Tres habuit dentes, pariter quos expuit omnes,
> ad tumulum Picens dum sedet ipse suum;
> collegitque sinu fragmenta novissima laxi
> oris et aggesta contumulavit humo.
> ossa licet quondam defuncti non legat heres:
> hoc sibi iam Picens praestitit officium.

> Three teeth Picens had, which he spat out at the same time
> while he sat next to his own tumulus [tomb];
> and he collected in his lap the latest fragments from his slack-jawed mouth,
> and buried them in a little mound of earth.

Once he is dead, his heir will not have to gather up his bones:
Picens has already performed that service for himself.

(8.57)

But the most scorn was turned on women who apparently wore replacement teeth
in public:

Cum sis ipsa domi mediaque ornere Subura,
fiant absentes et tibi, Galla, comae,
nec dentes aliter quam Serica nocte reponas,
et iaceas centum condita pyxidibus,
nec tecum facies tua dormiat, innuis illo
quod tibi prolatum est mane supercilio,
et te nulla movet cani reverentia cunni,
quem potes inter avos iam numerare tuos.
promittis sescenta tamen; sed mentula surda est,
et sit lusca licet, te tamen illa videt.

You yourself are at home, Galla, but you are being made up in the middle of Subura [Rome's slum]. Your hair is manufactured in your absence.
Nor do you lay aside your teeth at night any differently than you do your
silk dresses, and you lie packed away in a hundred boxes. Nor does your
face sleep with you. You flirt with an eyebrow that is brought to you in
the morning.

(9.37: ll. 1–6)

(The poem goes on to critique other body parts, of Galla and of the speaker
himself).

Nostris versibus esse te poetam,
Fidentine, putas cupisque credi?
sic dentata sibi videtur Aegle
emptis ossibus Indicoque cornu . . .

Because of my verses, Fidentinus,
do you think you are a poet, and want to be believed?
In the same way Aegle imagines she has teeth,
having bought them in bone and Indian horn.

(1.72.1–4)

Thais habet nigros, niveos Laecania dentes.
Quae ratio est? emptos haec habet, illa suos.

Thais has black teeth, Laecania snow-white ones.
What is the reason? This one has bought teeth, the other her own.

(5.43)

Dentibus atque comis—nec te pudet—uteris emptis.
Quid facies oculo, Laelia? Non emitur.

You use teeth and hair that are bought and you are not embarrassed.
What will you do about your eye, though, Laelia? They don't sell them.

(12.23)

Martial describes a socially undesirable male guest picking his teeth at a banquet:

stat exoletus suggeritque ructanti
pinnas rubentes cuspidesque lentisci,
et aestuanti tenue ventilat frigus
supine prasino concubina flabello,
fugatque muscas myrtea puer verga.
[. . .]
A youth stands by and supplies
red feathers and strips of mastic [wooden toothpicks]
to him as he belches, while a reclining concubine
makes a cool breeze for him with a green fan,
and a boy keeps off flies with a myrtle branch.

(3.82.8–12)

Another epigram also refers to toothpicks in social banqueting:

You sent me at the Saturnalia, Umber, all the
gifts that came to you in five days: a dozen
three-leaved tablets and seven toothpicks [*dentiscalpia*],
with which in addition arrived a spoon, a napkin.

(7.53)

The speaker is here referring to trifling goods sent to him, where in fact he would have preferred silver!

Other references to teeth in Martial's epigrams include a man's "biting" humor seen in a metaphorical rough tooth:

Iocis Paulos:
robiginosis cuncta dentibus rodit.

[One may outdo] . . . Paulus in humor: he gnaws at
everything with his scabrous tooth.

(5.28.6–7, translation after Bailey 1993, vol. 1: 381)

There were other references to teeth and dental troubles only some of which are understood today, since (perhaps fortunately) we cannot know all the terms of daily slang in the Roman streets. In an obscene context Aelianus explains that for an entire month his lover, the fair "Glycera had the toothache" (11.40). In the introduction to *Epigrams* Book 12, Martial greets his friend Priscus, and notes that among the various difficulties noted he could add to this the nice political metaphor of the "tartar of municipal teeth" [*municipalium robigo dentium*]" (12, preface). (*Robigo*, which must mean tartar here, is white, a term normally used for "mildew," a serious problem affecting crops and food supplies. Romans kept the goddess Mildew at bay with special offerings and festivals like the *Robigalia*.)

> Lentiscum melius: sed si tibi frondea cuspis
> defuerit, dentes pinna levare potest.
>
> Mastic is better; but if a leafy point [twig]
> is not available, a feather can polish the teeth.

(14.22)

Regarding dentifrice, Martial says (to an old woman):

> Quid mecum est tibi? me puella sumat:
> emptos non soleo polire dentes.
>
> What do you have to do with me? Let a girl take me up.
> I'm not accustomed to polishing bought teeth.

(14.56)

(Crawfurd (1914: 23) interprets this as the toothpaste speaking to an old woman with dentures, but there were undoubtedly double entendres in the perception of Martial's crowd.)

One mention of dentistry (apparently) links it with cosmetic services, like removing a slave's brand:

> Totis, Galle, iubes tibi me servire diebus
> et per Aventinum ter quater ire tuum.
> eximit aut reficit dentem Cascellius aegrum,
> infestos oculis uris, Hygine, pilos;
> non secat et tollit stillantem Fannius uvam,
> tristia saxorum stigmata delet Eros;
> enterocelarum fertur Podalirius Hermes:
> qui sanet ruptos dic mihi, Galle, quis est?
>
> Gallus, you order me to serve you day in and day out,
> going three or four times through your Aventine neighborhood.
> Cascellius extracts or repairs a painful tooth,
> you Hyginus burn the hairs that infect the eyes;
> Fannius doesn't cut but relieves a discharging uvula;
> Eros can wipe out the pathetic brands of slaves;
> Hermes is thought to be the Podalirius of hernias:
> but tell me, Gallus, who is it who heals the broken ones?

(10.56)

This off-handed mention, written about 80 CE, of a dentist named Cascellius, then practicing dental extractions and "restoring" ailing teeth perhaps on the Aventine hill in Rome (a major residential neighborhood),[14] implies that a dental specialty existed in medicine at this time. In the same context a series of other specialties are noted, suggesting that at that time dentistry was but one of many pseudo-medical specialties plied mainly for cosmetic purposes.

Martial, in his jibes, generally equated doctors with undertakers, noting that they ply the same trade as gladiators and military captains, only under different names (*Epigrams* 8.74, 1.30, 1.47; See Crawfurd's 1914 survey of Martial's comment on the medical profession). In some of Martial's examples (6.78, 8.9, 8.74), the doctor noted appears to be an oculist, suggesting the mortal dangers inherent in receiving treatment from any of the medical professionals of that day.

That *iatroi* (Greek: "doctors") did not practice barbering is suggested by Martial's note (1897: 609) that barbers' instruments included one used to cut the hair, another good for long nails, and a third for rough chins (no mention is made of the use of this shaving razor as a surgical tool or instrument for bleeding).

Marcellus of Side (Marcellus Sidetes): first century CE

Born late in the first century CE at Side in Asia Minor, Marcellus wrote during the reigns of Hadrian and Marcus Aurelius in the second century; his long medical poem in Greek survives in two excerpts, *On Lycanthropy* and *On Remedies Derived from Fishes*. The latter (see editions of 1851 and 1888) preserves just 101 lines naming fish species, some of which were used in dental prescriptions.

Pedanius Dioscorides (Greek Dioskourides): first century CE

Dioscorides was a Greek physician attached to the Roman army. Along with the works of Soranus, Dioscorides' encyclopedic herbal, *De materia medica*, is known as a major source of pharmaceutical data (Riddle 1987: 40–41), translated from his original Greek into Latin in 1526 and used in Europe as a pharmacopeia. His information pertains principally to oral medicine rather than dentistry, and need not be reviewed here. A number of the plants discussed by Dioscorides can be shown to have been known in Etruria, for instance *millefolium*, used to treat toothache (Pliny *Natural History* 24.152; see Turfa and Becker 2013: 869–870; Harrison and Bartels 2006, Harrison and Turfa 2010 and references therein).

Soranus of Ephesus: c.80–ca.140 CE

Soranus was born in the Greek city of Ephesus, now in western Turkey. He studied medicine in Alexandria (Egypt), a major medical center, and subsequently practiced in Rome, probably during the reigns of Trajan (98–117) and Hadrian (117–138). Soranus' biography of Hippocrates is the first known on the father of ancient medicine.

Soranus' treatises on acute and chronic diseases, written in his native Greek, probably reflect the level of medical knowledge of his time, based on centuries of accumulated experience. These texts were adapted into Latin by Caelius Aurelianus (q.v.). Soranus certainly was familiar with basic dental treatments. He is best known for his long treatise on *Gynaecology*; he noted that the standard tooth forceps as well as a bone forceps (4.11.63) could be used in the delicate obstetrical procedure of dealing with an impacted fetal skull (Soranus 1927: 142).

Suetonius: Gaius Suetonius Tranquillus: c.70–c.140 CE

The famous biographer of the early emperors was aware of the importance (or not) of good teeth for the image of a ruler, noting that Augustus had teeth that were widely spaced, small and scaley (*dentes raros et exiguos et scabros*: *Life of Augustus* 79.2).

Lucian: Lucianus: c.115–after 180 CE

Lucianus (Lucian) was a Greek satirical author, born in Samosata (now Samsat) on the Euphrates River in ancient Syria (now Turkey). Eighty of his prose works have survived, covering a wide range of topics, from the mythological to contemporary events, philosophy and more. He certainly was not a physician or a dentist, yet, perhaps surprisingly he downplayed the potentially lethal aspects of the physicians of the period. Lucian probably suffered from gout, and he offers a long list of preparations that can be taken for that ailment (1961b: 339–341), but concludes that they all fail to provide relief. Lucian indicates that each doctor (*iatros*) who used ointments in attempts to effect his cure had failed (1961b: 348–349). These same *iatroi*, described as poor Syrians, also did bleeding, using a hemispherical scalpel (Lucian 1961b: 366–367). This evidence indicates that both ointment application and bleedings were done by the same practitioners.

Lucian's works include one of the rare late references to fastening, or binding, teeth with gold (χρυσίῳ) (Lucian 1961a: 168–169), which some authors have translated as "gold *wire*" although the word is simply "with gold." Lucian could be referring to gold bands, in the Etruscan style, rather than the Near Eastern gold wire appliances. In his *Professor of Public Speaking* (*Rhētarōn Didaskalos* 24; the Latin *Rhetorum praeceptor*), Lucian's protagonist says he pretended to love a rich woman of 70 years with only four teeth remaining in her mouth, and those fastened with gold.

γυναικὸς ἑβδομηκοντούτιδος τέτταρας ἔτι λοιποὺς ὀδόντας ἐχούσης, χρυσίῳ καὶ τούτους ἐνδεδεμένους.

A seventy-year-old woman who had only four teeth remaining and all of them fastened with gold.

(Lucian 1961a: 169)

Waarsenburg (1991a: n. 9, 1994: 320, n. 982) suggests that this reference of Lucian may be the last known Roman literary reference to the ancient gold appliances.

Like Martial's epigram, this reference to a female wearing some type of dental appliance demonstrates the continued association of socially active women with dental appliances. It may reflect the use of the Eastern type of dental wiring rather than an Etruscan-style gold band. The Greek term ἐνδεδεμένους, "fastened," comes from the verb ἐνδέμω, meaning "to wall up in/ make for oneself in a permanent place," which unfortunately does not betray any details about the gold fasteners themselves. While it is possible that a specific aspect of the Etruscan tradition in dentistry continued within Roman society, the context noted by Lucian may suggest otherwise.

Lucian's *Rhetorum praeceptor* (Lucian 1961a: 168–169) is believed to have been written after 179 CE (Daremberg and Saglio 1918: 1679). That healthy teeth were associated with beauty, and not just youth, is reflected by the ridicule that the Syrian character named Simylus directs at Polystratus as being old, and also as having only four teeth in his head (being ugly).

So, with Lucian's satire and social commentary, we have the last reference to actual dental appliances, linked to real people—although the extant examples of these, whether wire or band-types, must be dated more than a generation before his writing. We seem to lack nearly all physical traces of those false teeth worn by the courtesans and other socialites of Late Republican and early Imperial Rome.

Galen (Aelius or Claudius Galenus): 129–after 210 CE

Galen spent over 40 years of his life in Rome and became physician to Emperor Marcus Aurelius; his copious medical writings were derived in large part from earlier authorities. The massive works of Galen include two volumes that each contain extensive information on dental matters. *De compositione medicamentorum secundum locos*, book 5, includes two chapters specifically relating to dentistry; the brief chapter 4, *de dentium affectibus* (Galen 1821–1833, reprinted 1965, XII: 848–853), and chapter 5 of *de gingivarium curatione* (ibid. 853–893). As with Soranus and other earlier medical writers, the primary concern in dental matters is with the gums. Subsequently, other aspects of dentistry more specifically concerned with caries and extractions are noted. Periodontal and related treatments and procedures also are discussed throughout an additional work by the pseudo-Galen known as *De remediis parabilibus*, I: chapters 7–8 (Galen 1821–1833; reprinted 1965, XIV: 354–364).

The suggestion that Galen, and Archigenes (who practiced in Rome slightly earlier, during Trajan's reign), had recommended the "drilling" of a hole into the pulp chamber of black (decayed? dead?) teeth (cf. Bennike and Fredebo 1986) has not been verified by archaeological/anthropological research. The *index rerum* of Kün includes no reference to the drilling of teeth (Niels Bruun, personal communication, March 8, 1994). The lack of any reference at all to the use of gold bindings or fastenings in Galen's works suggests that by this period, contemporary with that of Lucian, such dental appliances were going out of style.

Talmudic writings: c.300–400 CE

A fairly extensive series of references to ancient dentistry and dental appliances may be found in the Talmud and associated commentaries (see Gauval 1958; Weinberger 1948: 96). While the origins of these texts may date to the sixth century CE, most of the early extant documents are much later in date.

Despite the existence of a series of Eastern Mediterranean/Levantine wire dental appliances (Becker 1997, see Catalogue W-1 to W-6 and Chapter 4), not a single example of these "Hebrew" appliances has been identified in the archaeological record. Asbell (1942: 3) offers some useful data that will be summarized here (also, see Asbell 1941) for the insight they provide regarding manufacture and use of these appliances. All of the references in the following paragraph derive from Asbell (1942).

The Talmudic writings suggest that by the Late Hellenistic period Hebrews were making some type of dental appliances (*Shabbot* 64b, 65a; also *Palestinian Shabbot* VI: 5). The materials involved appear to have included gold, silver and wood (*Shabbot* 65a; *Palestinian Shabbot* VI: 8c). This is the only written reference to the use of silver in these appliances, and only one example (Tura El-Asmant, no. W-5) of a silver appliance has been recovered. References to these *schen zahar* ("gold, false") teeth distinguish them from a removable type, *schen-tothebeth*, which according to Rabbi Zera (279–320 CE) were not to be "carried" on the sabbath (Talmud, *Nedarim* 66a, 66b). The Palestine Talmud (*Shabbat* VI: 8c) notes a young girl who was ashamed to ask a *nagor* ("turner" (of wood as well as ivory); or perhaps an artisan) to make her another (appliance) of ivory. The term *Rarash*, or worker in wood, stone or metal, also is found associated with this "craft." An exhaustive study of Talmudic dental references would require specialized language skills and is best left to others. Greek or Roman origins for these dental practices have been suggested, but a Near Eastern association is more likely.

Marcellus Empiricus of Bordeaux: c.400 CE

Probably most of the medical wisdom of the era, including all that Celsus had gathered and in approximately the same order, was recorded (or transcribed) by Marcellus Empiricus. Chapter 11 of *De Medicamentis* deals with disorders of the lips and gums, while the following chapter (Marcellus Empiricus 1968; 1889: 119–127) goes on to discuss dental pain and the treatment of both teeth and gums. One of the remedies from chapter 12 (12.41) may be summarized as an example of the kinds of prescriptions that may have had pharmacologically effective ingredients:

> Crushed together, 5 peppercorns the size of a bean with an equal weight of gall-nut, galbanum, and foam of saltpeter [*Schaumsaltpeter*], pounded then kneaded with honey until it achieves the texture of wax, taken with warm water relieves the pain of decayed and aching teeth.
>
> (Marcellus 1968, XII, 41)

Galbanum is commonly defined as a yellowish to green or brown aromatic bitter gum resin, containing an essential oil, and can be derived from several Asiatic plants such as Sulphur wort (*Peucedanum galbaniflora*, see Manniche 1989: 132), and *Ferula galbaniflua*. Galbanum resembles asafetida, which today is used for medicinal purposes similar to those described in antiquity, as well as being used in incense. The pharmacologically active elements in the combination of galbanum, pepper, and gallnut, or in any part of them, may actually relieve toothache.

Marcellus' data on dental extraction seem to derive from Scribonius' works, while some of the treatments for toothaches (such as earthworms boiled in oil) are parallel to Pliny's *Natural History* (1963: 30.23). The end of this chapter notes some dentifrices, such as burned pig bones, and the entirety of Chapter 13 is devoted to this subject (see also Grimm 1847, 1855). The works of Marcellus Empiricus clearly demonstrate the development of treatments of oral disease within the larger context of Roman medicine.

Caelius Aurelianus: ca. 380?–c.450 CE?

Caelius, the Latin adapter of Soranus' texts, appears to have been born in Numidia (Northern Africa), probably early in the fifth century CE. Caelius was one of a large number of medical authors active at the end of the fourth or the early part of the fifth century CE. Whether any of Caelius' information on dental disorders derives from Soranus is uncertain, but probable. Professor Scarborough (personal communication to Becker) notes that Drabkin's idea (Caelius 1950) that Caelius Aurelianus "translated" Soranus' lost works *On Acute Diseases* and *On Chronic Diseases* has been seriously questioned by present specialists (Dysert 2007).

Caelius subsumes his discussion of periodontal problems and toothaches under chronic diseases (*On Chronic Diseases* 2.4: Caelius 1950: 610–621). The primary concern of these authors was with periodontal treatment since they were aware that the primary cause of dental loss appeared to be gum inflammation and the atrophy of the surrounding bony tissue. Astringent mouthwashes were prescribed and a long list of possible varieties of these rinses are listed. Subsequently, Caelius also reviewed the ancient medical writers as well as their lists of recommended pharmaceuticals. Caelius also noted that trimming of the gums, using a *pericharacteron*, sometimes might be necessary.[15]

Most significantly, Caelius advises that teeth which are sound (not decayed, injured (broken?), or loose) not be pulled simply because they ache—sound advice, since we now know this could be due to periodontal disease, sinus infection, or any of a number of other problems. The presence of some sound teeth among the many decayed examples at the Temple of Castor and Pollux clearly suggests that sound teeth were sometimes extracted for reasons that Caelius may have thought inappropriate (e.g. "women's complaints," as suggested elsewhere; Becker 1983). Even when teeth clearly were decayed, Caelius recommends that every attempt be made to keep them. Should this not be successful, Caelius later reviews procedures for pulling those teeth that are loose and require little force to extract them (*On Chronic Diseases* 2.27; 4.3; 5.63; 5.66).

Greek anthology

Medical aspects of the *Greek Anthology*, a Late Antique compilation of a variety of ancient inscriptions and literature of all periods, have been summarized by Rolleston (1914). The better known authors are included in the following summary, but a quote from Macedonius Consul[16] (11.374) gives the impression that dental appliances had become part of common knowledge by late in the Roman era:

> Τῷ ψιμύθῳ μὲν ἀεὶ λιποσαρκέα τεῖνε παρειήν,
> Λαοδίκη. . .
> μή ποτε δ' εὐρύνῃς σέο χείλεα. τίς γὰρ ὀδόντον
> ὄρχατον ἐμπήξει φαρμακόεντι δόλῳ;

"Make your fleshless cheeks always smooth with white lead,
Laodice . . .,
but never open your lips wide, for who by cosmetic fraud shall fix a row of teeth there?"

> (*Palatine Anthology* 11.374, after Paton 1956: 248–249)

Aetius of Amida: mid-fifth to mid-sixth century CE

This early Byzantine author (see Aetius 1935: Book 8) appears to have copied his meager dental information from Galen or Soranus (see Milne 1907: 135). By the Late Roman period medical knowledge in general within the "Christian" world was largely derived from earlier findings, with little or no new information being added to the ancient texts. Within a few centuries this information was to diffuse into the regions being brought into the Islamic tradition where it was maintained and, in many cases, expanded.

Paul of Aegina: c.625–690 CE

The vast amount of medical data recorded by Paul's *Medical Compendium* (1844) largely repeats or summarizes the accumulated wisdom of the ancients. Tall teeth are cut down with a *smilioton*, probably a type of file, and scaley concretions are removed through the use of a scaler, file, or even the scoop of a *specillum* (Paul of Aegina 1924: 66).[17] The gum or soft tissue (*gingevus*) surrounding those teeth that are to be extracted is cut down to the boney socket. Then the tooth is grasped with the *odontagra* (a "gripper," not a "puller") to shake (rock) it loose, and then it is extracted, possibly implying that removal should be accomplished only using the fingers as earlier authors recommend (this passage of the *Medical Compendium* (6.28) is taken from the earlier text of Celsus, q.v.)

Fragments of bone lodged in depressed fractures of the skull following traumatic injury also are to be removed with the fingers, if possible, or an *odontagra* or *ostagra* (bone forceps), indicating a preference for the more delicate tools first (Paul of Aegina 1924: 139). The same *odontagra* or *rhizagra* ("root gripper") could be used to remove a weapon imbedded in the flesh, from which the shaft has broken off (Paul of Aegina 1924: 131). Milne (1907: 138) suggests that the bone lever that Paul (6.106) describes as being seven or eight finger-breadths in length also could have been used as a tooth lever. This technique seems highly improbable.

Coptic Medical Papyrus: ca. 800–900 CE?

That Greek medical traditions were transmitted into the Islamic and Coptic world is not surprising. The text of the *Coptic Medical Papyrus* (Dawson 1923) provides information relating to both the treatment of dental pain, such as using red and yellow vitriol mixed with alum, as well as how to use herbs in the extraction process. Hellebore and gall are applied to the aching tooth to loosen it (deaden the pain?); or a mixture of plants including acacia and wild rue could be applied. The actual removal of the tooth would be by the fingers, reflecting the best aspects of ancient dental practice. Note that no references to dental prostheses appear in this text or in any of the later writings relating to dentistry until nearly 1,000 years later! The single possible survival of the ancient dental tradition of making prostheses lies in the works of Albucasis, and it is to his work that we now turn.

Albucasis (Abu-al-Qasim): c.936–1013. (Abū 'l-Qāsim Khalaf ibn 'Abbās al Zahrāwī)

Albucasis (also Abu al-Qasim, etc.) probably was born near Córdoba where he became a renowned teacher and the greatest surgeon of the Islamic world. Much of his classic text the *Kitab-at-Tasrif* (*The Method of Medicine*) derives from Paul of Aegina, but his additions led it to become the most commonly used surgical text in the Western civilized world (see Spink and Lewis 1973).

The important place of Albucasis in the history of medicine, and in particular his critical and original observations regarding ancient dentistry, has been secured through the translation of his impressive opus using two early Arabic manuscript versions (Spink and Lewis 1973: 272–295). His observations on the scaling and the extraction of teeth are particularly detailed and accompanied by drawings of an impressive range of instruments specific to these tasks. Regarding extractions he is particularly illuminating, although one of his statements regarding the extraction of a broken root may be a distortion of the ancient texts. The details of his narrative are of particular importance as the illustrations of instruments presented in the two versions of his manuscript that were consulted by Spink and Lewis reveal a serious lack of detail. Albucasis offers a section on wiring loose teeth, including the possibility of successfully implanting a patient's own tooth. He also notes use of wiring a false tooth into place in cases where this would be useful. The entire section is reproduced here with the note that the procedure described was in use in dental textbooks into the middle of the twentieth century. Spink and Lewis (1973: fig. 76) reproduce two related illustrations of this process from the Huntington copy of the manuscript. While Spink and Lewis (1973: 292, n.) find the Huntington illustrations "beautifully carried out, and [that they] show clearly how this procedure was executed," Becker finds them vague and useless and suggests the absence of any value may reveal why the Marsh manuscript omitted them.[18]

> When the front teeth are loosened by some blow or fall and the patient cannot bite upon what he is eating lest they fall out, and you have without avail treated them with styptic medicines, the technique in this case is to bind the teeth with gold or silver wire. Gold is the better, for silver oxidizes and corrodes after some days, but gold remains forever in its state and does not suffer this change. The wire should be moderate in thickness in accordance with the distance between the teeth. The method is to take the wire and run it doubled between two sound teeth; then with the two ends of the wire you weave between the loose teeth, either one or several, until you bring your weaving to a sound tooth on the other side whence you began; tighten it gently and judiciously till they do not move at all. You should tie the wire at the root of the teeth lest it slip. Then with the scissors cut off the two ends of the wire remaining over, and bring them together and twist them with forceps and hide them between a sound tooth and a loose tooth so as not to injure the tongue; then for the future leave them thus bound. But if it comes undone or breaks, bind them with another wire; so may he have the use of them all his life. This is a figure of the teeth and the manner of interlacing two sound and two loose teeth, as you see.
>
> After one or two teeth have fallen out they may be restored in their place and bound in as instructed, and become permanent. This can be done only by an expert and gentle practitioner. Sometimes a piece of ox-bone may be carved and made into the shape of a tooth, and placed in the site where a tooth was lost, and fastened as we have said, and it will last and he will get long service from it.
>
> (Albucasis, in Spink and Lewis 1973: 292, 294)

The text of Albucasis provides the best evidence that this aspect of the scholarly tradition in medicine that had been developing in ancient Rome had passed into the hands of these tenth-century Islamic scholars (see Rosenthal 1960). From the Arabic universities in Iberia to those far to the east, the traditions of ancient medicine were translated, recorded, and amplified. Much of this information appears to have diffused, with Islam, east towards India, as well as having been preserved for re-entry into Renaissance Europe.

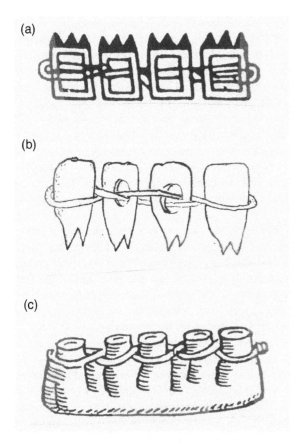

Figures 1.4a–c Tooth ligation as recommended by Abu al-Qasim (Albucasis):
(a) as it appears in the Latin translation by Gerhard of Cremona
(from Hoffmann-Axthelm 1970: fig. 6, from a copy in the City
Library of Bamberg); (b) the ligation as interpreted by Becker;
(c) as it appears in the Latin manuscript in the Laurentian library in
Florence (after Hoffmann-Axthelm 1970: fig. 7, *Flor. Laurent.*).

The late antique period and beyond

Allbutt's idea (1921; see Hoffmann-Axthelm 1970: 85) that dentistry fell into
neglect until the time of the supposed medical renaissance during the life of
the famed surgeon Ambroise Paré (1510–1590, see Packard 1921) is slowly
changing as evidence from the Byzantine period becomes more available
(e.g. Scarborough 1985). Continuities in Roman dental skills through the Late
Antique and Early Christian periods are now being clearly documented. For
instance, Künzl and Weber (1991) have been able to provide a classification
for all of the then-known types of Roman forceps. Ralph Jackson (personal

communication 1994) suggests that, "while none has a fully explicit dental association . . . the circumstantial evidence is sufficiently conclusive to indicate that the forceps *were* used to extract teeth, though not every example was necessarily intended solely for that task." Jackson also notes that the "notched jaw" on a newly identified, then unpublished, example that came from an extensive *instrumentarium* believed to have been found in Asia Minor or Syria, might have been more specifically for dental extractions (cf. Jackson 1993).

The decline in the tradition of Etruscan gold dental prostheses by the first century BCE accords with the conclusion that this was a cosmetic, and *not* a medico-dental concern. Medical information was continually propagated during the succeeding centuries but prostheses were not a part of it. That Albucasis preserved the written tradition of dental ligation reflects the use of this technique to preserve living teeth in place, and not the decorative purposes served by ancient Etruscan prostheses.

By the time of Paré (1510–1590), who began his career as a provincial barber's assistant, the ancient texts were not only still known, but continued to be used. Whether medical skills improved over the intervening centuries is less evident. The more abundant surviving textual materials, however, offer us a general view of medical procedures, and some indirect means by which we can plot the course of dentistry as well. For example, the cleaning and sharpening of a surgeon's tools in monastic hospitals of the Byzantine period were among the duties of an individual who carried the title ἀκονητής (*akonētēs*) that Gautier (1974: 104–105) translates as "*un repasser*" ("sharpener"). The instruments under his charge included lancets, cauterizing irons, a probe, and most important for our study "a tooth forceps"("*un davier*," "dental forceps," a translation of the Byzantine Greek monastic document's ὀδοντάγρα, *odontagra*). Although any or all of these tools could have been used in dentistry, the specific identification of this forceps implies that surgeons probably extracted teeth among their many duties. This aspect of dentistry also was part of the repertoire of many other tradespeople and quacks.

The Late Roman literary tradition, which in dark humor equated the doctor and the executioner, can be found in the twelfth-century works of Theodore Prodromos (?–ca.1166; Krumbacher 1897: 749–760, 804–806). Prodromos was known to be close to the court circles of the Byzantine emperor John II (John Comnenus: 1118–1143) and his successor Manuel I (1143–1180). In Prodromos' play *Executioner or Doctor*, in which dentists are lumped with physicians, the tragicomic specialist breaks a patient's tooth during an extraction (Podestà 1947, in Kazhdan 1984: 50). Clearly the audience was aware of the serious dangers of an incomplete removal of a tooth. The play also tells us that physicians of that time practiced dental surgery. From the twelfth century we also have a discourse on dentistry written by Maimonides (Weinberger 1948: 96).

The first known illustrations of instruments that can clearly be identified as used in dental extractions date from the medieval period (as in the images of Saint Apollonia). Albucasis produced some rather crude illustrations in the late tenth century, but they remain the earliest drawings now known of specific dental tools. The pharmaceutical aspects of dentistry were significantly diminished in Europe at that time, although the Arabic world maintained many portions of the rich tradition, only briefly noted above. While scholars in the Arabic world may have maintained many aspects of medicine, including those relating to oral hygiene (Sterpellone and Elsheikh 1990: 267–274), there is no evidence that they sustained techniques involving gold or silver wire.

In the year 1310 a discussion of the qualities and virtues of some pharmaceuticals, or what now are identified as spices (*droghi*, in modern Italian) was offered by a Florentine appropriately named Zucchero di Bencivenni (Italian *zucchero* = "sugar"). Among those *droghi* discussed is only one recommended as a specific for dental infirmity, or for tooth maggots, reflecting the old "tooth worm" theory of dental decay. The ashes of rosemary, when placed in a green handkerchief and stroked over the teeth, cause the maggots (tooth worms) to exit, according to di Bencivenni (Ciasca 1927: 754, Document XVIII). That rosemary was a commonly available garden herb may be the reason that this remedy, rather than those exotic prescriptions requiring myrrh and similar imports, is the only one noted during this period. The purely magical aspects of this treatment reflect the impoverishment of dental procedures during the medieval period.

By the middle of the fourteenth century the medical faculty at the University in Florence was large and quite diverse. The guild to which they probably belonged (*Arte dei medici e speziale*) was one of the largest in the city, having over 1,000 members (Ciasca 1927: 748–758; Origo 1963: 298–300). Members of this guild were general practitioners, surgeons, dentists, and specialists in wounds, bones, stones and gravel (urologists?), and the eyes.[19] Dentists at that time were specialists, using "surgical" procedures distinct from the general cutting activities practiced by barbers.

Despite an apparent lack of development in the pharmacological aspects of dentistry, progress can more clearly be seen in the fabrication of hardware specifically fashioned for performing tooth extractions. In 1363 Guy de Chauliac (1298–1368), surgeon at Montpellier and to the Popes at Avignon, made note of the use of the tooth-pulling device called a "pelican." This term may have been used for an early form of dental forceps (pliers), which has a handle set horizontally and a lower jaw much larger than the upper. Instruments of similar form remain in use to this day. Hoffmann-Axthelm (1970: 85) believes that de Chauliac taught his students that missing teeth could be replaced by artificially constructed dentures, but that de Chauliac himself did not fabricate such appliances. Hoffmann-Axthelm suggests that ideas regarding dental prostheses were being quoted from Albucasis by de Chauliac, in his manuscript text of 1363, published in printed form in 1598.

In Florence, at the end of the fourteenth century, internal medicine remained under the aegis of the physicians, while barbers used their shaving razors for bloodletting as well as dentistry. Barbers also appear to have applied leeches and plasters, and been responsible for the external parts of the body, in addition to setting bones. These skills seem to be related to "hands on" activities, or those that involved physical contact with patients. The medical treatments and knowledge of physicians focused on "disease" as a philosophical and intellectual problem, to be understood and treated through reason. These physician-diagnosticians utilized the services of apothecaries and alchemists to provide the treatments they considered best. Their esoteric skills may have been reserved for a specific class of people, since there could also be found a flourishing population of folk and religious healers, with their own sets of remedies, plus various witches and quacks (Origo 1963: 299). In the spring of 1387 Maestro Naddino di Aldobrandino Bovattieri of Prato, in a letter from Avignon, indicated that Maestro Giovanni Banduccio should be informed that:

> earnings from his art are small here, the art of surgery being generally prac-
> ticed by the barbers; there are some surgeons here well trained in science
> and practice, but this counts for nothing as the honor and payment for these
> surgeons is the same as for a barber.
>
> (translated from Brun 1923: 224; see also Origo 1963: 34–35)

The red and white striped pole that has become the sign of the modern American barber is commonly believed to have evolved from the pole wrapped in bloody bandages of the barber-surgeon of the medieval period in Europe.

The slow but steady progress made in the development of tools to be used for dental extractions was not paralleled by developments in oral medicine. The twelfth-century translation by Gerard of Cremona of the works of Abenguefit (Ali Ibn al-Husain Ibn al-Wafid, an eleventh-century physician and pharmacologist from Toledo in the Moorish kingdom in Spain), were now available in printed versions (Abenguefit 1533). Tacuinus (Giovanni Tacuino da Tridino, 1492–1547, publisher of a number of Greek and Latin Classics) had available these ancient data when he wrote about those "*Praeparatoria Dentium, secunda Maymonem*" that gave comfort to "*gingiuas, & dentes*" (Tacuinus 1533: 89–90). These treatises were formulations, many of a magical or astrological nature, discussing the combinations of vegetables, plants and parts of animals commonly consumed that could be used to treat various diseases. The illustration (sketch) of the "*Praeparatoria Dentium*" may be of interest. Tacuinus (1532: 52–54) also translated a related work by "Bvhahylyha Bygezla." Sections XXVI and XXVII of the "*Tacvino Tabvlae particvlares*" (incorrectly listed as section "XXXI" in the index) deal with the mouth and teeth: "*Labiorem, & Dentium*" and "*Centium, Giniuarum, & Vuluae*" (the text is paginated in Roman numerals, with the following "*Tabvlae*" paginated in Arabic). These texts all reflect the continuing tradition of ancient writings on oral medicine; a tradition that lacks any reference to dental prostheses and remains largely apart from the practice of dental extractions.

Dental hygiene, in the form of toothbrushes, tooth powders and pastes, as well as toothpicks, was a concern throughout the fifteenth and sixteenth centuries (Pederson 1978). The aesthetics of clean teeth during this period (d'Errico *et al.* 1986) appear to derive from the earlier Roman tradition, but evidence for this continuity is lacking. Also during the first half of the sixteenth century several advances in the technology of dental extraction appear in the literature. A drawing made by Giovanni d'Arcoli (below) in 1542 shows an instrument with a hook-like device, apparently to fit over a diseased tooth to facilitate its extraction. On this instrument is a tightening mechanism designed to allow the hook to grasp the tooth to be extracted. This type of tool would be best suited to the traditional rocking procedure used for loosening a decayed tooth prior to its removal. The actual extraction methods used during this period are not clearly defined in the literature, but they must have been much the same as they had been during the Roman period.

The beginnings of modern dentistry

A full separation between dentistry and the medical arts as now found in the United States of America took centuries to achieve. In much of Europe many specialties involving oral medicine and diseases of the face remain linked with dental surgery. In all cases the emergence of dentistry as a profession distinct from other branches of medicine and pharmacy can be traced to the 1500s from the literature alone. In that era, when dental pains were still believed to be caused by worms living in the teeth, bleeding and cupping continued to be considered as useful treatments for tooth decay, as were burning with a cautery and the direct application of acid to the tooth. In 1545 Walther Hermann Ryff (ca.1500–1548) of Nuremberg, who held a post equivalent to a Health Inspector, wrote a treatise on dental surgery that may be the first modern textbook exclusively treating matters of dentistry. Ryff's text (1545) *Die groß Chirurgei oder volkommene Wundtartzenei*, provides insights into the few advances then being made on this aspect of the field (see also Pfaff 1756). Nevertheless, curative dentistry or restoration involving the drilling of teeth and filling of prepared cavities remained rudimentary and rare while the replacement of missing teeth with single or multiple false teeth as well as full dental plates became increasingly common.

Ambroise Paré (1510–1590), often considered the founder of modern surgery (his knowledge of anatomy was augmented through extensive battlefield experience), was also involved in the production of dental appliances. His position as chief surgeon at the Hotel Dieu, the foremost hospital in Paris, and later as chief surgeon to the French kings, rendered his publications highly influential. From his origins as a humble barber's apprentice he must have learned a great deal about basic dental extractions before expanding his surgical activities. His text *De Chirurgie* (Paré 1564: 218) includes a figure that is labeled "*Dentz artificielles faittes d'os, qui s'attachent par vn fil d'argent en lieu des autres qu'on aura perdues*" ("artificial teeth made of bone, which are attached by a silver wire to replace those which have been lost") (see Figure 1.5). He illustrates five examples that are alike except for the number of teeth held within a base (see also Hoffmann-Axthelm 1970: fig. 8). Paré combined silver wire and other attachment techniques to produce a fixed partial denture that appears to have had at least some masticatory functions.

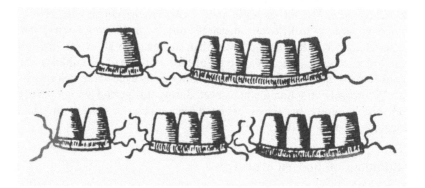

Figure 1.5 Examples of false teeth as indicated by Paré (1564: 218; after Hoffmann-Axthelm 1970: fig. 8). Paré illustrates five examples that are all alike, except for the number of teeth held in a base, with the citation "*Dentz artificielles faittes d'os, qui s'attachent par vn fil d'argent en lieu des autres quón aura perdues.*"

In Italy Paré's contemporary, Girolamo Fabrici d'Acquapendente (1533–1619), who founded the first permanent dissection theater where he taught in Padua, also was a surgeon-anatomist of some renown. Some modern authors (e.g. Baggieri 1998: 68) have associated d'Acquapendente with sixteenth-century advances in dentistry, but published evidence is wanting. Italian "dentistry" remained focused on the development of ever more elaborate dental appliances, such as the pure silver pair of dental plates that Weil Marin and Corrain (1986) date to the sixteenth century. The invention of porcelain dentures and replacement teeth is attributed by Mingoli (1953) to Giuseppangelo Fonzi (1768–1840) at the end of the eighteenth century (see also Weil Marin and Corrain 1986: 229).

The principal transitions to modern dentistry appear to be focused on developments that took place in France. These developments include Claude Jacquier de Gérauldy's recognition (1737) of the importance of the deciduous dentition in general dental health. His work appeared in a German edition in 1754 and remained a major text for half a century. Claude Mouton's (1746) study of artificial teeth included innovative work on swaging dental plates as well as insights regarding gold crowns and clasp bridges (see also Donaldson 2013: 162).

By 1600 genre painting by Caravaggio (*"The Dentist"*) and his followers commonly included remarkably detailed studies of tooth extractions and the many instruments used in this trade. While the title of Theodor Rombouts' (*c.*1597–1637) study of a molar extraction (1637) is titled "*El charlatan sacamuelas*" ("*The Charlatan Tooth-Puller*") the finely depicted practitioner's extensive set of dental instruments reveals the beginnings (or imitation) of a professionalized dental specialist (Colección Real, Museo del Prado P 01635: Sanchez 1972). The inclusion of portraits of dentists plying their trade among the works of the greatest artists of that period reflects a wide public interest in the care and preservation of the teeth. The specialized instruments incorporated as part of these scenes reveal that dentistry was coming into its own as a profession distinct from barber-surgeons and medical practitioners.

The construction of cosmetic "false teeth" during the sixteenth and seventeenth centuries was not limited to Italy, as suggested by an appliance said to have come from a Swiss tomb dated to about 1500 CE (Rath 1958: fig. 5). Unfortunately, Rath provides no information on the origin, owner, or even the source of his illustration. The date is too early for the mineral paste dentures that Hoffmann-Axthelm (1970: 85) believes came to replace bone or ivory false teeth by the early 1600s. Hoffmann-Axthelm bases this thesis on an illustration in Guillemeau (1598: 303). However, the artificial teeth illustrated by Guillemeau appear exactly like those depicted by Paré, his teacher, and were probably fashioned using traditional bone or ivory.

Pierre Fauchard (1678–1761) made major contributions to the field of dentistry (e.g. Fauchard 1728) and was an important figure in upgrading the professional status of practitioners. Under Louis XIV surgeon-dentists in France moved to a separate subdivision of the surgeons' guild, suggesting that in France formal dentistry had made a significant shift away from the hands of tooth pullers and barbers and into the realm of a medical specialty. Of interest is the note that women were allowed to practice dentistry in early eighteenth-century France, but that privilege was revoked during the mid 1700s, before Fauchard's death.

A brief note on the concepts relating to teeth and their preservation in Japan during this period may be of interest. A Japanese archaeological site has yielded several sets of teeth that had been lost before death, possibly due to periodontal disease or even combat. Of some 141 burials in a Samurai (warrior class) cemetery, 15 percent of those interred were accompanied by teeth that they had lost while alive (Oyamada *et al.* 2000: 8). Oyamada and his colleagues suggest that at least some of these teeth had been used to make dental pontics that were held in place with wire or thread, but no details have been published. Nor did the authors provide specific dates for these Samurai, whose class held power in Japan from the eleventh to the nineteenth centuries. More probably lost teeth were seen as part of the "body" to be buried as a means of keeping the corpse "intact." The advances made in early Chinese dentistry, specifically the early use of tin amalgam restorations, do not appear to have been adopted in Japan.

The first English language dental book, by Charles Allen (*The Operator for the Teeth*, 1685), appeared more than 100 years after Ryff's classic. This does not reflect a lack of regard for dentistry on the part of the English, as some might be tempted to suggest, but rather the multilingual nature of all scientific endeavors at that time. The many French language editions of medical and dental texts would have been purchased and read in England without need for a translation. Allen's volume reflects a trend for vernacular language use in England that included an English language Bible.

Rapid progression in the use of novel materials in the construction of false teeth occurred during the seventeenth century according to Hoffmann-Axthelm (1970: 85–87). By 1700 toothbrushes had become common household objects throughout Europe. Thus, popular interest in preventing dental decay preceded much of the development of improved instrumentation for the removal of decayed teeth. During the 1700s various forms of tools called "elevators" were perfected for the removal of incisors, canines, and root stumps. The dental screw, first illustrated in 1803, accomplished this task by turning the end into the root canal of the afflicted tooth and levering it out. Tooth keys for the extraction of teeth, first noted by 1742, were rapidly being developed as a simple and effective tool type. Bolsters were added to tooth keys by 1796, and a gum-protecting alteration became incorporated into most designs after 1816.

The archaeological evidence in Europe

Nearly all of the post-medieval data noted above is derived from published texts. Often there is a significant lag between an actual technological development or use of some aspect of material culture, and the time when this object is described in writing. Thus the use of a number of dental techniques, such as wiring, survived from antiquity but without being recorded in any European literature. The inception of methods for drilling and filling teeth, as well as for making prostheses, is documented by archaeological evidence at least a century before there are written accounts for many of these procedures. The dental prostheses known from the eighteenth century are far more complex and had considerably more functional capabilities than any of the ornamental Etruscan appliances and their immediate successors. For a better view of the foundations of modern dentistry, and one that provides a closer link with the past than previously believed, we must turn to the archaeological evidence.

Archaeological excavations within the church of Saint Hippolyte at Grand Sacconex (Geneva, Switzerland) recovered the remains of 259 individuals dating from the Late Middle Ages to the last half of the eighteenth century (Simon 1990). Epitaphs on the associated tombstones enabled considerable information to be recovered about many of the individuals represented in this sample, including two individuals of particular importance in this study. The deacon François-Bénigne du Trousset d'Héricourt, who died in 1761 at the age of 58 years, was originally from Paris. The lawyer Françoise-Jean Marihaure de la Salle, also from Paris, died in 1765 at the age of 63. The mouths of these two gentlemen held an assortment of bridges, ivory dentures, gold ligatures, and metal fillings, all extensively described and beautifully illustrated by Alt (1993, 1994, 1989). Marihaure de la Salle had dentures in both jaws, held in the mandible with gold wire (Alt 1994: figs 1, 2). Use of a scanning electron microscope (SEM) reveals that the maxillary bridge was carved from fresh, not fossil, ivory (Alt 1993: fig. 6; 1994: 69, figs 3, 4; Alt and Newesely 1994). The good deacon d'Héricourt also has a gold-wire splint identical to the ancient wire dental appliances from the Eastern Mediterranean (Becker 1997), plus a gold foil restoration, two fillings that appear to be tin, and a bridge incorporating a carved animal tooth (Alt 1994: figs 6–8). Alt notes that these discoveries confirm Fauchard's (1728) note that tin and gold foil, but not amalgams, were used in French restorative dentistry in the early eighteenth century.

As Alt (1994) points out, these sophisticated dental procedures had all been achieved prior to 1765. It seems likely that this dental work may have been done while these upper-class gentlemen were resident in or visiting Paris. Alt also notes that this evidence confirms the "contemporary descriptions in regard to therapy, material and manufacture in the times of Fauchard (1678–1761) and Pfaff (1713–1766)" (Fauchard 1728; Pfaff 1756).

Other finds of early "modern" dentures cited by Alt (1994) also come from in-church elite burials (Thierfelder 1987; Czarnetzki and Alt 1991). Early dental fillings are far more rare than dentures (Cohen 1962). Alt (1994, citing Chu 1858) believes that documentary evidence suggests that the technique of using tin-silver amalgams originated in China during the seventh century AD (Tang Dynasty; but see Czarnetzki and Ehrhardt 1990). Alt (1994: 69) also suggests that the original edition of Li's famous pharmacopoeia, which has appeared in dozens of editions since Li's death in 1593 (see Li 1596), includes a reference to this early use of amalgam for dental fillings.

Alt (1994: 69, citing Hoffmann-Axthelm 1981) believes that amalgam fillings in Europe date from at least 1528. Alt cites an archaeological example found in the mouth of Anna Ursula von Braunschweig und Lüneburg (1573–1601; see Riethe and Czarnetzki 1983, Czarnetzki and Ehrhard 1990) confirming the use of amalgam in this part of Europe before 1601. The same Anna Ursula is also said to have had a gold foil restoration in her mouth, the earliest documented use of gold as a filling material. In this case the historical documents appear to record this practice at an earlier date than can be confirmed by the archaeological record. Alt (1994: 69) suggests that Giovanni d'Arcoli notes the use of gold foil in restoring teeth in 1557 (d'Arcoli 1557, in Alt 1994: 69), but this edition of d'Arcoli is a very late reprinting of the first edition of this work (1493). The book by J. Stocker (1657), from the middle of the seventeenth century, is also cited by Alt. It seems possible that the use of amalgam fillings in Europe may have developed in the Germanic states, while tin and gold foil restorations originated in Italy and spread to France and then north towards Scandinavia.

Alt (1994: 69) suggests that these early restorations are seldom found because the methods used in the preparation of the cavities may have led to the loss of the filling. However, an "empty" prepared cavity in a tooth would be as easily recognized as a metallic filling. The rarity of archaeological reports of early dentistry reflects the relatively small number of excavations directed toward historical cemeteries and church locations. These are places where we would expect these types of dental work to be found. Excavations in elite burial areas from the period after 1500 CE should be reviewed for information on dentition and dental restorations. Even more rare is the publication of complete archaeological records from these contexts, and even studies of the related skeletal remains are rare.

The great variety of techniques and prostheses that burgeoned during the eighteenth and early nineteenth centuries is well illustrated by the study of the parishioners interred (often with nameplates) in the crypts of Christ Church Spitalfields, London (see Whittaker 1993 and Chapter 4 of this volume).

In 1998 and 1999 excavations were conducted below the parking lot of the Delaware Hospital, along West 12th Street in Wilmington, Delaware (USA). The Hospital had purchased the property in 1955 from the Catholic Church, which had purchased the land in 1852 for use as the Cathedral Cemetery (NO6308; 7NC-E-147). Interments there continued only until 1870, when a new area was opened farther from the expanding city. The nearly 3,000 graves recovered represent a locale of all classes, including Medal of Honor recipient Bernard McCarren. The skeletal remains and associated artifacts, including dental prostheses and restored teeth, have been reinterred in a mass grave in All Saints Cemetery (Newcastle County). The archaeological contract to MAAR Associates did not include study of the dental history represented by this 20-year time span at a period when modern dentistry was coming into its own. Relocations of cemeteries such as this provide fabulous opportunities for understanding health status as well as developments in specialized areas such as the history of dentistry. A tremendous opportunity to study types and extent of use of dentistry was lost. Had a specialist been allowed to review the materials, an important set of data might have been recovered, with the potential to improve dental care today.

By the 1870s techniques for drilling teeth to remove decay and to prepare a cavity for filling with amalgams and gold foil had become common in the Western world. Although such procedures can be extremely effective in preventing the spread of decay, cultural factors continue to lead many people to ignore decay until dental extractions are required. The procedures in use today for dental extractions differ to a surprisingly small degree from those employed by the experts in antiquity.

A major shift in modern dental technology was marked by the development in techniques for casting gold and other metals using the lost wax process to make inlays that could be cemented into slots in teeth prepared by drilling and cutting. Just how early this process was developed, perhaps during the second half of the nineteenth century, may be answered through archaeological recovery of early examples. The first account of this procedure was published by B. F. Philbrook of Denison, Iowa, who had rediscovered the process known as investment casting and applied it to the production of cast dental inlays. This presentation to the Iowa State Dental Society in Des Moines was published in their proceedings (Philbrook 1897). Whether or not William Henry Taggart of Chicago saw this publication remains a conundrum in the history of dental medicine. Some 10 years later Taggart (1907) presented a similar paper to the New York Odontological Society, which was published in their proceedings. Taggart also had developed instruments for producing these delicate castings and received several patents for their manufacture. At some point Philbrook's earlier work became recognized and the patents issued to Taggart were cancelled (Lamacki 2014). Cast inlays require a very different preparation of the tooth than is needed for inserting gold foil or silver amalgams. The inlays themselves require a very complex molding and casting operation to manufacture the actual inlay. Like dental crowns and bridges, inlays have an optimal range of gold alloy variation involving added copper to increase their strength. Platinum or palladium also may be added to the gold along with copper to increase strength, but these elements more commonly are added to provide the flexibility generally associated with removable bridgework.

Orthodonture or the treatment for the correction of irregularly aligned teeth, usually involving braces and sometimes surgery, first appears in the latter part of the nineteenth century. Orthodonture represents an important development in dental history that depends on a number of developments in various aspects of medicine and technology plus changes in cultural attitudes relating to what is considered as "good health" as well as personal appearance. Suggestions that any of the soft gold dental appliances fashioned by the Etruscans could have served to alter the arrangement of the teeth are based on fantasy. While the origins of orthodonture also remain to be studied in detail, only modern skills of dentistry as well as metallurgy can produce any repositioning of the teeth.

Despite many claims that orthodontia had been practiced in antiquity, the earliest suggestion that dental irregularities could be remedied dates from an early work by Pierre Fauchard (1728). His suggestions regarding methods that might be used to straighten irregularly erupted teeth include the use of a *bandeau*, a horseshoe-shaped device believed by some modern authors to have been able to expand the dental arch and allow teeth to rotate into desired positions. Fauchard's second edition (1746) was translated into English for its bicentennial by Lilian Lindsay (1946), Great Britain's first woman dentist to be trained at home, rather than in the United States. The lack of specific data in Fauchard's work rendered it a curiosity in the rapidly evolving world of modern dentistry.

The term "orthodontia" is generally believed to have been coined by Joachim Lefoulon, whose work was translated into English in 1844, quite soon after the French edition became available. Lefoulon (1844: 45) offers a very brief comment on the use of manual manipulation of the teeth to achieve a "better arrangement of the denture." He later returns to "orthodontosy [sic], vulgarly (and incorrectly) called dental orthopedy." Lefoulon's (1844: 99–115) chapter VIII, devoted to "orthodentosy," suggests that this "branch of dentistry was long in its infancy." The translator's use of different spellings did nothing to promote the use of the term offered by Lefoulon. Aside from describing earlier efforts to provide treatments for this problem in dental articulation, Lefoulon (1844: 107–108) recognized that no really effective treatment was then available. Soon afterward the first articles on orthodontics began to appear in dental journals, and books devoted entirely to the subject reviewed the many methods that were being developed in the second half of the nineteenth century.

Evidence for the use and acceptance of orthodonture among the American elite can be documented by an interesting literary reference. Edith Wharton, in *The Buccaneers*, her novel of young American heiresses sent to England in the 1870s to find aristocratic husbands (1938, Book 2, section 10) mentions orthodonture in an 1875 context, but with reference to events that took place in 1865. *The Buccaneers* remained unfinished at the time of Wharton's death in 1937; it was completed and published the following year. In her narrative Wharton (1938: 127), referring to events of about 1875, says: "Lord Brightlingsea cast an unfavorable glance on his daughter. ('If her upper teeth had been straightened when she was a child we might have had her married by this time,' he thought. But that again was Lady Brightlingsea's affair.)"

So Edith Wharton correctly recalled the situation of American orthodonture in the period around 1865 to 1875. Interest was growing, but was limited to those who could afford the costs, plus time and energy, to engage in the process of correcting what most of the rest of the world saw as part of the normal human condition. Becker well recalls his twentieth-century Italian colleagues ridiculing Americans for their open-mouthed smiles, often revealing the impressive results of American orthodontists. Today, younger and wealthier Italians see the correction of dental irregularities as part of maintaining good health.

Dental drilling and filling

While in Chapter 3 we note the skilled technique of drilling the replacement human teeth (or other tooth materials) to make the Etruscan dental appliances, this was a somewhat different procedure from drilling living teeth to treat cavities, or for other purposes. Fauchard's drilling of extracted teeth to make pontics (early eighteenth century, Gorelick and Gwinnett 1987a: 25) and the drilling of live teeth as preparation for restorations may be a re-development of ancient skills. This might also be considered as a new application of the skills, developed for other purposes such as fine arts, combining methods of drilling in stone and other materials with medical or decorative goals.

Gold foil fillings and silver amalgams placed into cavities prepared in human teeth now are well documented from early seventeenth-century archaeological contexts. Riethe and Czarnetzki (1983) also cite a number of early texts discussing these procedures. This evidence refutes the earlier assumption that dental drilling and filling of teeth in Europe did not develop until the nineteenth century (Powers 1988). Other texts suggest that such modern dental techniques were first used in America by James Gardette, in Philadelphia, by the end of the eighteenth century (Sissman 1968: 10–11), but this is nearly 200 years after the earliest known German examples. Dr. Eleazer Parmly appears to have perfected techniques of preparing cavities for gold foil fillings in the 1840s. His skill was noted some 50 years later (Smith 1894) because examples of his early work apparently were being documented near the end of the century as having lasted that long. Various mixtures—of gold, tin plus gold, and amalgam—were being tested by American dentists in the 1850s with increasing success.

Not only were dental skills rapidly enhanced through the use of new techniques, but the means by which these skills were disseminated were changing. Formal teaching and scholarly publication rapidly transformed the art of dental extractions in America. Around 1827 John Harris began to teach dentistry on a formal basis to a small group of interested students, including his younger brother Chapin (Dalton 1946). Chapin Harris's contribution to the professionalization of the discipline included publication of a volume on dental surgery (Harris 1839) that went through 13 editions and was not superseded until the end of the nineteenth century. A French translation also went into a second edition. Chapin

Harris, with Joseph Fox, also made significant contributions relating to the diseases of the teeth (1855) and to the conservation of decayed teeth.

A major advance came with Robert Arthur's publication, in 1854, of a description of the technique of filling teeth with "adhesive" gold, or gold foil under pressure. This technique had been invented by the seventeenth century or earlier, but no publication of it seems to have appeared prior to the mid-nineteenth century. An "adhesive" gold foil technique uses the process of cold welding to bond gold foil into a solid mass, under pressure, within a prepared cavity in the tooth. The specific origins of the gold foil technique warrant further research. It almost certainly had been in use for hundreds of years before being described by Arthur (1854).

The method of using gold as a filling material was practiced, if not actually developed, by Dr. Wilhelm Herbst of Bremen in the years around 1879 (Bennett 1885); he rapidly became extremely well known throughout the world due to his writings. This demonstrates the speed of information dissemination provided by the dental journals of that period. In April of 1884 a discussion of this new method appeared in the *Journal of the British Dental Association*. Soon after, this method was discussed in the *Dental Record* for 1885 (Vol. 5: 72–83), and then by Bennett (1885)—about the same time that Herbst himself (1885) was publishing a complete description. How much difference existed between these various gold foil techniques is not known, but the basic principal employed in the use of gold foils is similar to that which must have been employed in the fabrication of most if not all of the ancient Etruscan appliances and jewelry.

An archaeological clue to the developments in these techniques is provided by the discovery of a "gold dental filling" among the teeth of an individual interred in the nineteenth-century Canadian Prospect Hill Cemetery (Ontario) believed to date from before 1879 (Pfeiffer, Dudar and Austin 1989). An analysis of this "filling," whether of gold foil or a casting, would provide interesting data relating to the history of this aspect of dentistry in the United States. Much work remains for us to establish the details of these relatively recent developments in dentistry, which rapidly came to surpass anything that the ancient Etruscans could produce.

Modern ornamentation: inlays and replacement of healthy teeth

Maya tradition led to the drilling and inlaying of the teeth of nobles/royals for cosmetic purposes, and will be discussed in Chapter 4, but here we briefly comment on cosmetic procedures in today's world. Cosmetic drilling and filing of teeth prior to the nineteenth century are well known from African examples as well as from an impressive series from ancient Mesoamerica (Romero 1970, Gwinnett and Gorelick 1979; Becker 1992b). Examples of tooth filing, so common in ancient Mesoamerica, are also documented from twentieth-century Africa and Indonesia (Alt *et al.* 1990) as well as among the Inuit, or Eskimo (Schwartz *et al.* 1995). The decoratively filed teeth found on slaves or former slaves whose burials were recently excavated in New York City are believed by some (Harrington 1995: 14–15) to have originated while these individuals were part of their traditional cultures in Africa.

Sterpellone and Elsheikh (1990: 123) suggests that the use of purely decorative gold crowns on teeth in the USA and in Europe can be dated *c.*1900, noting that in Italy to this day a part of the population (unspecified) covers perfectly healthy teeth in gold. It is unclear whether he is alluding to a specific class, to gypsies, or to some other modern group.

Modi (1931: 9) notes that "jewelers" in India commonly drill teeth in order to insert gold or jewel studs, but indicates that this skill was not applied to restorative dentistry. The first use of dental drilling to prepare a cavity for the placement of inlays or other types of restoration remains unknown. No anthropological study of dental alterations among late twentieth-century ethnic groups as yet exists. However, newspaper and magazine reports frequently appear of diamonds and other precious stones being inserted into perfectly healthy teeth, in the style of the ancient Maya. "Paul, who is seventeen and lives in the Bronx, has four lettered gold caps on his top front teeth that spell out his name" (Anon. 1994: 41). By 1998 the fashion for decorative gold or jewel inlays had become so common in some parts of American as well as British society that a reference to "gold rapper-style teeth" could be used in a popular publication (Anon. 1998b: 108) with a contemporary audience understanding what was meant. In that year the British press briefly noted a Caribbean conch collector and dealer named Goldie with a photographic parody in the *Sunday Times* Style section (Anon. 1998a: 38). Goldie apparently has gold incisors and canines, or gold caps that cover them (Jason 1998). The parody in the *Sunday Times* provided photographs of three popular male actors, including the Hollywood film star Tom Cruise, with their smiles altered to include gold teeth.

Jamal Barrow, better known as the rap star Shyne, was described in 2001 as having jewel-encrusted teeth. The arrest of the 22-year-old rapper, who then was charged with attempted murder, provided photographers and their public with a glimpse of these famous teeth. But in the "politically correct" America of 2001 a "limit" was placed on advertisements employing these observations regarding these cultural behaviors. Toyota Motors Sales USA had distributed free postcards promoting their sport-utility vehicle identified as the RAV4. The postcard featured the close-up smile of a dark-skinned man on whose front tooth was appliquéd, in gold, a tiny RAV4. Toyota's foray into tooth art, fashionable in some corners of the black community, was distributed in clubs, coffeehouses, "and other establishments favored by the young and style-conscious," according to a company release (Boyer 2001: 62). Jesse Jackson denounced the promotional postcard as a ghetto stereotype.

In W. Somerset Maugham's short story "Honolulu" (1934: 136–137) the ship's mate named Wheeler, but called "Bananas," is described as "much darker than is usual in Hawaii. His upper front teeth were cased in gold. He was very proud of them." Just 13 years later John Steinbeck described the character Ernest Horton, a traveling salesman of novelty items, in the novel *The Wayward Bus*, as a disillusioned war veteran. Why he was disillusioned is not clear, but "His teeth were white and even except for the two front uppers, and these were glittering gold" (1947: 24). By the end of that century the deliberate removal of entire teeth for replacement with gold bridgework (Waters 1998) and the "decorative" capping of healthy teeth with gold had become more common in certain parts of American society. In America there is a general acceptance of the Hollywood style of dental capping where all the anterior teeth are crowned with porcelain to achieve the perfect, or at least a photogenic smile. The recent trend toward using removable gold covers as temporary tooth ornamentation has been reported by Glen Copestick (1998), who notes an association with the "street" industries of drugs and sex. The "Players Ball," held annually in Chicago and now with versions in Miami, Atlanta and other major cities, is described by *Wikipedia* as an annual gathering of pimps. Search engines used to find "Players Ball" will provide seekers with vast numbers of advertisements for "Pimp Daddy Costumes" as well as hundreds of manufacturers marketing decorative "grillz." These dental accessories come in an amazing assortment of shapes and colors, with gold being by far the most popular metal.

The modern somewhat extravagant examples of golden ornamentation of a smile by tooth inlays or replacements speak to some innate human interest in the teeth as a means of expressing status or identity, and this situation was already occurring, although rarely, and only among the women of the ruling classes, in Etruria prior to its takeover by Rome. Chapter 3 will present all the Etruscan appliances and the society in which they were developed and used, after a brief excursus explaining the fallacy of Egyptian origins for dentistry or dental appliances.

Notes

1 Although Professor Bliquez did not directly examine any of these dental appliances, he provides an essential compendium of the published data and an important review of the illustrations of these appliances that have been used, and abused, through the years (see also Emptoz 1987). The previous lack of detailed examination of the known pieces, and an absence of any careful review of the published literature, has resulted in the listing of several "examples," which are spurious. The present study may not solve all of the many problems generated over the past 100 years, but may point future scholars in a more useful direction.

2 We have only a few comments, and possibly one religious book (a calendar for interpretation of thunder omens—see Turfa 2012b) that survived because they were quoted or translated into Latin by Roman authors. Another calendar, in Etruscan, listing dates for religious ceremonies, was preserved when it was torn into strips to wrap a woman's mummy; collected in Egypt, it is now in the Zagreb Museum (see Bonfante and Bonfante 2002: 183–184 no. 67; Turfa 2012b: 23–24).

3 Treggiari (1979: 70) notes female crafters who worked "gold thread," but this was not strong enough to serve in dental applications. The rare finds of gold cloth/thread show that it was made by twisting thin, flat strips of sheet gold around a textile core spun from organic fiber such as silk, wool or animal gut. One precious fragment of what may have been a purple and gold cloak was found in the Etruscan François Tomb at Vulci (*c.*350 BCE). Late in the fourth century, a Macedonian royal tomb at Vergina, sometimes referred to as the tomb of Philip of Macedon, held a purple and gold tapestry made of threads of gold sheet wrapped around purple wool (see Gleba 2012: 227). The combination of gold and purple was certainly appreciated as a status symbol, but gold thread was strictly ornamental and could not have been employed in dental applications. We have no archaeological evidence from Italy or the western Mediterranean for the use of gold wire in dentistry as early as the use of gold bands in Etruscan Italy.

4 Hippocrates himself seems to have written few texts, but many of his students and subsequent physicians of the School of Cos recorded over 60 lectures, textbooks and essays; in addition to those manuscripts of the fifth century BCE, very many treatises on all fields of medicine were published under the Hippocratic Corpus, some as late as the Roman period (second century CE). The early corpus was probably assembled in Alexandria. It appears that the Aphorisms, whence came some comments on *Dentition* and the treatise *On Injuries of the Head* represent genuine, or early (fifth–fourth century BCE) works by or in the spirit of Hippocrates.

5 The only possible exception to extraction as the principal focus of ancient dentistry is the specious "implant" of a bronze scrap in a Nabatean male (age 40–50 years) from the northern Negev, *c.*200 BCE (Zias and Numeroff 1986b; Zias and Numeroff 1987. Powers (1988) more convincingly suggests that this is an accidental "implantation" due to burial conditions (see also the Zias and Powers discussion, 1989. Chandler (1989) provides an excellent summary of this matter (see Appendix III, no. 10).

6 In the field of *orthopedic* pain relief, Galen's "Olympic Victor's Dark Ointment" has been shown to be efficacious, disproving many attempts to disparage it. It has not been reproduced for commercial use, however, since the active ingredient seems to have been an opioid! See Harrison *et al.* 2012; Bartels *et al.* 2006.

7 A basket containing hemp leaves was excavated among stored supplies on the wreck of a Punic ship believed to have sunk off the western coast of Sicily (near Motya and Lilybaeum, modern Marsala) around the time of the Battle of the Aegates Islands, near the end of the First Punic War (241 BCE). The ship might have been a blockade-runner, as it was laden with cured meat and other supplies that could have been of use to the besieged Punic garrison on Motya. See Frost *et al.* 1981: 62–67, figs 23–27.

8 The use of pharmaceuticals in the Biblical world is well documented in Jacob and Jacob (1993); also see especially Newmyer 1993; and Crawfurd 1914: 23–24.

9 On the evidence of their naturalistic art, in the painted tombs of Tarquinia, the Etruscans were well aware of the colorful and painful effects of viper bites: see Hostetler 2004–2007, and images of demons such as Charu and Tuchulcha.

10 For a fascinating history of poisons in the Classical world and the personality of Mithridates VI king of Pontus, see Mayor 2010.

11 For substances of use as drugs in Etruria, see also Turfa and Becker 2013: 869–870; Harrison and Bartels 2006; Harrison and Turfa 2010 (antihelminthics) with additional references.

12 Celsus (VII, 5, 1–5) also includes data on removal of missiles from the human body, using techniques similar to those used in dental extractions. Paul and most other authors have similar data using the same techniques, suggesting that all of these procedures derive from the same medical tradition.

13 Milne's (1907: 137–138) suggestion regarding the origins of ideas propounded by Scribonius should be reviewed.

14 As brought vividly to life in the Roman, Late Republican-era mystery novels by Stephen Saylor (*Roman Blood, Catilina's Riddle*, etc.)

15 Later in this volume Caelius prescribes the use of periodontal surgery, suggesting that it be used only as an emergency measure. Quite probably two distinct situations are noted. Trimming the gums as a form of periodontal procedure, quite frequently used today, may have been recognized in antiquity as a means by which irritation could be reduced. Surgery to expose the jaw as part of tooth extractions, which Caelius and Soranus did not favor as a general rule, may have been seen as something to be avoided, if not absolutely undesirable.

16 Macedonius of Thessalonica or Macedonius Consul (*c.*500–560 CE) was a *hypatos* at the Byzantine court during the reign of Justinian (*hypatos*, translated as Latin *consul*, was a courtesy title for high-ranking courtiers at that time). His 42 epigrams that appear in the Greek Anthology were originally published posthumously (567 CE) by the scholar Agathios, in his collection the *Kyklos*.

17 Paul (6.28; in Milne 1907: 137) suggests that περισσοὶ ὄδοντες, often translated as "extra teeth," were filed down or pulled. Bliquez (personal communication 2001) points out that Francis Adams (1796–1861) has translated the Greek term as "supernumerary teeth" (see Adams 1844, 1849). Liddell and Scott's *Greek-English Lexicon* (Oxford: 1940 etc.) defines the term as "beyond the regular number or size, prodigious" or "out of the common, extraordinary, strange," a word in use since the time of Hesiod and the earliest recorded literature . . . so Paul's comment could be read as "extra teeth" or teeth that are exceptionally large in size or unusual in shape. Becker believes that he meant that any individual tooth that projected above the line of teeth would be filed down to provide better articulation.

18 Hoffmann-Axthelm (1970: 84–85) refers to a reference that he may have seen, supposedly taken from Abu al-Qasim, stating that Galen had carved a false tooth from cattle bone and attached it to other teeth by means of a gold "wire." Neither Hoffmann-Axthelm nor Becker have been able to locate such a statement among the writings of Galen. Quite clearly such an "observation" must derive from a secondary source confusing a known dental appliance with the writings of one of the ancient authors.

19 Painters (artists working with oil paints?) were also included in this guild, probably due to their need to learn the science of blending elements to make paints and varnishes (Origo 1963: 377, n. 20). This art of "formulation" may be reflected in the Roman Forum beauty shop by the presence of cosmetic and ointment jars.

2 Evidence from the ancient Near East

Correcting misconceptions

The Fallacy of Egyptian (or Greek) origins of dental prostheses

During the nineteenth century, and well into the twentieth, many scholars inferred that the origin of much modern technology could be traced to Egypt—after all, Egypt was an early inventor of many scientific advances, from writing systems to forms of astronomy, surveying, mathematics, architecture and medicine. This assumption, however, led to many erroneous interpretations of basic data that simply do not stand up to close scrutiny, and this is especially true for the field of dentistry and dental prosthetics. As Leek (1972) points out, there is no evidence whatever to indicate that dental technology relating to replacement teeth originated with the Egyptians. Even Masali and Peluso (1985: 56–57) recognize that there is a problem with the dating of the so-called Junker dental appliance from Egypt (from Gizeh, now in Hildesheim: it is probably a Hellenistic or Roman-era amulet — see Figure 2.1 and Appendix IV.B) although they accept the discredited ideas of Thoma (1917) and others who misunderstood Egyptian medicine. Masali's earlier paper (1980) offers a good, realistic impression of the extent of dental *pathology* in ancient Egypt (as well as a good bibliography, cf. Davide 1972). Egyptologist Roger Foreshaw (2010) has most recently surveyed the Egyptian evidence, from the papyrus texts to modern X-ray studies, and concluded that tooth wear and abscesses were frequent. He also states that no conclusive evidence of any sort of intervention can be found except for palliative, herbalist medication. There is virtually no evidence, certainly no physical evidence, of Egyptians practicing dentistry, in spite of the many mummies available for study.

The popular press still encourages us to look to Egypt as the origin of modern progress (and sometimes they are right!),[1] while in contrast many classically trained scholars, under the influence of Greek and Latin authors and with no other literature to correct this, still labor under outmoded notions that Greek civilization established the basis of all Western medical or technical progress. Many authors believe that there were Egyptian origins for various types of Roman technology, and others suggest that the Roman achievements in fields such as dentistry can be traced back to Greece. The idea that Roman dentistry developed from Greek foundations originated principally among scholars of Greek history, and their assumptions were probably strongly influenced by the reference in the

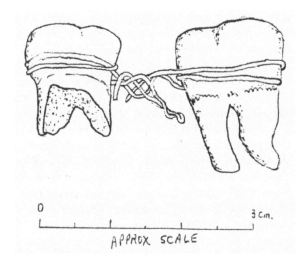

Figure 2.1 The Junker amulet (drawn by Becker, after Hoffmann-Axthelm 1970:
fig. 1), human teeth interpreted as if bound by a single gold wire (see
Appendix IV; a good photo is in Foreshaw 2010).

Odyssey (4.231–232), which extols the quality of Egyptian medicine (it says that
the Egyptian earth bears many drugs and every man is a physician—see Dawson
1953: 48; cf. Herodotus 2.77.3 on Egyptians as being exceptionally healthy). An
example of the Helleno-centric view is found in Sir John Boardman's suggestion (1980: 199–200) that goldsmithing in Etruria was the province of Greeks,
or that it copied Greek forms. (In fact, early Etruscan gold owes much more to
Phoenician/Levantine technicians: see Sannibale 2013 and Gaultier 2013.) Even
were we able to demonstrate Greek origins for other aspects of gold-working
technology, those gold-working skills do not apply in any way to the construction, and use, of Etruscan dental bridges. In the category of dental appliances, the
extensive archaeological evidence for dental prostheses in central Italy indicates
a non-Greek, Etruscan origin for them. Absolutely no Egyptian or Greek anteced-
ents or any other ancient parallels to these early Etruscan appliances are known.

The supposed evidence of Egyptian dental medicine:
ancient texts

The extensive modern literature claiming that the ancient Egyptians could make
gold fillings and use other dental techniques derives largely from nineteenth-
century allegations and outright fabrications of evidence. This erroneous belief
stems largely from the myth that all knowledge in ancient Greece and Rome derived
"from the Egyptians and the Phoenicians" (Guerini 1909: 69). Yet these fables were
recognized as fanciful as early as 1870 (Mummery 1870: 22). The absence of

dental prostheses in Pharaonic Egypt was recognized by Deneffe (1899: 54–56), who supported his position with data from Mr. Daressy (then conservator at the museum at Gizeh). Daressy confirmed what all careful scholars know, namely that those few reports of the use of dental prostheses in ancient Egypt are in error (see also Ruffer 1921).

John Nunn's brilliant survey of ancient Egyptian medicine provides the best description of the limited medical talents of the ancient Egyptians in matters pertaining to the mouth and dental treatments (Nunn 1996: 204–205). Nunn follows Ruffer (1920: 377) in noting the absence of any type of operative dentistry in ancient Egypt. The only potential indication of dental practice lies in some modern scholars' interpretations of a small number of written texts, all of Old Kingdom date (third millennium BCE). The texts have been taken to imply that dentists (possibly called *ibeh* or *ibhy*) formed a group that was separate from doctors (Nunn 1996: 118, 202). The Third Dynasty functionary identified as Hesy-Ra bore the title sometimes translated as "chief of dentists and doctors" (Nunn 1996: 124, fig. 6.4), but this unusual post may have placed him in a supervisory role for both specialties, emphasizing the fact that they were distinct medical fields. Nunn (1996: 119) also indicates that *ibeh* were distinct from *swnw*, who were doctors of the mouth.

Of the five "dentists" who Nunn (1996: 119) would identify in Old Kingdom texts, three are noted as *swnw ibeh*. Since there is no clear indication that these texts refer to oral surgeons, the *swnw ibeh* may have been physicians treating diseases of the mouth, and not tooth removers. Junker's (1927: 69) reading of Egyptian hieroglyphics, indicating the presence of a dentist in the pharaoh's court, is questioned by Leek (1972: 404), who finds no support for this argument, and follows Kaplony (n.d., I: 583, point 9) in suggesting that the title translated as "dentist" by Junker refers to a state office unrelated to dentistry.

Many years ago Ruffer (1920) had questioned the ability of the ancient Egyptians to perform dental extractions, and Nunn's insights appear to confirm that hypothesis. Nunn (1996: 203) infers from the skeletal evidence that dental caries were rare in Egypt prior to the first millennium BCE, suggesting that the discussion in *Papyrus Ebers* 553 and 554 probably does not relate to dental caries. Nunn concludes his discussion of "dentists" (1996: 205) with the general observation that "the papyri are silent on all operative aspects of dental care."

The frequent references found in various histories of dental medicine that ascribe the origins of dental appliances to the ancient Egyptians are simply spurious (cf. Quenouille 1977). This was recognized early in the twentieth century (Godon 1901), and repeatedly verified by careful scholars. Clawson (1933: 155, n. 18–24) provides a listing of "competent authorities" who conclude that there are no traces of restorative dental arts among the ancient Egyptians. He specifically notes Schmidt, Virshow [sic], and Mummery (1870) among these authorities. However, Clawson also notes that other writers, who he identifies as scholars unfamiliar with mummies, believed that the early Egyptians did construct dental appliances. These supposed believers include Perine (1883), Linderer (1851: 348; see the 1848 second edition), Purland 1857–1858, and Van Marter (1885c).

Even Guerini (1909) *inferred* the existence of dental appliances in ancient Egypt based on the supposed achievements of this culture (see also Ghalioungui and El-Dawakhly 1965: 54–55).

The thousands of mummies retrieved from Egyptian tombs ought to hold evidence of extractions or appliances, but all are equally silent. Many show evidence of poor dental health or even fatal abscesses, but none have filled, extracted or otherwise treated teeth.

The physical evidence—or lack thereof

In fact, Judith Miller (2008) was able to note the presence of caries during all periods of Egyptian history, but increasing in numbers as the diet increases in carbohydrates (thus worse in Late period and Ptolemaic and Roman times than during the Predynastic or Old Kingdom eras). She unequivocally states: "From the balance of the evidence provided by all research undertaken to date, it must be concluded that dental treatment only became a reality during the Graeco-Roman Period" (Miller 2008: 70; caries: 59, fig. 15). She surveys the famous medical papyri and finds that they deal with fractures and related issues, or else furnish prescriptions that are mainly for antiseptic mouthwash for the mouth and tongue, or for medicaments to be applied to encourage loose teeth to stay in place. As for extractions, she demonstrated that even in cases where a diseased tooth could have been removed with the bare hands, it remained, painfully, without intervention. From her survey of the literature and study of 500 Egyptian skulls in British collections, Miller notes that the neat holes through jawbones at the tips of tooth roots, taken by some modern commentators as evidence of surgical intervention to save a tooth with apical abscess (like a modern endodontist's apicoectomy), are actually the body's natural way of relieving pressure as the abscess eats its way through the bone and then drains. Foreshaw (2010: 73) also identifies these holes in the bone as natural occurrences in untreated abscesses.

No dental appliances that can be dated securely before 400 BCE have ever been found in Egypt: only in the seventh century BCE in central Italy do we find the first example of a true dental appliance (see Hunt 1975; Hoffmann-Axthelm 1985: 28–31, 38–39; Becker 1996; Ferguson *et al.* 1991). Although the earliest records now known anywhere in the world relating to any aspect of dental care are to be found in Egyptian medical papyri of the seventeenth and sixteenth centuries BCE (Badre 1986), these texts relate only to medical *treatments*, not to prosthetics (Leca 1971: 307–315). Leek (1967b: 52, following Dawson 1953: 49) notes that the information falls into two groups, one being "essentially medical in character" and the other "mainly magical or superstition" (Ritner 1993, Wilkinson 1994, Pinch 1995). Mesopotamia was no better off: the Old Babylonian clay tablets of the second millennium BCE either express magical approaches or offer the meager consolation of poultices applied to infected teeth or cloths wrapped around the aching jaw (Reid and Wagensonner 2014). Brown (1934) offers an excellent review of the relevant literature on dental medicine in Pharaonic Egypt, concluding that the claims to early Egyptian primacy in dental prosthesis technology are completely false. Weinberger's subsequent reviews of this material (1947; 1948: 77–81) as well as those of Leek (1967b) and Hoffmann-Axthelm (1985: 29–31) come to the same conclusion (see also Sigerist 1955: 277).

If there is no evidence, either physical or textual, for ancient Egyptian dental prostheses, why does a belief in them persist? The primary reason for the continuing fantasy is the poor quality of archaeological reporting involved in the publication of most of these finds, made long ago and then compounded by problems of curation and study. A second problem lies in frequent use of quotations from ancient Egyptian texts taken out of context. The semi-popular literature, such as trade journals (e.g. Harris *et al.* 1975 in the *Journal of the Michigan Dental Association*), frequently affirms the antiquity of the known appliances, but without regard for the archaeological documentation, which even for archaeologists can be difficult to find or to read. A fourth reason is that many finds of amulets and other objects have been confused with prostheses (see Appendix IV). The fifth major reason for writers to infer the existence of ancient Egyptian appliances derives from the presence of true dental prostheses, fashioned from wire rather than bands, that date from after 400 BCE, leading naive authors to infer, incorrectly, that earlier prototypes must have existed. This complex series of errors has led to poor inferences being drawn from the known early medical texts (see Ghalioungui 1971).

Many of the problems or fallacies in interpreting Egyptian medicine were generated by medical historians who themselves were unable to read the Egyptian documents. Dawson (1953) effectively summarizes the contents of known medical papyri and makes this situation clear. Leek (1967b: 52, n. 1) lists additional reviews of the relevant literature. No references to dental prostheses appear in any of the Egyptian texts, although a reference to tooth powder (dentifrice) appears in a text of Coptic or later date (thus, Late Antique, see Dawson 1953: 54). This tooth powder comment obviously derives from the Hippocratic corpus, and represents only a late copy of Greek medical documents, not indigenous Egyptian wisdom.

Medical Papyri with information on the mouth

The early Egyptian medical papyri are important for an understanding of the early history of dental "medicine." These texts attest to the recognition of disorders of the gums and mouth, and possibly of the teeth, during the New Kingdom (Eighteenth to Twentieth Dynasties, *c.*1550–1070 BCE), but they in no way relate to the history of dental prosthetics (Sigerist 1955: 346; Ghalioungui 1971, 1973: 119). Even the existence of professional dentists of any type in ancient Egypt has been questioned (Kornemann 1989).

The *Papyrus Ebers* (beginning of the Eighteenth Dynasty = *c.*1550–1500 BCE, but copied from earlier works, see Dawson 1953: 49) is the principal early Egyptian medical text to be cited, erroneously, as a reference to early dental prostheses. While it includes several tooth "treatments" (*Ebers* 553–555, 739–749) they all seem to focus only on periodontal problems, and are concerned with a pharmacological or herbalist approach, such as use of cinquefoil to alleviate toothache pain (Foreshaw 2010: 74–75). None involve the replacement of a lost tooth. In addition to accessing the ancient papyrus texts, one must translate them, and not all translations are equal. The von Deines *et al.* (1958a) translation is not commonly available, yet generally it is acknowledged as the definitive version. This is the translation used by Ghalioungui (1987) and others (see Nunn 1996: 30–31) who offer the most realistic interpretations.

Dawson (1938; 1953: 49–50) discusses the limitations of the Ebbell translation of this papyrus, particularly with reference to its translations of terms for herbs, drugs and diseases (see also Musitelli 1996: 210–211). For the purposes of understanding the relationship between the Ebbell translation of *Papyrus Ebers* and the history of dentistry, we quote from this translation below (but see Nunn 1996: 30). Section 89 of the *Ebers* text (Ebbell 1937: 103–104), which relates to treatments of the gums and oral problems (see also Dawson 1935, 1938), is presented below together with commentaries from Leek (see also Dawson 1953: 49, and references therein). Leek identifies and numbers these "remedies" as 11 separate treatments, and provides summaries (Leek 1967b: 52–53). The numbers listed here are those assigned by Leek (1967b). Ebbell's translation (Ebbell 1937) is quoted below, but readers are urged to consult the critical Dawson review in the *Journal of Egyptian Archaeology* (Dawson 1938). Comments appear in brackets. The parenthetical question marks are as they appear in Ebbell's translation. Information from Leek's valuable translation also is included in brackets.

Example of Egyptian dental medicine: *Papyrus Ebers*, prescriptions for teeth, mouth

1 "The beginning of remedies to fasten a tooth: powder of *ammi* /, yellow ochre /, honey /, are mixed together [Leek says "as a paste"], and the tooth is filled (?) therewith."
   [Leek uses "crushed seeds" where Ebbell has "*ammi*"]. (See Miller 2008: 63–64, Egyptian *mm* = an aromatic herb, although translated as the grain "emmer" by Ghalioungui.)

2 "Another: scrapings (?) of millstone /, yellow ochre /, honey /, the tooth is filled (?) therewith."

3 "To expel growth (?) of purulence in the gums: fruit of sycamore /, beans /, honey /, malachite /, yellow ochre /, are ground, pounded and applied to the tooth."

4 "Another to treat a tooth which gnaws against an opening in the flesh: cumin /, frankincense /, d3rt /, are pounded and applied to the tooth."
   Leek calls this a "septic tooth" and notes that all of these ingredients tend to be astringent. Leek (1967b: 53) also translates "*d3rt*" as colocynth, but Ebbell (1937: 133) offers a very different Egyptian term for colocynth. Colocynth (*Citrullus colocynthis*) is an herbaceous vine related to the watermelon and known from northern Africa and the Mediterranean. A powerful cathartic is prepared from the fruit. "*d3rt*" more likely identifies carob, according to Manniche (1989: 91).

5   "Another to fasten a tooth: frankincense /, yellow ochre /, malachite /, are pounded and applied to the tooth."

6   "Another: water /, š`ȝm /, likewise."

7   "Another to treat the gums with rinsing of the mouth: bran (?) /, sweet beer /, ⁻swt ḏh.wtj /, are chewed and spit out."

8   "Another to expel eating ulcer on the gums (i. e. *stomatitis ulcerosa*) and make the flesh grow; cow's milk /, fresh dates /, manna /, (it) remains during the night in the dew, rinse the mouth for 9 (days)."

9   "Another: inśt /, fruit of the sycamore /, yellow ochre /, sebesten [?] /, gum /, tj`ȝm /, bśbś /, balanites-oil /, water, likewise."

10 "Another to strengthen the gums and treat the gums: celery /, dwȝt [an unidentified plant]/, sweet beer /, chewed and spit out."
    Leek's summary of this passage uses the words for "making healthy" the teeth. Leek also states that the vegetable ingredients in recipe 10 include mandrake and a species of the genus *Potentilla*, which includes the rosaceous herbs called cinquefoils. These are abundant in temperate regions, and the genus name reflects the belief that they are "potent." However, the medicinal value, if any, is not clear. Manniche (1989: 76) describes *Ebers 748* as "a remedy to treat the teeth and fix them."

11 "Another remedy to treat 'blood-eating' (scurvy) in the tooth: ḳbw 1 *ro*, dȝrt 1/2 *ro*, gum 2 *ro*, fruit of a sycamore 4 *ro*, inśt 1 *ro*, water 10 *ro*, (it) remains during the night in the dew, rinse the mouth for 4 days."

Leek's (1967b: 53) translation conclusively demonstrates that the treatment for "fastening a tooth" (as in recipe 5) is a reference to a treatment of the gums, similar to modern periodontal treatment for loose teeth. Recent computerized tomography (CT) evaluations of mummies purport to identify small masses of foreign materials in or around the teeth. Until such "deposits" are removed and analyzed we cannot say how they may relate to the ancient Egyptian texts that discuss these medical procedures. Wade *et al.* (2012) published a recent find in which extraneous material seems to have filled a hole in the tooth of a man's mummy of Ptolemaic date from the Theban necropolis, but there is no indication of drilling etc., and other explanations are likely.

Leek (1967b: 54) also notes that dental commentaries in other papyri are similar, if not identical, to those in *Papyrus Ebers*; he provides a useful bibliographical reference (see also Dawson 1953). Leek's (1967b: 54) excellent summary of Egyptian terms for teeth and related anatomical features, and his discussion of some problems of interpretation, are valuable contributions to the literature (cf. Ghalioungui 1973: 118–119). We might expect to find oil of cloves in the Egyptian pharmacopoeia since today it continues to be used as a specific painkiller for extensive dental caries, but this spice (drug), which originally grew only in the Maluku (Maluccan) Islands, was not known in the West until at least Late Roman times. For the Egyptian pharmacopoeia see Manniche (1989: 76, 97, 104, 106, 123, 154), with several recipes for tongue, teeth, gums, or toothache.

Clawson (1933: 154) carefully discusses the famous *Edwin H. Smith Surgical Papyrus*, which is earlier than the *Ebers Papyrus* (Sixteenth–Seventeenth Dynasty, *c.*1500 BCE, the oldest treatise on trauma treatments). The *Smith Surgical Papyrus* takes a distinctly scientific approach but makes no mention of restoring lost teeth; it does record a case report in which a fracture of the mandible is described as untreatable (cf. Leake *et al.* 1953). Clawson suggests that if the Egyptians generally considered hard tissues of the mouth, like the jaw, to be untreatable there would be little likelihood that they attempted any remedies for dental loss.

Leek (1979; also Llagostera 1978) and many other scholars demonstrate that several of the items, which have been naively interpreted as examples of early Egyptian dental prostheses are nothing more than amulets and charms. Gray's (1967: 41, fig. 6) study at the Rijksmuseum in Leiden revealed a profusion of amulets tucked into the linen bindings of mummies. For example, Gray notes that "a small disk of solid gold" found "lying on the surface of the lips was removed" (see also Gray 1966). Naive readers have inferred that this disk was a gold dental prosthesis.

Leek (1967b) also reviews the details relating to the "Junker" amulet of gold wire with teeth found at Gizeh (see Appendix IV); it is often erroneously called a dental appliance in general works. (See also Foreshaw 2010: 74, fig. 3.) This belief that the ancient Egyptians made dental prostheses or fashioned gold "fillings" (e.g. Cigran 1893) also generates one of the most common types of spurious dental appliances (see Appendix III). A good example of the "creation" of a false prosthesis can be found in Weinberger's (1948: 77) review of the early dental literature. Weinberger erroneously suggested that Blumenbach, as early as 1780, believed that artificial teeth were being found in the mouths of mummies. Blumenbach (1780: 110), one of the notable pioneers of anthropology, actually discussed a mummy then located in Cambridge, but in fact, Blumenbach made no reference to dentistry in any form. Blumenbach certainly *does not* suggest the presence of false teeth associated with any mummy. Weinberger's interpretive error typifies the process by which inaccurate histories and false examples are created, because subsequent authors have merely repeated his statement without checking on its original context. Other false examples of Egyptian "dental work" include Platschick's (1904–1905: 238) statement that wooden teeth reportedly have been seen in the mouths of Egyptian mummies.

Even otherwise cautious scholars could fall into the trap of Egyptian primacy. Weinberger, whose first studies on these matters were published in 1934, also mistakenly believed that by 2500 BCE the Egyptians were practicing dental surgery. Although Weinberger (1947; 1948: 74–75) discounted most ideas concerning the practice of dentistry in early Egypt, he nevertheless accepted the amulet published by Junker (1929) as an example of very early dental wiring (Weinberger 1947: 180–181; see Appendix IV).

One aspect of Weinberger's confusion (1947: fig. 3) derives from two publications relating to a mandible from Giza (Peabody Museum, Harvard, inv. no. 59305) variously dated around 2200–2000 BCE (Thoma 1917: 329–330, figs 5, 6).

Hooton (1917) claimed that he detected evidence indicating that this jaw had been drilled by a "dentist," and unfortunately Sudhoff (1926: 15, fig. 15) as well as Weinberger (1947) and Ghalioungui (1973) accepted this conclusion.[2]

Weinberger's account was far from the first to create an erroneous report regarding supposed Egyptian gold dental appliances. Some false reports in the early nineteenth century may have been generated by the discovery in Italy, near the end of the eighteenth century, of at least one real ancient gold dental appliance (the Hamilton prosthesis, now lost: see Appendix I.A). In Italy, during the course of the nineteenth century, a number of dental prostheses were recovered from the Etruscan tombs, which were then being systematically stripped of their finer offerings. Interest in these discoveries probably stimulated various reports, all of them incorrect, suggesting the presence of gold dental appliances in ancient Egyptian tombs. Many of these claims cite as their source the text of the great Belzoni (1820), the early and colorful Italian explorer of Egypt. Yet even Weinberger in his review (1948: 78) of Belzoni's work demonstrates that the famous showman made no claims regarding the dental skills of the ancient Egyptians. Belzoni's book (1820), when scholars actually read it, confirms Weinberger's conclusion that Belzoni never suggested the presence of gold dental work among the ancient Egyptians. He merely mentions (Belzoni 1820: 172) that gold objects and gold leaf are found associated with mummies, but in no case are his, or any other finds, associated with their teeth. Early finds of amulets associated with Egyptian mummies have frequently been incorrectly interpreted, often from the time of their original discovery, and again by more recent observers lacking the inclination to verify these eighteenth-century findings of supposed Egyptian dental appliances (see Appendix IV).

While early Egyptian texts do refer to oral medicine, the treatments noted are entirely limited to pharmacological or magical procedures, as described above. Ruffer (1913, 1920) concluded that there was absolutely no evidence for any type of dentistry in early Egypt, and that even direct evidence for tooth extraction was absent from among the huge numbers of well-preserved skulls that were known (see also Musitelli 1996: 212; Sigerist 1955: 277, 371). Leek (1981) and other conscientious scholars conclusively dismiss the idea that an organized dental profession existed in Egypt during the third millennium BCE (cf. Ghalioungui 1971). As reviewed by Foreshaw (2010: 75–76), the dental health of even pharaohs like Amenhotep III and Ramses II was very poor and painful, yet even their mummies show no evidence of any sort of dental or surgical intervention. That the early Egyptians made extensive use of gold for decorative purposes is evident, but in no case was this technology applied to dental prostheses until centuries after the first examples had appeared in the Etruscan realm.[3]

Although Harris and Ponitz note the diverse views regarding the use of dental prosthetics in Egypt prior to 400 BCE, they cite only one popular paper (Harris, Iskander and Farid 1975) as their source for an earlier date for one of the appliances discovered there. This, the El-Qatta example (see Catalogue no. W-4), is clearly of Roman date (probably late first century BCE to first century CE) and is generally accepted as an actual example of the Eastern-type wire prostheses (see Chapter 4). Unfortunately, many authors simply fail to check either the modern works they cite (second-hand) or the ancient literary sources on which other references were allegedly based.[4]

The evidence we have assembled here clearly argues for the development of dental prostheses among the Etruscans; these ideas subsequently spread to Greece, Egypt, and the Near East at a time late in the first millennium BCE when trade and cultural exchange had reached a high level.

Near Eastern primacy in dental prostheses—a myth

As noted above, all available evidence from ancient Egypt indicates that Clawson (1933) and others are correct regarding the absence of dental prostheses in Egypt before *c*.400 BCE. Those few appliances found in that region appear to have been worn by subjects of the Persian or Ptolemaic kingdoms or by Romans buried in Egypt; the next nearest specimens geographically are two appliances of related type (W-1, 2) worn by residents of Phoenician Sidon to the northeast on the Levantine coast. Thus the supposed primacy of Egyptian or Phoenician dental appliances as suggested by Lufkin (1948) as well as Weinberger (1947) is nowhere supported by direct evidence. Popular writers, however, have often cited Phoenician expertise in gold (jewelry) working and the Orientalizing phenomenon of the eighth–seventh centuries BCE, when Phoenician and North Syrian luxury goods were distributed throughout the Mediterranean, along with the artisans themselves, as part of a commercial circuit for the acquisition of metals and other basic resources. It is generally accepted that Iron Age Etruscans in that period learned goldsmithing from Levantine visitors and immigrants (cf. Camporeale 2013: 888; Sannibale 2013: 108–126; Cristofani 1983; Gunter 2009: 161–162). Clawson (1934: 23–24) put it best when he stated that "contrary to the beliefs of various writers" (who he cited) "detached archaeological specimens of Egyptian prosthetic dentistry do not seem to exist." Nevertheless, fanciful stories of the ancient Egyptians using lost wax casting for "restorations" continue to appear (Chohayeb 1991), and can be expected to persist in the folklore of dental history.

A few other attempts to establish Near Eastern primacy in dental appliances have occurred over the years. Masall (1985) suggested that the Sumerians made early use of gold wires to hold teeth in place, as a post-mortem activity "related to the esthetics of embalming." This view lacks an awareness of basic dental practice in antiquity as well as in recent years (and embalming was not practiced in Sumerian culture either). Masali also believed that the ancient Egyptian examples were post-mortem additions (see Masali and Peluso 1985; Corruccini and Pacciani 1989: 61). In fact, no such "early" examples of gold-wire use can be documented in Mesopotamia. Guerini (1909: 28) suggests that the Egyptians may have decorated teeth with gold after death, but he correctly notes that they produced no dental prostheses.

To summarize the Egyptian non-evidence: Emptoz (1987: 546) provides an outstanding summary of the supposed evidence, including a reference to the tomb at Sakkarah of Khouy, whose title is sometimes translated as "the chief of doctors and dentists" (see also Leek 1967b: 55–56, Pl. X, 3). Hooton's (1917) suggestion that the Egyptians practiced dental surgery to relieve an abscess is elegantly dismissed by Leek (1967b: 56), and Miller (2008). Leek (1967b: 57) notes that not one of the more than 3,000 ancient Egyptian skulls that he examined showed any "sign of active human interference with the course of any dental disease." The creation and use of gold-band dental appliances, both bridges and braces, rests squarely with Etruscan civilization.

Notes

1 As in the cases of Archimedes' invention of the screw-pump and Julius Caesar's reform of the calendar, each acquired after a sojourn in Ptolemaic Egypt.
2 Weinberger (1948: 148) also accepted a common assumption that all prostheses of simple construction are Etruscan in origin, and that the more complex examples such as the Satricum appliance were made by Roman artisans (see Waarsenburg 1991a: 243, n. 12). This appliance is actually the *earliest* known, and while the town of Satricum was ethnically Latin, the technology, with gold band, is undoubtedly Etruscan.
3 The usual interpretive error is clearly seen in the work of Harris and Ponitz (1980). These distinguished Professors of Orthodontics at the University of Michigan conclude their brief review of "Dental health in ancient Egypt" with a "brief mention of the dental profession in ancient Egypt" (Harris and Ponitz 1980: 50). They erroneously believe that the *Ebers Papyrus* discusses the relief of dental pain, and that mention in that text of "how to fix loose teeth" is a reference to dental appliances. See, however, a recipe for relief of toothache, Manniche 1989: 104, on *Ebers* 741.
4 Harris (*et al.* 1975: 404) make a feeble effort to deny the conclusion reached by Leek through careful scholarship, indirectly citing Ghalioungui's (1973: 118) superficial study, a paper not even mentioned in their bibliography (see also Ghalioungui and El-Dawakhly 1965). The failure of Harris and his colleagues (1975) to verify the archaeological, as well as the odontological evidence, reflects the most common type of error that leads to suggestions of early dates for Egyptian dental appliances, and also to the "creation" of spurious examples of these dental pontics.

3 The dental prosthesis

A lost Etruscan invention

Introduction

This chapter presents the phenomenon of Etruscan dental appliances and suggests some possible social interpretations. In revisiting scholarly commentaries concerning these interesting pieces of ancient technology, we felt the need to point out misconceptions that have crept into popular understanding of this aspect of ancient medicine and technology, mostly because authors reworked earlier discussions without examining the actual artifacts or associated human remains. We also consider the general state of health and nutrition in Etruria during the first millennium BCE, when the various appliances were made and worn. Additional historical evidence appears in ancient literature and epitaphs and is augmented by evidence from Etruscan skeletons and anatomical models left as votives at the shrines of healing cults.

The evidence

The Catalogue (Chapter 5) presents full data on all Etruscan or Etruscan-style dental prostheses that are known to date, as well as the seven gold-wire appliances from fourth-century Hellenistic and Roman imperial-era burials in the eastern Mediterranean and Rome (see Table 3.5). We discuss significant details of these finds, and their place in Etruscan culture and the history of technology and medicine. We can consider a total of 21 Etruscan-type, gold-band appliances that are either extant and available for study, or (where lost or otherwise unavailable) well enough documented in published descriptions and images to facilitate comparison with extant pieces. Fourteen appliances come from Etruria proper (Tarquinia and environs, Orvieto/Bolsena and environs, Chiusi, Populonia), while four were found in burials in Latium (Satricum, Praeneste), Campania (Teano), or the *Ager faliscus* (Valsiarosa/*Falerii*). These fourteen are listed in Table 3.2. The last two appliances show the same design and techniques, but have far-flung provenances: Tanagra in Greek Boeotia, and, Sardis in ancient Lydia (Anatolia/modern Turkey). If genuine, they may represent Etruscans abroad—either itinerant Etruscan goldsmiths or female emigrées whose appearance marked them as different, and who died far from their native land.

All the Etruscan-associated appliances are constructed from gold bands, fashioned from flat strips rather than wire. Thirteen were designed as bands wrapped around one or more teeth; a further eight appliances have bands made into individual rings that have been attached in a linear series. The appliances range from those with one replacement tooth anchored to adjacent teeth (so three rings or spaces, the central one being the replacement tooth, as no. 3/Van Marter) to an impressive appliance (no. 12/Corneto II) made to span 8 teeth anchoring 3 replacements to 5 rooted, natural teeth. Most if not all of the bridges were inserted in the maxillary dentition, usually replacing central and/or lateral incisors. The "false" teeth are in some cases demonstrably human teeth with their roots trimmed, although whether they are the owner's own or someone else's cannot be ascertained with certainty. They vary in number from 1 false tooth (7 cases), to 2 (5 cases) or even 3 teeth (a single case, no. 12/Corneto II). Both band- and ring- designs could be used to insert replacement teeth (7 of the 13 bands and 5 of the 8-ring appliances were used to secure replacement teeth). The use of both types ranges over several centuries, from the most securely dated appliance, a band bearing a gold replacement for a left lateral incisor, from Satricum (seventh century BCE) to the Hellenistic period (fourth–third centuries BCE, three of band-type, one of ring-design)—but very few retain information on context, such as grave goods that might provide an approximate date for the wearer's burial.

Etruria: health, nutrition and evidence for dental concerns

The Sicilian historian Diodorus Siculus, citing an earlier author, Poseidonios, expressed the traditional Greek opinion that Etruria was wealthy and well fed:

> Not least of the things which have contributed to their luxury is the fertility of the land; since it bears every sort of product of the soil and is especially fertile, the Etruscans store away large supplies of every kind of fruit.
>
> (Diodorus Siculus 5.40.5)

As early as the Neolithic period (*c.*6000–2800 BCE), long before the culture that we recognize as Etruscan, the inhabitants of Italy had enjoyed a wholesome and varied diet, combining a wide variety of wild foods rich in vitamins, minerals and protein (from Cornel cherries to chestnuts, walnuts and acorns, wild birds, mountain goat, deer, and fish) with domesticated crops such as wheat and barley (consumed mainly as porridge). By the Bronze Age (*c.*2300–1000 BCE) olives and grapes were being developed to yield oil and wine, and so were domesticated livestock, the big three of the Mediterranean world, sheep, cattle and pigs (for surveys and references, see Turfa 2012b: 136–163; Turfa and Becker 2013). The high fiber aspects of this diet can cause significant wear on the teeth, from stone-ground whole wheat and tough food items, but it is much healthier than the later diet of complex carbohydrates like white bread. Increased dental loss has been posited from this change in diet. Many believe that the effects can be seen in the increased loss of teeth among the Etruscans and Italic populations that is noticeable in burials from about 600 BCE on. A single, but probably typical example is seen in the skull of a man from Archaic Chiusi, perhaps dating to *c.*600 BCE (see Figures 3.1a–c). This skull was acquired in the late nineteenth century by the University of Pennsylvania Museum, Philadelphia. The undamaged skull must have been buried in a chamber tomb that protected the body, a context that strongly suggests an aristocrat, perhaps one trained in sword-fighting or other activity that had left him with a broken but neatly healed nose; it had long been healed when he died at the age of 40–45 years. He had already lost several molars to decay and periodontal disease and his remaining teeth have deposits of heavy plaque (Becker *et al.* 2009: 78–79, no. 18). Like most of the ancient Italian population, however, he retained his front teeth lifelong—important evidence for evaluating the wearing of gold appliances.

Health in Etruria of the first millennium BCE was relatively good, to judge from the skeletal population, with a few oldsters (both aristocrats and farmers) afflicted with arthritis in backs and legs as a result of hard work and daily walking. A few children, in the years following weaning and loss of mothers' antibodies, showed poor tooth enamel and other effects of periodic infections

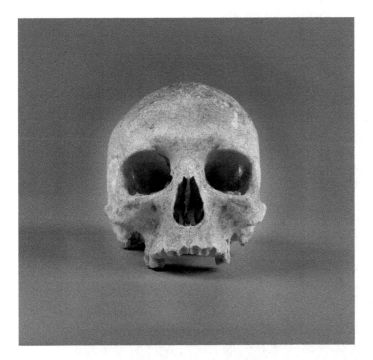

Figure 3.1a Skull of a swordsman from Chiusi, University of Pennsylvania Museum MS 1406, note attrition in mandible.

Source: courtesy Mediterranean Section, University of Pennsylvania Museum (neg. no. 256344).

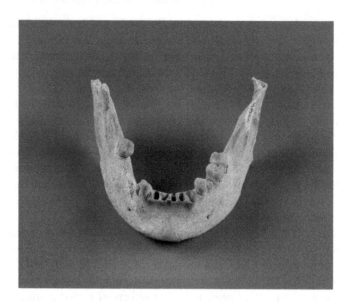

Figure 3.1b View of mandible showing antemortem loss of molars (anterior teeth were lost after burial).

Source: courtesy Mediterranean Section, University of Pennsylvania Museum (neg. nos. 256345, 290003).

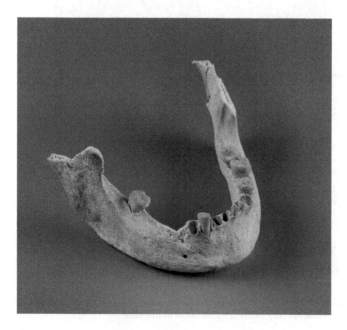

Figure 3.1c View of mandible showing antemortem loss of molars (anterior teeth were lost after burial).

Source: courtesy Mediterranean Section, University of Pennsylvania Museum (neg. nos. 256345, 290003).

or short-term episodes of malnutrition, perhaps the results of poor harvests and transient infectious disease/fevers. A special boy buried during the ninth century BCE in what would become the city of Tarquinia shows the traces of enamel hypoplasia that represent bouts of anemia. The cause of his death, around the age of 8–10 years, has been said to be a brain aneurism that may have earlier caused him to see and hear things that no one else could (Fornaciari and Mallegni 1997; Bagnasco Gianni 2013: 595). Some scholars have speculated that this child was the inspiration for the story of Tages, a famous prophet said to have been sent by the Etruscan gods (see Turfa 2012b: 178–179), but this can only be a hypothesis. Although it has been suggested, on the basis of dental deterioration, that the early historical populations of Italy, and the rest of the Mediterranean, routinely suffered bouts of malnutrition or poor nutrition caused by infections, parasites etc., this cannot be confirmed. Famine, food supply and "plagues" of infectious disease were a constant worry for most parts of the ancient and even the modern world. Whether these appear as dental hypoplasias or can be identified in any specific set of skeletal anomalies remains to be demonstrated. What we recognize as bubonic plague or childhood diseases such as chicken pox or measles cannot be inferred from skeletal collections. (In fact those particular diseases could not be supported by the small populations of Etruscan cities, and only appear later, during the Roman empire or later eras when enough infants were produced to form a reservoir of victims not yet immune.) Infectious diseases, though, must have swept through even the most rudimentary urban populations on a regular basis. That a wide variety of disorders were constant concerns is well expressed in a rare, surviving document, the *Etruscan Brontoscopic Calendar*, preserved in a Byzantine Greek translation of a Latin version published by a friend of Cicero in the last days of the Roman Republic (see Turfa 2012b for the first English translation of this text).

A few brief studies of Etruscan dentition include some information on malocclusions, tooth wear and attrition, as well as inferences on general nutrition, giving a picture of dental woes similar to ours today. Beyond the problems of dental health, Macchiarelli *et al.* (1995) have recognized biological traits and odontometric variations among various Italic peoples.

Epitaphs from Tarquinia and Volterra, from the fourth century and later, record the age at death, revealing that many people, both men and women, lived into old age (one man reached 106, and several were recorded in their eighties—but their skeletons have not survived: Turfa and Becker 2013: 861; Turfa in press). These data are confirmed by skeletal studies that reveal many people surviving well beyond 70 years of age, when the determination of age at death becomes less specific (Becker 2006). Survival into old age can also be documented among the non-elite (Vargiu and Becker 2005), where individuals are buried in simple graves. Members of the upper classes in Etruscan cities like Tarquinia and Orvieto could expect long, comfortable lives if they escaped the dangers of war or childbirth. Women who were missing a front tooth could expect to enjoy many years of displaying an ornamental gold-band replacement. Beauty in many cases is a visible token of a person's good health, and good health in antiquity would have been equated with fertility and the status of producing a family. Good or complete teeth would thus be a part of the phenomenon, as shown in a recent major Italian exhibition on *"Etruschi: Il privilegio della bellezza"* ("Etruscans: The privilege of beauty") (Rafanelli and Spaziani 2011; see Naso 2011).

An Etruscan noblewoman's dental health

A unique find allows us to compare physical condition with literary and/or artistic description: the terracotta sarcophagus of Seianti Hanunia Tlesnasa, a noblewoman from Hellenistic Chiusi. The lid bears her reclining portrait sculpture (Figure 3.2). Now in the British Museum (1887, 0402.1), her carefully preserved skeleton has furnished much information on health, daily activities, and dental health among the Etruscan aristocracy. Hanunia Seianti wife of Tlesna died between 250 and 150 BCE at 50 to 60 years of age (Becker 2002b; Stoddart 2002). Some specialists have suggested that in her youth she had suffered severe trauma, perhaps in an accident or fall, which left her with no broken bones but damage to joints on her right side, pelvis and spine that caused limping and later arthritis. They also believe that she sustained a temporo-mandibular joint injury (TMJ) that restricted jaw movement and led to lifelong dental woes, including bad breath, facial pain, chronic periodontitis, loose teeth and extensive tooth loss (Lilley 2002; Stoddart 2002; Swaddling and Prag 2002).

Some of Seianti's teeth (see Figure 3.3), such as the upper left first premolar, are extremely worn, from long life and also items in the diet. The malocclusion

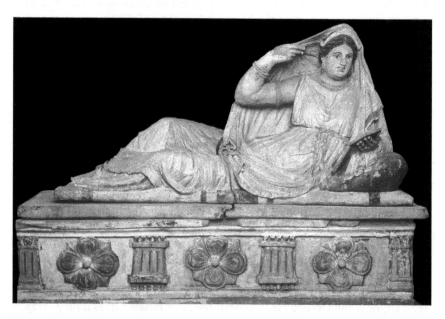

Figure 3.2 Sarcophagus of Seianti Hanunia Tlesnasa, Chiusi, terracotta, *c.*150 BCE.
Source: © Trustees of the British Museum.

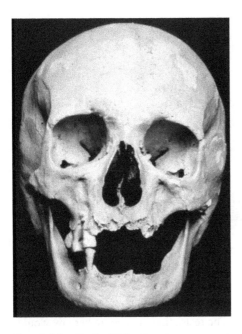

Figure 3.3a Skull of Seianti.

Source: photo courtesy The Manchester Museum and A. J. N. W. Prag.

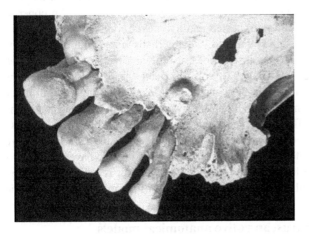

Figure 3.3b Detail: lesion in maxilla.

Source: photo courtesy The Manchester Museum and A. J. N. W. Prag.

caused by trauma is said to have led to irregular wear and a long-term chronic apical abscess of the upper left second premolar. The abscess from time to time built up painful pressure from pus that then drained through a hole in the bone and would

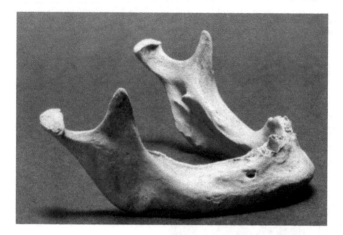

Figure 3.3c Mandible with antemortem loss of molars; anterior teeth lost
          post-mortem.

Source: photo courtesy The Manchester Museum and A. J. N. W. Prag.

have caused swelling of the cheek. The restriction in opening her jaw would have
made dental hygiene very difficult. Various teeth still had deposits of calculus, and
the upper left first molar had a carious cavity on its mesial aspect. Most of Seianti's
lower molars on both sides were lost years before death, and the bone had healed
completely and become smooth, like the jaws of elderly persons. An upper third
molar ("wisdom tooth") was impacted and had never erupted. (Impacted molars
were not uncommon in Italic populations, but perhaps more common among Italic
and Etruscan women was an absence of third molar development (Becker *et al.*
2009: 45 and Chapter 5, Table 5.12). Seianti's dental problems were mainly with
her back teeth. Like most Etruscans, she had not lost the all-important front teeth,
but the asymmetry of her jaw would have constrained her in speaking and eating—
although she could afford prepared foods that were easy to chew. Lilley (2002:
fig. 3.3b) has illustrated how post-excavation handling led to the modern insertion
of her canine tooth into the wrong socket, a practice that we have found in some
appliances displayed in museums. Although her portrait is believed to represent
her features fairly well, it does not show any signs of her injuries and disabilities.

Evidence of art: Etruscan votive anatomical models

An Etruscan phenomenon shared by neighboring Italic peoples is the dedication
of thousands of terracotta anatomical models of body parts as votive offerings
in sanctuaries across central Italy during the third–first centuries BCE (Turfa and
Becker 2013: 866–869; Recke 2013; Turfa 1994, 2004). The votives depict hands,
feet, heads and whole, dressed bodies, but also portray internal organs, sometimes in groups or shown as if revealed within a human torso. They represent the

healing of these parts in response to a vow made publicly by or on behalf of the sufferer. They almost never show any impairment or pathology. Among them are a few rare examples depicting a mouth with teeth or a head or bust in which the subject shows his or her tongue in an open mouth. The best-known examples of dental portrayals are from Latium and neighboring Italic regions, such as Carsoli, where models of the face from forehead through upper jaw show a boy (?) with open mouth revealing stubby upper teeth; the lower jaw is not present (Cederna 1951: 218, fig. 21) (Figure 3.4). From the sanctuary of the Sabine goddess Feronia, shared by Etruscans and Latins, comes a model of a lower jaw with a crudely modeled lower row of teeth incised with lines indicating 28 teeth, too many for *one* jaw (Baggieri 1996/1999: 93, fig. 10). Similar models are known from other votive deposits. At Praeneste the Sanctuary of Hercules received many different models depicting isolated mouths, lips, gums, and teeth, crudely modeled or molded (thus mass produced) (Baggieri 1996/1999: 40–41, figs 5–9, fourth–second century BCE). A surprising new discovery was revealed in 2012 outside the ancient Latin town of Lanuvium when the *carabinieri* apprehended clandestine excavators and confiscated offerings stolen from a cave with a vast deposit of anatomical models.[1] These terracotta sculptures included many heads that are cutaway to reveal only the neck, chin and lower jaw or mouth, perhaps indications of diseases of the mouth or sinuses (Atteni 2013). Again, none shows pathology or dental repairs, but they do attest to the concerns of many worshippers over the health of their mouths and/or teeth.

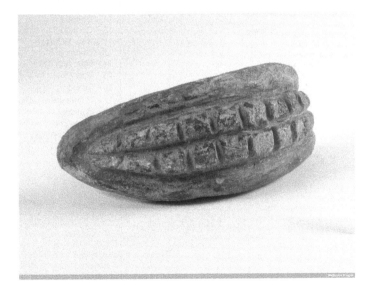

Figure 3.4 Terracotta anatomical model, mouth and teeth. Of a type found in the votive deposit in the sanctuary of Hercules at Praeneste/Palestrina, fourth–third century BCE (cf. Baggieri 1999: 41, fig. 8).

Source: courtesy of The Wellcome Collection (no. L0035826)

Etruria: the invention of dental appliances

Their Greek and Roman adversaries often identified all Etruscans (who they called *Tyrrhenoi, Tyrsenoi, Tusci,* or *Etrusci*) as a single ethnic group—and they are united by the use of their unique, non-Indo-European language, calling themselves *Rasenna* or *Rasna*. But archaeological evidence shows that regional, social and familial preferences resulted in quite distinct cultural styles and traditions for the denizens of different cities and regions. The most commonly recognized divisions are North–South and coastal–inland.

Southern Etruria, encompassing the major maritime cities of Caere (Cerveteri), Tarquinia and Vulci, is the source of the greatest number of documented dental prostheses. The area of central-northern Etruria is also represented by Chiusi and cities such as Bisenzio and Orvieto (ancient *Volsinii*), which developed around the volcanic lakes of Bolsena and Bracciano. Satricum and Praeneste, sources of two

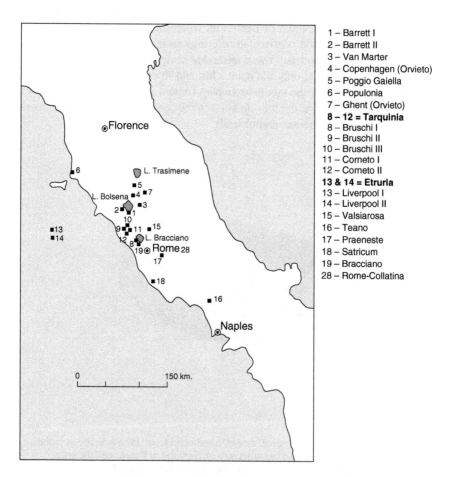

1 – Barrett I
2 – Barrett II
3 – Van Marter
4 – Copenhagen (Orvieto)
5 – Poggio Gaiella
6 – Populonia
7 – Ghent (Orvieto)
8 – 12 = Tarquinia
8 – Bruschi I
9 – Bruschi II
10 – Bruschi III
11 – Corneto I
12 – Corneto II
13 & 14 = Etruria
13 – Liverpool I
14 – Liverpool II
15 – Valsiarosa
16 – Teano
17 – Praeneste
18 – Satricum
19 – Bracciano
28 – Rome-Collatina

Figure 3.5 Map of locations in Italy of burials with gold dental appliances, marked by inventory numbers in the catalogue.

important prostheses, lie within the Latin-speaking region, and Civita Castellana (ancient *Falerii*) was ethnically Faliscan, another Italic cultural group similar to the Latins. Teano (*Teanum* of the Oscan-speaking Sidicini tribe) is a similar case, set in Campania near the Bay of Naples. Each of these communities followed patterns that can be recognized as predominantly Etruscan forms of art, religion and technology, practicing intermarriage with Etruscan states, even if only among the elite or wealthy. We might infer that some dental bridges arrived in the mouths of Etruscan or Italic noblewomen making dynastic marriages with neighboring ruling families. There remains the possibility that the wearers of dental appliances were actually non-Etruscans who had married into the great families of Etruria and wished to look the part, obscuring the gap where they had had teeth removed according to family or tribal traditions.

Gold dental appliances were widely distributed. Since inhumation burials became the norm in South Etruria one might ask if this behavior led to the preferential survival there of dental appliances. Finds, however, are

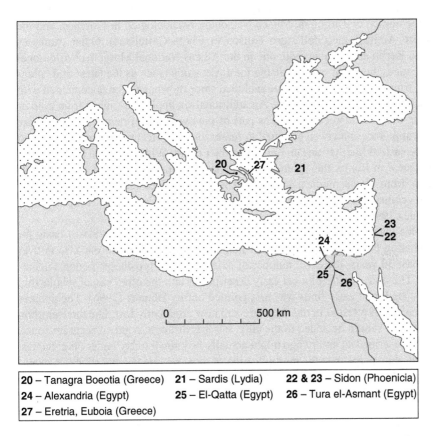

20 – Tanagra Boeotia (Greece)	21 – Sardis (Lydia)	22 & 23 – Sidon (Phoenicia)
24 – Alexandria (Egypt)	25 – El-Qatta (Egypt)	26 – Tura el-Asmant (Egypt)
27 – Eretria, Euboia (Greece)		

Figure 3.6 Map of locations beyond Italy of burials with gold or silver dental appliances, some band-type, some made of wire.

not uniformly distributed across the entire zone: there is an especially high concentration at Tarquinia. Also, no gold lumps or bits of appliances are known from any cremation to the north of this zone. If cremated individuals had been wearing these appliances, we ought to have found the evidence, even if cremations had been conducted at temperatures high enough to melt gold. It seems logical to assume that all examples came from buried bodies, and that appliances were not removed before burial. The Roman *Laws of the Twelve Tables* (see Chapter 1), in not requiring removal of gold appliances, imply that they were worn permanently, and not easily removed. Yet, of the hundreds of burials excavated to date, only about 20 have yielded gold dental appliances, including those few that are now lost. Clearly these artifacts were exceedingly rare.

The appliances

This study offers a catalogue (Chapter 5) of documented examples of gold-band dental appliances, built around Becker's detailed descriptions of 10 pieces held in 6 museums (Copenhagen, Liverpool, Villa Giulia in Rome, Museo Nazionale Archeologico di Tarquinia, Museo Nazionale Archeologico in Florence, and the Museo Archeologico dell'Agro Falisco in Civita Castellana). Other examples are in Berlin and Vienna, with one in the Athens National Museum.[2] Additional appliances, now lost or unavailable for direct study (such as the latest find, allegedly from Sardis in Anatolia) are included since they have been documented with descriptions and/or illustrations. An additional six appliances, made from gold or silver wire, are also considered as part of the evolution of dental history. These wire appliances had been assumed to represent dental technology as it developed in the eastern Mediterranean, Egypt and the Levant. With the recent find of a wire appliance in Rome, they point to the ancient origins of wiring in dentistry. We knew from Greek medical writers that it was practiced perhaps as early as the fifth century BCE through the first century CE (see Appendix I; cf. Emptoz 1987; Bliquez 1996).

This compendium of data on ancient dental appliances provides a basis for evaluating the range of variation in their construction. Despite our efforts over the past 30 years, the exact number of existing dental prostheses remains uncertain. The poor quality of most early descriptions and the often casual scholarship associated with early finds was first pointed out by Bliquez (1996). The number of appliances attested in old literature and now apparently lost, like the Hamilton appliance, should be added to the tally, but it is difficult to get an accurate count. Some described a century ago might actually be known today under other names. Rather than perpetuate the multiplication of data, we relegate questionable examples to Appendix I. Further confusion has arisen from the existence of modern copies of many pieces, a situation noted as early as 1909 (see Guerini 1909: 72). We provide a list of "copies" in Appendix II as a means of reducing confusion in future studies.

A summary of features of the Etruscan appliances: braces and bridges

For complete measurements and additional description, see the catalogue entries.

1 **Barrett I (lost)**: (Said to be from Etruria.) A simple, very narrow gold-band appliance, designed to loop around no more than three anterior teeth, probably the two central incisors and a lateral incisor. It was probably about 0.2–0.3 mm thick and varying from 1.2–1.6 mm across the flat surface, constructed from a strip of gold sheet approximately 53 mm in length, possibly with the overlapping ends fused to form a continuous, oval band. When in place it may have been an ornament, but it may also have been intended to stabilize a loose tooth at the center of the band. It is now slightly misshapen due to post-excavation handling. (See Figure 5.1.)

2 **Barrett II (lost)**: (Said to be from a tomb in the Capodimonte necropolis of Bisenzio.) A tomb group associated with this burial contains vases of *c*.500–480 BCE. A simple, narrow gold-band appliance, constructed from a strip probably about 0.2–0.3 mm thick and varying from 2.0–2.5 mm across the flat surface, and approximately 60 mm long (after ends were overlapped and fused). The length of the band suggests that it was designed to loop around the crowns of no more than four anterior teeth; most likely the four incisors, in order to stabilize one or two loose teeth at the center of the band. It may alternately have been purely ornamental. A post-interment alteration derives from the pinching of the band to hold for display three teeth that may or may not be those of the original wearer; they are not the teeth originally attached by the appliance in this position. (See Figure 5.2.)

3 **Van Marter (lost):** (Said to be from a tomb at Lake Bolsena.) This three-ring appliance was constructed from gold strip folded into a squared configuration. It probably originally held one replacement incisor, anchored to a central and a lateral incisor. The squared outline of the central "ring" helps prevent the modified, or false, central incisor from rotating in its socket. Like those two preceding examples, it is today known only from its published description and illustrations. (See Figure 5.3.)

4 **Copenhagen (believed to be from Orvieto):** Associated with objects of *c*.500–490 BCE from the necropolis of Orvieto. This "three-ring" appliance has lateral loops carefully fitted to the original and surviving dental crowns (left central incisor and right lateral incisor) and a sharply rectangular central gold unit in which the false tooth (not recovered) was attached. (See Figures 5.4a–d.)

5 **Poggio Gaiella (Region of Chiusi)**: Excavated in the necropolis of Poggio Gaiella near the city of Chiusi, associated with objects of the fourth–third centuries BCE. This elaborate appliance appears to have been crafted to surround eight teeth, presumably from around both first premolars and all teeth in between. Two strips of gold, varying in width, were used in its construction. After recovery this appliance appears to have been much manipulated

in order to mount it into a skull for display, resulting in some separations of the welds, and minor distortions of the contours. The alveolar margins of the skull, which is believed to be a relatively modern young adult, reveal no areas that would require bracing from a dental appliance, and this may be another case of the modern mounting of appliances in more photogenic skulls. (See Figures 5.5a–k.)

6   **Populonia (lost)**: Excavated from a destroyed tomb in the San Cerbone necropolis of the city of Populonia, said to be of the fourth century BCE. Generally described as a four-ring appliance, with a rivet through one of the (central?) rings, this piece is poorly documented and no longer available, having been lost in the 1966 Florence Flood of the River Arno. (See Figures 5.6a–c.)

7   **Ghent (said to be "from near Orvieto"—missing since World War II)**: This appliance surrounded four teeth, almost certainly the maxillary central incisors. It may have been used as an ornament, or perhaps to stabilize one or more loose teeth. The width of the band is unusually uniform. The manufacture is unusual in that two separate strips of gold, of unusually uniform width, were used to form the appliance, a pattern similar only to the longer Poggio Gaiella appliance. (See Figures 5.7a–f.)

8   **Bruschi I (probably from Tarquinia or adjacent territory)**: This simple band was formed from a strip of relatively uniform width, about 74 mm long, with its ends overlapped for a length of about 3 mm and fused. The location of the weld is, unusually, quite evident as indicated by a slight expansion of the width. This is another example generally believed to have surrounded the left canine and three incisors, including the right central. (See Figure 5.8.)

9   **Bruschi II (from Tarquinia, now missing)**: This was a four-ring appliance with a single rivet though one of the center loops, similar to the Populonia pontic. This is yet another example generally believed to have surrounded a canine—right in this case—and three incisors. If this placement is correct the replaced tooth would have been the right central incisor. (See Figure 5.9.)

10   **Bruschi III (from Tarquinia)**: This band appears to be fashioned from a single long (about 83 mm) strip of gold into an oval into which four braces (dividing strips) have been fitted and fused to create five tooth spaces. The elongate "rectangles" of these openings suggest that this appliance had been flattened, creating its unusual length (cf. Corneto I). The sizes of these openings clearly suggest that one canine as well as all four incisors were held by this appliance, with no indication that any replacement tooth was involved. (See Figure 5.10.)

11   **Corneto I (lost)**: Probably excavated in a Tarquinian necropolis in 1876–1877. The five spaces of this "braced" oval band are believed to have surrounded all four maxillary incisors and the left canine, in a construction remarkably like Bruschi III, but with a single rivet securing a replacement or cut-down central right incisor. (See Figure 5.11.)

12   **Corneto II (lost)**: Possibly excavated around 1885 in a Tarquinian necropolis. This impressive appliance of seven attached rings, spanning eight tooth

spaces, is perhaps the most complex of all the known Etruscan bridges. Three teeth are replaced, using three gold rivets. Both central incisors are replaced by the major feature, an elongate "ring" into which an animal tooth or piece of ivory has been inserted. This false insert was held in place by two rivets, as if the two sections were separate teeth; a replacement (not surviving) for the left first premolar was also riveted in place. The right lateral incisor and canine served as anchor teeth on one end, the second premolar on the other. (See Figure 5.12.)

13 **Liverpool I**: Collected before 1857, perhaps from excavations at Vulci. This single band, an apparently seamless oval, surrounded all four incisors, and may have been formed from a piece of gold that was expanded to shape rather than cut from a sheet. It has two cut-down human central incisors, possibly the teeth removed from the owner, riveted into the center. (See Figures 5.13a–g.)

14 **Liverpool II**: Collected before 1857, perhaps from excavations at Vulci. This single band, once surrounding all four incisors, is considerably more gracile than the band of Liverpool I. The construction appears much the same, with two rivets in the positions where the centers of the central incisors would have been; two lateral incisors conserved with it may be those of the original owner. (See Figures 5.14a–g.)

15 **Valsiarosa**: Excavated in the Valsiarosa necropolis of *Falerii Veteres*, from Tomb 2, dated to the fourth century BCE. This appliance surrounded all four maxillary incisors, and provided a modified or false tooth for the right central incisor. None of the teeth, rooted or replacement, survive. By the 1880s this appliance had been mounted in a modern human skull for display, photos of which are in circulation, although the display has been changed now. (See Figures 5.15a–e.)

16 **Teano (not available)**: From Tomb 18 of the Fondo Gradavola necropolis of Teano (*Teanum*) near the Bay of Naples, associated with grave goods of the fourth to third centuries BCE. This six-ring stabilizing appliance, anchored on the canines, appears to have a unique construction. A basic six-loop construction appears surrounded by an exterior layer of gold, as if a retention band had been placed outside the ring series. Photos show it with three or four crowns in place. (See Figure 5.16.)

17 **Praeneste**: A sporadic find from the necropolis of the Latin city of Praeneste, by 1885 displayed in Palazzo Barberini, Rome. Simple band surrounding all four maxillary incisors, with two rivets securing replaced or replacement central incisors, probably teeth removed from the owner and filed down. The canine displayed with this appliance may derive from the same person, but that tooth was not originally serving as an anchor tooth for the band. (See Figure 5.17.)

18 **Satricum**: Excavated from a tomb within Tumulus C of the Borgo Le Ferriere necropolis of the Latin town of Satricum, probably buried no later than *c.*630 BCE. This gold appliance is the only known example in which the replacement tooth also was fashioned from gold and fused to a very thin band

that surrounded five dental spaces. Almost certainly, all four incisors and one canine were enclosed by this band, but which canine cannot be determined. This appliance also is the earliest example known, probably made between 700 and 650 BCE. (See Figure 5.18.)

19 **Bracciano**: Acquired or inventoried *c*.1990 by the Vienna Museum of Natural History and said to have been excavated from a seventh-century BCE tomb near Lake Bracciano. This simple gold-band appliance, of somewhat mysterious provenance, spans three dental spaces and holds in the middle a surviving cut-down right central incisor. Both anchor teeth also survive; a feature most unusual in Etruscan chamber tombs. Given the questionable origins of this example one should note that the gold of the band was much thicker than found in most bands, and the gold rivet rather large. (See Figure 5.19.)

20 **Tanagra**: Said to be from a tomb of the fourth–third century BCE at Tanagra in Boeotia, Greece. This is a gold-band appliance designed to surround six maxillary(?) teeth; almost certainly the four incisors and both canines. The two long loops that were heat fused at the "center" were formed from two original strips (each nearly 25 mm in length and the ends overlapped for about 6 mm and fused to form an elongated oval. Then the bands were welded to form a single appliance (compare Poggio Gaiella). Given the apparently unusual flexibility of the alloy used for this example, the fitting must have been extremely delicate. The possibility that this had been a mandibular appliance, related to the Eastern wire appliances, cannot be ruled out. (See Figure 5.20.)

21 **Sardis (unverified)**: Said to have been excavated from a tomb near the ancient city of Sardis in Turkey, dated by a woman's grave goods to the third century BCE. Preserved in a skull said to be female, this is an unusual mandibular prosthesis formed from a single strip of gold said to be 48 mm long hammered into a loop to surround all four incisors. The central incisor sockets appear to have been fully absorbed, perhaps after the appliance was made, and both central incisors are riveted replacements made of human or bovine teeth. Details of the tomb context are cast into doubt because of the apparently illegal excavation/collection of the burial.

Characteristics of Etruscan appliances

In 1910 the Italian scholar Ettore Gábrici was among the first to note clearly that gold dental appliances were an Etruscan and not a Roman or Egyptian invention, when he wrote of the gold appliance found at Teano: "*credo che sia penetrato nella Campania per mezzo degli Etruschi*" ("I believe that it reached Campania through the agency of the Etruscans" Gábrici (1910: cols. 44–45; Bonfante 1986: 250). Strictly speaking, the earliest attested appliance does not come from Etruria proper, but from the seventh-century necropolis of the Latin town of Satricum, south of Rome. The art and architecture of Latin Satricum show a distinct Etruscan flavor during this period before the rise of the Roman state. Possibly this complex and sophisticated dental appliance was made early in the seventh century, since

630 is the estimated time of its wearer's burial (no. 18). This demonstrates that the skills used to fashion dental prostheses from bands of gold were established at least as early as the mid-seventh century BCE. Most other gold-band appliances were found within the Etruscan sphere of Italy, but two that are largely identical in technique have been linked to Greece (Eretria) and, according to unverified reports, to Sardis in Anatolia. If these two are genuine and correctly identified as to context, they may represent the burial of an Etruscan or Italic ethnic, perhaps a foreign bride, in a Greek and a Lydian community. The alternate possibility of an itinerant Etruscan goldsmith has also been suggested.

Etruscan appliances all are based on the use of flat gold bands, not wire, even though Etruscan jewelry frequently employed gold wire. The wire had to be painstakingly twisted and worked from strips of sheet gold. Filigree and cloisonné granulation (see Gaultier 2013; Sannibale 2013) were known, but this technology was not employed in the fabrication of dental pontics or restorative dentistry. The much wider and more easily visible gold-band appliances had the potential added benefit of providing impressive fashion/status statements, which may imply that their use was related to other cultural traditions such as dental evulsion, the deliberate removal of teeth. In the earliest example, Satricum (no. 18), use of a flat band enabled a gold-replica tooth to be fused in place. Later examples show that bands enabled cut-down real or artificial teeth to be riveted in place (see Craddock 2009).

Ancient dental appliances fashioned from gold wires only appeared centuries after the first band appliances. Until recently wire appliances were archaeologically known only from the eastern Mediterranean, especially the Levant and Egypt. Our previous belief that wire appliances originated, by independent invention, in the Ptolemaic or Roman-era Levant (Becker 1997) has been altered by the find of a single example (no. W-7) from Rome of the second century AD (Minozzi *et al.* 2007). Dentures and braces employing gold (or silver) wire involved a technology completely different from that used by the Etruscans. The find in 2000 of an Imperial-era appliance in Rome at last resolves the conundrum posed by literary references to false teeth from the days of Cicero, Caesar and the early Empire. Now we have a single wire construction from an excavation in the Collatina necropolis, on the outskirts of ancient Rome. Until the emergence of this prosthesis it appeared that modern authors had incorrectly translated references by Roman medical authors such as Celsus to wire prostheses (Andre-Bonnet 1910: 46).

To return to Etruria: After 600 BCE, the general availability of gold prosthetic devices in central Italy is indicated by a thin but steady stream of surviving examples. Telling references to such appliances survive in the Roman *Law of the Twelve Tables* (see Chapter 1) of the fifth century BCE. While believed to be much older, it was written down some two centuries after the oldest extant dental appliance (no. 18) was made. Considering that such appliances are likely to be found only in the richest tombs, we probably should be amazed at the number that did survive. None have been recovered during the past 75 or more years, and few came from properly conducted excavations (but see nos. 19 and 21).

Etruscan dental devices were anchored to sound teeth and provided the means for replacing as many as three missing teeth. The most complex example now known (Corneto II, no. 12) straddles eight tooth spaces and probably replaced three teeth. All known Etruscan/Italian appliances were fashioned from gold, which had to be sufficiently malleable to be fitted into a human mouth. In state of the art analysis (Liverpool I and II, nos. 13–14) dental bridges had the same alloy for both rivets and bands. To date very few definitive tests have been conducted to determine such details of construction. In the seventh-century Bracciano example (no. 19) of murky provenance (Teschler-Nicola *et al.* 1998) both band and rivet are said to be over 92 percent pure gold, suggesting that the gold had been specially refined (see Becker 2003).

All dental appliances were worn on various combinations of the front teeth, most often to span the four incisors. They were sure to be noticed by bystanders. While the primary intent in fashioning dental bridges may have been the decorative replacement of missing teeth, thereby providing the wearer with a uniform dental line, the golden smile must have been an important goal. An incidental function was to hold the remaining teeth in position. The claims of some authors (e.g. Capasso 1986: 55) that the Etruscans tried to *close* a space between missing teeth are not supported by the evidence: a gold band cannot provide the forces necessary for this purpose. Such an effort would be medically counterproductive as it would cause the sound teeth in the dental arch to loosen, shift and create articulation problems.

Gold bands, on the other hand, can also provide the benefit of holding loosened teeth in place, as well as serve as a support for the cosmetic replacement of lost teeth. Clearly, in those cases where we find only a simple gold band without rivets, we may infer that it had been intended to stabilize loosened teeth, probably because of irreversible periodontal disease ("receding gums"), or possibly until healing after a blow.

Our difficulty in determining the function of simple gold bands derives from the larger problem of examining these artifacts out of context. In particular, the lack of information regarding the skulls in which the appliances were found leaves us without the most basic contextual evidence. If we had the skulls of those who wore these appliances, then identification of alveolar bone loss in mandibles fitted with suspected "braces" would serve to verify this inference. The problem is exacerbated by examples such as the Poggio Gaiella appliance (no. 5) and others where the skulls and jaws used for museum display of these artifacts are not those of the ancient wearers of the prostheses but modern replacements.

Most of the relevant data regarding the dental health of the Etruscans has been embedded within skeletal reports (cf. Becker *et al.* 2009: table 6; Becker 1993a; Turfa and Becker 2013: 870–873; see also Kron 2013). Several studies now in progress should provide extensive documentation for rather good dental health, and a pattern of tooth loss that begins only in late middle age. Preliminary studies by Becker at Tarquinia, corroborated with small samples from Vulci, Narce, Chiusi, Orvieto and Montebello (Becker *et al.* 2009) indicate that dental loss invariably begins in the molar area, and only gradually affects the anterior dentition

(Figure 3.1 illustrates this). Presumably this was an issue of hygiene: molars are often poorly cleaned and affected by decay and periodontal disease. Further, we note that all 86 extracted diseased teeth from the Roman Forum *taverna* were molars (well, one was a premolar), again demonstrating that even in a Roman, second-century CE population loss of front teeth was rare. These data should confirm the evidence that incisor loss was quite rare among the Etruscans; findings that in turn support the belief that some special situation—deliberate tooth evulsion—may have stimulated Etruscan manufacture and use of some dental pontics.[3]

Ancient metallurgy and the origins of modern dentistry

Available materials are often determining factors in the efficacy of dental treatments, and this certainly applies to Etruscan appliances. Some 2,000 years ago, the encyclopedist Pliny noted the ease with which gold can be cold-worked (Humphrey *et al.* 1998: 207–208; Craddock 2000c: 233), but at the time of his writing (shortly before his death in the eruption of Vesuvius, 79 CE), the Etruscans had been masters of gold-working for over 600 years. Gold in its purest form is the most malleable of the eight precious metals. The ability to purify gold, by parting it from other naturally occurring metals, originated about the time that Etruscan metallurgy was entering a literal golden age. The malleability and stability of gold made it ideal for fashioning dental appliances. These features explain why gold is still used for medical and dental applications today.

Pure gold (Au) is extraordinarily stable, never tarnishes, and is extremely malleable (Nutting and Nuttall 1977).[4] Also important, but perhaps not a subject of overt concern in antiquity, is the fact that gold is non-toxic. The use of other metals in the mouth would have led to problems (still noted today) of irritation and intoxication. A major question relates to the ability of the Etruscans to separate the silver that is often as much as 25 percent of naturally occurring "gold." The natural metal is actually an alloy, electrum, a mixture of gold and silver that always includes less than 2 percent copper. The silver content can be as much as 45 percent. The process of "parting" the gold from the silver in natural electrum is believed to have developed in Lydia in Turkey *c.*560 BCE, and legendarily has been linked to the personage of Croesus the king of Lydia. An earlier date for a similar development in gold refining in Etruria is actually possible, based on the composition of the earliest gold dental appliances.

Electrum is the name for all natural alloys of gold, in nuggets and other forms, as well as any artificial blends of gold and silver. "Almost all gold occurs naturally containing some silver . . . typically . . . between about 5 percent and 40 percent by weight" (Ramage and Craddock 2000b: 11). Silver can comprise as much as 45 percent of natural electrum, but levels below 20 percent are so rare that Vaûte (1995) suggests that all such alloys must have been intentionally generated. Almost certainly any gold that contains less than 5 percent silver or other metals has been purified, and most gold over 800 fine (800 parts per 1,000) has been specially processed to achieve that high percentage of gold. Copper is the only other metal found in natural gold above trace levels, but rarely occurs in amounts greater than 1 percent or 2 percent. Thus gold alloys with copper levels above 2 percent are almost certainly human products. The total weight of the platinum group elements (PGE) in natural gold alloys is far less than 1 percent by weight (Ramage and Craddock 2000b: 13; for details see Craddock 2000c: 238–244). For an understanding of the variations in strength of the various alloys see the Copper-Gold Phase Diagrams provided by O'Brien (1989: 253, fig. 12.6) or by Pingel (1995; also Martinelli and Spinella 1981). Various modes by which concentrations of copper might vary in ancient gold alloys are discussed by Ontalba *et al.* (1998: 856).

Pure gold (24 carat) is 999 fine or 99.9 percent gold. Gold at 22 carat (916 fine) has 91.6 percent purity, and proportionally decreases to 12 carat or 50 percent gold (500 fine). Gold can be rolled and/or drawn into thin wire, or hammered into a foil as little as 0.08 micrometers thick (3.33×10^{-6} inch). A small ring of gold, or loop of gold, can be cold worked by hammering into a large, seamless band similar to the more common form of Etruscan dental appliance.

Etruscan appliances in which a long band has been overlapped and heat fused to form a loop are rare: this signals the Bracciano appliance (no. 19) as being unusual. But except for Bracciano, and now the two Liverpool appliances, the available database lacks specific studies of the elemental composition of appliances. The Bracciano example is said to range from 92.2 to 98.6 percent gold, a much higher percentage of gold than would occur naturally (Teschler-Nicola *et al.* 1998). This reveals that the metal employed had been refined quite carefully, far more than any other sort of Etruscan gold object. The analysis of the Liverpool appliances confirms the deliberate refinement of gold by Etruscans.

Significant deposits of gold are known from Ireland, the Iberian Peninsula, Germany, Egypt and India. Evidence for prehistoric sources of gold in Europe is summarized by Lehrberger (1995: 129–131 for Italy). In most cases the ancients recovered gold from placer deposits, water-born or alluvial secondary deposits. The structure of these deposits and the geochemistry of gold are summarized by

Table 3.1 Uses of different gold alloys in *modern* dental practice

Gold casting	VHN*	Au	Pb	Ag	Cu (±)	Used for:
Type I	59–90	83.0	—	11.5	5.5	Small inlays, low stress
Type II	90–120	77.0	1.0	13.0	9.0	Most inlays, single crown
Type III (Hard)	120–150	74.0	4.0	12.0	10.0	Most crowns and bridges
Type IV (extra hard)	(Achieved by adding 2.0 to 7.0 Pt)					Partial dentures
	Quenched 150 min Hardened 220 min					

Source: adapted from O'Brien 1989: 306, table 15.2; and Martinelli and Spinella 1981: 27, fig. 2.4. Note that heat treatments are critical in controlling variations in the qualities of these gold alloy castings.

*Vickers hardness number. Brinell hardness numbers also can be used to indicate resistance to wear or to indentation.

Morteani (1995). The limited archaeological evidence for ancient gold mining was collected by Weisgerger and Pernicka (1995). Historical Etruria grew rich on the mining of metals, and parlayed the iron trade into an international commerce with the iron-poor Aegean and Near East. Deposits in the metal-bearing zones of Etruria[5] include some gold and silver, but we have no indication that these were exploited in the Etruscan period—it may well be that the Etruscan gold appliances used imported metal from Iberia or Egypt (see for mining Giardino 2013, with full references; also Giardino 2010: 146–150, Italian mines 149–150). Craddock (2009: 369–393) provides a basic treatment of ancient gold sources and technologies.

Aspects of the recovery and working of gold in ancient Europe are described by Morteani and Northover (1994), while prehistoric metallurgy of gold and silver has been reviewed by Raub (1995). Many authors offer insight into the significant developments in smelting procedures that appeared late in the European Iron Age (*c.*1000–800 BCE), a period during which human cremation also was a widespread custom.[6] At some point after 1000 BCE, smiths learned that gold alloys can be freed of their base metals by cupellation, a process that removes the copper by adding lead and heating to a high temperature (modern metallurgists prefer 1100°C). This forms a lead oxide run-off known as litharge but leaves the gold and silver ("noble metals") behind.

Various techniques now can be used to separate gold from silver in a simple (to metallurgists) process known as "parting" (Craddock 2000b; Bachmann 1995.) Early parting technology has been identified in Anatolian Lydia *c.*560 BCE, based on recent studies of a gold-working shop excavated at King Croesus' capitol of Sardis (Ramage and Craddock 2000a). Panned electrum "dust," as well as any natural gold alloy, can be parted by a process called cementation. This involves collecting natural electrum and beating or rolling it into foil sheets. These are then layered with common salt (NaCl) or any other salt (natron, alum, etc.) within porous earthenware vessels. A simple wood-fired furnace can generate and sustain the 600 to 800°C temperatures needed to effect the metallic separation, temperatures at the low end of those already used in funeral pyres. In the metallurgical process a period of several days of heating causes the chlorine gas generated from the salt to combine with the silver in the electrum foils, forming silver chloride vapor. Much of this condenses out in the walls of the vessel or of the furnace ("kiln") and can be recovered. The gold content of the natural electrum foils, commonly about 70 percent by weight, can be concentrated or raised to over 99 percent by this process. Silver and gold mines, associated smelting refuse, and ceramic vessels believed to have been used in this process have been studied at ancient Iberian sites, where Phoenician commerce had stimulated the already developing mining and metallurgical industry (Rovira and Renzi 2013; Renzi *et al.* 2009, with references).

The silver passing out of these electrum foils can be recovered by crushing the clays of the pots and the furnace and subjecting the resulting "ore" to common smelting by incorporating lead in the process (cupellation). Ramage and Craddock (2000b) indicate that this molten metallic mixture of lead holding some

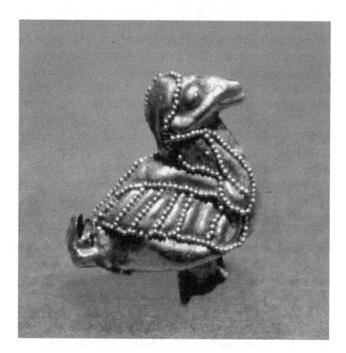

Figure 3.7 Etruscan gold-work in the form of jewelry, a constructed bird ornament decorated in granulation technique, *c.*650 BCE, from Cerveteri, University of Pennsylvania Museum MS 3350 (H. 1 cm). Compare the massive brooch covered with such birds, from the "princely" Regolini Galassi Tomb of Cerveteri (see Sannibale 2008a).

Source: University of Pennsylvania Museum. Courtesy Mediterranean section.

silver could be converted, at around 1,000°C, to a lead oxide from which the liquid silver would separate. Not employed in antiquity were other techniques familiar today such as mercury amalgamation, fire assaying or use of reagents such as strong acids (Craddock 2000c; cf. United States Customs 1998).

The casting of a hollow gold tooth by an Etruscan goldsmith *c.*630 BCE (actually somewhat earlier, since that is its burial date)—the Satricum appliance (no. 18)—required considerable metallurgical skill. The working of the gold to create this tooth may have been entirely dependent on the smith's ability to refine the metal to a relatively high purity. Craddock discusses (2000a) variations in the composition of gold alloys and how these differences influenced the final products in antiquity. Since a great deal of effort went into the separation of gold and silver from natural electrum it was apparently only done for special cases, namely dental appliances. While Craddock (2000b; Ramage and Craddock 2000b) suggested that maintaining standards of Lydian electrum coinage stimulated development of this technology, the evidence of refined Etruscan dental gold now appears to be earlier.

Non-destructive analyses of gold objects

To address the various questions concerning the use of gold in Etruscan "dentistry" we ideally would like to develop a program of extensive testing. A beginning has been made in the analysis of metals in Etruscan artifacts with XRF (X-ray fluorescence) and SEM (scanning electron microscope) techniques. (See Cowell's (1977) review of the theory and mechanics of XRF.) The XRF technique is a non-invasive means of determining the composition of the surface of objects made from earth-obtained materials such as metals and ceramic soils. Vast numbers of other types of gold objects have already been studied (West *et al.* 2012; Musílek *et al.* 2012; Guerra 2008; Morteani and Northover 1994). For the use of these analytical techniques at excavations see Donais and George (2012). The analytical sections of Ramage and Craddock (2000a: chapters 5–10) provide the ideal model for investigating the metallic composition of the surviving Etruscan gold appliances. At present limited data only are available for the Bracciano appliance (no. 19), and complete analyses for the two appliances in Liverpool (nos. 13–14). Future testing will enable us to evaluate possible differences between the metallic composition of the pontics as distinct from the bands/braces that may have been therapeutic in function.

XRF readings only reflect elements present on the surface but burial conditions may cause elements to leech or migrate to the surface. Cowell (1977: 76) cautions readers regarding the use of X-ray fluorescence to analyze archaeological objects as the composition below the surface would be difficult to evaluate since several processes can effectively enrich gold levels at the surface of the object without causing it to peel away (cf. Demortier 1986; Demortier, Morciaux and Dozot 1999). XRF effectively penetrates only 0.01 to 0.1 mm beneath the surface depending on the specimen. Since the bands used in Etruscan appliances are so thin, however, they are good candidates for such analysis.

Ion beam analysis (IBA) also has been applied to the study of the elemental composition of ancient gold artifacts (Demortier 1995, 2000). Denker and Maier (1999) discuss the use of faster protons to achieve deep penetration without damaging the artifact, and have achieved success at depths up to an impressive 4 mm. For studies of metals using scanning electron microscopy (SEM) see Meeks (2000).

Etruscan expertise in gold-working

Analysis of gold objects from the so-called Etruscan princely tombs does suggest that the Etruscans could purify gold at an early date (early or mid-seventh century BCE). The techniques for the manufacture of dental appliances were simple compared to those used during the seventh century and later for fine jewelry (casting, construction, hot-bonding or reaction soldering, filigree and wire-making, granulation etc., see Giardino 2010: 71–110; Echt and Thiele 1994; De Puma 1987; Formigli 1983).

Parrini *et al.* (1982: 118, n. 4) noted problems in the XRF study conducted by von Hase (1976) of the surfaces of jewelry from the mid-seventh-century

Bernardini tomb at Praeneste. Mello *et al.* (1982: 549) examined two gold bracelets from seventh-century Etruscan Vetulonia "metallographically and microanalytically to determine how the filigree wires were joined" and found high copper concentrations at the "joints" (joins) of the wire that suggest a form of welding was used (see above). Of interest here is their finding that the wires used were composed approximately of 69 percent gold, 28 percent silver, and 3 percent copper. These proportions suggest possible admixture of copper, but the objects also might be entirely fashioned from natural electrum. Years of comments on the granulation process itself, including the experimental recreations of Nestler and Formigli (1994/2001) have generated an impressive literature, but this skill was not employed in ancient dentistry.

A completely different but related technology emerged about two centuries after the Etruscans began to make gold pontics (Becker 1997). By the later fifth century BCE, wires of gold or silver were used (see Nicolini 1992; also Carroll 1970, 1972) where ligation techniques enabled the stabilization of loose teeth. Variations of this wiring were also used to hold a replacement tooth in some jaws. Replacement of a lost tooth is the function of the single known wire example from Italy (Rome). The earliest known wire pieces are from fifth–fourth-century Phoenician Sidon; others represent Ptolemaic and Roman Egypt. The Greek, Hippocratic medical text mentioning wiring of loose teeth is dated in the late fifth century. We now suggest that the archaeologically recovered example from Rome confirms the literary evidence for gold-wire dental appliances in Italy of the Late Republic and early Empire. Possibly the tradition of ornamental appliances of the Etruscans evolved into the development of wire prostheses in Italy for which we have yet to excavate the earliest examples. Alternatively, wire systems may have emerged in Phoenician or Greek regions and spread into the Roman world. The use of gold-wire ligatures remained a fundamental procedure in dentistry into the second half of the twentieth century. Comparative information on the composition of the gold in all the Etruscan prostheses could permit us to generate the basis for a possible chronology of types of appliances.

Analysis of the gold in Etruscan dental appliances

The two appliances in the Liverpool World Museum have recently been studied according to new techniques for precious metals analysis: unfortunately, as with many nineteenth-century collections, they lack context. It is likely that they were excavated early in the nineteenth century in a necropolis of the city of Vulci. Some precious items made their way from the Bonaparte excavations at Vulci into the collection of Joseph Mayer, the Liverpool goldsmith whose museum forms the basis of the Liverpool World Museum today. It is no longer possible to date these appliances precisely, but it is evident that the technology of constructing and fitting the gold bands was in practice as early as the mid-seventh century BCE, the date of the excavated Satricum example (no. 18).

The two Liverpool pontics were transferred to the University of Liverpool for testing by scanning electron microscopes with energy dispersive spectrometry

(SEM-EDS), by Matthew Ponting and Pablo Fernández-Reyes of the Department of Archaeology, Classics and Egyptology (see Appendix VII for their 2015 report). The extremely high purity of the gold in both appliances (approximately 98 percent), and the similarity of the composition of the two rivets in each to the sheet of gold forming the appliance were striking. The extremely low silver and copper contents of all these items reveal an extraordinarily high ability to separate native electrum into silver and gold. The purity of the gold rivets allowed them to be hammered to neatly fit into the gold bands, thus firmly securing the false teeth in place. In fact, the purity of the gold in the Liverpool examples exceeds that of most gold artifacts of the Mediterranean cultures of the first millennium BCE. If the other appliances could be tested by the new SEM-EDS method, the results might well show that Etruscan metallurgy—in the case of gold refining at least—exceeded the standards of other cultures. Why did other metallurgists not create gold of such purity? They simply had no need of it, and no use for such malleable gold, since they never had to make and fit delicate bridges in the mouths of imperious aristocrats!

The oft noted dental appliance from Satricum (no. 18) is unique in having a hollow gold tooth attached to a narrow supporting band that suspended the false tooth between healthy teeth. The Satricum "tooth," a replacement for an upper central incisor, appears to have been made in two parts that were welded/fused. (Demortier (1988) thought it was welded, but this may reflect his ignorance of the process or a translation problem.) The use of a gold replacement tooth as a fabrication technique seems never to have recurred. The use of organic materials for the replacement teeth, such as the wearer's own real teeth that have been cut down, seems to have become the norm (Liverpool I, no. 13, is a fine example). The construction of the Satricum appliance is of interest for comparison with techniques used for jewelry in Tartessic (Phoenician-influenced Iberian) and Mesopotamian goldsmithing of about the same period (cf. Piette *et al.* 1986).

Etruscan ornaments did not use such malleable gold. Von Hase (1976: 229–233) provides XRF analyses for six Etruscan objects. The results of his 16 tests suggest that all were fashioned from natural electrum. Echt and Thiele (1994: 439) published metallurgical analyses for two Etruscan gold fibulae (ornamental "safety pins"), from Comeana and Volterra; each was tested on at least four surface locations. Considerable variation was found in the gold content of various sites, but there was no indication that this had functional significance in terms of hardness or flexibility. In a review of similar studies of artifacts, Formigli (1983) found that the reported silver content in items studied before 1983 ranged from 15 to 37 percent, with copper varying between 0.1 and 10 percent. The silver content seems to fit with the use of unaltered electrum. Where high levels of copper are noted, Formigli (1983: 322) believes that it was added. Morteani and Northover (1994) have enormously expanded the list, but thorough analyses of the metals in dental appliances are only now beginning.

Gold used in modern dentistry is far from 24 carat (pure, or 999 fine). Dental uses of gold vary in requirements, and can range from as low as 10 carat to around 16 carat (alloys of roughly 40 percent and up to 65 or 70 percent gold;

O'Brien 1989: 303). Martinelli and Spinella (1981: 27) give the normal range at between 64.1 and 88.4 percent. The proportions vary widely according to individual suppliers. Even at 64 percent gold, the 36 percent copper used in the alloys of a modern dental appliance poses no health risk. Ancient Etruscan appliances (certainly those tested) had gold levels far higher than these modern norms, and thus the Etruscan appliances posed no danger to health (*pace* Baggieri 2001). Only when an appliance directly touches gingival tissue is there a possibility of contact irritation. As has been revealed (Becker n.d. a), the Etruscan band examples only used what we now call sanitary or "hygienic pontics," or those that do not touch the gum. These were designed to surround the crowns of the teeth, but not to rest on or have contact with the gingival regions. The later use of wire appliances reveals that the people making dental appliances learned that gold and silver in contact with soft tissue did not create irritation such as resulted from copper or iron.

An analysis of Etruscan jewelry by Mello and colleagues (1982) led Menconi and Fornaciari (1985: 94) to assume that electrum was used in Etruscan appliances. Baggieri and Allegrezzo (1994: 5) make reference to an X-ray fluorescence study conducted on the Valsiarosa appliance by Giovanni Ettore Gigante and Roberto Cesareo (Dipartimento Energetico, Università di Roma "La Sapienza"). It indicated the presence of silver and copper, and possibly iron traces; the iron, they suggest, reflects a later contamination. This contamination may well derive from the brown-colored mounting material, possibly wax or glue, used over 100 years ago to attach this appliance to a modern mandible for display. Traces of this material were still evident on the specimen when it was examined by Becker around 1990 (see no. 15.)

The Bracciano appliance (no. 19) was subjected by Teschler-Nicola and her colleagues (1998: 61) to "analysis from ten different regions of the Bracciano gold band, including the rivet." The X-ray they published (1998: 62, fig. 6) indicates that the rivet (2.5 mm in diameter, cf. Becker 1992a) is far greater in diameter than any other appliance. Their analysis of the metals, employing a JUEOL-6400 scanning electron microscope "equipped with a KEVEX energy dispersive system (EDS)," found that the gold content, by weight, ranges from 92.2 to 98.6 percent (Teschler-Nicola *et al.* 1998: 64, table 2). In only two of these 10 surface samples is the gold level below 95.3 percent, the third lowest level, with the median falling between 97.2 and 97.6 percent. Although Teschler-Nicola (*et al.* 1994a and 1994b) suggest that this could be panned gold, this would be an exceptionally high purity for natural gold. This level of purity implies that an effective parting of gold from its natural electrum alloy may have been involved. The silver content in this appliance is indeed low, varying from 0.7 to 7.0 percent, with the median falling between 2.1 and 2.2 percent. Copper levels in these 10 tests range from 0.2 to 0.8 percent (median between 0.6 and 0.7 percent). The precise locations of the tests on the Bracciano appliance are not indicated, however (Teschler-Nicola *et al.* 1994b, 1998), leaving us without the exact copper content of the rivet, information that could reflect the true skills of the Etruscan goldsmith. If the rivet is from "Location A9," with <0.2 percent copper, that might suggest that it did not have copper added to provide strength. This corresponds with the findings for the Liverpool appliances in which the rivets were of similar composition to the bands.

It is possible that the peening of the ends of the rivet in the Bracciano appliance and the working of the band to attach the overlap (Teschler-Nicola *et al.* 1998: 62, fig. 7) caused differential migration of specific metals, in effect altering the ratios at those sites. This possibility could be explored if the 10 test locations can be assigned to specific points on the appliance. If the surface levels of gold have been "enriched" then the proportions of gold to silver (and copper) in the Bracciano appliance would be within the range of high quality, naturally occurring placer (secondary) gold,[7] as suggested by Teschler Nicola *et al.* (1998: 61, following Hartmann 1982). No "parting" would have been needed to raise the purity of the gold.

Menconi and Fornaciari (1985: 92) mention the Bruschi III (no. 10) dental appliance in the Museo Nazionale Archeologico Tarquiniense and discuss the findings of its gold content. They believe that it contains 65–75 percent gold, with a silver content of 22–35 percent and copper at 0.5–3 percent (Menconi and Fornaciari 1985: 94). This would suggest that natural electrum had been used to fashion this appliance—if the data derive from direct testing of the appliance itself.

Today even more sophisticated analytical techniques are available (e.g. Ontalba *et al.* 1998). A paper examining the "biocompatibility" of Etruscan dental appliances provides graphs of XRF tests of three examples in the Museo Nazionale Archeologico Tarquiniense (Baggieri 2001). Only Bruschi I (no. 8), identified by Baggieri (2001: 324–325, graph 1) as "T-A," was analyzed in this study. Baggieri claims that the test revealed 30 percent silver and 5 percent copper, but does not indicate how these figures were derived (cf. Baggieri and Allegrezza 1994: 5). Baggieri (2001: 325–326, Graph 2) indicates a high silver (Ag) count for Bruschi I, while stating that the Satricum appliance (no. 18) has only 7 percent silver, and 2 percent copper according to readings taken from the point of a *saldatura* (weld). He believes that the Valsiarosa appliance (no. 15) has 13 percent silver, and 5 percent copper (2001: 327–328, graph 3; cf. Becker 1994a, 1999b). For possible results of tests on the Bruschi III appliance (no. 10), see Menconi and Fornaciari (1985).

Gold parting in Etruria

The data on the gold content of the Etruscan dental appliance now in Vienna, the Bracciano example (no. 19), are consistent with its having been fashioned from purified or "parted" gold and not from natural electrum. (An unlikely alternate possibility is that the Bracciano appliance is actually a modern forgery.) The purity of the gold in the Bracciano appliance contrasts with the findings of Menconi and Fornaciari (1985) for the dental appliances from Etruscan Tarquinia. They, like Baggieri, find that the proportions of the gold alloys are closer to naturally occurring electrum. The new data generated for the two Liverpool appliances, however, certainly show very low silver content and thus imply the purification of the gold for both the gold bands and the rivets. A complete XRF or SEM study of all extant appliances by the same team would be completely non-invasive and could resolve this issue, and perhaps demonstrate Etruscan primacy in the refining of gold, a technique driven by the unique, Etruscan need for easily worked material for dental insertion.

Fitting Etruscan appliances in the mouth

A dental bridge fashioned from relatively pure, malleable gold, whether assembled from a series of rings, or as a single long loop, could be fitted into the mouth with ease. The rings at the ends of the series could be secured around the living, "anchor" (or "post" or "abutment") teeth by the simple technique of firmly pressing down the malleable gold around the natural and secure teeth that served as "posts." Among such examples of "pontics" or bridges we find interesting variations in the ways in which the replacement teeth could be held in place. One technique uses the gold of the ring surrounding the replacement by pressing it firmly around the "tooth" being used for insertion into the appliance. More commonly a rivet was used to hold the false or replaced tooth within the bridge. The techniques were never combined for redundancy.

Obviously, all appliances fitted with rivets held replacement teeth, although some have lost the "tooth" itself. One example (Corneto II, no. 12) includes a replacement for two teeth that is carved from a single piece of material, possibly an animal tooth. Each side of this double-tooth is held by a separate rivet. In order to avoid slippage of the appliance, the "loop" ends of the gold band would be best fitted around the widest point of the anchor teeth, which is some distance above the soft tissue of the gum. This is the case whether the gums are healthy or if they have been permanently affected by periodontal disease. If an appliance were fitted closer to the soft gum tissue, where the diameters of the anchor teeth are smaller, the excess length of the band needed to pass over the widest point of the tooth would have to be reduced to achieve a tight fit, by bending or crimping the band—making it more likely to work loose. If fitted around the tooth at the widest diameter, the band would be pinched in place by the sound teeth between which the extreme ends of the loops would pass. Having the sound anchor tooth and its neighbor gripping these loop ends and thus locking the entire bridge into place has obvious benefits. The insertion of the gold strip of the pontic between two healthy teeth might cause some problems in dental articulation. Even though the gold sheet may be no more than 0.1 mm thick, the slight shifting of the teeth might be annoying for a short period of time (a few hours to a few days, depending on sensitivity). The adjustment could generate a problem in the alignment of dental cusps. Such misalignment might cause greater pressure or shock to be focused on certain teeth, perhaps resulting in headaches for the person who has had the appliance inserted.

An interesting aspect of the simple technology of Etruscan dental appliances: the gold rivets traverse the false or replacement teeth via a horizontal

Table 3.2 List of appliances: pontics or braces?

Appliances with rivets/ replacement teeth	Appliances with no rivets or apparent replacements
6 Populonia	1 Barrett I (Etruria)
9 Bruschi II (Tarquinia?)	2 Barrett II (Bisenzio)
11 Corneto I (Tarquinia)	5 Poggio Gaiella (Chiusi)
12 Corneto II (Tarquinia)	7 Ghent (Orvieto)
13 Liverpool I	8 Bruschi I (Tarquinia?)
14 Liverpool II	10 Bruschi III (Tarquinia?)
15 Valsiarosa (Falerii)	16 Teano
17 Praeneste	20 Tanagra (Boeotia, Greece)
19 Bracciano	
21 Sardis (Anatolia)	

Appliances with replacement teeth, no rivets

3 Van Marter (Bolsena?)
4 Copenhagen (Orvieto?)
18 Satricum—gold tooth

hole drilled completely through the replacement.[8] The rivets also pierce the gold band, but the holes may be made in the strip of soft gold by simply piercing it with an awl. If the band was pierced from the interior surface the gold expressed would form a collar that would surround the heads of the rivet, which were then peened in place.

Drilling in antiquity

The Etruscans' ability to drill holes through real (dead) teeth has wider implications. This part of the fabrication of false teeth derives from drilling processes that were long in use for working gemstones and items from ivory or other hard materials. Appliances nos. 3, 13, 17, 19, 21 (Van Marter, Liverpool I, Praeneste, Bracciano, Sardis) retain replacement teeth made of human teeth; quite probably the person's own, recycled teeth. Seven others had replacements made of some non-metallic materials (Corneto II is said to be animal tooth), now lost. Only the Satricum appliance, the earliest dated example, used a specially made, hollow gold tooth. Those appliances that incorporated teeth or ivory required drilling that demonstrates the technological ability of the Etruscans to perforate these materials. These Old World drilling techniques long predate the Classical period and the dental appliances (Gambier and Houet 1991).

Etruscan drilling techniques parallel in many respects the skills used in dental decoration practiced in the New World by the ancient Maya in Central America. By the fifth century CE, the Maya had developed complex ornamental tooth filing patterns, and also perfected mechanisms for cementing finely crafted stone inlays (of jade, pyrites, etc.) into cylindrical holes drilled into living teeth. Maya "inlaying" activities were purely cosmetic procedures (Gwinnett and Gorelick 1979).

The Maya had been drilling and carving jade for centuries before applying these skills to cosmetic dentistry.

In Europe three distinct types of hand drills were well developed in antiquity for use in various remarkably delicate procedures (Milne 1907: 126–128). In contrast to modern practices, in antiquity drills were not employed for the cleaning of dental caries as a preparation for therapeutic filling with restorative material (cf. Bennike 1985: 175–182). Medical boxes containing folding bow drills used to power trephination tools (for use on the skull) are known from ancient Rome (Künzl 1982: 84–85). Bow and other drills must have been commonly used in surgical procedures long before Etruscan and Roman practices. Aside from possible evidence for a remarkably early use of a drill on a Neolithic person from Denmark and some prehistoric New World examples, no application of the drill or of metal tools to the preparation of cavities in living teeth can be documented in Europe until the end of the fifteenth century CE.

Gorelick and Gwinnet (1987a: 39) questioned why drilling technology was insufficiently developed before the nineteenth century to permit its application to modern types of dentistry. In fact, centuries earlier, some success with the preparation of cavities for filling with various materials already had been achieved (see Chapter 4). Despite the fact that ancient cultures may have had the technological potential for creating an appropriately clean site for the installation of gold foil or other fillings, the several technical aspects of this procedure were not brought together until the modern period. More significantly, where cultural expectations of dental decay and loss are based on centuries of tradition, the very idea of trying to do something about the features of "life" inhibits any attention to changing the situation.

Suggestions that lead fillings ("stoppings" in British English) were used by the Romans in the extraction of severely decayed teeth have never been demonstrated. Many of the basic materials and means were available to the Romans to successfully repair decayed teeth, but this was never done. The combination of skills needed for basic dental repair in the cleaning and filling of drilled cavities was not developed until after 1800 CE. Until about 1250 CE, even gold foil technology (see Hunt 1975) had not progressed to the point of inserting a foil implant. The skills needed to fill cleanly drilled cavities were not brought together for use in dentistry until after 1700 CE. To a large extent the lag between the development of the technology for drilling and the filling of teeth relates to cultural rules, or to cultural concepts regarding beauty. The importance of a complete set of teeth, perhaps enhanced by a bit of gold, stemmed from cultural factors, which may have generated the Etruscans' desire for the use of these decorative and/or cosmetic devices.

Functions of Etruscan dental prostheses

Detailed examination of Etruscan gold dental appliances enables us, in the words of Andrew Wallace-Hadrill (1990: 149, on Pompeii) to "focus on luxury as a social process." Etruscan dental prostheses were designed to be cosmetic, with ornamentation as their main goal (Becker 2001). Traditional views (Sudhoff 1926: 85; Hoffmann-Axthelm 1970: 83; Menconi and Fornaciari 1985: 94) postulate a variety of reasons for Etruscan use of dental pontics, including supposed improvements in speech by filling the gap from missing front teeth. Some of the simple band types of these appliances could have been functional, for instance Poggio Gaiella, Populonia, Ghent, Bruschi I and III, and Teano (nos. 5, 6, 7, 9, 10, 16). These conceivably were designed to stabilize, and thus preserve, loose teeth. Of course, the functional aspects may have been enhanced by the ornamental. Some Eastern Mediterranean wire appliances were certainly designed to stabilize loose teeth (see Chapter 4); we may infer that some Etruscan appliances served functional as well as decorative purposes.

Appliances designed to fill a gap left by lost teeth would also serve to maintain the remaining teeth in their correct places. Such a bridge would assure continued proper articulation of the teeth and their continued efficient function. While this is one of the principal goals of modern orthodontics this function may have been entirely incidental in Etruria. Almost certainly the functional aspect of maintaining tooth alignment was unknown to the makers and users of Etruscan dental appliances. Pacciani and Corruccini (1986; Corruccini and Pacciani 1989, 1991) suggest, based on studies of burials, that Etruscans had relatively few cases of malocclusion. This is typical of the pre-modern world. Their study of collections of Etruscan skulls (none with prosthetics) led them to suggest that an appliance made from soft gold could have been used to realign the teeth of an Etruscan, or even to direct teeth into the gap caused by a lost tooth, but this is not tenable because of the materials used: soft gold appliances are incapable of providing the forces needed for modern orthodonture.

All known Etruscan bridges or braces provide for replacement or the stabilization of teeth in the anterior portion of the dental arch, perhaps 8 of those catalogued spanned the 4 upper incisors. (See also Guerini 1909: 75–76; Capasso 1985: 52; Hoffmann-Axthelm 1985: 39; Bliquez 1996). The idea of replacing back teeth remained beyond the interests, as well as the abilities, of ancient craftsmen.

Women only: sex and tooth size

Becker's metric findings, derived from studies of the relative sizes of teeth and jaws, show that all the Etruscan/Italic wearers of dental prostheses were female. (Wire appliances are another matter.) Luigi Capasso (1986: 55) first suggested in print that all were female, indicating vanity as the primary motive. The nearly complete lack of archaeological data deprives us of contextual information for evaluating the gender of the wearers. Some teeth believed to be from the owners remain associated with these appliances; others have "rings" or openings for individual teeth now missing. Both elements enable us to measure the opening and infer the size of the teeth (cf. Becker 2000a: 61, table 5.1).

Sexual dimorphism, size variation by sex, within any specific population has long been recognized as an important feature of human diversity parallel to that seen in other species. Sex variation has been recognized in Paleolithic

Homo sapiens at least since the Middle Pleistocene (Arsuaga *et al.* 1997). Some scholars (Enachesco *et al.* 1962) believe that size and sex differences can be detected even in neonates. The use of odontometrics to determine sex had its beginnings in England (Goose 1963; Kieser 1990), also in America (Garn *et al.* 1967). Ditch and Rose (1972) expanded on the work of Goose (1963) by demonstrating that differences in human tooth size provide 93 percent accuracy in the evaluation of sex. They found incisors less diagnostic than molars, with canines showing the least dimorphism (also Kieser 1990: 67–70). Kieser (1990) indicates how chromosomal effects influence the transmission of these differences. Other scholars were less successful in recognizing human sexual dimorphism in teeth, but did have some success using discriminant function analysis with molars. Rösing *et al.* (1995) have perfected their original research. Improved statistical techniques have enhanced predictability and now almost all teeth can be successfully used to evaluate sex. Stermer Beyer-Olsen and Alexandersen (1995) found, for a medieval Norwegian population, that the "left maxillary first molar facio-lingual dimension, was not only the best discriminator in sex assessment but also the tooth most often available for study." Maxillary first molars are the tooth preferred by Becker for evaluating sex, but are not always available.

Kieser's (1990) findings were replicated in studies of a central Italian Iron Age population at Osteria dell'Osa, Latium (Becker and Salvadei 1992; Salvadei 2002), and also at an Imperial-era necropolis near Rome (Manzi *et al.* 1997). Most of the early work on dimorphism in dentition has been summarized by Rösing *et al.* (1995); Prossinger (1998: 501) provides a means by which dimensions of missing teeth may be inferred.[9] Rösing's (1980) research on infant tooth size was successfully adapted by Molleson (1992) for her study at the Romano-British site, Poundbury. In Japan, Funatsu *et al.* (1997) demonstrated that sexual dimorphism can be identified through crown diameters even of deciduous teeth (also Kondo *et al.* 1997). Kieser (1990: 65–67), however, found that in his Caucasian sample, the adult anterior maxillary teeth, particularly the mesial-distal lengths, offered the best data on the extent and patterning of sexual dimorphism (Scott and Turner 1977; also Harris 1997). This is not the case with most other studies, where first molar dimensions are best correlated with sex.

The Etruscan population of the Iron Age and Archaic periods certainly displayed overall (skeletal) sexual dimorphism, with women who were generally very gracile, with delicate faces and distinctly small teeth. They were tiny in stature, often under 5 feet in adult height while men might be almost a foot taller (Becker *et al.* 2009: 100 and table 4). These estimates of stature derive from long bone dimensions (Becker 1999e), which also aid in the evaluation of sex. The data demonstrate that sexual dimorphism was common in Italy from the Iron Age through the Roman Empire, so we should be able to rely on tooth size as a gauge of the sex of appliance wearers. We conclude that the Etruscan devices (especially the Copenhagen, Valsiarosa, Bruschi III, both Liverpool examples) were designed for *women* only (Becker 2000a: 61, table 5.1). The meager archaeological evidence bears this out: all preserved skull remains are female.

Why the need for replacements?

Etruscan dental appliances require the presence of relatively healthy "anchor" teeth to support them. It would be very unlikely that natural ante-mortem loss had taken place among the women wearing appliances, or that only one or two central incisors would be lost through periodontal disease, with no effects on the adjacent teeth. Similarly, accidental trauma and the resulting loss of anterior teeth are rare in most cultures (Lukacs and Hemphill 1990; also Merbs 1968), and virtually unknown among the Etruscans.

The cosmetic aspects of Etruscan dental appliances appear to be the principal and probably only concern of their users. The lack of any attempt to provide molar replacements also reflects the finding that this technology was never intended to provide enhanced chewing ability (Hoffmann-Axthelm 1985: 78; Menconi and Fornaciari 1985: 94; Bliquez 1996). Only adults were considered appropriate subjects for the expenditure of effort needed to secure a gold prosthesis, just as today gold inlays and foil fillings are only used for adults who will benefit from the considerable durability of such work.

The few cases of direct evidence confirm that these Etruscan dental appliances were worn by women, for ornamentation, and this probably correlates with gender-specific dental evulsion. Had the simple Etruscan gold bands been used for functional reasons one might suppose that at least some would have been worn by men, nor is use by men confirmed in ancient literature. One may infer that the use of these appliances by women acted as a disincentive for men to wear similar devices. In contrast, the wire appliances of the Hellenistic-Roman period in Italy, and particularly those of the eastern Mediterranean, *were* functional, and the limited evidence indicates that *at least* one Levantine wire example (Ford, no. W2, from Sidon) was worn by a male. The corpus of these eastern Mediterranean examples is too small (at seven) to go beyond this observation. Functional differences between wire and strips of gold may be the important variable.

Why wear a dental appliance? The public roles of Etruscan women

Varieties of decorative tooth filing and chipping, the drilling of teeth for ornamental inlays, and other cosmetic procedures involving the teeth are found throughout the world (Milner and Larsen 1991). There is no region where these activities have not been closely correlated with gender roles. Today we may infer that where women use such cosmetic procedures they normally appear in public in groups that include members of both genders, as is now common in the Western world. These public behaviors are not acceptable, however, in most of the countries in the Islamic world, nor in many other cultures where genders are segregated. The Classical literature makes it clear that indiscriminate mingling of the sexes was strictly avoided throughout much of the ancient Mediterranean region.

Unlike the Greek and Roman cultures, however (see Økland 1998), Etruscan society did not segregate women from men at public gatherings such as religious festivals, funerals or banquets. In fact women enjoyed an important place in Etruscan urban society (summarized by Rathje 2007, 2013). Most evidence derives from the placement of artifacts in women's graves in Etruria, the Faliscan territory and parts of Latium during the eighth–sixth centuries BCE. The deposition of banquet equipment, such as punch bowls on stands, wine amphorae, decorative drinking cups and symbolic ornaments such as miniature cheese graters worn pinned to the dress, attest to women's roles during life, such as hosting banquets (Turfa 2005: 17–18, 104 no. 34).[10] As early as 580–575 BCE, Etruscan artists depicted wives reclining beside husbands at formal banquets. Privileged females are depicted reclining to dine in the terracotta frieze of a monumental building at Poggio Civitate (Murlo) near Siena. The palatial structure's wooden beams were decorated with scenes of gods and goddesses and the activities of the ruling class, including the reclining banquet with both sexes represented. One diner clearly has a female chest and drinks from a Greek-style cup while the bearded men hold hemispherical drinking bowls. A younger figure, playing the kithara, also may be female (see Rathje 1989; 2013: 825–826).

The painted tombs at Tarquinia show the next phase of this phenomenon, with aristocratic men reclining on Greek-style couches to dine, while their wives modestly sit on chairs beside them. The Tomba Bartoccini (c.530–520 BCE) is the earliest known example of women on chairs, following Greek custom (Steingräber 1986: 286–287 no. 45, pl. 35). Soon after this period, the wives, some of them depicted as bleached-blondes (or are they real blondes? the scholarly debate continues), are again depicted reclining beside their husbands. These couples are served food and drink by attractive young male and female servants while special performers entertain. (See Figure I.1, *Tomb of the Leopards*.) At Tarquinia, at least 22 tombs of the late sixth to late fourth centuries BCE show women and men dining in public. One last monument, the fourth-century Tomb of the Shields, depicts richly dressed ladies seated on chairs rather than reclining with their husbands. It probably implied that the ladies had enjoyed a Greek-style education. One painted tomb at the city of Caere and another at Orvieto also feature reclining couples (Steingräber 1986 *passim*).

The *Tomba delle Bighe* (Tomb of the Chariots, c.490 BCE) at Tarquinia (Figure 3.8) actually shows men and women seated together in bleachers watching nude athletes and chariot races, although the banqueters who recline in another scene are all male (Steingräber 1986: 289–291 no. 47). Such images during the sixth–third centuries BCE referred to a funeral feast with overtones of the kingdom of the dead (Bonfante 1981; De Marinis 1961).

During the Hellenistic period (c.300–31 BCE) sculpted sarcophagi or urns with reclining men and women on the lids were favored to recreate the image of a family banquet in mixed company (see Figure 3.9). The Volterran Inghirami Tomb was arranged with urns aligned as if the male and female effigies were conversing at a family dinner (Haynes 2000: 370–371, fig. 292). Annette Rathje (2013: 826) notes: "In fact, the presence of women stresses the significance and power of family. It is very interesting that women are not represented as mothers on these occasions."

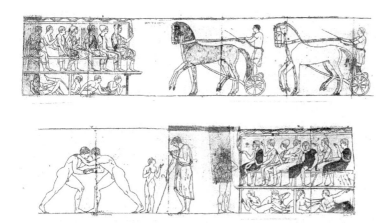

Figure 3.8 Fresco from Tomb of the Chariots, Tarquinia, early fifth century BCE, sampling of scenes: men and women sitting together at public funeral games, after an antiquarian sketch (see Steingräber 1985: 290–291, figs 80–82); originals now faded, in Tarquinia Museo Archeologico Nazionale.

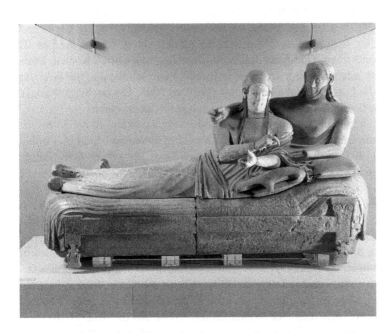

Figure 3.9 *"Sarcofage des Époux,"* now in the Louvre, Paris. Painted terracotta "Sarcophagus of the Spouses" from Cerveteri, Rome province, Italy, 520 BCE. A wineskin among the couch pillows was a hidden symbol of the couple's devotion to the cult of the wine-god, Fufluns (Bacchus/Dionysos). A closely related sarcophagus, from another tomb of this family, is in the Villa Giulia, Rome.

Source: De Agostini Picture Library. G. Dagli Orti/Bridgeman Images.

The sixth-century BCE Tarquinian "Tomb of the Baron" depicts an Etruscan priestess in rituals together with men old and young (Steingräber 1986: 283 no. 44). At Tarquinia and Chiusi, women with aristocratic names, wearing rich costumes and/or placed in prominent positions in the composition, appear in tomb paintings (Steingräber 1986: nos. 44, 48, 53, 25). Etruscan acceptance of women as the equals of men, appearing in public situations, was a behavior repugnant to ancient Greek authors. (Athenian women were constrained from participating in many public ceremonies.) Greek commentary on the supposedly unnatural social behavior of Etruria is known from numerous written works (see Rowland 2001), including Theopompus (in Athenaeus' *Deipnosophistai* 12.517d–518b) and Diodorus Siculus (5.3).

The dress of Etruscan women included calf-length skirts and sturdy boots to facilitate walking, along with functional hats, cloaks and parasols. These items, depicted in many works of art, supported freedom of movement, travel, and consequently ready access to society in general. This is paralleled by depictions of affluent women in chariots and wagons in both tombs and artistic representations, known from as early as the Iron Age (see Bonfante 1994, 2003, 2013; Amann 2001). There is even early evidence (seventh century BCE) for women owning commercial workshops, such as the pottery factory at Caere-Cerveteri run by "*kvsnailise*"—"Slave of the woman of the Cusna Family" (Colonna 1993; for critical analysis, see Benelli 2016). At late seventh-century Poggio Civitate, a burned building held a cache of *tesserae hospitales*—ivory tokens used as ID cards by businessmen. One ivory fragment, depicting one or two women, bears on the reverse a tantalizing inscription restored by one scholar as "[*mi veleli]as vheisalna[ia]* = I am of Velelia Feysalnai" (Wallace 2008: 189 no. 80; p. 5 no. I). If correct, the uncommon name indicates an active business*woman*.

Variations in the relationship between gender interaction and ethnicity in various parts of ancient Italy are the subject of papers in a volume edited by Cornell and Lomas (1995). The evidently high status of *Etruscan* women (see Nielsen 1986, 1989; Gasperini 1989; Spivey 1991: 64) and the extent of their cosmetic concerns (as documented by Rallo 1989a, 1989b) extended to their use of dental appliances. A recent exhibition assembled the many aspects of "*Etruschi: Il privilegio della bellezza*" (Rafanelli and Spaziani 2011), presenting female iconography, aesthetics and concrete evidence of beauty products and procedures, including use of dental appliances (Naso 2011). Women in the Italic zones of Italy, for example, the Daunian ladies whose incised stelai depict their ornate tattoos, intricate textiles and jewelry, certainly enjoyed social freedom and formal public display of status, but the phenomenon of dental appliances never operated in southern or Adriatic Italy (see Norman 2009, 2011a, 2011b, 2012, 2016).

We cannot gauge the significance of Etruscan gold dentures from art, since virtually no "normal" people, certainly no aristocratic women, are depicted with open mouths, whether in banquets or other situations. A quick survey of Etruscan art shows an odd blend of naturalism and pattern, with detailed renderings of fine apparel and nature in the background—but certainly no images of golden dentures. The only female creatures with open mouths or teeth showing are the Gorgon Medusa, depicted in the antefixes of the Portonaccio Temple at Veii (*c.*500 BCE, Brendel 1995: 244, fig. 170), or animals such as the wounded Chimaera of Arezzo whose mouth is open in a humanized expression of pathos (*c.*350 BCE, Brendel 1995: 326–327, fig. 248). Animals and monsters show savagery or suffering by their open mouths. A sort of grimace or perhaps a shout is rendered with open mouth and visible (but normal) teeth of the dueling warriors on the Sassi Caduti Temple at *Falerii, c.*480 BCE. A horrific scene from the Seven Against Thebes shows Tydeus savagely biting into the skull of his enemy Melanippos, on the terracotta *columen* plaque that decorated the gable of the temple of Uni-Astarte at Pyrgi (*c.*460 BCE) (Brendel 1995: 246, fig. 171; 234–235, figs 163–164). Warriors who are dying or in a berserk state may show teeth, but never polite members of society.

Greek prejudice and Etruscan equality

From the earliest period of Etruscan culture there appears to have been no gender avoidance associated with dining. Even the occasional one-of-a-kind urn, as early as the seventh century, depicts male and female (probably the married heads of a household) together, seated on chairs or stools. By the sixth century BCE these early formalities shifted to depictions of couples reclining, as the eastern Mediterranean tradition of the male reclining banquet was adapted to Etruscan society (Amann 2001: 146–166, 171–173).

Perhaps the best known reclining images are two sixth-century terracotta sarcophagi from tombs at Cerveteri, each depicting an Etruscan couple; one now in the Louvre and the other in the Villa Giulia Museum (Haynes 2000: 214–215, fig. 176; Brendel 1995: 230–231, figs 158–160; Amann 2001: pl. 33). (See Figure 3.9.) The wives dip out perfume for their husbands who drape an arm about their spouse's shoulders. Each woman has distinctive clothing, jewelry and hat. At other cities, such as Vulci and Chiusi, tombs have been discovered in which similar compositions depict a couple on the lids of sarcophagi or urns.

Etruscan gender relationships are described by the pictorial evidence and by foreign authors. For more than a century most "modern" authors relied on writings by Theopompus, a fourth-century Greek historian. His description of the Etruscan way of banqueting was preserved in the second century CE by Athenaeus of Naucratis, in *Deipnosophistae ("Dinner-table philosophers")* (1961, vol. 5: 328–333 (Book XII, 14, 517d–518b); see Amann 2000: 177–179; Müller 1841–1872, Vol. 2: frag. 204; also Nielsen 1988–1989: 71).

> Theopompus . . . says that it is customary with the Etruscans to share their women in common.
>
> Further, they dine, not with their own husbands [alone], but with any men who happen to be present, and they pledge with wine any whom they wish.
>
> (Athenaeus 1961, 5: 329; see also Müller 1841–1872, I: 315)

Theopompus also has been quoted as saying that Etruscan women take care of their bodies, and exercise nude with one another and with men, perhaps influenced by the Athenian view of Spartan women (cf. Scheffer 2007: 45, n. 46).

Athenaeus (*Deipnosophistai* 1.23d) preserves one other remark, a short quote from a lost work of Aristotle, the *Nomima Tyrrhenōn (Customs of the Etruscans)*: "the Etruscans banquet with their wives, reclining under the same *himation* [cloak]" (see Amann 2000: 176, 184). (A fourth-century sarcophagus from Vulci, now in Boston, depicts this probable marriage ritual of husband and wife beneath the groom's cloak,—grossly misunderstood by Greek observers: Haynes 2000: 290, fig. 233.)

In addition to reclining with their husbands in the presence of others and even *speaking* with others (making toasts), Etruscan women are labeled as displaying other social and implicitly sexual oddities. Among the many Etruscan behaviors that scandalized the Greeks was their mode of depilation (Athenaeus *Deipnosophistai* 12.517–518, see Connor 1968; Livy *Ab Urbe Condita* 1.57; Diodorus Siculus *Bibl.* 5.40; Athenaeus 1961, 5: 332–333).[11] Nielsen (1998: 69, 75) summarizes the literary sources relating to Etruscan women, also citing *Deipnosophistae* Book III, 38: 153d.

More can be brought to bear in the interpretation of these images. McKechnie (1989: 152–153) indicates that only Greek *hetairai* (courtesans) were permitted to be everything that a Greek "wifely woman was not allowed to be—seen in public, present at dinners, property owning and mobile." These freedoms are documented in a fourth-century Greek legal transcript: "The defendant Neaera drank and dined with them [the men] in the presence of a large company, as a courtesan would do" (Lefkowitz and Fant 2005: 73–82). McKechnie's notes (1989: 169–170, n. 131) indicate that *hetairai* also had access to the best Greek wines that generally were denied by male Greeks to their own wives (see Loraux 1993). The exclusion of polite Greek women from feasts dates from at least the Archaic period, as suggested by Murray (1990). The ethnocentrism of those Greeks, when observing Etruscan couples together in various contexts, led them to the prejudicial conclusion that the Etruscans were lacking in appropriate social behaviors (see Bonfante 1981, 1984, 1994).

Gender segregation and ethnographic parallels

Gender segregation, a form of that category of behaviors that in anthropology is termed "avoidance," involves specific cultural rules requiring respectfully avoiding specific sets of interactions with categories of people of opposite gender who are not kin, or who are assigned to specific kinship groups (e.g. "father's sisters"). These rules help to minimize stresses in cases of ambiguous social obligation. One of the most common "avoidance" rules around the world (cross-cultural) involves the relationship between a man and his wife's mother. The well-known and normal stresses in this relationship are specifically avoided by rules in some cultures including complete avoidance (do not speak with, look at, dine with). In contemporary American society, aspects of this "avoidance" survive in its weakest form. What is called a "joking avoidance" in anthropology refers to those weak avoidance relationships in which minor stresses between affines (relatives by marriage) of opposite gender are subjects to be laughed at or ridiculed—like "mother-in-law jokes."

A number of sets or types of gender avoidance were practiced by Greeks and Romans but not by the Etruscans. A well-documented ethnographic parallel comes from modern-era Hawaii. In traditional Hawaiian culture men did not dine in public with women. The arrival of Captain Cook and his crew in 1778 created an interesting problem in retaining, or deliberately invoking culture change. In a deliberate act to force one aspect of culture change on his people King Kamehameha II, shortly after the death of his father in 1819, ate a public meal attended by women. This deliberate breach of an essential taboo was an effort to lead his people (force them) into what King Kamehameha II believed would be a path to modernization. Not surprisingly he soon after ordered a destruction of the holy temples and a burning of the statues of the gods. These acts, perpetrated (or conducted) by the King led to vast changes in traditional Hawaiian society. Various forms of avoidance have remained common in Middle Eastern, Oriental, and other late twentieth-century cultures. In the twenty-first century these avoidances are perhaps best known from Afghanistan and much of the traditional Muslim world. The daily newspapers document the fight between traditions and the modern world.

Etruria and Rome, additional evidence on social customs

Fayer (1994: 396–397) notes that for Roman children, the legal age of puberty for females was the end of the twelfth year, and the end of the fourteenth for males (see also Kajava 1994). These age grades also relate to the status of women in Italy in general. Etruscan society also distinguished women, from birth (to judge from rare infants' epitaphs), with an individual first-name (*praenomen*) such as Larthia or Thanchvil (Tanaquil). This indicates something about their status in contrast to that of, say, Roman women, who by the end of the third century BCE no longer (if ever, in some cases) had a *praenomen*. The individual, given name had been replaced by the generic *gentilicium*, the name of the clan or extended family (thus all daughters of Marcus Tullius Cicero would be called Tullia, etc.—see Kajava 1994: *passim*, including 89–90 and 98–99). The nature of name assignment reflects strongly on status, and may enable us to infer other aspects of the social workings in the society. Noble, or simply affluent, Etruscan women—those who inscriptions show owning businesses, making votive offerings, or receiving epitaphs, could be given two- or three-part names like those of men, and each girl received her own first name, different from any siblings. Another emblem of equality may be the *bulla*, a bubble-amulet worn in Rome only by free-born boys, but in Etruria and some Italic cultures (e.g. the Picenes of the southern Adriatic) worn by girls and women as well (see Turfa 2005: 20, 34 n. 34).

The gender differences between Etruscan and Roman society are quite evident in the tradition of the public banquet. Pedar Foss, in his dissertation (1994a: 45–56), summarized the literary evidence for "Age, Gender, and Status Divisions at Mealtime in the Roman House," (1994b; also 1995). A famous literary example comes from Pliny the Younger, nephew of the great Pliny who died at Pompeii. Pliny (*Epistula* 4.19) does not allow his wife to participate in (all male) poetry readings, but he does allow her to conceal herself from the male participants behind a screen. She is allowed to be "present" and listen, but must not be seen. Such seclusionary screens, extremely common in the Near East during the nineteenth and twentieth centuries, have great antiquity, and examples are known at Pompeii and Herculaneum, in fabric or wood, or represented in wall paintings. Portable screens of wood and fabric provide a means of segregation even in the simplest housing, but usually remain archaeologically invisible. A contrasting image is that of Trimalchio's wife in Petronius' *Satyricon*: she, as a freed woman, a former working member of society, most certainly participates in the famous banquet. Bradley (1998: 38, 47) offers contrasting behavior among women of the Roman imperial families. In Etruria exclusion of females was never an issue.[12]

The reason for dental appliances: tooth evulsion?

The need to use gold limited dental appliances to the affluent or privileged, but since we do not see the phenomenon among other Mediterranean cultures (until the later wire appliances), we must wonder why only the *Etruscan* elite practiced it. One explanation that may fit the meager extant evidence will seem even stranger to modern Westerners unfamiliar with the anthropological literature. The process of tooth evulsion, often described under the ethnocentric heading of "dental mutilation," commonly involves the removal of one or both central incisors of the maxilla and/or mandible. Less common is the further removal of lateral incisors, and even more rarely the canines are included in the process.

The teeth replaced by Etruscan appliances almost invariably are incisors, certainly always the front teeth. Yet the front teeth, incisors and canines, are the last to be lost in old age. (Old skulls may be missing the incisors now, but this comes from post-mortem tooth loss as the bone dries out and teeth loosen. It is easy to tell the difference between an old, healed, socket and one that held a tooth up to the time of death.) During the first millennium BCE and into the Roman Imperial era, anterior teeth would have been the last to be lost to dental disease. Front teeth are not normally lost—barring accidents or sports injuries like modern rugby, or rare cases of brawling, like (perhaps) a man whose body was preserved at Herculaneum.[13] For Etruscan women of the ruling class to lose a front tooth should have been very rare. This strongly implies the *deliberate* removal of healthy teeth by these particular Etruscans; the gaps were soon filled with rather ostentatious "artificial" teeth, either their own teeth with the roots cut off, or replacements carved from other materials (Becker 1995c). This process of dental evulsion—the deliberate knocking out of healthy anterior teeth, usually performed without replacement—is well known in the archaeological (Kennedy *et al.* 1980 on prehistoric India) and ethnographic literature (see Puccioni 1904: 387–388) and is a custom known even today in many parts of the world (Pietrusewsky and Douglas 1992; Merbs 1968, on Arctic groups).

Ornamenting teeth through filing, common in many cultures, seems like a relatively mild process when compared with the deliberate removal of an entire tooth, or a series of teeth. Tooth removal, also known as "dental ablation," is reported with regularity in the anthropological and archaeological literature (cf. Milner and Larsen 1991: 363–364) despite being difficult to identify in ancient skeletal populations. The rarity of this custom in ancient Italian populations may be a function of poor skeletal preservation and recovery. The rarity also might be correlated with such customs as removing a finger joint on the death of a kinsman. The practice of finger-amputation until recently was part of some mourning rituals among the Gende people of Papua New Guinea. In the words of Laura Tamakoshi (personal communication to M. Becker, January 7, 2016), "Both men and women did it but women more often, in part to show that they hadn't caused the death through sorcery and that they were overwhelmed with sorrow." (For illustrations, see http://hand411.com/ritual-finger-amputation-in-papua-new-guinea/, consulted July 1, 2016.) What has yet to be studied is the distribution of tooth evulsion and finger joint removal, to determine if they have overlapping zones of activity.

The list of modern, recorded ethnographic examples of tooth evulsion is extensive (Hrdlicka 1940, for Siberia and America; Suzuki 1982: 38–39, for Okinawa; Cook 1981, for Eskimo examples). Singer (1952) reviews dental ablation from "recent" (modern) groups in Africa. Pietrusewski and Douglas (1992) offer a complete study for traditional Hawaiian society where the custom was part of mourning rituals and has only recently faded.

Sub-Saharan Africa: possible modern parallels

Removal of front teeth has in some cultures been considered aesthetically pleasing and a sign of ethnicity and/or status; in the modern world, however, immigrants to Europe and America are sometimes conscious of a stigmatizing effect. In Sub-Saharan Africa, ritual tooth avulsion has been documented for at least 1,500 years (Morris 1993). Scholars conjecture that it may have begun as a response to tetanus infection: removing a tooth allowed the patient to be given nourishment while s/he suffered "lockjaw." Many generations later, there is no tetanus treatment problem, but rituals have developed to mark the eruption of permanent teeth—by forcibly removing the front teeth as a coming of age ritual. Studies of eighteenth-century burials of enslaved Africans in America have identified some individuals who had undergone cosmetic/ritual tooth extraction (Handler 1994). Until very recently, however, the extracted teeth were not replaced, and the distinctive "Cape Flats Smile" this caused was considered desirable (Morris 1998).

Among the Dinka and Nuer of Sudan, and numerous other African populations, ritual dental extraction was practiced for centuries, and has been studied in recent refugee populations. See Willis *et al.* 2008 for additional references. They state that the condition "has been associated with adulthood, beauty, tribal identity, sound production, and soft food consumption," noting that "as many as nine cultures of Southern Sudan removed anterior teeth during their recent history and specific extraction patterns have become inextricably linked to tribal identity" (Willis *et al.*

2008: 121). Two to eight incisors/canines were extracted, and descriptions of the procedure and its ideology were obtained from (male) patients who sought restorative dentistry once they had settled in the US. In the study, "Refugees reported changes that they considered important to successful resettlement—the ability to eat, speak, and look like members of the host community" (Willis *et al.* 2008: 123). The Sudanese People's Liberation Army outlawed the practice in 1986–1987 to counter ethnic discrimination and genocide, but some groups are believed to still practice ritual extraction.

Willis and colleagues (2008) found that "Contrary to historical accounts, anterior dental extraction is not restricted to males; rather anterior tooth extraction was also performed on females and was essential for the transition to adulthood." For boys the procedure was an affirmation of manhood and they did not cry; one man stated "If the mandibular teeth were not extracted, he could not talk to older boys or any of the girls; he would be considered immature." Extractions were performed by a special individual, the *naak*, with a knife-like implement, and were done rapidly and without anaesthesia.

Agbor *et al.* (2011) studied extraction in populations in Cameroon, interviewing traditional healers and their patients, finding that the most frequent reasons for tooth extractions were ritual extractions and infant tooth mutilations (removal of the tooth germs, see Kikwilu and Hiza 1997; Accorsi *et al.* 2003; Jamieson 2006). Their article gives a good impression of the problems of retention of broken roots and infection that could have affected ancient tooth evulsion. Over half the traditional healers interviewed understood that a successful extraction had to remove all of a tooth's roots; there was wide use of analgesic and anti-inflammatory plants.

Tooth evulsion in ancient Italian populations

The phenomenon seems to be especially deep-seated in Italy, attested as early as the Neolithic period (*c.*6000–2800 BCE). Recently, John Robb (1997b) has applied some interesting statistical techniques to a limited skeletal sample to infer this ancient behavior among Neolithic Italic peoples (see also Milner and Larsen 1991). The loss pattern of anterior teeth, noted in several Italian skeletal studies, has been extensively documented (see Robb 1997b: 665, fig. 2), although exceptions can be identified (Becker 2000c: 61).

We also may rule out violence as a cause of Etruscan incisor loss (cf. Robb 1997a) because of the pattern of loss. Patterns of violence that result in cranial injuries reflect the predominantly right-handedness of most culprits who will inflict injuries on their victims' left sides. This would suggest that the loss of single incisors in Etruscan women, if incurred through violence, would be primarily left central incisors. In fact, just the opposite is true, since where only one incisor is replaced by a dental pontic it invariably is the *right* central incisor. Given the dominance of right-handedness, might the choice of a right incisor represent the action or selection of the woman herself? Did she perhaps point to her tooth with her right hand to consent to the operation as a form of sacrifice?

The possible participation of young Etruscan females in athletic events might be suspected as a regular source of anterior tooth loss, although in the absence of sports like softball etc., the opportunities available to them do not seem likely to have caused such injuries. A lack of first-hand biological evidence prevents us from determining if long bands (about a third of the appliances) served as stabilizers for loose teeth or purely as ornamentation.

Analyses of dental loss patterns are rarely reported in skeletal studies (but see Verger-Pratoucy 1966—prehistoric; Pérez-Pérez *et al.* 1992—medieval Spain). At Tarquinia, where five (25 percent) of the known dental appliances were found, recent research provides us with important information regarding normal dental loss patterns. Becker's skeletal studies of the Etruscan population of the second half of the first millennium BCE (Becker 1990, 1993a, 2000a, 2002b, 2005a, 2006, 2007) revealed that *molar* loss, due to decay, generally began after age 40. Anterior teeth in this population were rarely lost prior to age 60. Periodontal problems, though generally extensive at ancient Tarquinia, seldom reached a degree that might cause loss of the *anterior* dentition prior to age 75 or 80. These findings are corroborated in the small skeletal samples from central Italy now in the University of Pennsylvania Museum (Becker *et al.* 2009: table 6). For the Iron Age through Hellenistic periods, of 11 individuals with front teeth still in place at time of death, 3 were male, and 8 were female. Only one small elderly lady, cremated and buried at Chiusi around 600 BCE, had lost her (lower) front teeth (both canines and a central incisor) almost certainly before death; she had several other dental problems including caries (Becker *et al.* 2009: 72–74, no. 14). (Unfortunately, such samples are few in number, and limited to those levels of society affluent enough to have provided expensive burials for family members.)

North African prehistoric parallels for dental evulsion

One of the earliest known cases of tooth evulsion dates from the Upper Capsian period (Paleolithic/Old Stone Age, *c.*15,000 BCE) of Algeria. An individual had 6 incisors deliberately removed (4 upper and the 2 lower central; Vallois 1971: 204; see also Suzuki 1982: 38). Briggs (1955: pl. 9, 11; based on Briggs and Margolis 1951) provides information from the subsequent North African Mesolithic (Epipaleolithic), indicating that dental ablation can be recognized in almost every population studied, suggesting that the custom was widespread in that region in prehistoric antiquity; it continues to the present. Borgonini Tarli and Repetto (1985: 26–27) also discuss the skeletons that Briggs presented from Taforalt in eastern Morocco and Afalou-bou-Rhummel in Algeria. Briggs suggests that there were variations among these cultures, with some removing only one incisor and others apparently removing all the incisors as well as canines. Briggs (1955: 82–85, pl. XVII) also believes that the evulsion was done between 8 and 11 years of age, or when these teeth had just erupted. If he is correct, these patterns of evulsion were culturally dictated as the child's coming of age was the determining factor, rather than a gesture of mourning prompted by a random death in the family. Brothwell (1963: 120, fig. 47c, also 130) reproduces a drawing of one skull (Morocco: Mechta 8) illustrated by Briggs (1955) showing evulsion of the maxillary incisors. (A whole range of African examples of "avulsions" are listed by Alimen 1957: 339–340.) Jackson (1915) notes several possible examples from Neolithic Britain.

Davide (1972: 583) offers evidence of evulsion from Sudanese mummies. In the ancient Sudan, examples of mandibular incisor evulsion (all four) are known from the Meroitic culture (*c.*300 BCE–400 CE) in the Nile valley. In modern Sudan evidence for evulsion has been gathered by Verger-Pratoucy (1985: 129, also 1968, 1975). Modern Somali men immigrating to America after 2000 often have bridgework made to replace teeth ritually removed when they were younger and at home. Keith (1931) reports that at the late prehistoric (Natufian or Epipaleolithic, 13,000–9800 BCE) caves at Shuqbah in the Judaean hills, 4 of the 5 skeletons in which the palatal area was recovered have evidence of tooth evulsion. These findings from the Levant indicate that this custom extended beyond North Africa, and back into deep antiquity.

China, Southeast Asia: parallels for dental evulsion

Some descriptions from ancient China support other interpretations for the practice of dental evulsion. Ethnographic observations tie the practice to major life events such as puberty or marriage, as well as funerary offerings. Kanaseki (1962: 201) reviews the data. Regional variations are of particular interest; some ethnographic reports attest the practice as early as the Han Dynasty (206 BCE–220 CE), thus nearly contemporary with the Meroitic African evidence cited above. Among the Han themselves the custom was not practiced, although it was known to them (Kanaseki 1962: 202). In other areas of China one or both maxillary central incisors commonly had been removed from males at puberty (age 14–15), and one central incisor of females was removed when they married. Kanaseki's overview reports that the practice of ablation was centered in four districts of southwest China and that all of the practitioners were from various tribes of the Liao and Miao, or among the Li people on Hainan Island. In Wu-ch'I Province, Hunan, the upper right central incisor was removed from females at the age of 15 or 16. This also may have been the age of marriage. In two different areas of the Miao tribe to the south, there is evidence for the removal of two teeth from females before their weddings. However, in Yen-chiao, Szechwan Province, two teeth were removed from the children of the family on the death of their parents. Tooth ablation is also noted in areas of Japan during the Jomon Period (12,000–300 BCE: Hideji 1986; Fujita 1998; Morimoto 1998).

Archaeological evidence from Southeast Asia also indicates the considerable antiquity of dental ablation. Tayles (1996) notes that *c.*4000–3500 BP a high proportion of individuals were missing their anterior teeth. The symmetry in this pattern leads Tayles to suspect deliberate ablation. Many more examples of the phenomenon are buried in notes within the ethnographic literature. The behavior has been relatively common throughout the world. In contrast to the Etruscan situation, however, there is no evidence associated with the Asian or

African examples for the cosmetic replacement of the teeth, until emigration in the modern period.

Europe: Italy, central Europe

Although well documented in the world literature, Etruscan/Italic tooth evulsion had remained unknown prior to the studies of Etruscan gold-band appliances. We infer evulsion as a factor associated with the documented 12 cases in central Italy, and perhaps an expatriate lady in Sardis, who lost one or more front teeth. (Other Etruscan and Italic women who wore gold appliances as braces or ornaments benefitted from the same technology, but perhaps for different reasons.) This would identify the Etruscan evulsion behavior as one of the few examples known from Europe later than the prehistoric period (cf. Whitehouse 1992). Robb's (1997b) meta-analysis of skeletal material from the Italian Neolithic confirms that tooth evulsion was being practiced then, noting, too, that only females were involved. Anterior dental loss that is not easily explained is documented in a few additional cases of burials found in Italy. We will return to the Italian Neolithic below.

At Metaponto (a Greek colony in southern Italy) a high status Roman tomb of the fifth century CE was excavated in the "Castrum 1979" project. Tomb 6 held the remains of an adult male, 2 females and 2 children (Becker 2000c: 61). The principal adult female manifests significant anterior dental loss before death. Although there is some decay in her molars, where we might expect her to have lost teeth, there is no loss of the posterior dentition. Several possible explanations for her anterior tooth loss may be posited, among which is dental ablation.

Medival evidence from Europe may include the wife of Prince Spytihněv I (kingdom of Bohemia, 895–915). Her date of death is not known, but she was buried in a church on the grounds of Prague Castle. Preliminary review of the bones of the principal female in the grave of Prince Spytihněv I (a second woman remains unidentified) indicates an extremely robust woman who died in her fifties (Becker 2000b: 344, *passim*; Becker 2016, in press). All 32 of her teeth had erupted and were in place at death except the mandibular right central incisor and the maxillary right central incisor, lost well before death. Post-mortem damage to the mandible makes the evaluation of time of loss of the lower incisor a problematical endeavor. This unusual maxillary incisor loss may have been accidental, but the possibility of evulsion should be considered since there remained no trace of accompanying injury at the time of study.

Ritual dental ablation is associated with status ranking in some of the ethnographic literature. In most examples dental ablation appears in relatively egalitarian or tribal societies rather than low level states (like the cities of Etruria). One possibility suggested by Morimoto (1998) for incisor ablation is that it renders impossible the performance of certain female tasks that require the use of the teeth as tools (preparation of leather, textiles, rope). Ablation would restrict an elite female from joining in such work, requiring some other agent to perform these tasks.[14] In these cases the deliberate removal of teeth would signal high status, demonstrating the family's ability to provide additional resources.

Like Chinese foot binding, the removal of an ability to perform specific tasks could only be sustained by those whose families had servants or slaves to perform "their" work. Still, we have no indication that Etruscan women, at any level of their society, performed tasks that required the use of their teeth. Nor would Etruscan women, like Tunisian women today, have used their teeth to hold a veil over their faces. What other ritual explanations could have applied?

Mourning sacrifice as an explanation

Frazer's (1910) insightful observation, based on familiarity with the literature from southern Asia, that dental ablation was a sign of mourning remains one of the best general explanations for this behavior. Pietrusewsky and Douglas (1992) provide the most extensive consideration of the cultural "reasons" for the removal of teeth and summarize historical evidence for mourning ritual in old Hawaii. Although the custom had disappeared early in the 1800s, in Hawaii the removal of a tooth was "a sign of mourning for the death of a loved one (*manewanewa*). It also was a sign of respect for the death of someone else's kin, or respect for the death of a ruler." One tooth at a time seems to have been the normal ablation rate, but with many deaths by the time of maturity few men retained any of "the front teeth on both the upper and lower jaw" (Ellis 1979: 120, cited in Pietrusewsky and Douglas 1993: 255). There is some question as to whether the entire tooth was removed or just the crown was knocked off. No archaeological evidence has yet been presented to address this question. In general, ritual ablation seems to be a late feature of Hawaiian culture, and not uniformly practiced by all groups there. Ablation also appears to have been rare or entirely absent throughout the rest of the Pacific, perhaps because ablation emerged with the development of complex social classes on Hawaii.

We cannot yet determine whether the mourning aspects of tooth evulsion can be considered as parallels to the cutting off of finger joints on the death of a relative as documented, even recently, among many tribes of the New Guinea highlands (Gardner 1963). Paleolithic evidence of the practice may also appear in the hand outlines painted on the walls of European caves: some are missing phalanges (Groenen 1987, also Snow 2013). Abundant evidence of Etruscan funerals is depicted in painting and sculpture, including some bizarre practices (whipping, intercourse, defecation, a bleeding prisoner bitten by a dog), but no mourning rites like tooth evulsion appear. In Etruscan society, tooth evulsion might instead reflect some puberty or marriage ritual(s), paralleling (with no direct relationship of course) the rituals known for early China. Note that, as in Etruria, in many of the ethnographic parallels the right maxillary incisor is the tooth of choice.

Leprosy: an unlikely candidate

Readers may imagine another possible etiology: the natural loss of upper central incisors is one of many symptoms that accompany infection with *Mycobacterium leprae*: leprosy! Leprosy (Hansen's disease) causes rhinomaxillary changes (*facies leprosa*) that are pathognomonic (highly characteristic) of the disease (Anderson and Manchester 1992, Anderson *et al.* 1994; Møller-Christensen *et al.* 1952, Møller-Christensen 1961). These changes include the development of a hare-lip, or appearance that looks like a rabbit (from *lepus*, Latin "hare"). Leprosaic changes in the bony tissue of the central maxillary area lead to very early loss of the upper central incisors (Roberts 1986), soon followed by loss of the lateral incisors. However, these alterations make it unlikely that the adjacent teeth could have supported a dental appliance. Furthermore, there is no evidence for the presence of leprosy anywhere in Italy during the first millennium BCE (see Turfa 2012b: 190 n. 119). True leprosy probably arrived in Italy from the Near East sometime after 500 CE, some 500 years after the last apparent use of dental appliances in Etruria. The only example of leprosy that Becker has seen in Italy was in a burial in Cremona dating from between 1300 and 1400 CE (Becker n.d. e).

Functional theories and Etruscan dental appliances

Hoffmann-Axthelm (1985: 78) suggests that the use of dental appliances, in addition to their cosmetic value, may have helped the wearer to maintain normal speech. The deliberate removal of teeth in the first place suggests that these pontics probably had no purpose other than ornament. If the pontics were to fit properly and safely, they would not have been easily removable like jewelry (*contra*, Menconi and Fornaciari 1985: 94). The Talmud, which includes discussions concerning the propriety of a woman wearing a gold tooth on the Sabbath, does imply removability for Late Antique prostheses. Rodkinson's translation of the Talmud (1896, I: 125–126) provides these important data: "as for a metal or a golden tooth[,] Rabbi permits a woman to go out with it, but the sages prohibit it." The discussion continues of "A metal or a gilt tooth" with the following summary: "The difference of opinion only concerns a gilt tooth, for a silvered tooth is unanimously permitted." These lines imply that in Late Antique Jewish culture, silvered and gilded dental items were both removable and ornamental (see also Lufkin 1948: 48). This reference is the only clue we have from the ancient literature to the use of silver as well as gold in dental appliances in Late Antiquity, and both may refer to a metal tooth that has been plated rather than made from pure gold. Alternatively, these references may describe replacement teeth wired into position, for which we have only one piece of archaeological evidence, a single silver wire example (no. W-5, Ptolemaic, from Tura El-Asmant).

The "false" teeth placed in the Etruscan bridges were often fashioned from actual human teeth with the roots cut off (nos. 3, 13, 16, 17, 19, 21). Bliquez (1996: n. 15) suggests that the individual's own teeth, that he believed to have been loosened by periodontal problems and removed by a specialist (cf. Becker 1996), could have been used (see also Guerini 1909: 71–73, 79; Deneffe 1899: 78; Casotti 1947: 669).[15] We agree with Bliquez's sequence except that we suggest that, instead of damaged/lost teeth, healthy teeth were deliberately removed (ablation). The use of one's own teeth, or "recycling," would guarantee a correct color and size match. Bliquez (1996) concludes that recycling the teeth of the wearer is certain in the Praeneste example (no. 17), now in the Villa Giulia. The authors of papers on appliance no. 19, Bracciano, also believe it to have been re-cut from the wearer's original tooth.

Capasso's (1985) suggestion that the teeth of previously deceased individuals might be used as replacements in living persons seems improbable, but see Chapter 4 for the grisly phenomenon of "Waterloo teeth," presumably the stimulus for such interpretations of ancient material. A tooth extracted due to decay could not be used as a substitute in a bridge, but ivory or other products might in some cases serve better than using a recycled human tooth. Bliquez (1996) dismisses Van Marter's suggestion that living teeth might be transplanted from one individual to another, citing a sixteenth-century source as possibly the "first *testimonium* to the practice" (Paré 1585, vol. 17: 26, 621c). That this absurd practice continued among French dentists through the later 1700s is a testament to supposedly modern efforts to restore teeth by methods that simply did not work.

The epigrams of Lucillius and Martial (see Chapter 1) indicate that in Roman dental appliances various substitutes for human teeth could be employed, such as bone or ivory. As just noted, the Corneto II example (no. 12) is said to be carved from the tooth of an ox. The replacement teeth of Liverpool II are missing, as if they had been made of a more fragile material (such as ivory?) than the rooted teeth, which have survived, but this is only conjectural. Brown (1934: 1160) erroneously believed that wood was used for the dentures of President George Washington. Scholars may have incorrectly attributed the use of wooden teeth to the Romans because of Martial's *Epigram* 2.41.7, which actually says that a woman's remaining *real* teeth were *the color of* pine-pitch or boxwood, rather than "made of pine and boxwood" (see Bliquez 1996: Text 10). In the case of George Washington, none of his bridges had a wooden base (Becker n.d. f; see Chapter 4).

The makers of appliances

A good dentist also needs to be an artist. Many aspects of culture, society, and technology were involved in the phenomenon of constructing Etruscan bridge-work. While Etruscan gold-band bridges may have been produced by goldsmiths and perhaps ivory workers, the later, therapeutic wire appliances are the only type mentioned in the medical literature. Lufkin (1948: 48, quoting from Asbell 1943: 4) notes that two types of restorations are cited in the Talmud: the *shen thothe-beth*, which he interprets as an inserted tooth of metal or wood, and the *schen* [sic] *zahav*, a gold or silver shell or crown meant to cover a mutilated or blackened natural tooth. Becker believes that Lufkin's interpretations are fanciful. We have no archaeological evidence for any type of appliance in the eastern Mediterranean other than wire prostheses.

The Talmud indicates that both types of appliances were made by a *naggar*, a worker in wood or metal. A hollow shell type of false tooth only appears in the early Satricum appliance (no. 18), but it is not constructed to fit over a damaged or decayed, rooted tooth, but instead replaces a lost tooth. Etruscan goldsmiths would have fitted or applied the devices as a branch of cosmetology, with only incidental therapeutic value. They would have been quite independent of practitioners who performed extractions—and are not known for ancient Etruria—or physicians who prescribed remedies for diseases of the mouth. Since the predominant reason for the tooth loss among the Etruscan women who wore gold pontics was probably social rather than medical, the cosmetic solution, using gold of greater than 10 carat, would not have required medical intervention. We are even uncertain if the injury resulting from ablation would have had to heal before replacement could be begun.

Etruscan designs and techniques of manufacture

Etruscan gold-work, especially jewelry, has long been recognized for its artistic and technological complexity (see Cristofani and Martelli 1983: 8–16; Gaultier 2013) (see Figure 3.7). Gold dental appliances from central Italy show some of the same metallurgical techniques in their individualized production that are seen in various ornaments from rich tombs. Etruscan appliances basically consist of a long oval band made from a single strip or pellet of gold, or are fashioned from a series of rings each formed from a short gold strip. The oval bands could be formed in either of two ways. One is to take a lump of gold and to pierce it, and then to draw it out by hammering or beating into a rough oval band. By trimming off any excess along the lateral margins, a uniform oval band can be produced (cf. Liverpool I, II, nos. 13, 14). Alternately, a thin piece of gold could be hammered out into a long strip and then formed into a closed oval by joining the ends by fusing or welding. (Soldering, placing molten metal between the two surfaces to be joined, would not be as reliable for use in the mouth, and does not appear in the extant examples.) Fusion by true welding depends on actually melting and mingling both metal surfaces to be joined.

As noted in Chapter 1, future studies of the metals in the gold alloys used for these appliances may help us to understand more than the technology. We may be able to determine conclusively whether the Etruscans had the ability to separate gold from the silver in the natural alloy (electrum) as much as 100 years before the process can be documented in Lydia. To date, gold recovered from the Sardis excavations of a foundry of the time of Croesus, provides the earliest documented examples of the industrial parting process (see Ramage and Craddock 2000a), although the Satricum and Bracciano appliances are older and the two Liverpool appliances might be seventh century also.

For Etruscan examples, a welded band, formed into an oval to closely surround the teeth in question could include one or more false teeth riveted toward the center, as in the Liverpool I example (no. 13). The lateral extremes of the oval band, flanking the false tooth (or teeth) serve as loops to anchor the bridge over the wearer's surviving teeth. For the loop-and-ring series types the lateral loops could anchor the appliance. Central loop(s), often rectangular in section to minimize rotation and obviate the need for a rivet, could each fit tightly over a false tooth. While some authors believe that this type of device could only be used to stabilize loose teeth (Deneffe 1899: 78–80; Bliquez 1996: item "H"), this is not the case. The gold of each link could be pressed tightly to hold a false tooth firmly in place, as is evident from several examples (see our nos. 3, 4, 16).

Quite probably the skilled Etruscan artisans could estimate the size of a tooth, or the length needed for a band, sufficiently well to be able to cut a piece of gold from which they could stretch a flat collar. Certainly there was no need to take a wax impression and make a working model of each tooth on which to fit each loop, as Weinberger (1948: 123) suggests, on analogy to modern procedures. Quite possibly the different widths of the known Etruscan gold bands may relate to the skills of the makers. Alternately the wider examples may have been permanent and the narrower examples designed to be removed. Once again we must note that loss of context has robbed us of the chance to settle such questions.

An historical analysis of the phenomenon of Etruscan dental appliances

The Etruscan appliances derive from a very different, and earlier, tradition of gold-working, and it is only with Late Republican and early Imperial Rome, the first centuries BC and CE, that we see practitioners who certainly did pull teeth and prescribe for oral problems. Over a century ago, several scholars (Northcote 1878: 172–173; Lanciani 1892: 353) noted a fragmentary tombstone of an ancient Roman believed to be a dentist and said to be named Victorinus or Celerinus (only the ending *–inus* is preserved for his name) (see Figure 1.4a). He was buried in the Cyriaca cemetery on the via Tiburtina above the basilica of San Lorenzo fuori le Mura. The supposition that he might have been a dentist derives from the depiction on this stone of a forceps, possibly an instrument of the dental trade (cf. Laviosa *et al.* 1993: 132, fig. V6). His tombstone states, in Greek, that he paid for the monument himself, so we may assume that he was proud of his profession. Lanciani and Northcote also illustrate two inscriptions from the Roman catacombs. One, in the Cemetery of Calepodius (Figure 1.3b) is of an "Alexander" and is carved with a forceps and a tooth. Another, uninscribed (Figure 1.3c), is apparently of a surgeon, with a relief of similar forceps among his many instruments; it was excavated by De Rossi in 1851 in the Catacombs of Praetextatus (Northcote 1878: 172–173; Lanciani 1892: 353 with line drawings; Jackson 1988: 119). Bliquez (2015: 206–207; 239–241, fig. 65) discusses the medical texts that name instruments for extractions, illustrating an imperial-era forceps from Germany. The numerous medical/surgical kits known from antiquity, however, never include the specialized tools that were needed by the goldsmiths who constructed Etruscan-type dental appliances (Künzl 1982; Bliquez 1994). Nor do we find any literary evidence to suggest that dental appliances were fashioned by medical practitioners. It seems that Etruscan culture had a unique place in the use of dental prostheses, and unique social reasons for both their use and the phenomenon that caused elite women to wish to replace lost front teeth. The appliances themselves largely belong to the realm of technology, specifically, metallurgy and goldsmithing.

In central Italy by 600 BCE, the use of false teeth in the form of simple bridges was being occasionally practiced by women of high status (cf. Becker 1990;

Sterpellone and Elsheikh 1990: 59). The gold tooth of the earliest dated appliance (Satricum, no. 18) was cosmetic in function, displaying, whenever the lady opened her mouth, a profusion of gold and of technological expertise. All the other known replacement teeth in these appliances were either modified human teeth or carved from animal teeth or other materials to look like natural human teeth.

The surviving appliances cover a wide spatial and chronological span. Of the meager genuine corpus that archaeological excavation and nineteenth-century collectors have vouchsafed us, we can infer that each surviving appliance was made by a different artisan, most likely on the commission of one woman, or her family. Thus the corpus assembled here probably represents 21 different "patients" and a like number of artisans, ranging over a span of 5, possibly 6 centuries, (seventh to second century BCE). We may be certain of several cities/regions where such devices had been obtained or used, including Bisenzio, Orvieto/*Volsinii*, Bolsena (perhaps), Chiusi, Populonia, and especially Tarquinia in Etruscan territory, as well as Latin Satricum and Praeneste, Faliscan *Falerii*, and Teano, in Oscan Campania. These Italic settlements all maintained strong economic, social and political connections to Etruria.

Several appliances never held replacement teeth and may have been made to stabilize loose teeth by anchoring them to firm ones (Barrett I and II, Poggio Gaiella, Ghent/Orvieto, Bruschi I and III, and Teano, nos. 1, 2, 5, 7, 8, 10, 16). Thirteen, however, served as bridges to insert, essentially permanently, replacement teeth in the front of women's mouths. These represent several regions: Etruria: Orvieto (probably: no. 4), Bracciano, Populonia, Tarquinia; Faliscan *Falerii* (Valsiarosa), Latin Praeneste and Satricum and Oscan Teano. Some other examples have uncertain provenance, but are probably from southern Etruria (Tarquinia, and/or Vulci). We suspect that Vulci was the likely source for the Liverpool appliances. If genuine, then the find from Sardis in Turkey marks the farthest distribution of such devices.

Some of the pontics known today may represent an Etruscan or perhaps Italic custom that was not described in surviving art or literature or known from any evidence beyond these appliances. (Some Neolithic burials of women with missing front teeth might possibly furnish a precedent for the tradition in Italy.) It seems likely, based on the dental health of the known Etruscan skeletal populations, where front teeth are seldom ever lost before advanced old age, that some women of the upper-class living in central Italian cities had one or more teeth deliberately removed, but then replaced with showy gold-band prostheses. A few others got similar devices simply as ornaments or to strengthen loose front teeth. As Danielle Gourevitch (2007: 8) points out, if these appliances were purely functional and used for eating, they ought not to have disappeared after the Etruscan period: Romans, including many men, could have benefitted from such appliances—but the Etruscan gold-band bridges and braces never reappeared after the late first millennium BCE. Instead a wiring system replaced them and it, in turn, disappeared in Late Antiquity.

It appears that, in mid-first-millennium central Italy, certain elite families had a tradition of tooth removal for certain of their daughters or wives, possibly to mark puberty, marriage or some other *rite de passage*, or perhaps some other major landmark in the family's life such as mourning the death of an important relative. To judge from our limited number of samples, Tarquinia might have been the epicenter of this custom, since 5 of the 21 known appliances were found there. The distribution of appliances from north to south, however, suggests that dental appliances of various types were a general feature of Etruscan culture also occasionally found in neighboring Italic regions. Prosopographic evidence, involving the epitaphs of hundreds of Etruscans, demonstrates that Tarquinia was one of the cities where the aristocracy, including the *Hulchnie/Holconii* family known from Etruscan and Roman sources, regularly sent offspring to marry into the leading clans of other cities. At least four of the women with Etruscan-style dental bridges were buried in family tombs in the Italic regions just beyond Etruria proper. Did their golden smiles represent a shared belief system, or perhaps exogamy practiced by noble families who might marry daughters off to the ruling class of other regions? Such dynastic marriages are attested in some burials of the Iron Age and Archaic periods, where the costume and biochemistry of the bones attest to an important man or woman raised elsewhere.

Were Etruscan dental appliances really worn by Etruscans? (A suggestion by Turfa)

This question cannot be conclusively answered based on the meager archaeological evidence, but it raises an important issue. The number of known gold-band dental appliances is surprisingly small, with a mere 19 examples found in Italy (and only 2 others abroad), and they are distributed over several centuries in time. Yet the number of affluent burials already discovered in Etruria and central Italy and reasonably documented must be in the thousands, hundreds of them still containing sarcophagi or urns that once held human remains. Over 4,400 Etruscan epitaphs, not quite half of them for women, have been preserved from family tombs, most for the period of the fourth–second centuries, which overlaps the timeframe of the dental appliances. Even allowing for the depredations of tomb robbers and the possibility that simple gold bands were melted down and seldom sold to collectors in their original condition, the tiny number of appliances must signal a very unusual situation. Is it possible that they were worn not by Etruscan noblewomen like Seianti Hanunia Tlesnasa, but were produced as an Etruscan fix for a non-Etruscan social dilemma? What if a woman, perhaps of the ruling class of an Italic tribal domain, such as the Picenes, Daunians, Peucetians or Messapians of southwestern and central Italy, who had undergone a ritual of tooth removal, married into an Etruscan aristocratic family?

Examples of *Etruscan* exogamy and immigration are already known (on "social exchange" by exogamy, see Bartoloni 2006). For instance, during the eighth century BCE (era of the legendary Romulus and Remus), the Iron Age population of the future city of *Gabii*, in Latium, welcomed a foreign—Etruscan—prince to be their leader. He was buried in Osteria dell'Osa Tomb 600 with full military and civic honors, symbolized by his Villanovan distinctive arms, armor and lavish banquet equipment (De Santis 1995). Associations with a different emerging culture imply Sardinian-Etruscan exogamy. During the ninth–seventh centuries BCE, nearby Sardinia was in constant contact with Etruria, and probably shared artisans and religious cults with the mainland. (Lo Schiavo 2002; Camporeale 2001: 37; 2013; Delpino 2002). It appears from finds, in Etruscan women's tombs, of tiny metal charms in the form of goldsmiths' tools and other ornaments, that metal craftsmen from Phoenician-controlled Sardinia married into the Etruscan families of Populonia (Babbi 2002; Bartoloni 1991: 109–113; Bartoloni *et al.* 2000: 526).

Another potential category of evidence for exogamy in the proto-historic period preceding the advent of writing in Italy is the distribution of a number of distaffs of unique design and execution. During the eighth and early seventh centuries, several women in Etruscan and Italic necropoleis (at Veii, Verucchio, Volterra, Cerveteri, Tarquinia, Vulci, Bisenzio, Sasso di Furbara, Narce, Capena, Rome, Este, and Novilara) over a period of about two generations were buried with a finely constructed bronze distaff. These distaffs were very desirable objects, attributed to a single workshop in Etruscan Felsina (Bologna), yet they are found in burials of several cultures. Their wide distribution may reflect a previously unrecognized and sophisticated trade network or diplomatic circuit, but is more reasonably explained as exogamy: women learn crafts such as textile manufacture from their mothers, and tend to take their personal techniques and tools along with them. (See Gleba 2008: 110–113 type A1; cf. Turfa 2005: 82–83, no. 3; Turfa 2009: 529, no. 18.) Perhaps our estimation of exogamy in Italy is a bit skewed: examples of Etruscans buried away from their home cities, such as men's crested helmets or women's ornaments and tools, may be easier to identify than evidence of Italic ethnics abroad. One Italic (Latin) custom seems to have been burial of a woman who had been a mother with a large metal ring placed over her skirt/ abdomen (see Iaia 2007). Etruscans would have been recognizable abroad by their distinctive costume: for the women, colorful, tailored dresses and elaborate boots with up-turned toes, and by their brooches, the "leech"-shaped *fibulae* (essentially large safety pins) with swollen curved bows. Such fasteners have been identified in Greek sanctuaries and in burials across the central and western Mediterranean and beyond (see Turfa 2012b: 214–215 for more on this).

Blonde women occasionally appear among the aristocratic matrons banquet ing in the tombs of Tarquinia, and also as servant girls in the same scenes (Tomb of the Shields, *c.*350 BCE, Steingräber 1986: figs 146, 147). There are many plausible explanations for their hair coloring, but one would be a non-Etruscan ethnic origin.

In the Cannicella necropolis of Orvieto, for example, a tomb built around 550 BCE was inscribed for its "founder," almost certainly a head of a household, named Katacina: this is a Celtic, Gaulish name (*ET* Vs 1.165). The right to own land, even the mere "footprint" of a tomb, is assumed by scholars to have been a right of citizenship, so Katacina was probably a Gaul, who long before the famous invasion, had emigrated to the Etruscan city of *Volsinii* and been granted citizen ship. *Volsinii* would one day pay dearly for the practice of slavery, when its freed slaves took over the city, leading to conquest by Rome (263 BCE), but in the sixth century society seems to have embraced outsiders of various ethnicities and social classes. Recent excavations in the Campo della Fiera, site of the famous religious sanctuary, the *Fanum Voltumnae*, have unearthed a fine stone-carved base for a votive offering, inscribed with the name of its rich donor. She was Kanuta, a freed slave of the Larecenas family, now the wife of Aranth Pinies, whose name is linked to one of the great ruling families attested in this and other major cities such as Tarquinia (Stopponi 2013: 637, fig. 31.7). Etruscans must have relished happy endings as much as we do.

Other, earlier examples of outsiders embedded in Etruscan families or Etruscans in Italic and Greek families, include the burials of the eighth-century Greek colony of Pithekoussai (on the island of Ischia in the Bay of Naples). There were many families with mixed marriages between Syrian, Phoenician, Etruscan, Greek, Daunian or Campanian Italic men and women—to judge from the burial rituals and special objects (Etruscan brooches or bucchero vases, Daunian painted pottery, Syrian unguent flask, buried in graves containing Greek painted pottery or Greek inscriptions—see Ridgway 1992: 52–54, 67–77, 111–118; 2000). The graves of numerous children of these couples attest many who may have succumbed to the local malaria.

Obviously, the number of foreign, perhaps Italic, brides in Etruria was not great in any one generation; neither is the number of dental appliances. What if a few women had entered Etruscan society who had been born and raised in one of the Italic tribal societies, and had undergone some form of ritual tooth evulsion? Once in the atmosphere of banquets shared by men and women (married couples), in a society where women circulated freely, might they have felt disadvantaged? The gap-toothed appearance that was so respected in their homeland was now a liability. It is tempting to recall the analogy to the modern refugees from Africa, whose facial expressions have been severely altered by tooth evulsion: when they join American or European societies, they seek remedies such as dental implants in order to fit in as new citizens (see Morris 1998; Willis *et al.* 2008; Agbor *et al.* 2011: in some cases, implants and surgery were donated by researchers in return for documentation of the immigrants' dental histories).

The practice of dental evulsion as a life-marker, for puberty, marriage, mourning, etc., seems not to have been common in Italy, but it had been known in several Neolithic communities of the Adriatic shore and central Apennine regions (now Apulia (especially Foggia), Basilicata, and Abruzzi (Chieti, L'Aquila, Pescara)). John Robb (1994a, 1994b, 1997b) has studied the burials of Neolithic Italy and in 30 female cases identified 8 clear-cut examples of adult women who had one or more incisors removed in life. Their burials are scattered across a wide swathe of southwestern and central Italy: Basilicata: Cala Colombo (2 women); coastal and highland Abruzzi: Catignano (Pescara) (1 woman); Grotta Continenza (L'Aquila, 2 women); Lanciano (Chieti) (1 woman); Apulia: Fonteviva (Manfredonia, 2 women). One more case was identified in an old find that could not be sexed, from the great Neolithic town-site of Passo di Corvo (Foggia, Apulia) (Robb 1997b: 660; see map in Robb 1994a: 31, fig. 1). At Catignano, one woman aged 40–50 years had a healed skull fracture that was probably the reason for her two (!) healed trepanation surgeries; she had periodontal disease, caries and apical abscesses and had lost some molars and premolars, but her front teeth were in place—except for an upper right lateral incisor, which had been deliberately removed years earlier (Robb 1994b). In Robb's sample, another older woman (50 years), at Lanciano, had a similar profile of poor dental health and loss of molars and premolars, and two extracted incisors (Robb 1997b). Robb (1997b: 663) suggests that "between a quarter and a half of Neolithic women would have lost incisors or canines during life" due to social traditions. In a compelling set of arguments, Robb (1997b: 664–668) found no collateral damage to indicate domestic violence, and no particular pattern of occupational wear, or poor dental health: the oldest individuals had the worst dental health, but they had much more time in which to neglect hygiene and/or to undergo a tooth ablation ritual. Citing other ethnographic parallels, Robb supposes a social ritual such as commemorating, by the removal of a tooth, mourning, initiation or *rites de passage*. Of course there is no evidence of replacement of teeth in the Neolithic women. Robb suggested the importance for many cultures of creating a cosmetic or aesthetic effect, visually marking the ethnic identity of the woman so treated.

The burials range in time from Early through Final Neolithic, especially the fourth–third millennia BCE. There is thus a wide gap of perhaps two millennia between them and the creation of the Etruscan dental appliances, but studies of relevant human remains for the interim period are scarce—indeed, finds of Italic cemeteries of the Bronze Age and early Iron Age are relatively few to date, so we cannot argue against the continuity or revival of the practice of dental ablation from lack of evidence. Recent studies of Iron Age/seventh–sixth-century BCE Daunian women's images, incised on their grave stelai from the region around Manfredonia, have demonstrated the likelihood of such body modifications as tattooing of the hands on these figures who wear richly decorated and accessorized costumes (see Norman 2011a, 2011b, and 2016. For Etruscans in Italic Campania, see Cuozzo 2013.) The evidence in favor of dental appliances for foreign brides in Etruscan society is only circumstantial, but seems logical, given human nature and traditions of tooth evulsion popping up all over the world at different locations and times. Only in modern, Western society, and in early Etruria, has there been a confluence of both the social impetus and the technological capacity for creating prosthetic devices.

Technical and social aspects

The technology of these appliances is intriguing. Those who produced appliances were extremely talented artisans, probably also possessed of significant "people skills," considering the need to interact with the (aristocratic) dental patient in the lengthy process of construction, insertion and adjustment. The several different goldsmiths who made the Etruscan band appliances probably never knew of one another, nor would they have been trained to make these prostheses, other than learning how to work as goldsmiths. The *earliest* known appliance, the Satricum gold band, has attached to it a gold tooth. This was crafted sometime before *c.*630 BC, when its owner was interred in Borgo Le Ferriere Tumulus C (see Waarsenburg 1991a, 1994). It is the only appliance that features a replacement tooth fashioned from gold, and Turfa believes that it illustrates the idiosyncratic nature of these artifacts. Becker suggests that there was an evolutionary development over the centuries, beginning with a false tooth in gold (Satricum) and progressing to riveted replacement teeth in other, more natural materials. Whether re-use of the wearer's own teeth preceded the use of other teeth or materials cannot now be determined. All of Etruria must have had knowledge that such things could be made, but each artisan worked according to his (or her) own designs and methods. Skills would have been passed on through apprenticeship and observation.

It is important to remain critical of the presentation and interpretations of past finds. Just because an appliance is/has been exhibited in a human skull/jaw does not prove that this was the original owner's skull. Becker's detailed anthropological study of the two surviving skulls now associated with dental appliances (Valsiarosa-*Falerii* no. 15, and Poggio Gaiella-Chiusi no. 5) shows that neither skull is that of the woman for whom the appliance was made! Each one was probably selected by a nineteenth-century preparator as a more attractive or complete example than the original find (if any bones were found) on which to display the gold bridgework. Nor need the skull and appliance be a close match. The Poggio Gaiella appliance was made for an upper jaw, but sometime after excavation was crammed into a mandible, and may have been broken in the process. The Valsiarosa example, likewise designed for an upper dentition, some time ago was inserted into some other woman's *lower* jaw where it long preserved the glue or wax used to force the attachment. This early effort at conservation and display has since been corrected. We also suspect that in several other cases, where human teeth are associated with an appliance, the teeth used may not be the owner's originals (Becker 1994a, 1994b; also Torino *et al.* (1996: 124). The Teano appliance (no. 16) is a notable exception. The teeth surviving all seem to have been original to the appliance and from its original owner.

The recent report of a band-type dental appliance said to have been discovered in a tomb at Sardis (Turkey), now in a private collection in the Ankara area, is published in place within the female skull in which it was claimed to have been found (Sardis, no. 21). The importance of this find is twofold. First, if genuine, it appears to remain attached to the original teeth and they are securely located in a mandible associated with a complete skull. Thus we may have a unique example of the person for whom the appliance was made. Second, the appliance is unequivocally attached to the *mandibular* incisors. Again, if real this would be the first sure example of an Etruscan-type prosthesis in a *lower* jaw. Unfortunately, the looters have deprived it of its historical context. It may have indicated the emigration or dynastic marriage of an Etruscan woman during the early Hellenistic period. If the skull is not that of an Etruscan woman, it may signal a parallel development of dental prosthetics in the Eastern Mediterranean, or the perambulations of an Etruscan-trained goldsmith. (DNA evidence could also be very informative, but of course the specimen has not been removed to a laboratory, and may be contaminated or deteriorating.)

Apart from the curious examples of appliances from Boeotia (Tanagra, no. 20) and possibly Anatolia, the distribution of Etruscan dental prostheses ranges from Populonia on the northern coast, through several major cities of central and southern Etruria. It also extends south and east through the Faliscan and Latin zones down to Campania (Teano), where Etruscan influence and settlement were certainly strong in the later Iron Age and Archaic periods (cf. Cuozzo 2013). The distribution seems concentrated in the region of Tarquinia, where 5 of the 21 examples have been identified. The territories of Orvieto-Vulci-Bolsena/Bisenzio are essentially neighboring and have furnished 3 to 5 examples. We may base some speculation on the numbers of finds with provenance while being mindful that, with such a small sample, a single new discovery could radically change the picture. The distribution may be focused on what de Marinis (1961: 116–117) identified as the Tarquinian artistic region. Certainly this is the area famous for colorful images of women banqueting, in monumental painted tombs of the sixth through fourth centuries BCE. While the prevalence of cremation in some northern areas like Chiusi and Volterra might have eliminated some evidence of dental appliances worn there, we might have expected some evidence to have emerged by now, if the custom was routinely practiced there. (The Poggio Gaiella appliance may have been associated with a Chiusine family that practiced inhumation.) Funerary sculpture in these cities bears out the participation of women in the banquet, but the archaeological data suggests that dental appliances were rare there. We must keep in mind, however, that no images of women with mouths open or exposed teeth occur among the funerary or other portraits of Etruria.

For Etruria we have only the archaeological evidence for the use of gold dental appliances. In contrast, good literary documentation exists for the use of other types of dental appliances of the succeeding eras, in Roman literature and in the literature of Late Antique Talmudic culture, where no actual examples of appliances have yet been identified unless the Judaic texts are referring to wire prostheses. Greif (1918) offered an interpretation of dentistry as practiced in the Eastern Mediterranean based on texts from the Bible and Talmud. The Talmudic corpus, compiled centuries after the Etruscan appliances were made (and buried with their owners), indicates that artisans and turners (workers of wood or ivory) of the Jewish Diaspora produced dental appliances for women and in the same materials (gold, silver). As in the case of ancient Etruria, these artisans were *not* doctors.

The individualized activity of isolated goldsmiths and their clients makes it difficult to discern a smooth evolution of prosthetic technology, and the few cases that are well dated chronologically do not illustrate a single sequence of development. It appears that appliances developed early and with rapidity, implying that a few talented goldsmiths carried their craft to unusual heights. Developed as ornamentation, the design of gold-band appliances ceased after Etruscan culture began to wane as the elites among these people became subsumed into Roman society. The Late Republican–Early Imperial Latin authors reveal the ongoing use of some sort of dental appliances by affluent women. We have, on one hand, examples of early Etruscan appliances, both bridges and braces, but no literary references to them. On the other hand we have Roman writers satirizing the vanity of women wearing false teeth, but with only one actual Roman example; a wire appliance of the first–second century CE (Collatina, no. W-7, see next chapter). One may conclude that Etruscan skills in gold-working, and in particular their ability to make seamless gold bands, and to form a delicately crafted series of rings or loops, enabled them to make dental prostheses of unusual quality and efficacy. The importance in Etruscan society of the status and role of women, who appear to be the principal, if not the only, beneficiaries of these skills, must have been a significant variable in the use of these appliances.

Of the five dental appliances linked to Tarquinia, two were bands (or braces) acting as simple stabilizers of loose teeth and three held false teeth in place. Other braces were found at Chiusi, Orvieto (probably), Teano, and Tanagra in Greece. Of the 8 stabilizing appliances, 6 were the long-band type, and 2 were formed from individual rings. The distribution of the 13 appliances holding replacement teeth was about even in terms of technique: 7 were formed of bands, 6 were ring types. Judging solely from the condition and design of the pontics, 7 of the 13 wearers had lost a single front tooth, almost always an upper central incisor. Five women had to replace two front teeth (Tarquinia, Praeneste and Sardis, plus the two Liverpool examples). Only one person, also a resident of Tarquinia, had lost three front teeth to be replaced with a ring-type pontic utilizing carved animal teeth.

The choice of ring- or band-design for inserting replacement teeth was about even, perhaps reflecting the decision of the goldsmith. Ring construction would serve well to brace loose teeth, but the difficulty of fabrication and insertion may be why only 2 of the 8 examples used that form. The majority of designs are the familiar, simpler bands. Apart from the foreign finds at Greek Tanagra and Lydian Sardis, the outliers spatially were at Populonia, the northern and only coastal city of Etruria, and Teano, an Oscan enclave north of the Bay of Naples. Both are ring designs, Populonia to replace one incisor, and Teano a long stabilizing band. The possible examples from the region of Orvieto and Lakes Bolsena and Bracciano (nos. 1–4, 7, 19) are almost evenly divided between ring and band designs, and between functions: replacement or stabilizer. But, with the possible exceptions of the 2 examples now at Liverpool (nos. 13–14) and the 5 from Tarquinia (nos. 8–12), none of the appliances can have been made by the same craftsman.

What were these people doing with their teeth to cause loosening? The lack of even the most basic skeletal data related to ancient dental appliances leaves us in the realm of speculation. Given our knowledge that natural loss of incisors for Etruscan women was highly unlikely, we have to consider that this handful of gold appliances has alerted us to some tradition of considerable importance but for which even a simple description, let alone rationale, has been lost along with any Etruscan literature. The evidence clearly attests to the fact that Etruscan gold-smiths of the first millennium BCE were capable of performing specialty projects like replacing or bracing strategic teeth. They had the design capability as well as the metallurgical skill. The really unusual aspect of this uniquely Etruscan phe-nomenon is the *cause* for replacing someone's front teeth—what life-changing event(s) caused these women to lose or sacrifice their front teeth? The gold in their smiles was a testimony to their family's affluence and power, and perhaps, too, a reminder of some special sacrifice made by the woman, her own version of the bravery of a man in battle, perhaps, offered for some landmark in her life or her family's posterity.[16]

Notes

1 LazioTV1, October 24, 2012: "Scoperto un nuovo sito a Lanuvio, sorpresi 4 tombaroli," www.youtube.com/watch?v=Nxo9WMJlhzQ (consulted August 2, 2016).
2 Following Becker's studies of the known appliances, Turfa has examined and measured the Liverpool appliances, thanks to the kind help of Cynthia Reed, goldsmith and archaeologist, Dr. Georgina Muskett of the Liverpool World Museum and Dr. Margarita Gleba (McDonald Institute for Archaeological Research, Cambridge University). With Cynthia Reed, Turfa has also viewed the appliances on display in the Museo di Villa Giulia and Tarquinia Museo Nazionale.
3 Molars seem to be the first to go in many populations and all periods. For example, the medieval and early modern "population" buried between 1120 and 1539 at the site of the medieval priory of St. Mary Spital ("Hospital," now the London area of Spitalfields) showed the highest frequency of loss to first molars, then to second and third molars, due to the high frequency of carious lesions in these teeth (Connell 2012).
4 Hardness 2.5–3 (Mohs); specific gravity 19.3; melting point 1064°C. One gram of gold can be beaten into a sheet 1 meter square—see Giardino 2010: 145–160 for full description.
5 Especially the Colline Metallifere ("Metal-bearing Hills") and Tolfa region near Cerveteri, and the region bordering Bisenzio and Narce, also areas where a dental appliance has been found.
6 Certainly early Etruscans and Italics were aware of the effects of the high heat of a pyre (temperatures of over 900°C; see Becker 1998b) on metals, for they usually did not consign precious metals and bronzes to the fire, preferring to bury them intact. Only a few fibulae, probably used for modesty in securing garments on the deceased, and the rare status symbol, perhaps clutched in the hand, like a woman's ornamental distaff, might be burned on the pyre. See Becker *et al.* 2009: 103–104, for metal objects deliberately reserved from the pyre, in burials at Vulci and Narce.
7 Placer gold can be mined from stream beds or panned as nuggets from streams.
8 A "rivet" to secure a false tooth should not be confused with a "pivot" tooth. In English the term "pivot tooth" generally is understood to indicate that a "post" of metal has been inserted into the surviving root or stump of a tooth prepared to serve as the mount for a false crown (see Appendix I.E). Baggieri and Allegrezza (1994: 5) use the Italian term *pernino*, a technical term for a small pin. Since this device requires that both ends (heads) of the rivet be hammered down to expand the gold rod over the margins of the holes through which it passes, a more appropriate term in Italian might be *ribattino*.
9 Mallegni *et al.* (1980) searched for sexual dimorphism in the seventh- to sixth-century BCE population of a necropolis at Pontecagnano, Italy. This team evaluated dental size and asymmetries, but averaged the data prior to analysis rather than presenting individual measurements (Mallegni *et al.* 1980: 113). As one would expect, the averaging resulted in homogenizing the findings and failed to document dimorphism. Since the primary measurements were not provided, Mallegni's information cannot be retested.
10 Cheese graters became a symbol of the punch of hot wine, spices and cheese served to banqueting warriors, as attested in the *Iliad* and imitated in Iron Age-Archaic Italy: see Turfa 2005: 103–104, no. 34; Ridgway 1997.
11 The comment about Etruscan women shaving their bodies may be another Greek fantasy. Curiously, a fragmentary skeleton shipped from a tomb at ancient *Falerii* (Civita Castellana) to the University of Pennsylvania Museum in 1900 included a sample of cloth and hair from the skull; the excavator's accompanying letter noted that the intact

skeleton when revealed still retained both head and pubic hair. Overnight most of the skeleton disintegrated and only the skull, a sample lock of hair and fragment of the head covering were saved. See Turfa 2012b; Becker *et al.* 2009: 64–67.Vases date the tomb *c.*350 BCE, just the era of Theopompus.

12 The Cortona Tablet, a bronze plaque recording a mortgage and sale of land, names a woman among the participants (Bonfante and Bonfante 2002: 178–183; Benelli 2002), while several "princely" tombs of Etruria and neighboring regions held chariots or carts belonging to powerful women (Galeotti 1986–1988); even occasional burials of the proto-Etruscan, Villanovan culture (ninth–eighth centuries) included a model ship in the funeral of a woman, believed to indicate her control over a real longship in life (cf. Hencken 1968: 30–31, 48, 136, pls. 76–77). In contrast to other regions, there seems to have been a high rate of literacy among women in Archaic Etruria, when the alphabet was still a novelty elsewhere. (Turfa 2012b: 215–216, 220–223; see Rallo 1989a, b.)

13 The 40-ish soldier, carrying a sword and digging tools, was on the beach trying to right a boat for escapees when he was struck down by the flaming cloud of 79 CE; his missing three incisors led Luigi Capasso to surmise that he had lost them in a fight (Capasso 2001: 249–258, no. E26).

14 While there is no evidence of Etruscan female skeletons with such tooth-wear, one man's teeth show excessive wear of the upper incisors, interpreted by Mallegni *et al.* (2005: 84–85, fig. 6) as evidence that this sailor used his teeth in spinning and repairing rope. He died tragically, his arm stretched out to his dog, both trapped by a spar when his small cargo ship sank in a storm in the harbor of Etruscan Pisa during the reign of Augustus. Lazer (2009: 218) discusses evidence for lifestyle or "industrial use of the teeth" in the human remains found at Pompeii, noting with caution Capasso's (2001: 1042) identification of 18 cases at Herculaneum of possible fishermen with worn teeth. Liston (2012: 134–135, fig. 9.3) indicates use of anterior teeth to hold fibers during spinning as a possible reason for excessive wear in the skeleton of an Early Iron Age woman buried in Epirus, Greece.

15 Although it is more likely deliberate evulsion, as periodontal disease would have affected potential anchor teeth, making the pontic unusable.

16 If women of other classes, not able to replace lost teeth with gold, did engage in the practice of tooth evulsion, how would we know it? We lack Etruscan literature and direct archaeological evidence for commoners is sparse. The skeletal data that would provide the best, if not conclusive, evidence for dental evulsion simply has not been recovered, and little effort is now being made to change the needed field techniques. As Robb pointed out, the custom of tooth evulsion, undertaken for whatever reason, was in operation in parts of Italy as early as the Neolithic period. We do not find many skeletons missing their front teeth in the common burials of first-millennium, i.e. Etruscan, central Italy but that's because almost no skeletal material is recovered. Robb noted (1997b) that the women with ablated teeth seemed to be slightly older at death, perhaps indicative of a different status or of better than average access to resources. He also noted that trepanation was much more frequent in men than women in those same populations, perhaps reflecting a different form of (sacrificial?) ritual for males. More documented finds of human skeletal remains could significantly affect our understanding.

4 Dental appliances and dentistry after the Etruscans, to the present day

The later use of dental appliances by Romans is known from several references in ancient literature, ranging from the fifth-century BC law code of Rome to poets of Gold and Silver Age Latin such as Horace and Martial (see Chapter 1), yet, with one exception (no. W-7), there is no firm *archaeological* evidence to illustrate this (see Bliquez 1996). So familiar were the tropes of Romans with "false teeth" that Guerini (1904) surveyed the Latin literature and later erroneously suggested (1909: 100) that by the Late Republic full sets of removable dentures were being produced, a fantasy that Bliquez (1996) rightly dismisses. The earlier gold-band appliances appear to have been made by and for Etruscans or their Italic (especially Latin and Faliscan) neighbors, whose cities came to be absorbed into the rapidly expanding Roman state. The Roman false teeth satirized by the poets might have been developed from Etruscan technology that by the Late Republic (last centuries BCE) and Empire was centuries old, but none of that type have yet been found. The seven wire appliances of the Hellenistic and Roman era are quite different in technique.

We really should expect to have found more than a single example of the Roman dental appliances by now. Surely a *need* for bridges often arose, but if a *demand* had existed, then later examples ought to have appeared in archaeological contexts. Some prostheses may have been removed before burial, but most of those known have been looted from graves and Roman law actually permitted the burial of gold dentures with the corpse. The reasons for the extinction of Etruscan-style dental appliances appear to lie with changes in the cultural demand for these items, and not in the decline of gold-working technology.

A survey of the seven wire appliances from Rome and the Eastern Mediterranean/Levant

W-1. Sidon I (sometimes labeled Gaillardot): from a fourth-century tomb at Sidon, one of the great cities of Phoenicia, found on the skeleton of a woman. Gold-wire pontic, approximately 34 mm long in its present condition, was used to replace both of the wearer's own mandibular right incisors using wires that pass through two holes drilled front to back (buccal-lingual) in each tooth.

Three widths of wire (generally) surround all six teeth, and were tightened by running wires between the teeth and then pulling the external horizontal wires in towards the center. Where and how the ends of the gold wire were tied off is not indicated by any illustration. (Figures 5.22a–b)

W-2. Sidon II (sometimes labeled Ford, or Torrey): from an anthropoid sarcophagus (a type reserved for elite nobility) found in a Sidonian tomb, on the skeleton of what was said to be a middle-aged man. This gold-wire retention device was woven around and between six teeth, probably the mandibular canines and incisors. The detailed pattern of this wiring, made from a single gold strand over 100 mm long, offers a paradigm for how the Sidon I (Gaillardot) example was made. (Figures 5.23a–b)

W-3. Alexandria (lost?): from a tomb of the Roman era at Alexandria, Egypt, first century CE. Thin gold wire, a millimeter or less in diameter, has been used to stabilize a mandibular left lateral incisor by binding it to the two adjacent teeth. No holes are drilled in any tooth; the wire may now be incomplete. (Figures 5.24a–c)

W-4. El-Qatta (current location uncertain): found in a millennia-old Egyptian mastaba tomb that had been re-used in the Roman era. The two pieces of gold wire that are assumed to have been part of the same appliance now are associated with three maxillary teeth. A right canine is surrounded by two loops of gold wire, twisted closed at the distal side. A right lateral incisor is surrounded by a single loop of wire, which then passes through a hole drilled laterally through a right central incisor that has been cut down for replacement in this jaw. The appliance probably originally encircled the now-missing left central incisor for use as the other anchor tooth. The fact that the root of the drilled tooth has been filed down suggests that it was intended to re-place a central incisor in the Etruscan fashion. (Figures 5.25a–d)

W-5. Tura El-Asmant (current location uncertain): found in a Ptolemaic necropolis south of Cairo, perhaps on the skeleton of a young man with very poor dental health. This Etruscan-like bridge supports a replaced maxillary right central incisor, with root filed down, between its natural adjacent teeth. The re-placed tooth has had two holes, one above the other, drilled through the mesial-distal aspects. A single silver wire, about 75 mm long, passed around one anchor tooth, with both ends then passing through a single hole in the re-placed tooth and dividing again to surround the opposite anchor tooth where it was then twisted closed. A second silver wire, of similar length, passed in the opposite direction at the level of the second drilled hole and parallel to the first wire, similarly passing around the opposite anchor tooth and tied off with a twist. These two wires at no point were in contact. (Figures 5.26a–d)

W-6. Eretria (not available): from the fourth-century BCE tomb of a woman(?) in a necropolis outside the city of Eretria. The poor original drawing and subsequent unavailability of this gold-wire appliance render difficult any efforts at description. This appears to have been a classic use of wire to stabilize loose teeth, but whether the four teeth apparently depicted were original to this artifact is another of the many unknowns. (Figures 5.27a–b)

W-7. Collatina (Rome): excavated in a tomb of the Collatina necropolis on the edge of Rome, worn by a woman in her fifties of the first–second century CE. Her body had been incompletely cremated (a common condition in this era) but preserved the appliance. This simple gold-wire dental prosthesis holds one re-placed tooth, a right central incisor, in an otherwise normal mandible. It is fashioned from a single length of gold wire, less than 1 mm in diameter, with an estimated length of perhaps 100 mm. The wire passes around two teeth on each side of the single "replacement" or re-placed tooth. The replaced tooth is held in place by one (or two?) wires passing through a mesial-distal hole. (Figure 5.28)

In most of these cases, while the appliances had been found on the wearer's skeleton, it appears that only in the recent case of the Collatina discovery in Rome (W-7) were the complete human remains preserved for study. Four of the seven appliances, nos. W-2, -3, -4, and -6 (Sidon II, Alexandria, El Qatta and Eretria) functioned to stabilize teeth that must have been loosened in the jaw; only three, Sidon I, Tura El-Asmant and Collatina (W-1, -5, and -7), actually anchored false teeth (probably those of the wearer, returned by drilling and fastening with wire to live teeth). The use of gold wire to consolidate loose teeth sounds like the procedure for trauma detailed in the Hippocratic corpus (*On Joints* 32) and reiterated by Celsus (*De medicina* 7.12.I.F), although the skeletons have not been described or subjected to testing such as radiography or MRI to determine any other evidence of injury. The ancient medical texts are silent on the notion of replacement of the owner's lost teeth in this fashion. (See Chapter 1 for these texts.) The practice of wiring loose teeth was obviously known to the Greek world, although we find the physical evidence of its practice nearly simultaneously in the Levant, with the Phoenician burials of the fifth–fourth century BCE and in Eretria in Greece; the practice, and the related technique of wiring in replacement teeth, continued into the Ptolemaic and Roman eras. The Collatina (no. W-7) appliance was well preserved in the mandible of a middle-aged woman with periodontal disease, in spite of her body being cremated (the requirements of fuel and time for a thorough cremation seem to have led to many such situations). If this thin wire appliance could survive cremation, then the fact that we find so few of them may imply that the use of gold appliances in any era was quite rare, and that the Roman satirists who mocked them were reaching pretty far for their laughingstocks.

The Levant and the Islamic world

While complex dental bridges seem to disappear in the Mediterranean sometime during the early centuries of the Christian era, a parallel, although uncommon, use of *wire* devices began sometime around or after 400 BCE in Egypt, the Levant and the eastern Mediterranean and continued into the era of Islamic dentistry. The wire appliances are listed in Table 5.11 (see Chapter 5), and only seven are known. No actual Hebrew examples are known, yet there is rich textual evidence for their use in this culture, although the origins of such dental appliances are less clear. The extensive data from Talmudic literature, formulated since the Babylonian captivity (about 586 BCE), clearly indicates that dental appliances were well known among the ancient Hebrews (see Nobel 1909; Engelmayer 1964; and Preuss 1971: 329–333). The *Sabbath Rules* of *c.*300 BCE are believed by Hoffmann-Axthelm (1970: 82) to mention dental replacements of gold, silver, and natural materials. He also interprets these texts to indicate that such appliances were worn only by women.

The Jerusalem Talmud (*c.*370–390 CE) and the Babylonian version (352–427 CE), which is now accepted as the general standard, refer to teeth made of (bound with?) silver, while the Mishnah notes teeth made of gold (Preuss 1971). Zias and Numeroff (1986b: 66, n. 7) conclude that, because the Talmud discusses dental prostheses under the category of women's ornaments, this indicates that the Hebrews were maintaining the tradition of using dental bridges for cosmetic purposes. The archaeological evidence for dental wiring in the eastern Mediterranean suggests that these Hebrew appliances may have been primarily functional.

The source of the Hebrew tradition in dental prostheses is unclear, and we cannot determine whether it followed a tradition of earlier Phoenician wire appliances, or if the Hebrew technology was influenced by the gold-band techniques that the Etruscans developed in Italy. Wire as well as ribbon appliances can be used for cosmetic and also functional purposes. Most of these skills appear to have been lost in the Western world by Late Antiquity.

The use of gold or silver wires, rather than bands, to brace teeth or hold replacement teeth in place appears to be a Near Eastern or Eastern Mediterranean technique. Examples of wiring indicate that this was a wholly separate tradition from the Etruscan band appliances, both in technique of manufacture and in goals. Wire appliances from the Eastern Mediterranean world appear to have been continued in the Hebraic medical tradition, which in turn was absorbed within the Islamic world. Dechaume and Huard (1977: 20–26, pls. 5, 6) summarize the history of Arabic dentistry. Their illustrations from manuscripts (1977: pl. 6, fig. a) of Arabic wire appliances, however, are sparsely referenced.[1] Brown (1934: 829), citing a biography by Muhammed Ibn-Sad, notes that Othman, the third Calif of Islam (574–656 CE), is said to have had false teeth fastened to his own teeth with gold. Presumably the attachments were made of gold wire. The Arabian method of ligating loose teeth with gold or silver wire is described by Abulcasis *c.*1100 CE (Brown 1934: fig. 2, from the Leclerc translation of *De Chirurgia*, 1861, fig. 63).

Islamic dentistry, including the wiring of teeth, appears to have spread to India with the Muslim expansion in the twelfth century (Guerini 1909: 30, figs 5, 6; Brown 1934: 835). Grawinkel (1906) provides a particularly useful review of Indian dental medicine, with illustrations of wired teeth (see also Casotti 1927: 626, figs 2–3). The usual pair of figures illustrating "Hindu" wired teeth are reproduced by Karl Sudhoff (1926: 52, fig. 35). Modi (1931: 10) notes that in India the ligatures used to stabilize loose teeth or to create pontics continued into modern times. Modi (1931: 10) also states that, even in 1931, "there are some jewelers who specialize in the operation." Of particular interest is the implication of jewelers or goldsmiths, since we have seen that goldsmiths had been responsible for the Etruscan prosthetics.

China and amalgams

These methods of wiring or tying teeth spread from India to China, and continued in use at least into the nineteenth century. Kerr (1894: 198) reports the late nineteenth-century use of a section of bone cut from an ox femur to imitate 3 to 4 lost teeth, held in place by copper (?) wire passed through holes drilled in either end of the pontic, and tied to sound teeth. The going price for this Chinese bridgework at that time was 25 to 30 (American) cents.

Much more sophisticated dentistry was practiced in China at a very early period. Dental fillings, made from a tin-silver alloy, are noted in a Chinese text of 659 CE. The precise composition of this material was recorded as early as 1505. By the end of the sixteenth century amalgams were in common use in China. The formula for these, involving a tin-silver amalgam, may be the same one that was brought to Europe from China in 1826 (see below; Czarnetzki and Ehrhardt 1990: 326).

Renaissance Italy and Europe

Arculanus (Giovanni of Arcoli, a professor of medicine at Bologna, Padova and Ferrara, 1412–1484) in his *Practica* (1480) is believed to have referred to the use of gold foil to fill carious teeth (cf. Dechaume and Huard 1977: 26; Muratori 1968; Bazzi 1968).[2] Most authors accept that Italian dentists of the fifteenth century were aware of this technique. By the fifteenth century the simple gold foil technology was available, and appropriate theory regarding the etiology of dental decay was in place (the notion of cleaning out the "tooth worms"). The possible use, or even the consideration of the use of such a technique, by Arculanus would be the earliest Western literary reference to any type of gold filling technique.

Another early report of the use of gold in any aspect of "early modern" European dentistry is Tallat von Vochenberg's 1530 publication (Figure 4.1), which speaks of filling teeth with gold (chapter 5, pp. 22–23 q.v.). Verification of the use of a gold amalgam in dental fillings in the late 1500s is now available through archaeological evidence from a site, the Johanneskirche, excavated in Crailsheim, Germany (Czarnetzki and Ehrhardt 1990: 326). Thus the written evidence correlates quite well with the documented use of gold in some form (for the ruling classes) by the end of the 1500s, a period that predates the commonly known use of gold as a dental filling material by over 200 years. The development of modern uses of gold in dentistry continues to be an attractive area for research.

The use of both gold foil and tin amalgam fillings before 1600 in Europe has been documented through an examination of the teeth of Anna Ursula (1572–1601) daughter of Duke William the Younger of Brunswick-Lüneburg and Dorothea of Denmark, who died in 1601 and was buried in Crailsheim (see also Chapter 1). Her right first upper molar had both types of fillings. Czarnetzki and Ehrhardt (1990) suggest that the amalgam may have been compounded according to a Chinese prescription that may date back to the seventh century CE (they cite Li 1596 and Hung-Kuan-Chih 1954). Czarnetzki and Ehrhardt (1990) also note

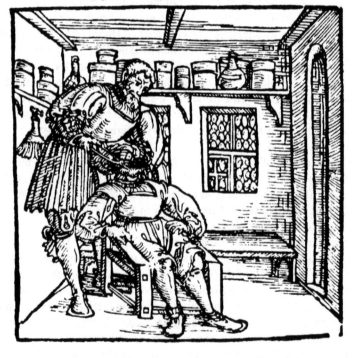

Figure 4.1 Woodcut, frontispiece of Johannes Tallat von Vochenberg's *Artzney: Buchlein der kreutter, wider* [sic] *allerlei kranckeyten und gebrechen der tzeen.*

Source: Auspurg: H. Steiner, 1530. Alamy, image BJW915.

that the use of gold foil to fill tooth caries, documented here for the later sixteenth century, was described in a Latin dissertation more than a century earlier (Stocker *et al.*1657). The practice of using gold foil was well known by the late 1700s.

In the West, after the Middle Ages, the traditional art of tooth pulling became the core of the rapidly expanding field of dentistry (see Šmelhaus 1938, 1939). The first modern mention of artificial teeth derives from Guy de Chauliac, who around 1363 wrote a medical treatise that was published using the new printing-press technology in 1478. Much of his work is directly taken from Abulcasis and other Arabic writers (Brown 1934: 836, 959; see also Geist-Jacobi 1899; Casotti 1933, 1935). The development of modern bridges and plates appears to relate to de Chauliac's work, as demonstrated by the archaeological discovery of a bridge dating from the sixteenth or seventeenth century, cited by Czarnetzki and Alt 1991. A replacement for the maxillary incisors carved from hippopotamus (?) tusk had been wired into place in the mouth.[3]

Ambrose Paré (1585) noted the replacement of lost teeth, by various means, at the end of the Middle Ages (Dechaume and Huard 1977: pl. 48, fig. 2). Paré's writings (see Dechuame and Huard 1988; see also Chapter 1, Figure 1.5) plus these recent archaeological discoveries indicate that simple wiring practices, at least, were retained in the European dental repertoire (see Cohen 1959: 776). The best archaeological evidence confirming Paré's (1585) written description of dental practices derives from a series of graves, and corroborating documents, from the Church of Saint-Hippolyte in Grand Sacconex [sic] near Geneva. Ivory bridges spanning, or replacing, up to nine teeth were found held in place with gold wires. Other complex gold wires were used to hold six or more loose teeth in place (Alt and Newesely 1994). The identification of the types of materials used in these bridging appliances, whether ivory, hippopotamus tusk, or bone, has been discussed by Cohen (1962).

During the Renaissance we find clear evidence for the revival of several other aspects of dental skills (see Piperno 1910), together with the development of new techniques and a scientific approach to dentistry. By the 1600s the manufacture of false teeth had become a major business in many parts of Western Europe, apparently relating to Renaissance developments in aesthetics and technology. Periodontal disease has long been recognized as one of the common disorders associated with aging. By the early seventeenth century Ben Jonson (1607) has his comic figure Volpone refer to the problems associated with receding gums, a common symptom of periodontal disease, in the context of his description of a quack cure-all. The character notes that the use of this "powder" purportedly kept Venus young because it:

> clear'd her wrinkles, firm'd her gums, . . . in age
> restores the complexion; seats your teeth, did they dance
> like virginal jacks [musical keys], firm as a wall; . . .
> (*Volpone* Act II, scene ii: 227, 235–236)

An earlier reference by Volpone's dwarf, descriptively named Nano ("Dwarf" in Italian), has him note that good health includes being "Stout of teeth, . . ."

(*Volpone* Act II, Scene ii: 187) and clearly reflects these virtues as among the more generally desired human characteristics. This mirrors the tragic, aging aspects of periodontal disorders, which are all too common now as in antiquity. By 1600 preventative treatments were no more effective than those used by the ancients, but the production of replacement dentures had become a major industry and some restorative treatments were being used.

The seventeenth century was also witness to some significant developments in dental prosthetics (Platschick 1904–1905: 243; Casotti 1933, 1935 provides some good illustrations). These new types of prosthetic devices, in the form of full sets of dentures, had become quite commonly employed by the beginning of the eighteenth century. Fauchard, the great French technician for whom the museum of l'Ecole Dentaire de Paris is named, was among the outstanding early practitioners of this art.

The eighteenth century and later

During the eighteenth century, when we see the decline of the tooth-worm theory of dental decay (Gorelick and Gwinnet 1987b), numerous published documents attested to a variety of procedures for the replacement of lost teeth. Wired dental prostheses became generally available by the 1750s (Duval 1808). The well-known silversmith-patriot, Paul Revere, is much less well known for his gold-work, which included the fitting of false teeth. Revere advertised in the *Boston Gazette* (September 19, 1768) that he could refasten false teeth that had become loose (Verger-Pratoucy 1995). Whether he was using gold wire or adjusting an anchorage is not known, but the procedure suggests that enterprising goldsmiths were involved in this aspect of dentistry in colonial America just as they had been in ancient Etruria.

Prosthetic devices included those supposedly made in 1796 by John Greenwood of Philadelphia for President George Washington of the new United States of America. Four examples of Washington's dentures, together with his last extracted tooth, are housed in the National Museum of Dentistry in Baltimore (Sutter 1996: 19; Becker n.d. f; also see Appendix II.E). Most of these appear to have utilized wiring techniques rather than gold bands. Greenwood's appliance is said to have been carved from the tusk of a hippopotamus, into which human teeth were fixed in place with gold rivets similar to those used by the Etruscans (Sissman 1968: 11, fig.).[4] It has become a trope in modern American history to say that George Washington had wooden teeth, but despite other descriptions that suggested wood was employed, none extant are of wood (instead they are of ivory and gold: it seems that Washington had more than one such appliance fashioned for himself).[5]

By 1793 sophisticated porcelain and gold appliances had been introduced to the public in London (Dubois de Chemant 1788, 1797 (English translation); see also Dechaume and Huard 1977: pls. 49–53). No traces of these eighteenth-century porcelain replacements, or of any appliances from this era, are as yet known from the archaeological record. A large cemetery recently excavated in

Wilmington, Delaware by MAAR Associates includes a number of individuals with dentures or pontics, but most of the graves date from the nineteenth century (Ronald Thomas, personal communication). None of the pontics from this site have yet been studied, but eighteenth-century examples may be among them. The nineteenth-century appliances also warrant review.

Published advertisements for "dentures" of this period are plentiful, providing good evidence for their presence and variety. Obviously, specific details regarding the form of the appliances are today lacking, although we do know the approximate costs of some English examples, taken from a list of fees dating from 1781 (Purland 1858, II: 492). These fees included the costs for "constructing and fitting an artificial tooth with silken ligatures" (at "0/10/6," that is, no pounds sterling, 10 shillings and 6 pence), "ditto with gold-wire fastenings (0/15/6)." The cost of fitting a "human tooth" in place was 2/2/0, while "ditto with gold-wire fastenings" was 2/7/0. (Presumably the "human tooth" was that lost by the original owner, but other possibilities come to mind . . . and the human teeth set into the Liverpool I appliance (no. 13) may have been trimmed from incisors larger than those of the small woman who was to wear them . . .)

Duval (1808: 9–10) indicates that French dentists of his day were aware of the ancient, Classical medical literature on the use of "gold wires" to fasten an artificial tooth in place. "Wire" was commonly used in dental appliances from the seventeenth through nineteenth centuries in France and the nearby regions of Europe. The fabrication of the complex prostheses being produced in the 1800s, however, had required some time to be redeveloped from their Classical prototypes. By the mid-nineteenth century functional appliances held in place by gold wires or fiber "thread" had become common for those who could afford the price (Hockley 1858).

Note that the use of gold-wiring techniques did not end in the nineteenth century. Gold wiring to stabilize teeth loosened by alveolar bone loss (from periodontitis) continued into the late twentieth century despite the development of numerous alternative treatments. The use of "A-splints" as a pattern or technique of gold wiring to reduce mobility in loosened teeth was a common clinical procedure taught in modern dental schools in recent years (see Baumhammers 1971; Ash and Ranfjord 1982).

One phenomenon of early modern dentistry seems to have been the era of "Waterloo teeth," a brief time when dentures were fashioned from human teeth not the wearer's originals. (Figure 4.2 illustrates an upper denture from England with such human teeth.) The name was applied when, after the Battle of Waterloo (1815), entrepreneurs were found to have combed the battlefield removing healthy teeth from the bodies of the dead soldiers.[6] Such a source of healthy, young men's teeth was a rare occasion. Soon, fortunately, new methods were developed to produce ceramic replacement teeth, preferable for many reasons to those removed from corpses.

Among those interred in the crypt of Christ Church Spitalfields, Eliza Favenc of Greenwich, who died 1809 aged 27, had an early gold foil filling, with subsequent (secondary) decay, since the cavity could not have been made

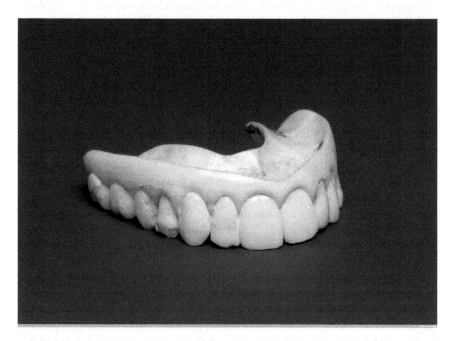

Figure 4.2 Upper denture, ivory with human teeth (Waterloo teeth), England, 1810–1860.
Source: courtesy of The Wellcome Collection, inv. L0058131.

sterile (see Whittaker 1993: 54, fig. 4.3 (2872)). This was one of only two early examples of restorative dentistry found among those buried in the crypt. Another discovery was the set of upper and lower dentures of one of the congregation buried probably between 1812 and 1847: the base plates were carved of ivory. The teeth were "Waterloo teeth" fastened to the plate with gold pins (see Whittaker 1993: 59, fig. 4.11 (2238)). The denture was contoured to fit around remaining teeth (upper lateral incisors) and over remaining roots of some lost teeth. For the lost molars, the ivory was simply carved into occlusal platforms, marked with an X. Rotating rivets held springs in place to help keep the dentures in place.

Ancient cases employing drilling: with or without filling

Modern-style gold inlays, as well as the use of gold foil and other materials for the filling of prepared dental cavities, were known in Europe by 1600 (Riethe and Czarnetzki 1983), long before written references to these aspects of dentistry had appeared in English. While there are similarities between many of the techniques used to manufacture ancient Etruscan dental appliances and the more recent use of gold foil, the two procedures are radically different. The human ability to drill holes in ivory, teeth, and even the hardest known stone is many thousands of years old (see Alt 1989). Fine drilling using thin reeds and small diameter sticks has a long history and has been applied to all types of materials including hard stones such as jade. Given the drilling capabilities of peoples around the world it is not surprising that we have evidence for the drilling of a hole into a live (*in situ*) maxillary molar from a Danish individual from *c.*2,000 to 3,000 BCE (Bennike 1985: 176–182; Bennike and Fredebo 1986: 81–87). The reason why these Neolithic people performed such a procedure is not known, but the drilling has been verified by Bennike using scanning electron microscopy and then by experimental replication. Why no other example of dental drilling has been known from European contexts prior to the sixteenth century we cannot say.

Andrea Cucina *et al.* (2001) report finding two examples, dated to before 9,000 BP, of human permanent molars each with a tiny hole on the occlusal surfaces from a site at Mehrgarh in Baluchistan, Pakistan. Both molars, from two different males, appear to have been drilled, perhaps using a stone-tipped drill according to Cucina, although a wooden stick with abrasive powder is more likely. These two adults had all their teeth in place at death, excluding the possibility that these were suspended or post-mortem procedures.

In contrast, the two "borings" that Hooton (1917) saw as evidence of therapeutic dental intervention in Old Kingdom Egypt, often cited as evidence for Egyptian operative dentistry, are actually common pathological features (apical abscesses) unrelated to any medical procedures (see Sigerist 1955: figs 14–16; but note the contradictory conclusion in fig. 17). Leek (1972: 404–405) compares these two features to the common sinuses found in numerous mummies, all caused by dissolution of the bone in the apical regions of those teeth after infection caused the death of the dental pulp and root. This opening of a hole in the bone of the jaw is often the response in cases of untreated abscess. (See also Miller 2008: 67–69 and figs 16 and 20).

Turner (2000) discusses "Dental transfiguration" in the American Southwest and provides a useful bibliography. However, to date we have but a single prehistoric example of possible therapeutic dental drilling from that region. About 1025 AD someone at the Fremont Site in Colorado drilled a human canine on the occlusal surface to relieve pressure from a periapical abscess (White *et al.* 1997; Anon. 1997; but see Koritzer 1968; St. Hoyme and Koritzer 1971).

Einhorn (1973: 521) refers to an example of "therapeutic tooth-filling" in the mouth of a skeleton from the St. Louis mound culture that is dated to 900–1200 CE, although no specific report on the archaeology of this "find" has yet been published. Schwartz (*et al.* 1995) report finding a drilled tooth from Alaska, dating from the period between 1300 and 1700 CE, which also is said to have been bored to relieve the pressure from an abscess. They conclude that this was a therapeutic treatment based on their belief that no "ritual" drilling is known from any Arctic group. In fact, some of these procedures appear to differ considerably from the cosmetic labial filings and drillings known from elsewhere in the New World, such as in the state of Illinois (see Milner and Larsen 1991: 364), but the Alaskan example may be part of a cultural tradition rather than a medical matter.

Maya dentistry: a note

The elaborate drilling performed by the ancient Maya of Central America in order to put inlays into the labial surfaces of the teeth required considerable skill. These drilled inlays are in addition to the filing of the tooth to create innovative profiles. The technology used to achieve the drilled sockets for the inlays had been perfected long before the Maya Classic Period (*c.*250–900 CE) through the drilling and carving of complex jade artifacts. Becker (1999c) had studied a number of examples in archaeological Zone 6B at Tikal, Guatemala associated with the residence of a middle class family of dentists. All of the adult males recovered from that family burial had elaborate inlays on a par with, or superior to, the inlays found among the elite in the largest temples.

The Maya royal family were distinguished by dental inlays of jade and amazonite, as seen in the teeth of Nuun Ujol Chaak (Figure 4.3), whose burial (24, Lot 18, field no. 12K-174) was excavated by the University of Pennsylvania expedition to Tikal, Guatemala. Nuun Ujol Chaak, also known as Shield Skull, was one of the later kings of Tikal (*c.*657–679 CE). On his death, his son Jasaw Chau K'will built the enormous Temple 33 in the center of the front row of the great North Acropolis temples of Tikal and interred his father in what we identify as Tikal Burial 24. Jasaw Chau K'will himself was later interred beneath Temple

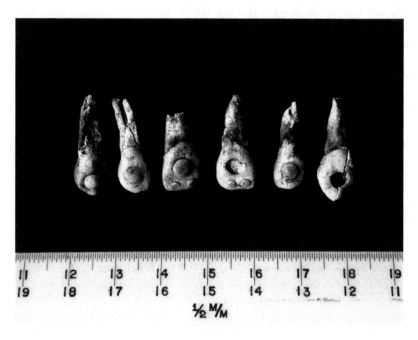

Figure 4.3 Maya dental inlays of jade and amazonite: teeth of Nuun Ujol Chaak, excavated in Guatemala, Tikal burial 24, Lot 18, field no. 12K-174.

Source: courtesy of The Tikal Project of the University of Pennsylvania Museum, neg. no. 62-4-754.

I at Tikal. Several other rulers were also given elaborate dental inlays, which required the drilling of surfaces in the living front teeth.

Of comparative interest is the report (Arlen Chase, personal communication) that the incidence of dental inlays among the ancient Maya inhabitants of Caracol, Belize, is much higher than at Tikal, Guatemala (see also Lancaster 2001). Guillermo Matas, DDS, of Guatemala is now engaged in research regarding Maya dentistry in general, for which there exists a considerable literature that awaits the results of data from Tikal, Caracol, and many other sites more recently excavated.

Notes

1 Dechaume and Huard 1977: plate 6A provides three drawings from manuscripts: figure A-top is attributed without details to "MS 91. Tüb.," which must mean *Berlin Manuscript* (or folio) *91*, housed in the Universitätsbibliothek Tübingen, Germany. (See Hamarneh and Sonnendecker 1963: xii.) Figure 6a-lower left is cited "Channing," probably John Channing's edition of the manuscript of Abulcasis (1778). Figure 6a-lower right is attributed "Argelata 1531" and might refer to a later edition of the book *Chirurgia* by anatomist Pietro d'Argelata (died 1423) first published in Venice in various editions (1492–1499).
2 Arculanus also described the *pelican* instrument for tooth extractions.
3 Since at least the Late Bronze Age, hippopotamus "ivory," actually the tusks or canines, has been used and traded in place of elephant ivory; the prime ancient examples in this trade come from the Phoenicians and their ancestors, the Canaanites. The famous Uluburun shipwreck, a Canaanite vessel that sank off the Anatolian coast, was carrying unworked hippo tusks in its royal cargo, dated *c*.1300 BCE. See Pulak 1998, 2001: 37–39.
4 Dentures are in the collections of the National Museum of Dentistry, Mt. Vernon, and elsewhere, and have been exhibited at various venues by the National Institutes of Health. Websites (with correct information) include: www.dental.umaryland.edu/museum/index.html/collection/ also www.mountvernon.org/digital-encyclopedia/article/false-teeth/ (both consulted February 15, 2016).
5 Another website claims that Washington had tooth transplants of healthy teeth bought from his slaves: www.pbs.org/wgbh/pages/frontline/shows/jefferson/video/lives.html (consulted February 15, 2016).
6 Waterloo teeth: see the website of the British Dental Association: http://britishlibrary.typepad.co.uk/untoldlives/2013/07/smiling-with-dead-mens-teeth.html.
   For illustrations of newspaper adverts for such teeth: www.bbc.co.uk/dna/ptop/A5103271, a BBC blog, "Smiling with Dead Men's Teeth" (consulted June 27, 2016), comments on Waterloo teeth, noting (note 3) "The Etruscans, who were making beautiful false teeth in the seventh century" were the only past culture to do so, "but the art seems to have died out along with their civilization." It notes a price of 2 guineas (approx. $300) offered in 1782 for an incisor. The battlefields of the American Civil War also furnished teeth from corpses. Also abundant illustrations are available from www.bbc.com/news/magazine-33085031 and www.historyhome.co.uk/c-eight/france/teeth.htm (consulted February 25, 2016). Molleson and Cox 1993 *passim* illustrate some of the congregation buried at Spitalfields, London, who had Waterloo teeth. See Chapter 1.

5 Catalogue of Etruscan and Roman-era dental appliances

PART I: CATALOGUE OF ETRUSCAN AND ROMAN-ERA
GOLD-BAND DENTAL APPLIANCES

Three examples that may be in Buffalo, New York: the Barrett and Van Marter appliances

Background: history and identification

Dr. William C. Barrett, an editor of the *Dental Register* and first Dean of the Dental Department at the University of Buffalo, was friend and colleague to Dr. James Gilbert Van Marter, who was practicing in Rome, Italy during the 1880s. Barrett received his DDS from the University of Pennsylvania in 1881 and became a founder of the dental school at Buffalo *c.*1891. The source of details of Van Marter's life and training in dentistry and how these two came to correspond, remain unknown. Van Marter was to obtain three Etruscan dental appliances, which eventually came to his friend's collection in Buffalo, New York.

In the January 1885 issue of the *Independent Practitioner*, Waite (1885a: 508) refers to an article by a Dr. Van Marter of Rome (probably Van Marter 1885a).[1] This suggests that by 1885 Van Marter had made drawings of the two prostheses then in the Corneto (the old name for Tarquinia) Museum (nos. 11–12). This information may have stimulated Barrett to ask Van Marter to act as his agent in the purchase of other examples from the Etruscan tombs then being systematically stripped of their offerings.

Van Marter's letters to Barrett describe the excavations of tombs in the area of ancient Tarquinia, claiming that gold dental prostheses were often recovered. During this important period in the history of dentistry, with the creation of formal schools and professional societies, there was great interest in dental hygiene as well as dental history. By 1886 Van Marter had located and sent two appliances to Buffalo. After the first (Barrett I, no. 1) arrived, Barrett requested that another be purchased for him, together with any archaeological materials from the same tomb. This prescient concern for archaeological context reflects the scientific orientation of these medical practitioners. The second dental appliance

(Barrett II, no. 2) that Van Marter purchased for Barrett is described in a letter of 1886. A third appliance that appears to have been sent to America, now identified as the Van Marter example (see no. 3), may have been excavated about 1889 during the period of systematic mining of major Etruscan tombs (Becker 1999a).

Both Barrett gold appliances are simple bands, within which only some of the teeth appear to have survived. It is possible that teeth were added to the Barrett I appliance in order to provide some verisimilitude to this artifact. The records suggest that three teeth were with the Barrett II appliance when it was sent to America. The third appliance, the Van Marter, held an original false tooth. The reason for Barrett's purchase of a third example may have been to own a true pontic with a false tooth, as he already had two simple band "retainers." The source(s) for these three appliances was always unclear and remains largely unknown since they had disappeared by the time of Barrett's death in 1903 (but, see Becker 1999a).

Some confusion arose in the late nineteenth century between that first pair of appliances owned by Barrett and the Liverpool pair (nos. 13–14). The confusion apparently derives from W. H. Waite's note (1885a: 508) indicating that Waite had borrowed both (Liverpool) pieces in 1885, and exhibited them before two unnamed New York dental societies. The pair must be the same two brought to Hereford, England in August of 1885 (Waite 1885a: 508): thus, the Liverpool pair, and not the Barrett pieces. Mr. Spence Bate, of the British Dental Association (Western Branch) suggested using funds at hand to illustrate these pieces, inasmuch as *The Independant Practitioner* "did not circulate largely in this country." The resulting drawings (Waite 1885a: facing p. 512) clearly depict the Liverpool pair of dental appliances collected by English goldsmith Joseph Meyer in 1857 (nos. 13–14).

Edlund (1981) found that Barrett's books and dental instruments had been bequeathed to the University at the time of his death in 1903; while his "Etruscan relics" were given to the Buffalo and Erie County Historical Society, where she examined the three vases. They were a small jug, a *plumpe Kanne* (beaked jug) in impasto, imitating bronze vases with palmette handles, and a bucchero ovoid oinochoe with animal heads framing the handle. A date *c.*500 BCE fits these surviving vases, and presumably the burial with the dental appliance.

A cursory search of *Publications of the Buffalo Historical Society* for the years around 1903 did not locate any information regarding the Barrett estate, but subsequent findings may explain this failure. The estate, or parts of it, did not formally become part of the collections until 1930 (Edlund 1981). The present locations of these three important examples of the history of dentistry remain unknown. The following descriptions are based on published illustrations and descriptions studied by Becker. Dunn (1894), in discussing the Italian appliances, stated that, by the early 1890s, five examples were "lost," presumably indicating that they had been sold or given to private collections. If this was Dunn's meaning, the three examples of appliances sent to Dr. Barrett might account for most of those described as "lost."

1 Barrett I

Present location: unknown (lost with Barrett Collection; Buffalo, New York).
Type: simple band (3 spaces).
Origin: Etruria.
Jaw part: maxilla, 1I plus (I1, I2?).
Date: if Van Marter's (1886: 59) description of grave goods is correct, possibly
    500–475 BCE.
Sex: female? (based on size of teeth/jaw).
Dimensions: L. 20, W. 1.2–1.6 mm.

Description: narrow band to stabilize three teeth. A simple, very narrow gold-band
appliance, perhaps 0.2 to 0.3 mm thick, varying from 1.2–1.6 mm wide. It was
designed to loop around no more than 3 anterior teeth, probably the 3 central incisors and a lateral incisor. Length as illustrated approx. 20 mm, with a buccal-lingual

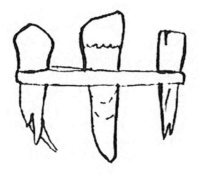

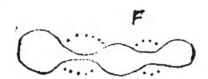

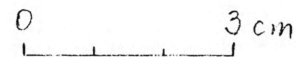

Figure 5.1 The Barrett I appliance, two views drawn after Farrar 1888: figs 6 and 8.
        View with dotted lines suggests the locations of the teeth originally bound
        by the appliance.

distance approx. 6 mm. The total length of the gold strip is calculated at 53 mm, after the overlapping ends had been welded. Published information suggests an elongated oval, with a constricted or pinched center that reflects post-interment affects. When in place it may have been ornamental, but may have been intended to stabilize a loose tooth at the center of the band. The tooth crown, from which the root has decayed, may be from the same tomb, even from the owner, but this cannot be confirmed.

References

Becker 1999a.
Edlund 1981.
Farrar 1888, I: 33, figs 6, 8.
Naso 2011: 151, no. 10.
Van Marter 1885a, 1886: 59.

History and context

Van Marter (1886: 59) describes the source of this appliance as a tomb of the sixth century BCE (but see no. 2) "or about one hundred years prior to the dates of the oldest partial denture which *I sent you last year*" (emphasis ours). Van Marter's comment suggests that around 1885, the year before he sent the "entire" collection of artifacts recovered from an Etruscan tomb to Barrett (see Barrett II), Van Marter had already sent him the first gold dental appliance. Van Marter's published statement, quoted in full under Barrett II (no. 2), is clarified by reading Farrar's 1888 publication, which describes the two Etruscan appliances sent to Barrett at his address in Buffalo, New York.

The Barrett I piece was excavated prior to Barrett II that has been more extensively described. Our only description of the Barrett I example comes from John Nutting Farrar. Farrar practiced dentistry in New York City but, like Barrett, came from upstate New York. Farrar may have seen both Barrett pieces in Buffalo; however, Barrett appears to have carried these artifacts to various other cities to show his colleagues. Lacking data on the other appliances then known in Italy, and intrigued by these early examples of restorative dentistry, Farrar illustrated his brief text on ancient dental gold-working technology with the two examples that were near at hand. This decision is quite fortunate for us, as today this record provides the only information that exists for this one of the two Barrett pieces.

J. N. Farrar was one of the pioneers of orthodontic practice, concerned with both the cosmetic and functional aspects of bridgework used in orthodontics (Farrar 1905). The Etruscan pontics that he examined had only cosmetic purposes, but may have had at least incidental orthodontic functions since the replacement tooth served to hold the living teeth in place. Simple band appliances could have served the ancillary function of sustaining normal dental articulation by stabilizing loose teeth and/or maintaining normal tooth positions. In no case could they have served to shift the position of teeth, a complex aspect of orthodontics sometimes claimed for Etruscan appliances by recent commentators (Corruccini and Pacciani 1989; Torino *et al.* 1996).

Description

Van Marter's description of the Barrett I appliance (1885a; cf. Van Marter 1885b and c) is not very clear, nor is his illustration of much use in delineating its form. Van Marter's vague description (1885a) was used by Helbig (1886: 25), and provided Bliquez (1996) with an indication of the type of appliance that was once, and still may be, in Buffalo (see also Sterpellone and Elsheikh 1990: 139).

2 Barrett II

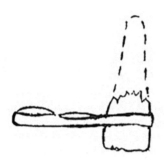

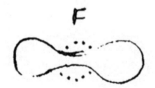

Figure 5.2 The Barrett II appliance, two views drawn after Farrar 1888: figs 5 and 7. The dotted lines suggest the locations of the teeth originally bound by the appliance.

Present location: unknown (lost with Barrett Collection; Buffalo, New York).
Type: simple band (4 spaces).
Origin: Bisenzio (ancient Visentium); necropolis at Capodimonte on western
   shore of Lake Bolsena.
Jaw part: maxilla (possibly 2I–I2).
Date: fifth century BCE? (Helbig 1886; see also Edlund 1981).
Sex: female.
Dimensions: 25 by 2.0–2.5 mm

Description: simple, narrow gold-band appliance, probably about 0.2 to 0.3 mm
thick and varying from 2.0–2.5 mm wide. The length of the band appears designed
to loop around the crowns of no more than 4 anterior teeth; most likely the 4
incisors. Length as illustrated approx. 25 mm, with a buccal-lingual distance of
about 6–7 mm. The total length of the gold strip is calculated at 60 mm, after the
overlapping ends had been welded. Published information suggests an elongated
oval that, as originally illustrated with two constricted or pinched areas, held three
teeth in place. These constrictions appear to hold in place three teeth introduced
post-excavation. This post-interment alteration depicts the band as binding these
teeth, probably not original to the appliance, at the neck or lower on the root,
which would have been impossible. When in place it may have been only ornamental, but it may have been intended to stabilize one or two loose teeth at the
center of the band.

References

Becker 1999a.
Bliquez 1996: 2654. Bliquez's appliance "R," fig. 28.
Cigrand 1893: 60n (cites Van Marter 1886).
Edlund 1981.
Farrar 1888: 33, figs 5, 7.
Helbig 1886: 25–26.
Koch 1909: fig. 5.
Naso 2011: 150, no. 1.
Sudhoff 1926: 86, fig. 52 ("*nach Guerini*," but clearly a photograph of a poor copy).
Van Marter 1886: 59–60, fig. 3.
Waarsenburg 1991a: 242, n. 5 (no. 14).
Weege 1913, Vol. II: 371.
Weinberger 1948: 125, fig. 41: 4 (from Sudhoff).

History and identification of context

Van Marter stated:

> The most recently opened and the oldest Etruscan tomb yet discovered in
> Italy was lately excavated at Capadimonti [sic], near the Lake of Bolsena.
> The entire contents of this tomb, including three teeth bound together
> with a band of pure gold, gold spiral rings for the side hair, silver finger

ring, necklace of amber and glass, arm band, bronzes, vases, etc., etc., I take pleasure in sending you by first express. The part of the find of interest to our profession is the three teeth, a drawing of which I send you herewith. (See fig. 3.) This tomb belongs to the VIth Century BC, or about one hundred years prior to the dates of the oldest partial denture which I sent you last year.

(Van Marter 1886: 59)

From Farrar's comments one cannot tell if both Barrett dental appliances came from this tomb or from two separate tombs. Van Marter cites only one appliance. Other information indicates that two separate tombs were the sources.

Farrar (1888: 33) also says that the excavation took place in 1886, and that the entire contents of the tomb were bought by the American dentist Dr. William Carr. Perhaps Farrar simply made an error in the name, but it is more likely that he was noting the name of another intermediary in this transaction. Farrar notes that the tomb contents subsequently were presented to "W. C. Barrett, and now constitute a portion of his private museum. The specimens in this collection are more especially interesting to the dentist [including carious molars]." He continues:

Besides these teeth [the molars], there were three that were bound together with a gold band; also the crown of another (central), bound with a similar device. Figs. 5 and 6 illustrate the two specimens, and show the relation of the bands to the teeth in side view. In Figs. 7 and 8 the plain lines show the top view of the bands detatched [sic] from the teeth as they appeared when I saw them. When in use, however, these bands were undoubtedly bent as shown by the dotted lines. These bands were probably bound to the teeth with gold wire as shown in Fig. 9 [where Farrar illustrates the Sidon I example, see no. W-1]. The tomb contained other antiquities, a list of which is given below, as evidences of the high rank held by the occupants of the tomb, and to show that consequently these specimens of denture were probably of the best that the period afforded.

(Farrar 1888: 33)

Farrar lists artifacts supposedly recovered with this piece (also Helbig 1886; Edlund 1981):

two spiral gold rings;

incised hair ornaments;

one silver finger ring;

necklace of lapis lazuli and pure amber;

bronze plaque nearly 2 feet in diameter, with lions' feet and sea horses in full relief;

one large bronze vase with ear pieces representing the Taurian Jove;

bronze ornament, evidentally an armour-piece for the head;

bronze wine-strainer;

silver "fibrilla" [sic];

two bronze cups;

four earthen jugs (two finely molded);

two vase handles with carved head and tail pieces.

Weege (1913, II: 371) lists a gold dental appliance recovered from a tomb in Capodimonte, but whether it is the Barrett II piece or yet another remains uncertain. Also of importance in Weege's text is the reference to a piece that Van Marter says was sent to Barrett during the previous year, about 1885. This "partial denture which I sent you last year" (Barrett I), as we now know, was an actual appliance, not simply information concerning that appliance.

The Barrett II appliance must have been recovered late in 1885 or in 1886, because the associated tomb goods were described by Helbig in an 1886 publication (see also Edlund 1981). Helbig (1886: 25) suggests that the appliance is from one of the "*tombe a fossa che furono scoperte in uno strato inferiore a quello teste' descritto,*" ("trench tombs discovered in a lower stratum from that described") Helbig (1886: 26) dated the earlier tomb to the sixth century, based on comparison with Attic vases from a tomb at Tarquinia. This made the Barrett I appliance the earliest dental appliance then known. Edlund (1981) identifies three surviving artifacts as dating *c.*500 BCE and probably from the tomb with the appliance. The list of tomb contents sounds like a mixture of types of the sixth through fifth or fourth centuries, as expected for a family tomb with multiple depositions. Only in 1898 was an earlier dental appliance discovered at Satricum (Satricum, no. 18).

Barrett's estate supposedly was divided between The University at Buffalo and the Buffalo and Erie County Historical Society (see Edlund 1981: 82). Although he died in 1903, the acquisition is reported to have become official only in 1930, possibly being considered as a loan until that time. Since Barrett's widow died about 1925, these vases may have remained in her possession until her death. If all the Barrett materials remained with his widow, the gold appliance or appliances, as well as other valuable items, may have been sold or otherwise lost from the collection between 1903 and 1925.

Aside from the three vases noted by Edlund, all other pieces from this tomb including the dental appliance, remain missing. Mrs. Mildred F. Hallowitz, History of Medicine Librarian of the Health Sciences Library (SUNY-Buffalo) provided Edlund with information regarding the bequest of artifacts to the School of Dentistry. One item, a bronze situla, has been noted as possibly being sent to Dresden, but (according to Becker) there may be some confusion between the Barrett tomb bronzes and other bronzes from this tomb that Helbig (1886) notes went to Dresden.

The Albright-Knox Museum in Buffalo, New York, which focuses on modern art, also holds a small collection of ancient artifacts. It is located across the street from the Erie County Historical Society, to which some of the Barrett collection was bequeathed. The enormous warehouse of the Erie County Historical Society, opened in 1990, contains vast numbers of boxes awaiting inventory. We may hope that three Etruscan gold dental appliances are among these holdings.

Description/identification

The earliest illustrations and descriptions leave much to be desired; each commentator offered a slightly different location and description of the teeth. Farrar illustrates this second Barratt appliance as if it were a mandibular prosthesis. Although this could be the case, it would be very unlikely (but, see no. 21). The teeth depicted appear to be a second premolar, canine, and central incisor, with one space between each where a first premolar and lateral incisor would be expected. Farrar's illustrations of Barrett II show a simple gold band that extended over five tooth spaces. This band may have been used to stabilize loose teeth rather than hold a false tooth in position. At least one of the 4 teeth surrounded by this appliance was lost after death, assuming that the remaining 3 teeth depicted by Farrar actually were original to this band (which Becker doubts).

Helbig suggests that this prosthesis, encompassing the upper left lateral incisor-canine-premolar, was worn by a "young woman," a "*giovinetta*." He clearly, and correctly, indicates that the band might only have served to hold a naturally loosened canine in place. The canine is less likely to be loosened by a blow or peridontal disease than either of the adjacent teeth, but Helbig is essentially correct. Koch (1909: 16, fig. 5) offers a very rough sketch, possibly taken from Van Marter, and erroneously illustrates it as mandibular.

Weinberger (1948: 125) accepts Farrar's conclusion that this appliance is mandibular (I1, C., and PM2) but completely errs in suggesting that it has rings with spacing bars where the PM1 and I2 are missing. The very narrow gold band appears to have been pinched together in the two spaces where no teeth were present, probably after recovery from the tomb. This appliance should be compared with Bruschi I (no. 8), a thin band from Tarquinia that has been pinched together (probably recently) in the center, where it once embraced a tooth. (Note that Bruschi I is also described incorrectly as having a spacer "bar" separating "two rings.")

3 Van Marter

Present location: unknown (perhaps in Buffalo, New York?).
Type: ring series (3), with central false tooth.
Origin: Lake of Valseno (Bolsena?), near Rome.
Date: 600 BC (?) according to Van Marter.
Jaw Part: maxilla?
Sex: female ??
Dimensions: 25 by 4 mm (estimated from published drawing).

Description: constructed of gold rings welded together to replace right central incisor with reworked human tooth (not cut from a central incisor). This three-ring appliance, with the central loop altered to a more rectangular configuration, is approximately 5 mm deep. The squared outline helps prevent the modified, or false, central incisor from rotating in this socket. The lateral rings as depicted in the drawing, the only extant record, appear similar but one may have been designed to surround a central incisor and the other for a lateral incisor, the teeth that served as anchors for a postulated replacement incisor.

References

Becker 1999a.
Naso 2011: 150–151 no. 4.
Van Marter 1889: 261.

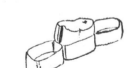

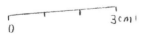

Figure 5.3 The Van Marter appliance (drawn after Van Marter 1889: 261).

History and identification

This dental prosthesis had been "buried" in the literature for over 100 years until recovered in the course of this study (Becker 1999a). Only a drawing and brief description, published by Dr. James Gilbert Van Marter (1889), preserve it for us. It is only fitting that this example be named for him.

In 1889 or shortly before, while Van Marter resided in Rome, he recorded that this dental appliance had been "taken from an Etruscan tomb lately opened not far from Rome on the lake of Valseno" (Lake Bolsena; Marter 1889: 261). This appears to be the third and final Etruscan dental prosthesis sent to Dr. Barrett in Buffalo, assuming that the publication date of 1889 accurately reflects the date of discovery. The two earlier examples sent to Barrett derive from tombs excavated around 1885–1886. The discovery and *purchase* of three gold appliances by Van Marter in this five- year period reflects the considerable extent of excavation of rich tombs in Etruria during the 1880s.

Fortunately, Barrett appears to have arranged publication of the note written by Van Marter, and illustrated this brief notice with a drawing slightly larger than life size. In many aspects this piece is similar to the Copenhagen example (no. 4), but here the replacement tooth appears to have survived while the post teeth did not, exactly the reverse of the situation with the Copenhagen example (Becker 1992a).

Description

Van Marter states that the rings of this specimen are welded, with no joints evident, as would be the case were the rings soldered together. While not explicit in his description, Van Marter certainly meant welding, which is exactly how the Copenhagen example and all of the other ring-series appliances appear to have been assembled. The anchor (or post) teeth to which this bridge was attached are depicted as missing, with only the central ring holding a "tooth." Van Marter (1889: 261) describes this replacement tooth as "a bicuspid, turned one-fourth round on its axis." This may have been meant to replace a large central incisor. Although Van Marter's illustration shows this appliance in a "mandibular" position, the "tooth" appears to be a large right maxillary example or, more likely, a carved false tooth. Becker suggests that this may have been intended to replace a maxillary central incisor and not the PM1 (possibly bridging the spaces I1–I2, rather than C–PM1–PM2). This latter series would be very unlikely (replacing a first premolar).

From the illustration it appears that the replacement tooth is held in position like a gemstone, in a fashion similar to that of the Copenhagen example (Becker 1992a, 1994b; no. 4). That is, the "ring" is rectilinear and holds the replacement by pressing the gold band to conform to the contours of the tooth. In its construction the Van Marter piece is closest in type to the Copenhagen bridge.

4 Copenhagen

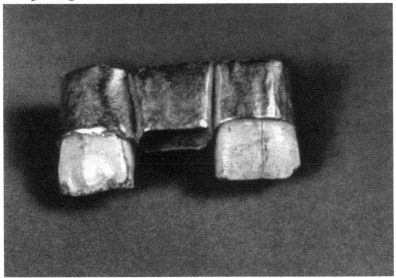

Figure 5.4a The Copenhagen appliance, frontal view.

Source: courtesy of the National Museum of Denmark, Copenhagen.

Present location: National Museum, Copenhagen (Deptartment of Near Eastern and Classical Antiquities), inventory no. 8319.
Type: three welded loops, no rivet.
Origin: Orvieto (via Riis 1941: 161).
Jaw part: maxilla, 1I–I2.
Date: *c.*500–490 BCE or slightly later, based on ceramic associations.
Sex: female.
Condition: deteriorated somewhat since photographs were published.
Dimensions: 21.6 by 5.5 to 6.2 mm.

Description: "three-ring" appliance with lateral loops carefully fitted to the original and surviving dental crowns (left central incisor and right lateral incisor) and a sharply rectangular central gold unit holding a false tooth, not recovered. The three units have buccal-lingual distances that range from 5.1 to 6.7 mm.

References

Baggieri (1998: 69) gives provenance *"Volsinii"* (modern Orvieto).
Becker 1992a, 1994b, 1995a, 1997, 1999b: fig. 3.
Bliquez 1996: 2656–2657, fig. 56. Bliquez appliance "W."
Johnstone 1932a: 132n, pl. 94:17–18.

Marvitz 1982: 49.
Naso 2011: 151, no. 6.
Pot 1985: 38–39.
Poulsen 1927: 47.
Riis 1941: 161.
Villamil 1994.

(b)

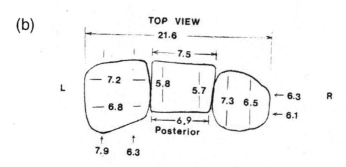

(c)

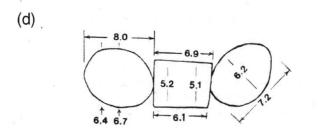

(d)

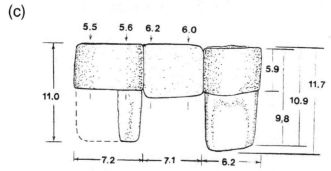

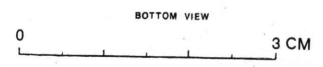

Figures 5.4b–d Views of the Copenhagen appliance, drawn by Becker.

History and provenance

The National Museum of Denmark has an excellent photograph of this appliance (Negative no. M 194; FOI 132). The catalogue card states that it was received as a gift, in 1924, from the Ny Carlsberg Foundation, and that it comes from Orvieto. Riis (1941: 161) believed this because he thought it was one of "a number of gold objects—said to have come from the same grave as [a] censer" and other items. The censer is listed by Riis (1941: 79, pl. 15.3) as item B4, which came to the museum from the same source as several Attic vases, "the amphora of the Affector, the Oltus cup, the hydria of the Berlin painter," etc. Riis believed that these items formed a mixed group, probably from different tombs rather than a single context, at Orvieto. Thus Riis clarifies Frederik Poulsen's (1927: 47) statement that the Copenhagen dental appliance came from a grave (no site named) that included these famous vases plus five bronze vessels; the last batch of materials includes *"Einige Goldsachen, die sich jetzt im Nationalmuseum von Kopenhagen befinden,"* "some gold objects," which must include the gold-band prosthesis. (The Affector painted between *c.*550 and 530 BCE; Oltos worked *c.*525–500 BCE, and the Berlin Painter from 500–460 BCE, leaving a wide chronological range—if we accept that these Attic (Athenian) vases were deposited with the person wearing the gold bridge.)

Description

Three gold rings held a central, false tooth, and two living "anchor" teeth. The surviving central incisor crown had been complete, but was damaged while on exhibit and the fragment lost before this study began (Figure 5.4a shows the appliance prior to damage.). The lateral incisor crown is largely intact. No portion of the false or replacement tooth was recovered.

Fashioned to be worn in the upper jaw of an adult female, this prosthesis was made using a complex variation of the simple band technique, welding a series of individual "rings" or small loops, each of which is fitted to a single tooth. This is only one of at least four construction variations now known (see Van Marter, no. 1).

The size of the teeth can be estimated from the empty gold rings, and must have been made for a woman of distinctly small stature.

Construction

To make this appliance, three separate straps or bands were fashioned and welded into three small loops. Then these three rings were welded into a series. Alternatively, each seamless ring may have been produced by expanding a small piece of gold by rolling and hammering. The left loop was fitted to the upper left central incisor (1I), the loop on the other end fitted to the right lateral incisor (I2). These sound teeth served as the anchor or "post" teeth to which the bridge was attached to hold it in place. The rectangular central loop held a false tooth (now missing). No rivet is needed in this design since the false tooth was held by the same method by which a gemstone is fixed in its setting. A circular band was fitted with the false tooth in the same fashion that a goldsmith would make any bezel setting. The rectangular setting would prevent rotation and facilitate a good fit, then the false tooth would be secured in place by pressing the gold tightly, as with the gold of the lateral loops.

Each loop is seamless, and all are joined at their adjacent surfaces by invisible welds made after each had been shaped. Each loop was custom designed (form fitted) to encircle one dental element. The lateral loops were curved in such a way as to conform to the base of each anchor tooth's crown, with specific fitting done after the false tooth had been set in place and the appliance was ready to be inserted.

The replacement tooth in the Copenhagen appliance would have reproduced only the "crown," its "base" cut into a rectangular shape, which would remain stable in its collar and unlikely to slip. This series then forms the bridge, of a design remarkably similar to modern examples. The lateral bands were fitted to the living teeth by simply pressing the soft gold band securely around them. The construction of this appliance indicates that it was meant to be a permanent fixture. (The roots of the anchor teeth have dissolved, probably during burial.)

The widths of the three gold bands vary significantly, the variation exaggerated by the bending and fitting needed to adjust each band to a specific tooth, either natural or false. This resulted in the appliance being much more effective than those bridges that incorporate only a single long band. Viewing this unit from the rear, the mesial divider (the midline of the skull) would pass between the left and center dental elements. The left element, surrounding the central incisor, is a band worked to a thickness of about 0.3 to 0.4 mm. The thickness of the central element is closer to 0.3 mm, and that of the lateral incisor is under 0.3 mm, possibly 0.2 mm. These variations indicate a gradual thinning of these bands, perhaps because a single long strip was the source of all three units and this source was thicker at one end than the other. This might only reflect random variation, slight bends or disturbances that occurred after death, or attenuation that occurred during the fitting process.

The breadth of the gold bands also shows minor variations. The center of the anterior surface of the left unit measures 5.8 mm high along the entire front (labial) exposure. An encrustation of modern glue obscures the rear surface. The height of the band forming the central unit is 6.1 mm.along the lingual surface, continuing to the front (labial) surface on the medial side. This strip broadens toward the midline where it is some 6.5 mm high. The right unit is formed from a band slightly less than 6.0 mm high at the lingual-distal corner but widens to 6.1 mm at the labial-distal corner; it continues to broaden across the front of the tooth to 6.3 mm at the labial-mesial corner. Variations may be due to changes effected in the gold band during close fitting rather than from variations in the original gold strip(s).

The left unit is relatively oval in plan at the lower margin, but nearly square at the top where it surrounded the widest aspect of the tooth. The central unit is nearly a perfect rectangle in plan at top and bottom, with the lower aspect slightly smaller than the upper. The right unit is a very irregular square at the upper side and an irregular oval at the lower edge.

The probability is that the gum would recede away from contact with the replacement "tooth" and that a new element would have to be fitted from time to time. This could be done with relative ease, or at least as easily as the removal of the entire device from the adjacent teeth.

Human remains with the appliance: dentition

Marvitz (1982: 49) illustrated the crowns of the anchor teeth when they still appeared to be intact within the lateral loops of the bridge. Both roots and most of the dentine, however, probably had disintegrated in the tomb. When examined in 1989 the tooth on the left (1I) in the Marvitz photograph was badly fractured, and what appears to be translucent glue covered much of the rear of these teeth as well as the gold band. The damage and glueing may have resulted from its display in an exhibition held about the time that Marvitz (1982) published. Much of the neck area of the 1I is preserved within the gold band; the exposed area is now largely missing except for the labial-mesial aspect of the enamel.

Both anchor teeth are worn down into the dentine along their articular or cutting edges, but there is no trace of secondary enamel replacement in the dentine area. The lateral tooth (the I2, which shows very little recent damage) has some tiny chips along this surface reflecting continued biting of hard materials or coarse elements. The entire I2 crown is intact; a trace of shoveling[2] (1 on a 0–4 scale) is evident. A major question regarding the permanence of this appliance involves the probability of its trapping decay-causing particles. The adverse long-term effects, and the probability that the gold bands would be distorted and loosened in days if not months, leads us to wonder if appliances of this design were intended to be worn continuously or if they were inserted only on special occasions.

Maximum diameters of these teeth cannot be measured directly but may be estimated from the inner dimensions of the enclosing gold-work. (Approximate crown heights: right lateral 10.9 mm, left central 11.5 mm.) Shoveling appears along the left lateral margin of the lateral incisor, and may exist as a trace along the damaged medial margin. The extent of the damage to the labial surface of the central incisor is such that no observations regarding shoveling can be made. The relatively small size of these teeth and the gap bridged by this appliance implies that the wearer was female.

Age determination by degree of wear requires a comparative population, and is less effectively applied to anterior teeth. The individual represented by these teeth appears to be over 30 years of age, but probably under 50 years of age.

5 Poggio Gaiella

Present location: Museo Archeologico Etrusco, Florence (inv. no. 11782).

Type: single complex "band," now in two pieces, spanning eight tooth spaces.

Origin: Poggio Gaiella in Città della Pieve (7 km south of Chiusi, 50 km southwest of Perugia).

Jaw part: originally probably maxillary, 1PM–PM1. This appliance was not original to the mandible in which it was displayed where it surrounds the mandibular 1PM–PM2 (nine tooth spaces) of a jaw from which the 2I was lost, possibly during recovery.

Date: uncertain (see Rastrelli 1998). Menconi and Fornaciari (1985: 93, 94) offer a date of the fourth–third century BCE, but without supporting archaeological evidence.

Sex: female, age 25–40 years.

Dimensions: L. 42; W. 2.82 to 3.3 mm.

Description: This elaborate appliance was crafted to surround eight teeth, from around both first premolars and all teeth in between. Two strips of gold were used, varying in width from 2.82 to 3.29 mm, with a median width of 3.16 mm. The thickness of the strips ranges from 0.12 to 0.17 mm, with a median of 0.14 mm.

Two separate strips of gold are shown in Figure 5.5a. The sequence by which the form of the original piece was reconstructed is shown in two illustrations (Figures 5.5b4) providing two interpretations of its construction. One band some 90 mm long passes along the labial side of the central six teeth, then curves into complete circles at each end to form loops surrounding the premolars. The buccal aspect is 42 mm long, welded at either end to the loops formed from the labial element. This could have been done at the same time that the lateral loops were welded. A center weld stabilized the appliance between the central incisors.

After recovery this appliance was much manipulated in order to mount it into a skull for display, resulting in some separations of welds and minor distortions. The alveolar margins of the skull, believed to be a relatively modern young adult, reveal no areas that would require bracing from a dental appliance. This may be another case of the modern mounting of appliances in more photogenic skulls.

References

Baggieri 1998: 67 (the popular basis for his 1999 essay)

Baggieri 1999 (an error-filled essay)

Baggieri 2001: 323, pl. xxxviih (repeats his 1999 essay)

Becker 1995a, 1996, 1999b: 44, fig. 1.

Bliquez 1996: 2646–2648, "D," also "E," and possibly "F" (see Bliquez 1996: 2647, n. 5, also figs 5–9.)

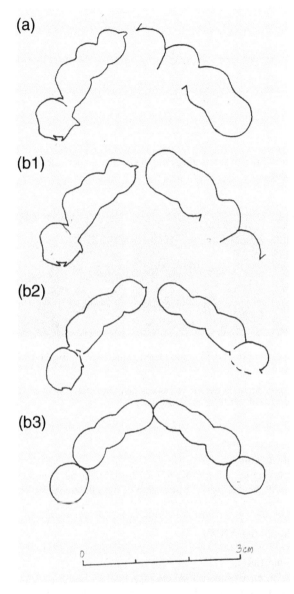

(a)

(b1)

(b2)

(b3)

0   3 cm

Figures 5.5a–b3 Views of the Poggio Gaiella appliance: (a) schematic drawing of the superior view of the configuration of Poggio Gaiella as it now rests in the display mandible; (b1) Becker's reconstruction of the Poggio Gaiella appliance in its correct orientation, (right half inverted and reversed); (b2) Poggio Gaiella, damage in course of "repair"; (b3) Poggio Gaiella, as reconstructed by Becker.

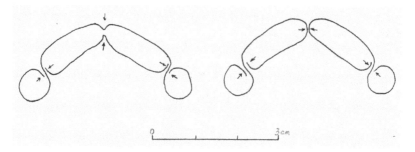

Figure 5.5b4 Variant possibilities of fabricating Poggio Gaiella, if not made using four-ring technique.

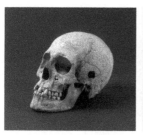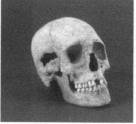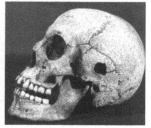

Figures 5.5c–e Photographic views of the Poggio Gaiella appliance, as displayed in a modern skull.

Source: courtesy Soprintendenza Archeologica per la Toscana and Lawrence J. Bliquez. (Florence Museo Archeologico neg. nos. 23530, 23528, and L. J. Bliquez.)

Bobbio 1958: fig. 14 (after Casoti 1957).
Capasso 1986: 52–55 (with 3 figures).
Cassoti 1927: 627 (illustrates copies only); 1947: 671–672; 1957:105, fig. 5; and 1958.
Corruccini and Pacciani 1989: 61–62, figs 1, 2 (text derives from photographs, not direct examination).
Dunn 1894: 4 (fig.).
Emptoz 1987: 557, 558, fig. 20 (no. XXIV).
Frassetto 1906: 156.
Ghinst 1930: 407 (after Dunn 1894).
Hoffmann-Axthelm 1985: 78, fig. 65 (not in 1981 edition).
Laviosa *et al.* 1993: 131, figs V4 and V5. The two color plates from the Soprintendenza Archeologica della Toscana (Firenze) are the best now available.
Menconi and Fornaciari 1985: 93: figs 3, 4. (Location called "Chiusi," p. 94.).
Naso 2011: 150, no. 3.
Penso 1984: figs 143–145?

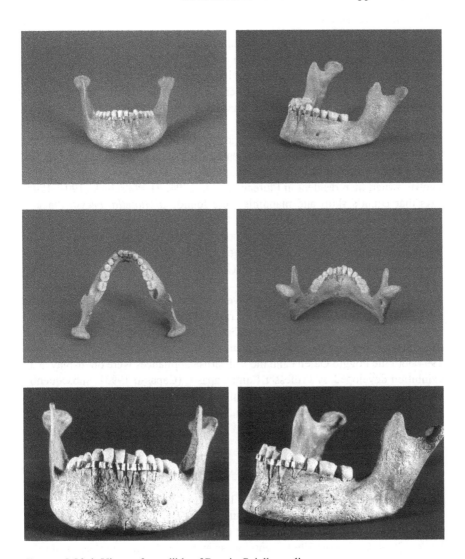

Figures 5.5f– k Views of mandible of Poggio Gaiella appliance.

Source: courtesy Soprintendenza Archeologica per la Toscana and Lawrence J. Bliquez. (Florence Museo Archeologico neg. nos. 23523, 23524, 23526, 23525, and L. J. Bliquez.)

Platschick 1904–1905: 239, fig. 2 (from "Giojella").
Sterpellone and Elsheikh 1990: 140, fig. 68.
Torino *et al.* 1996: 120–121.
Torino *et al.* 1997: 536–538.

History and provenance

The ancient necropolis at Poggio Gaiella, a hill south of ancient Chiusi (Etruscan *Clevsin*, Latin *Clusium, Camars*), was the city's largest, with tombs of the Orientalizing and Archaic periods. Unfortunately the exact context from which this appliance was recovered remains unknown. Anna Rastrelli (1998) presents an impressive summation of the history of excavations in Chiusine necropoleis.

A report on the excavations at Poggio Gaiella appeared only a year after the last of the Casuccini "excavations" at nearby Città della Pieve (Braun 1841). The earliest known account of the Poggio Gaiella appliance was written by its first known owner, then resident in Florence (Dunn 1894: 4). Platschick (1904–1905) says that Dunn's skull and mandible were found "*a Giojella, presso* ["near"] *Chiusi.*" Dunn donated this appliance and the skull on which it had been mounted to the museum in Florence (Corruccini and Pacciani 1989: 61); the exact date of this transfer remains unknown. The Poggio Gaiella appliance and associated skull were in Florence in 1957, where Casotti (1957: 105, fig. 5) saw them in Sala XLIII of the Archaeological Museum.

The breakage into two pieces may have been a result of trying to fit it around the teeth that are present in the mandible. Frassetto (1906: 156) studied 15 Etruscan skulls, 2 of which came from Poggio Gaiella. His data may enable us to tell if the skull that now has this dental appliance in it is one of these 15. In January of 1994 both the Poggio Gaiella and the Valsiarosa appliances were on display at an exhibition developed by Professer Luigi Capasso (Capasso 1993). Subsequently the Poggio Gaiella appliance and the skull were returned to the storage area of the Museo Archeologico Etrusco in Firenze, where Becker made this study in March of 1994.

Description: the skull and mandible

This is the skull of a female (cf. Becker 1993a), but not the person for whom this appliance was made. Only a few measurements (in mm) were taken to confirm this sex evaluation. Mandibular molar dimensions also provide evidence: see Becker 2014; cf. Kieser 1990. Dental wear is minimal, but complete closure of the basilar suture confirms the age at more than 21 years (cf. Baggieri 1998: 67). Externally the cranial sutures appear to indicate an even greater age, perhaps about 40 years (cf. Corruccini and Pacciani 1989). Studies of the Etruscan population at Tarquinia (Becker 1990, 1993a) suggest that external closure of the cranial sutures commonly occurs at a relatively young age (see also Becker and Salvadei 1992). The minimal evidence of periodontal disease plus the configuration of cranial sutures indicates that she was about 25 years of age, if not older, at her death. An extensive review of the dentition confirms the estimated age at death (Becker 1995a).

The condition of the mandibular dentition yields evidence that the appliance was not made for this mandible. This mandible now has only three incisors in place. The modern restoration of the jaw failed to leave an empty socket for the 2I, which was lost post-mortem, (see also Sterpellone and Elsheikh 1990: 126).[3] A central incisor (1I) now "fills" both left incisor spaces, but this 1I appears discolored or darker than the surrounding teeth and may not be original to this mandible. The shifting of the mandibular teeth during the conservation process has produced a closing of the gap left by the "missing" tooth, causing the opening of spaces between the other teeth.

The Poggio Gaiella appliance spanned a maxillary 1PM to PM1 in the person for whom it was designed. After recovery from a tomb it had been placed in a mandible for which it was not made. Dunn, implying that this "appliance" was found *in situ* around eight teeth, indicates that "*i bicuspidati*" were included within the appliance. Dunn's reference cannot be interpreted as indicating that all 4 premolars were bound (10 teeth), but may have meant that only the premolars on one side of the jaw were held in the appliance. The two pieces or parts of the band are now placed so that the 2PM of this mandible is not encircled and since an incisor is missing, probably only recently, the appliance now extends to include the PM2. Dunn's observations suggest that the appliance had been set into this mandible before he acquired it. The "excavator" may have rudely set this appliance into a skull obtained (from a modern context? see Becker 1993a) specifically as a showpiece.

Becker's examination of the configuration and sizes of the extremely distorted pieces of this appliance suggests that it originally extended from a maxillary left first premolar across the front of the mouth to the right first premolar. This interpretation would include spanning two premolars. Thus Dunn may have evaluated this appliance correctly, with the problems of the present placement arising only after he had donated the Poggio Gaiella appliance to the museum. As to Dunn's belief that this prosthesis was worn in a mandible, we suggest the following scenario. The original skull did not survive and Dunn made his evaluation either on the basis of the configuration of the appliance or perhaps the location in a mandible as he first saw it before it was purchased. The distortions now evident in the appliance (extreme bending and folding, plus breaks), and the damage that renders an easy evaluation impossible, suggests that the appliance was forced into the mandible of an intact skull derived from an unknown source, and after some teeth were lost.

Clearly, at some time before Poggio Gaiella came into Dunn's possession a great deal of damage had been done to this delicate gold appliance. In addition to the bending and springing of the long sections of the band, the band appears to have been torn, and several welds have separated. Among the breaks may be one at a point where these two parts had been joined. All the evidence indicates that this appliance had not been associated with a mandible articulated with a complete skull at the time of discovery.

Description of the appliance

Detailed examination of the two pieces of this dental appliance suggests that the two elements were joined as shown in the illustration. Both pieces of the appliance are so ill-fitted to the teeth of this display mandible and so badly bent that there is no possibility that they match the teeth of this restored mandible. More significantly, there has been no ante-mortem loss of teeth, nor any evidence of loosening of the teeth, which might require the use of a dental appliance, nor evidence for a blow, which might have had a temporary effect of loosening the teeth.

Beginning at the right end of the right unit (cf. Platschick 1904–1905: fig. 2) is a sprung part of the appliance that was located behind the premolars of the display mandible, then pressed between the PM2 and M1. The unit is broken off after a sharp bend. A small "tail" under 2 mm long does not appear to have been connected with the loose end (width 2.82 mm), which extends back from the labial aspect of the right unit. This entire unit appears reversed, with the aspect now shown as mesial originally around a PM with the "tail" passing around the maxillary PM1. The portion of the band passing in front of this PM is continuous with the "divider," which would have been the piece of a small band that passed between the canine and the PM1. The most distal aspect of the right unit, as now seen, was welded onto the larger band of the left unit. Visual observation suggests that this "divider" was part of the PM1 ring that had been welded to the larger band, as is the case with the left unit.

At its closest point to the left unit this part of the right unit has a very sharp bend ending in another "tail." There is no indication where this may have attached. These two "tails" plus the divider seemingly welded to the front all may have connected to a piece of this unit now missing. It appears that three simple welds held four separate bands together.

Beginning at the most distal part of the left unit we find an extremely bent and folded "ring" now surrounding the 1PM, probably originally fitted to a canine. As we now see it this "ring" has a very peculiar double internal fold at the distal-lingual area, an equally peculiar "bump" at the distal-mesial portion, and a mesial part clearly formed by a very thin (0.13 mm) band, which had been welded in place. The weld on the labial aspect still holds, but the distal weld has separated. Microscopic examination might determine if this weld had once attached at the distal end of the "bump." The remainder of the left unit appears to be a simple ring (band) that probably spanned three teeth, the left canine to the left central incisor.

The Poggio Gaiella appliance presents an interesting variation of a simple four-ring prosthesis. Four rings would also require only three simple welds to fasten the units together in a series. One of the many reasons for doubting that this appliance was a single, long braced band is the fact that if it were one appliance it would be unusually long and be unique in being made in two parts. Braced bands loop over sound "anchor" teeth at either end in order to support loose teeth that are between the sound teeth. An effective means of securing the entire band would be to place braces (cross pieces) at either end to hold the band more firmly to the "anchor" teeth. With an unusually long appliance such as this, braces at either end would be essential. Stability could have been achieved by making two units, each carefully fitted with a braced area that would loop around a sound tooth (PM1's in this case) at the distal ends, and welding these two units together at the center. The center weld would reduce unwanted flexibility created by a long band, and would increase stability. We can "construct" a normal prosthesis if we reorient the various parts seen as they were mounted for display. Assuming that the mesial area of the right unit of Poggio Gaiella had been the distal portion, and if it originally had looped around a sound right first premolar (PM1) as an anchor tooth, the result would be a reasonably ornamental and probably functional appliance.

Two possible variant techniques of manufacture, using long bands, are possible, but unlikely. Although only three welds might be needed in either case, two of these welds would be "complex"; that is, they would have to weld two different sets of units together at the same time. Close fitting is much more difficult when long bands are used. Given all these possible variations, the Poggio Gaiella appliance is likely a variation of a simple four-ring prosthesis.

Ghinst (1930: 407) believed that the Poggio Gaiella appliance was intended to support teeth loosened by periodontal disease. This is a reasonable assumption, but Ghinst says that he based his conclusion on alveolar resorption evident in the mandible (also Emptoz 1987). Either the Poggio Gaiella appliance was in a different mandible prior to 1930, or Ghinst seriously erred in his evaluation of the health of the alveolar margin of this skull. Quite possibly the person for whom the Poggio Gaiella appliance was made did have periodontal difficulties, but there remains the basic problem of whether this appliance was actually found in this skull. Unfortunately, "*Les photós que nous présentons ici illustrent nos hypothèsis*"—do not appear in Ghinst's publication. His statement may refer only to photographs that he had shown as illustrations at the congress where his paper was read. Unfortunately these are not known to have survived. Capasso's (1986: 53) illustrations (reversed?) indicate that the appliance has recently been in two pieces, as does a reverse print shown by Corruccini and Pacciani (1989: fig. 2).

Measurements

Detailed measurements may be of some aid in determining if these two elements are from a single dental appliance. Dr. Jacopo Moggi-Cecci (Università degli Studi, Firenze) provided the use of an extremely accurate, illuminated sliding dial caliper (Mitutoyo Digimatic 500–110 electric). The two pieces of this appliance, as they are mounted in this mandible from PM1 to PM2, have a maximum "length" of 41.76 mm. If we draw a straight line as a tangent to the curves of the two most distal parts and then a line perpendicular from the most anterior aspect, that perpendicular line measures 20.41 mm long. The two elements may be considered individually as the right and left, with reference to their present position as displayed in the unrelated mandible.

The widths of the "right" band and its parts vary from 2.82 mm to 3.23 mm. The thickness of this ribbon of gold varies from 0.12 to 0.15 mm. The "left" unit varies between 3.02 and 3.33 mm wide, while the thickness of the gold strip varies from 0.12 to 0.17 mm. The more narrow aspects of the right unit are under 3 mm wide and are found at the mesial part of the appliance. The more narrow aspects of the left unit, while wider than the right, also appear toward the mesial aspect. Poggio Gaiella may have been constructed in a similar fashion to the GHENT appliance (no. 7), as a single complex band, somewhat more elaborate and longer than the GHENT appliance. These detailed measurements indicate that Ghinst (1930) was the most accurate in his appraisal of the width of this appliance (see also Casotti 1957). Less specific estimates are provided by Menconi and Fornaciari (1985: 94 = 0.20 to 0.25 mm) and by Tabanelli (1962: 92 and pl. 49). Emptoz (1987) offers only the vague estimate of 4.5 mm.

The very length of this band suggests that it was not purely decorative, implying that the anterior teeth of the person for whom it was made had actually been loosened by periodontal disease, or a blow. Periodontal disease would be expected in a relatively mature person of at least 30 to 40 years of age. Also, the uniform width of the band reinforces the conclusion that this was a functional prosthesis. It also might have been designed to support teeth that had been loosened by a blow, in which case a mandibular placement also would be possible. If true, this would be the best evidence from Etruria to suggest that dental appliances were used as a therapy for teeth loosened by accidental trauma as well as for cosmetic purposes.

Casotti (1947: 672, 1957: 105) offered a complex, but fanciful, description of how this appliance was held in place, concluding that the two pieces had once been "wired" together and otherwise manipulated to serve as an orthodontic corrective device to close "gaps" between the teeth (also Capasso 1986: 54). Not only is this a fanciful observation, but the fictitious goals of such a device would be counterproductive. Moving the teeth only would have disrupted their dental alignment and loosened them all. Casotti (1957) later noted which teeth were present when he examined the supposed Poggio Gaiella skull. He did not recognize the post-mortem loss of a mandibular incisor, leading him to speculate that the appliance was meant to close a "gap" supposedly created by the loss of the maxillary I2 (also Pacciani and Corruccini 1986: 55, fig.). However, no tension can be provided by any of these ancient appliances, and therefore there is no possibility that any prostheses could have altered the position of teeth (cf. Torino *et al.* 1996). Most devices served only inadvertently to maintain spaces between natural teeth.

This appliance is commonly confused with the more simply constructed band that had been in the Florence collections (Cat. no. 84467 and listed below as Populonia). Waarsenburg (1991a) points out that Ghinst's (1930) description of the two "pieces" in Florence actually describes the very same example (see also Penso 1984: figs 143–145).

6 Populonia: buried at Populonia (missing: lost in Florence Flood 1966)

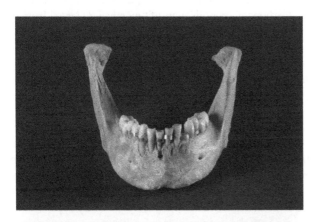

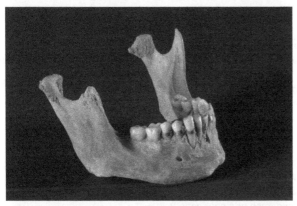

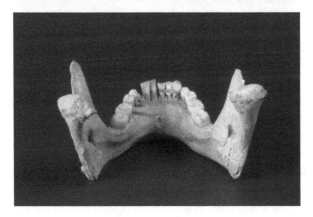

Figures 5.6a–c Views of Populonia appliance, set in a human mandible.

Source: courtesy Soprintendenza Archeologica per la Toscana (Florence Museo Archeologico neg. nos. 20055, 20056.20057.)

Present location: Museo Archeologico Etrusco, Florence, inventory no. 84467. Said to have been lost in the 1966 flood.

Type: four-"ring" series, with one rivet (at I1?), four spaces. Cf. no. 15, Valsiarosa.

Origin: Populonia, San Cerbone necropolis, part of "*membra disiecta*" from damaged tombs.

Jaw part: probably maxillary 2I–I2.

Date: fourth century BCE.

Sex: probably female.

Dimensions: approx. 25–30 mm long.

Description: generally described as a four-ring appliance, with a rivet through one of the (central?) rings. Original reports (Guerini 1894a, b) are insufficiently clear to distinguish this item from the Valsiarosa appliance (see no. 15, below), with which it has been often confused. Bliquez (1996) first revealed this and other problems created by authors writing without any primary study of the appliance (see also Waarsenburg 1991a).

References

Bliquez 1996: 2648, 2652, "F" and probably "O," figs 10–11.

Capasso 1985: 53. Capasso conflates the Populonia example with the Poggio Gaiella appliance (no. 5).

Casotti 1935: fig. 1 (reproduces Guerini 1894a: fig. 7).

Casotti 1947: 676 (668, 674–675: 3 cm long and 0.6 cm wide).

Emptoz 1987: no. XI?

Ghinst 1930: 406–407.

Guerini 1894a: 393, figs 1 and 2 (these illustrate the Valsiarosa example).

Guerini 1894b: figs 1 and 2 (show the Valsiarosa example).

Guerini 1909 (once again depicts the Valsiarosa example).

Hoffmann-Axthelm 1985: 78–79, Abb. 65.

Lufkin 1948, fig. 17 (photograph of a poor copy?).

Minto 1943, 183; pl. 48 fig. 1 (photo of mandible, but no appliance is visible).

Naso 2011: 151, no. 7.

Platschick 1904–1905: clearly confuses Populonia and Valsiarosa.

Tabanelli 1962: 92, 94–96, pl. 48, 52.

Torino *et al.* 1996: 120–121 (from Casotti 1947; cf. Becker 1994d).

Waarsenburg 1991a: n. 5, no. 1.

Weinberger 1948: 148, fig. 53 (Weinberger's fig. 41, no. 7 is either a copy, or the Valsiarosa example). Weinberger suggests that this is for mandibular I2–PM2.

History and provenance

The necropoleis of Populonia held numerous rich seventh–sixth-century tombs, many plundered during the nineteenth–twentieth centuries CE. Minto's brief publication (1943: 183) of items excavated in the vicinity of the Tomb of the Funeral Beds (1908–1909 and 1920–1921) lists several of the more spectacular sporadic finds, including:

quella singulare legatura dei denti, ottenuta mediante una sottile fettuccia d'oro, ritrovata in una mandibola di cranio (pl. XLVIII, 1), proveniente da una tomba ad inumazione distrutta, che richiama ad un esempio consimile riscontrato nella mandibola di un cranio, proveniente da una tomba etrusca di Città della Pieve, con dentiera legata in oro (R. Museo Archeologico di Firenze, Sezione topografica).

this unusual binding of the teeth, achieved by the use of a thin strip of gold, [was] found in a mandible of a skull (pl. 48, 1) that came from a destroyed inhumation tomb, which recalls a similar example, found in the jaw of a skull that came from an Etruscan tomb at Città della Pieve, with a denture bound in gold (Royal Archaeological Museum of Florence, Topographic Section).

Minto was referring to the Poggio Gaiella appliance, also stored in the Museo Nazionale Archeologico di Firenze. This may explain why subsequent authors have confounded the two items. The difficulty of seeing any appliance in the mandible illustrated in his plate 48 further compounds the problem. Tomb of the Funeral Beds at Populonia is an Archaic structure, but the gold jewelry from the same area of sporadic finds in the necropolis includes a number of pieces in fourth-century style, so the date of the appliance could be from the seventh to the fourth century BCE—the latter date was suggested by Ghinst (1930).

Analysis of past accounts

Ghinst says that this appliance is gracile (presumably meaning that it was found or displayed in a gracile mandible), involves 6 mandibular teeth, and that the mandible held 14 teeth. This appears to confuse the appliance with the skull in which it is mounted. Ghinst says that the appliance is held by "*un mince ruban d'or*" and measures "*larg. 2 1/2 mm env épais 1/3 cm*," passing from tooth to tooth "*sous forme de spire.*" He also says that the alveolus is strongly resorbed, suggesting "*un cas de pyorrhée traumatique*" but that this is difficult to see since there is earth still adhering to the neck of the teeth? ("*au colet*"). In many respects this description sounds like that for Poggio Gaiella. We are not at all certain that Ghinst actually saw either of these appliances, and suspect that his data also are derivative.

Regarding the confusion between Populonia and Valsiarosa, Weinberger's (1948: 125–126, fig. 41: 7) illustration for Valsiarosa (no. 15) looks more like a copy of the Populonia piece. Weinberger cites Deneffe (1899: pl. 3, no. 1), Sudhoff (1926: fig. 45), and Farrar (1888: figs 1 and 2) as his sources. Weinberger's illustration appears to show a copy that may also be illustrated by Lufkin; it resembles an industrial casting rather than any known appliance.

Weinberger's photographs of the Populonia appliance clearly indicate a very common type that bound four maxillary incisors. However, for reasons unknown he states that it is a mandibular prosthesis (I2–PM2), and his illustration and text

(1948: 148, fig. 53, right) incorrectly suggest that the PM1 was replaced by a false tooth, held in place by a rivet. Weinberger's caption for the copy (fig. 41: 7) also says it held a premolar. The chamber pierced by the rivet appears to be square, while the other three are more ring-like (although somewhat distorted by their archaeological past). Three rings were formed, one each for the two left teeth and for the right anchor tooth. The chamber for the false tooth appears to have been formed by connecting the flanking rings with two short strips of gold welded in place.

Later in his book Weinberger (1948: 148, fig. 53) describes the original of what is supposed to be the Populonia example, and includes two "original photographs" said to be in the "author's collection." These appear to show the original appliance in Florence. These may be photographs of the piece which Guerini (1894a: 393) noted during his visit in Rome: *"je trouvai dans celui de Pape Luigi un appareil en or . . . "*

Guerini's poor drawing of a gold appliance of four "rings" with the central pair somewhat quadrangular, indicates that one central ring has a rivet. Although his fig. 1 depicts the central pair of rings as quadrangular (cf. Copenhagen appliance), in fig. 2 they are circular. Guerini's drawings also make these four rings appear to be a graded series, small to large, with the riveted example the second largest.

Guerini's (1894a) "Papa Luigi" museum in Rome is, of course, the "Museum of Pope Julius," the Villa Giulia Museum, devoted to Etruscan antiquities. Guerini (1909: 70) offers a correction to his earlier (1894a) identification.

Waarsenberg (1990) suggests that 4 or 5 specimens often said to be in Florence are "probably only one specimen." Many of the phantom pieces have been created from the photographs of the (apparently) two different inventoried examples once identified at the Museo Nazionale Archeologico in Florence. In addition, *copies* of at least one piece may be creating some of the confusion, as Waarsenburg explains. Other specious "specimens" of dental appliances have emerged in Florence (see Appendix III, no. 6, below) as the result of misidentification of copper-stained human teeth as "gold crowns."

7 Ghent (lost)

Present location: unknown: lost during German occupation of Ghent in 1940s.
Type: complex band forming three "loops," the central of which is double size (and surrounded two teeth). Spans four dental spaces; no rivets.
Origin: Orvieto (ancient *Volsinii*).
Jaw part: maxilla, probably 2I–I2, rather than the commonly believed 1I–C (now attached to a suspect or added canine).
Date: sixth century BCE or later (estimated).
Sex: female?
Dimensions: L. 27, W. 2.8 mm.

Description: This appliance surrounded four teeth, almost certainly the maxillary central incisors. It may have been used as an ornament, or perhaps to stabilize

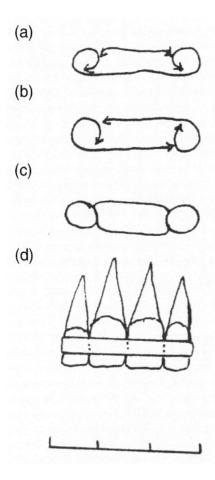

Figures 5.7a–d Drawings of the Ghent appliance (said to be from Orvieto, now
lost), by Becker: (a) and (b) construction technique; (c) plan of the
applicance, to scale; (d) labial surface of the appliance showing how
it would brace the four incisors.

one or more loose teeth. The width of the band is unusually uniform. An unusual
manufacturing technique using two separate strips of gold, a pattern similar only
to the longer Poggio Gaiella appliance (no. 5). Ghent, like Poggio Gaiella, may
have been constructed in one of two ways. A strip approx. 39 mm long could
have been rolled at both ends and tacked to form the lateral loops, with a second
strip only 17 mm long then welded to form the back portion of the appliance.
Alternately, two identical strips, about 28 mm in length, could each have been
rolled at one end, then that "loop" welded to form a "9" (each loop to surround
one anchor tooth) before having the long end of each of the pair welded to the
loop of the other. This final welding created an elongate opening to surround the
two central teeth.

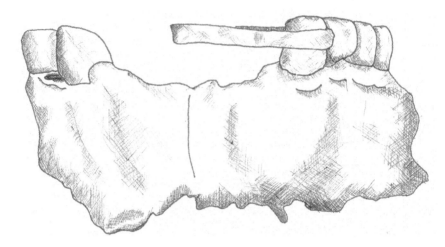

Figure 5.7e Appliance from Orvieto, now lost, side view, as illustrated by Guerini 1909.

Source: drawing by Tim Downs (timdownslocations@verizon.net).

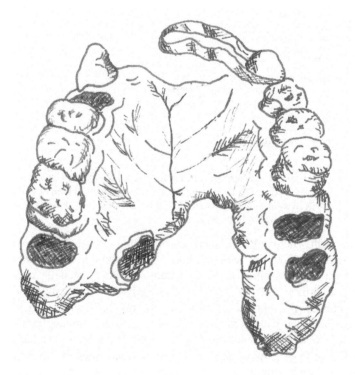

Figure 5.7f Appliance from Orvieto, now lost, view from below, as illustrated by Guerini 1909.

Source: drawing by Tim Downs (timdownslocations@verizon.net).

References

Bliquez 1996: 2646, "C," figs 3–4.
Boissier 1927: 29, fig. 5.
Casotti 1947: 673–674, fig. 3 (from Guerini 1909: fig. 21).
Cavenago 1933: fig. 1.
Dechaume and Huard 1988: fig. 4B3, lower. Photograph may show a copy (see Appendix II.D).
Deneffe 1899: 59, 63–67, fig. 1 (probably the original appliance).
Emptoz 1987: 557, fig. 19 (no. XXII).
Guerini 1909: 74–75, figs 21, 22.
Lufkin 1948: Fig. 21.
Sudhoff 1926: 84–85, figs 48–49.
Tabanelli 1962: 93 (not at all useful).
Waarsenberg 1991a: n. 5, no. 12.
Weinberger 1948: 123–125, fig. 41: 1.

History and provenance

Emptoz (1987), in a review of the early literature pertaining to the Ghent piece, concludes that this appliance together with an associated maxilla come from Orvieto. Boissier (1927: 29) clearly errs when he says that the Ghent appliance came "from Tarquinia, near Orvieto." Deneffe's (1899: 59, 63) estimate of date, 600–500 BC, is based on the dates of the famous stone masonry tombs and their original depositions at the Crocifisso del Tufo necropolis of Orvieto (also Sudhoff 1926: 84).

Soon after its discovery this appliance was purchased by Ghent University, Belgium, and by 1899 it was in the Ghent University Museum. It *may* be the only one recovered with a portion of the original associated skull. Skull and appliance were together in 1899, although a more photogenic skull easily could have been chosen for display, as happened with the Poggio Gaiella and Valsiarosa appliances.

Description

Deneffe (1899) offers the most complete description of the Ghent appliance, derived from the original, rather than a copy as appears to be the case with his other descriptions. It disappeared during the German occupation of Ghent in the 1940s.

Much of the maxilla in which the Ghent appliance was seated had been lost by the time of Deneffe's photograph (1899: pl. 1). Assuming that this facial fragment is actually part of the skull of the owner of this appliance, much can be determined from this photo. Possibly all 16 teeth of this maxilla were in place at the time of death, but the 3M, 1PM, 2I–I2, M2 and M3 appear missing in the photograph, probably lost *post mortem*. If this is a retention band for loose teeth, as we believe, there need not have been any loss of teeth before death.

The Ghent band appeared attached to the right canine as a post, and would then have attached to the left central incisor in order to support loose incisors.

However, its configuration suggests that it actually spanned the four incisors (2I–I2) rather than following an asymmetrical pattern. The incisors commonly are lost post mortem, and the Ghent appliance must have been placed on this canine to hold it in place for display (see Cavenago 1933: fig. 1).

Deneffe's (1899: 64) description is both complex and contradictory. First he says that this appliance is a single oval, with three rings each built from two lengths of band attached at each end to post teeth. He gives the total length of the appliance as 26 mm, noting that the *central* band is 1.5 cm long and 0.6 mm wide (thick). This indicates that the central opening, formed by the long arms of the ribbons, is 26 mm long, or just the width expected of two broad, female central incisors, with the smaller openings at the ends conforming to expectation for the size of lateral incisors. Deneffe describes the breadth of the gold band as 3 mm, but where it encircles the post teeth, at the ends, it is 3 mm broad. However, Deneffe notes that the appliance is 5 mm broad in the rear, and notes this variation of 2 mm (1899: 67). He later states that the band and the "partitions" are a bit more than 0.5 mm thick.

Sudhoff (1926) estimates the width of the band at 4 mm, a figure copied by Emptoz, who also incorrectly states that it has rivets. Weinberger (1948) describes the gold along the mesial surfaces of the anchor teeth as "partitions." Only discovery of the actual prosthesis could confirm this evaluation (see also "The Ghent copies" in Appendix II).

The Tarquinia series (nos. 8–12): history and provenance

In the village of Corneto, today recognized as ancient Tarquinia (Etruscan *Tarchna*, Roman *Tarquinii*), during the end of the nineteenth century, two separate collections of archaeological materials included Etruscan dental appliances. One belonged to Count Bruschi and included three Etruscan dental appliances. Dasti (1878: 386) indicates that the private "Museo Etrusco nel Palazzo Bruschi Falgari," was open to anyone requesting admission. This rich collection was assembled by the Contessa Giustina Quaglia Bruschi Falgari, one of the important women antiquarians/archaeologists of the nineteenth century. Dasti (1878: 386) says *"sia smalti oggetti in oro, de'quali molti esseguiti artisticamente con rara perfezione"* ("there are enameled [sc. shiny] objects in gold, of which many were artistically executed with rare perfection").

Two other dental appliances found their way into the Corneto Museo Civico, which opened in 1878. Excavation of tombs at Tarquinia was at its height throughout the later nineteenth century into the twentieth (see Leighton 2004: 10–24). The number of dental appliances in Corneto is reported differently by early authors, depending on when they saw these growing collections, which were merged into the new national archaeological museum (today Museo Archeologico Nazionale Tarquiniense). In the move, some pieces either were not actually transferred or subsequently disappeared. The quality of early descriptions and illustrations is uniformly poor, which prevents us from determining with certainty which pieces came into the two original collections, and in what years. We also cannot determine when some items were last seen. The general confusion even renders difficult an exact count of these examples.[4]

In 1992 only one appliance was on display in the Museo Archeologico Nazionale Tarquiniense (Bruschi I); another was in storage (Bruschi III); these two are described from Becker's observations. Among these five examples, the similar Bruschi III and Corneto I are frequently confused, and they continue to be difficult to distinguish in most reports. Van Marter (1885a) saw Corneto I and II in the Corneto Civic Museum, and says that he received certificates from Dasti attesting to the dates when these tombs were opened. Why Van Marter sought such documents is not known; his papers might furnish a trove of information regarding this matter as well as other aspects of Etruscan archaeology.

An example of the problems created by the early reports is an anonymous note in the February 1885 issue of the *Journal of the British Dental Association* (p. 123), referring to Van Marter's publication of the previous month (1885a) and describing:

> An example made of rings of gold [which include] the first bicuspid "and two centrals" said to be carved from animal teeth [probably Corneto II]; a second example which has 2 lower incisors, both said to be natural [Corneto I?].

This second example, said to be Roman, is dated to 400 BCE without explanation. Waite (1885a: 316–317) subsequently, and unfortunately, stated that the two examples in Liverpool are so similar to the pieces (from Corneto) described by Van Marter (1885a), and repeated in the *Journal of the British Dental Association*, that they need not be illustrated. All of this is further confused by Waite's (1885a: 508, 512) relation of his then recent trip to the United States, during which he may have seen the two appliances then owned by Barrett.

Guerini (1894a: 393) also notes that he saw (only?) two appliances in Corneto, presumably the pair then in the Civic Museum. Dunn (1894) describes two appliances in each museum. Deneffe (1899: 77–78) suggests that two pieces were in the Civic Museum at Corneto in 1899, and that three were still in Count Bruschi's possession. This implies that Count Bruschi acquired the third appliance between 1894 and 1899. Deneffe, however, describes only two of the three pieces that he said were in the Bruschi collection (Bruschi I, and a second less clearly identified). The fifth Tarquinia appliance now is believed to have come into Count Bruschi's collection about 1894. Platschick (1904–1905: 239), following Dunn (1894) says that only four pieces were in the two museums in Corneto, three of which were maxillary and one mandibular. Platschick does not list Bruschi I, probably because he did not see any examples, and only repeats what Dunn reported.

Deneffe (1899) implies that Corneto I as well as a second prosthesis from Tarquinia had been among the eight appliances copied (see Appendix II.A) for the Ghent University Museum. Deneffe also thanks Helbig, as the "*Directeur du Museé Comunal de Corneto*," for permission to copy two appliances, and then (1899: 82) thanks Count Bruschi for his permission to copy, for the Ghent collections, the three prostheses in his possession. In fact, copies of all five of the Tarquinia pieces were made for the Ghent collections (Ghent copies nos. 4–8, see Appendix II.A). Moltesen (1987: 242) documents the fact that Helbig was, for some time, Honorary Inspector of Excavations at Tarquinia. Helbig certainly facilitated the copying of these prostheses.

Waarsenburg (1991a: 243, n. 11) suggests that it was Helbig (1877: 64) who provided a fifth-century BCE date for one of the Tarquinia appliances. We have very little other information useful in establishing specific dates for these pieces.

Today we can account for only two of the five examples that had been in the two earlier collections. In June of 1991, when Becker studied the two examples now in the Museo Archeologico Nazionale Tarquiniense, staff suggested that the three pieces that now cannot be located were lost during the transfer of items to the then-new national museum system collections around 1916.

8 Bruschi I

Present location: displayed in Museo Archeologico Nazionale Tarquiniense, formerly in association with two teeth. Previous collection of Count Bruschi-Falgari, Corneto.

Type: simple, narrow band spanning four spaces (not three spaces as commonly reported).

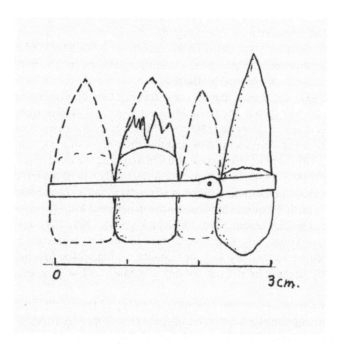

Figure 5.8 Tarquinia appliance: drawing of Bruschi I appliance, by Becker.

Origin: region of Tarquinia (?)—also said to have been found at Cerveteri (Guerini 1909: 74).

Jaw part: maxilla, four spaces. Probably spanned all four incisors, but Guerini and Deneffe took the presence of a left canine (not original to the appliance) to infer its use as in Figure 5.8).

Date: possibly fifth century BCE (see Waarsenburg 1991a: 243, n. 11).

Sex: female.

Dimensions: L. 32; W. 2.0 mm. Gold band: W. 1.9 to 2.2 mm; Th. less than 0.20 to approx. 0.25 mm; total L. of gold ribbon estimated 74 mm. Weight 2.5 g.

Description: simple band, formed from a strip of relatively uniform width, with slight variations from 1.9 to 2.1 mm, and about 74 mm long. The ends of the strip, which is 0.20 thick, were overlapped for a length of about 3 mm and welded. The location of the weld is, unusually, quite evident as indicated by a slight expansion of the width.

References

Baggieri 1998: 68 (popular basis for his 1999 essay).

Baggieri 1999: 38–39, fig. 7, top pair (numerous errors, details omitted).

Baggieri 2001: 324–325, pl. xxxviia and graph 1.

Bliquez 1996: 2649–2650, 2654, figs 15, 16, 37 #7 (prosthesis "I" and also "S" figs 29–30).

Brothwell and Carr 1962, fig. 3 (illustrate only a copy).

Casotti 1947: pl. 1 (copy of Guerini 1894a: fig. 8).

Cataldi 1993: 125 (mentioned, not illustrated).

Deneffe 1899: 81–82, fig. 7 (from a copy).

Emptoz 1987: 556, fig. 18 (no. XXI). See also p. 557, no. XXIII.

Guerini 1894a: 394, fig. 8 (of a copy?).

Guerini 1894b: fig. 8 (see 1894a).

Guerini 1909: 74, fig. 20 (looks like a copy; see figs 23, 24 for possible original).

Hoffmann-Axthelm 1981: fig. 65 (not in 1985 edition).

Lufkin 1948: fig. 22 (cf. fig 23; data copied from Guerini 1894a, 1894b and 1909.

Menconi and Fornaciari 1985: 94, 97, fig. 10 (perhaps the best published photograph).

Naso 2011: 151, no. 8.

Rath 1958: fig. 3. Illustration secured by Rath from "Foto Istituto Scala, Firenze."

Sterpellone and Elsheikh 1990: 136, fig. 64 (two teeth in place, but depicted as mandibular).

Sudhoff 1926: 84, fig. 47 (his #8, on p. 85 with figs 51a and b, also appear to be Bruschi I).

Tabanelli 1962: 93.

Torino *et al.* 1996: 120.

Torino *et al.* 1997: 536.

Waarsenburg 1994.

Weinberger 1948: 125, fig. 41: 6 (from Sudhoff 1926).

Weiss 1989: fig. 29 (mislabeled). His suggestion that it is in the "Civic Museum of Corneto" indicates that his research, showing the appliance as mandibular, was long out of date.

History and archaeology

Guerini (1909: fig. 23) says that the Bruschi I appliance was "found in 1865 in a tomb by Cervetri [sic]" and that it then belonged to "Castellani's collection, Rome." (Much of the Castellani collection did in fact come from the Caeretan region and included gold jewelry.) Possibly the appliance was recovered from Cerveteri, located between Tarquinia and Rome, in 1865 and only later, before or around 1894, sold to Count Bruschi. No number is written on this piece, but the number "160" appears on a small white circular tag on the velvet backing in this display, possibly the velvet in use when this piece was in Count Bruschi's collection. It was in the collection of Count Bruschi-Falgari when Guerini (1894a: 394) supposedly first saw it, but was not noted by Dunn (1894), who lists only two examples of gold appliances in the Bruschi collection. Casotti's (1927: 628) note that only two appliances are in this collection appears to be copied from Dunn.

The Bruschi I appliance may have been acquired by Count Bruschi about 1894, or after Dunn had seen and published the two examples in the Bruschi collection. Deneffe's publication (1899) reveals that by 1899 Count Bruschi owned *three* examples, which apparently included this piece. This apparent increase in the number of appliances in Count Bruschi's collection reinforces the belief that Bruschi I was added to the Count's inventory *after* Dunn had examined Count Bruschi's holdings.

Description: the Bruschi I appliance and associated teeth

Becker first examined this appliance in 1991, in a laboratory in the storage area of the Museo Archeologico Nazionale Tarquiniense, in Palazzo Vitelleschi, Tarquinia. At that time the two teeth within this appliance were found to have a slight calcareous coating, not dental calculus but a deposit acquired during the centuries of burial underground. (Such deposits are not uncommon on inside chamber tombs, especially in the region of Tarquinia and Vulci.) The teeth themselves reflected the pattern of deterioration typical for teeth recovered from Etruscan tombs in this area (see Becker 1990). The roots are typically warped and cracked, with considerable damage in a pattern commonly seen on teeth from other "open" tomb contexts (i.e. chamber tombs where air circulates around the bodies). Unlike our findings with other dental appliances with which intact teeth may be associated, those few examples with teeth from which the roots have deteriorated are most likely to have been with the prostheses when they were found. The teeth with Bruschi I appear to be a maxillary left canine and a left central incisor, suggesting that the appliance may have spanned at least the left canine to the left central incisor. This placement is exactly what Guerini (1894a) and Deneffe (1899) both concluded, and suggests that the teeth now with the appliance were the ones seen by these two authors. This does not prove that these are the original teeth, nor that they are in their original positions. The wear on the teeth suggests that the owner was a mature female, perhaps 45–55 years of age, but we cannot be certain that the teeth represent the person who actually wore the appliance.

Examination confirmed that this appliance was worn in the maxilla, but the Bruschi I band probably spanned four teeth rather than three. The canine now in Bruschi I, rotated in its location, has a maximum length of 25.0 mm, with M-D breadth 7.2 mm and B-L width 8.3 mm. The surface is worn, but obscured by calcareous deposits. The left central incisor now within this band has lost much of its root, with the remainder measuring 17.6 mm long. The remainder of the root has fractured and was recently repaired. The incisor crown breadth is 8.6 mm and the maximum B-L diameter is 7.3 mm. This incisor has been worn evenly into the dentine, and no trace of shoveling is evident.

The thin gold band is a simple construction, for most of its length just under 2.0 mm wide varying from 1.9 to 2.1 mm (2.2 in one location, see below). Baggieri (2001: 324) gives the weight of the band as 2.5 grams. This is an unusually narrow band for Etruscan dental appliances, particularly if it had been intended to stabilize loose teeth. Its thickness varies from under 0.20 mm to about 0.25 mm at the point where it is welded. This wider section, near the medial aspect of the canine now placed within it, appears more globular (slightly wider and thicker), suggesting that a weld was made at this location by overlapping the ends of a long band. The total length of the original ribbon from which this band was formed is estimated at 74 mm. Baggieri (2001: 324) claims that microscopic examination of the exterior surface at 170 magnification reveals a line marking the junction of the welding and trauma to the band, which he attributes to damage from mastication. Becker notes that considerable damage is evident even without high magnification, but what is visible probably reflects excavation and subsequent handling. At the point of overlap on this gold band there also appears a tiny raised dot of gold, the function or origins of which are unknown. This "dot," of insignificant size and barely visible to a casual observer, would have been on the right labial side of the mouth. The maximum length of this appliance as it now exists, after distortion, is 24.5 mm, with the breadth at the inserted canine 6.1 mm, and at the incisor, 8.0 mm. The distance across the buccal and lingual aspects of the band, at the present compressed center, is about 1.6 mm. The actual maximum length of the oval band is shown in Figure 5.8, and demonstrates that the band had spanned four teeth.

This band certainly could not have held any false teeth, but could only have been used as a decoration, or to stabilize teeth loosened by a blow or by periodontal disease. Yet it appears too narrow to have served a purely decorative purpose, unless a discrete hint of gold was intended or the owner could not afford a more elaborate example. Severe periodontal disease in the area of the incisors has not yet been demonstrated as common among the Etruscans (cf. Becker 1990), but the incisor area is often involved in periodontal disease in other populations.

The loss of some of the teeth within this band (or perhaps they simply were not recovered in the excavation) led to its central area being deliberately pinched together to hold the remaining (or added) teeth "in place" within the band.

Critique of other published observations

Hoffmann-Axthelm (1981: fig. 65, but not illustrated in 1985 edition) shows what appears to be the Bruschi I appliance—a very thin band around an I1 and canine, with the center of the band (recently) bent to hold these teeth at the ends. Illustrations of this appliance generally depict two teeth, with intact roots, at the lateral ends of the appliance. Other descriptions of these teeth vary, probably because they derive from one or more copies that have included human teeth (incisors and/or canines).

The most common error associated with the Bruschi I appliance is to describe the pinched central area of this simple oval band as a "spacer bar" connecting two loops. This error obviously derives from naive evaluations of photographs, or possibly from flawed reproductions. Deneffe's description is roughly accurate. At first he notes that the gold band was pressed together in the center, but later Deneffe (1899: 82) describes this as a "*barre*" and a bar-like stricture is exactly what he illustrates. Becker suggests that Deneffe's 1899 illustration derives from a Guerini copy (see Appendix II). Emptoz (1987) repeats this error when he describes this piece as having "*une tige*" ("a shank") of gold. Emptoz even suggests that this "*tige*" may have supported a false tooth. Other authors repeat this erroneous "observation" when they state that a bar connecting two rings acted as a spacer bar, or by various other descriptions revealing that they have never examined the piece. The use of the term "wire" for this thin band has led other evaluators to suppose it resembles the Phoenician examples (e.g. the two from Sidon, nos. W-1 and W-2). Perhaps this is why Emptoz (1987: 557) infers that a sixth appliance could be found at Tarquinia; his example XXIII that he believed to be made of wire. Emptoz says that the example he assigns to number XXIII had been part of the Bruschi Collection, and mistakenly notes it as a gold-wire retention band. Clearly this confusion results from Emptoz's misreading of earlier descriptions and photographs, in which the unusually narrow band looks like wire.

Sudhoff, normally a careful observer, also created two examples from Bruschi I through the use of two different photographs, both shown without crediting their sources. Sudhoff (1921: fig. 47; 1926: 84, fig. 47) describes Bruschi I as coming from Tarquinia, and describes the maxillary left central incisor and canine in place. Later, Sudhoff (1921: figs 51a and 51b; 1926: 85, figs 51a and b) describes a supposedly different piece said to be from Caere, although he suggests that it might have been made in Tarquinia. Both illustrations seem to be of the same piece.

Weinberger (1948: 125, fig. 42: 2 and 6), following Guerini (1909) and Sudhoff (1921, 1926), also created two phantom appliances from this single example. One is derived from Guerini's figs 23–24 (Sudhoff's fig. 51) and the other from Guerini's fig. 20 (Sudhoff's fig. 47). The value of conducting primary research is nowhere more clearly seen than in these examples.

Guerini (1909: fig. 20) illustrates what is probably a very poor copy of the Bruschi I appliance, perhaps his own replica. He incorrectly shows it as if it were a "bar" extending between two rings. Guerini's (1909) description could be of another thin band (see Weinberger fig. 41: 2). Guerini's (1909) fig. 24 depicts another reproduction of this piece (possibly the Wellcome Museum copy, see Appendix II), further confusing the matter.

Most recently Baggieri (2001: 324–325) has presented data supposedly derived from an X-ray diffraction analysis of the Bruschi I appliance, which he identifies as "T-A," but a number of errors recur.

9 Bruschi II

Present location: missing since *c.*1916–1925. May have been transferred from
    Count Bruschi's collection to the Museo Archeologico Nazionale Tarquiniense.
Type: four rings, with a rivet in the only empty ring (1I?).
Origin: area of Tarquinia?
Jaw part: maxillary(?), probably 2I–I2.
Date: not known.

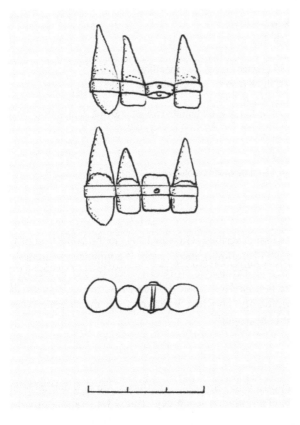

Figure 5.9 Tarquinia appliance: Drawing of Bruschi II appliance, three views, by
          Becker.

Sex: female ???
Dimensions: L. 29, W. 2.1 mm.

Description: This now missing piece was a four-ring appliance with a single rivet though one of the center loops similar to the Populonia pontic (no. 6). Early illustrations suggest a 7.0 mm rivet with a shaft length of 5.9 mm and a diameter of ca 0.75 mm. The peened heads of the rivet have diameters of 1.5 to 2.0 mm. Generally believed to have surrounded a canine (right) and three incisors. If correct, the replaced tooth would have been the right central incisor.

References

Bliquez 1996: 2652, "N," figs 21 and 37 (no. 6).
Bobbio 1958: fig. 11 (taken from the copy illustrated by Rivault 1953: fig. 4).
Brown 1934: fig. 4b.
Casotti 1947: 671, pl. 1, 7 (from Guerini 1894a: fig. 7).
Deneffe 1899: 80–81, fig. 6 (shown as maxillary).
Dunn 1894: 9, with figure.
Emptoz 1987: 555, fig. 16 (no. XVIII).
Guerini 1894a: fig. 7; 1894b: fig. 7.
Guerini 1904: 394, fig. 7.
Guerini 1909: 73–74, fig. 19 (sketch) notes it as maxillary.
Platschick 1904–1905: 241, fig. 8 (shown as mandibular).
Rivault 1953: fig. 4 (from a copy in Paris).
Sterpellone and Elsheikh 1990: 134, fig. 62 bottom (rough drawing copied from unknown source).
Sudhoff 1926: 81, fig. 44.
Weinberger 1948: 125, fig. 41: 3.
Woodforde 1967: fig. on p. 11 (sketch of rear view).

History

When the appliance was first described (Guerini 1904) in the collection of Count Bruschi-Falgari at Corneto (Tarquinia), the Bruschi II appliance presumably was excavated in the territory of Tarquinia, on land owned by the Bruschi-Falgari (which encompassed the famous Hellenistic Tomba Bruschi: see Vincenti 2009). Sudhoff (1926: 81) specifically says that it comes from the "*Gräberstadt von Tarquinii*," "the Tarquinia necropolis."

Description

The three earliest depictions of the Bruschi II appliance are in remarkable agreement as to details of its configuration, each depicting a four-ring appliance that seems to be welded together, with a single false tooth held in place by a rivet. As always one should not assume that the teeth depicted were original to the appliance. By 1894 the false tooth originally riveted in place had been lost, but three natural human teeth were then present. The replacement tooth may have been made of perishable material, although it is just as likely that all the original teeth as well as the replacement tooth dissolved in the tomb. Our depiction of this appliance is based *entirely* on the assumption that the canine shown in early illustrations was original to the appliance, which is not a likely pattern of manufacture. More likely this appliance spanned all four incisors, but that could only be confirmed by precise measurements, which are no longer possible.

Dunn's drawing (1894: 9) appears to show the lingual surface of Bruschi II in an inverted position, with the tooth size as depicted suggestive of the four incisors, and with the rivet for a false tooth at 1I. Dunn depicts rather wide rings, perhaps 5 mm wide (later copied by Platschick). Guerini's drawing (1894a: 395, fig. 7; also 1894b: fig. 7) suggests a buccal view of a maxillary appliance, with the tooth on the left being a canine. This would indicate that the replaced tooth was an 1I, as depicted in Figure 5.9.

Deneffe (1899: pl. III, 6) says that Bruschi II is a maxillary appliance, 3 cm long, a measurement only 1 mm longer than Becker's calculation from the photograph. However, Deneffe states that the band is 4 to 5 mm wide; in agreement with Dunn but twice the 2.1 mm estimated by Becker. Deneffe's photograph appears to show the lingual surface. Although the configuration of the tooth on the right is unclear, Deneffe specifies that it is a canine and that the appliance spans the 1I–C. Guerini (1909) depicts it thus. Sudhoff (1926: 44) copies Deneffe exactly. Deneffe's photograph, however, shows much more slender rings than those drawn by Dunn. The Deneffe illustration may be a copy and not the original. The width of the individual rings probably did vary, however, as each ring of Bruschi II may have been made separately before all 4 were welded together.

Based on an evaluation of the three teeth "in place" one might assume that the Bruschi II appliance was mandibular. These, however, could be modern replacements rather than originals. More likely this piece was worn in the maxilla, as suggested by most of the early observers. A medial tooth more recently depicted as present in this appliance does not appear to be the correct tooth for that location, and should thus be omitted (see photograph in Weinberger 1948: fig. 41:3; also Brown 1934).

The Bruschi II piece also is often confused with the Valsiarosa example. A copy of an appliance bridging four spaces (1I–C.), which appears to be a copy of Bruschi II, is in the Musée de l'École Dentaire de Paris (Rivault 1953: fig. 4; see copies in Appendix II).

10 Bruschi III (often confused with Corneto I)

Present location: Museo Archeologico Nazionale Tarquiniense.
Type: stabilizing band with four braces welded within to form five spaces (no rivets). Two spaces are now empty, three others held human teeth when Becker examined it, but all appear to be recent replacements.
Origin: Tarquinia area? (from collection of Count Bruschi-Falgari).

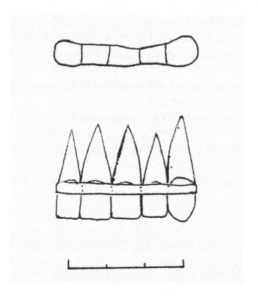

Figure 5.10 Tarquinia appliance: drawing of Bruschi III, a braced band for
stabilizing loose teeth, two views, by Becker.

Jaw part: maxilla? Possibly left canine to I2. Menconi and Fornaciari (1985) suggest that this spanned the maxillary 2PM–I1.
Date: Menconi and Fornaciari (1985) imply a second-century BCE date, but this is
unconfirmed.
Sex: female.
Dimensions: L. 36.8, W. 2.6–2.8 mm. See Table 5.1 below for additional
measurements.

Description: band apparently fashioned from a single long (about 83 mm) strip
of gold in an oval into which four braces (dividing strips) have been fitted and
welded to create five tooth spaces. The elongate "rectangles" of these openings
suggest that this appliance had been flattened, creating its unusual length (cf.
Corneto I). The sizes of these openings clearly represent one canine and all four
incisors. There is no indication of a replacement tooth. The gold dividing strips
are slightly narrower than the minimum diameter of the surrounding oval. The
teeth displayed with this appliance are not those of the original owner.

References

Baggieri 1998: 68.
Baggieri 1999: 38–39, fig. 7 lower (useful illustrations).
Baggieri 2001: 325, pl. xxxviid.

Bliquez 1996: "H," figs 13, 14 and 37 (no. 5).

Bobbio 1958: fig. 11 (copy, photo taken from Rivault 1953).

Casotti 1947: 673 (max. 2I–C.) with three teeth *in situ* (from Deneffe?).

Deneffe 1899: 79–80, fig. 5 (maxillary). Apparently a photograph of a copy with random teeth inserted.

Dunn 1894: 8–9, fig. on bottom of p. 8 (very poor drawing).

Emptoz 1987: 553? fig. 13?, no. XIII?

Guerini 1909: 70, fig. 15 (a copy that appears to be a "casting").

Menconi and Fornaciari 1985: 92, figs 1, 2 (fig. 1 depicts this with two teeth; p. 94, fig. 2 is an excellent "plan" view with no teeth in place) (Maxillary 2PM–I1?).

Micheloni 1976. Appliance belonging *"all'arcata inferiore"* thus mandibular, according to Torino *et al.* (1996: 119–120).

Naso 2011: 151, no. 9.

Platschick 1904–1905: 241, fig. 7.

Rath 1958: 12, fig. 3 (illustrations only).

Rivault 1953 (from a copy in Paris, see Appendix II).

Sterpellone and Elsheikh 1990: 135, fig. 63 (photograph has only two teeth in place).

Sudhoff 1926: 85, fig. 50.

Tabanelli 1962: fig. 50 (q.v. for teeth in place) (Mandibular C–I2).

Torino *et al.* 1996: 119–120. These authors accept this as a mandibular appliance, supposedly following Micheloni 1976.

Torino *et al.* 1997: 536.

Critical observations on the Bruschi III appliance and associated teeth

This appliance often is confused with Corneto I, which also spans five spaces, but has two rivets. Bruschi III appears to be a maxillary appliance, which spanned (included) five dental spaces, probably from the left canine to the right I2. This location is inferred from the size and relative positions of the "rings." The premolar seen within the band in 1991 certainly is a "display replacement" tooth not original to the appliance, and the other two teeth seen in 1991 also are recent additions. When Menconi and Fornaciari (1985) saw this appliance it had only two human teeth associated with it. Based on the two teeth that he saw and identified as mandibular, Baggieri (1998: 68, "T-B") believes it was worn in a mandible (Baggieri 2001: 325).

An appliance of this type would be unlikely to span 1PM–I1: probably it was placed around a maxillary canine and across all four incisors, as suggested by Tabanelli (1962). It was seen by Menconi and Fornaciari in 1985. This description is based only on Becker's provisional examination of this appliance, since Bruschi III then (1991 to 1995) was securely glued to a plastic sheet and displayed in inverted position; it could not be detached.

Bruschi III appears to have been formed by constructing a simple gold band into which a series of four braces, or internal cross-pieces, have been inserted by welding. The four braces partition off five separate spaces. The exact manner of construction is not clear. Becker (11 June 1991) identified all three teeth as maxillary, although they are not original to the appliance (cf. Dunn 1894: 8, fig.). All three are loose in the gold sockets: the teeth would fall out if placed right side up on the vertical display surface. The measurements listed below are approximate, but adequate for comparative purposes. The inference that two false teeth had been held in place by this appliance (Casotti 1947; Tabanelli 1962) is not supported by the sizes of the individual spaces, the shapes of the sockets or the breadth of the band (cf. Copenhagen). We also must agree with Deneffe (1899) and Bliquez (1996) that no false teeth were in this appliance. The three teeth "traditionally" displayed in this appliance might reflect only the remaining fragments in place when Bruschi III was first seen.

Description

The total length of this narrow band is 36.8 mm, spanning five tooth spaces from the left canine-I2). Each of the enclosing units formed within the band, also refered to as "rings," is somewhat warped or distorted from its original shape, but some are much more bent than others. Therefore, the estimates of the size of individual units must be inferred from the few measurements that could be made. All measurements are presented in Table 5.1.

The largest chamber appears to be the "ring" that would have held the suspected left lateral incisor (2I). This considerable mesial-distal length, however, has been created by a compression of the B-L diameter. The lingual surface is a single low curve, but the buccal surface has a bend toward one side that gives the appearance of two curves. The present B-L width is about 4.5 mm, but varies due to the bend noted above. The B-L dimension may even have been greater than the M-D, but what is presented here are only those lengths that could be measured and described.

The "ring" for I2 appears to be the second largest, and would be expected to be about the same size as that for the left lateral incisor (2I).

Table 5.1 Dimensions (in mm) for Bruschi III (measured while it was affixed to the display mount noted above)

Tooth space	M-D length*	B-L breadth*	B-L breadth**	Height of band ***	Thickness of band ***
I2	7.2	6.9	7.3 (est.)	2.7	?
I1	6.1	5.9	6.3	2.75	0.2
1I	5.3	5.3 approx.	6.2 (est.)	2.6	
2I	7.9	4.5 (bent)		2.8	
C	5.9	9.3 (est.)		2.7	0.25

   * Measurement across the interior surfaces of the "ring."
  ** Measurement across the interior surfaces of the "ring."
 *** Taken at the center of the lingual surface.

Table 5.2 Measurements of exterior surfaces of band Bruschi III

Between Teeth	I2/I1	I1/1I	1I/2I	2IC
Exterior	8.1	—	—	—
Interior Length	3.9(?)	3.8*	3.8**	4.1***
Thickness	—	0.2	—	—

   * The brace is narrower than the band (by approximately 0.1 or 0.15 mm only) on the "inferior" surface.

  ** This brace is wider than the encircling band to which it attaches, on the buccal surface, by at least 0.5 mm, and approximately 0.2 mm wider on the lingual surface (all these are on the inferior surface of the band, which is uppermost as it is displayed).

*** The brace between 2I/C is detached from the surrounding band at the buccal surface. An imperfect weld is suggested. At the lingual attachment the brace is about 0.1 mm higher than the band to which it is attached.

Measurements (B-L) were taken to the external surfaces of the band at the points where the four "braces" separate the anterior from posterior surfaces (includes the length of the brace and the thickness of the band. The thickness of only one brace could be measured as per Table 5.2.

The central socket or "ring" of this appliance, which would have surrounded the 1I, clearly is the smallest, as expected for a mandibular appliance. The socket for the 1I appears to have been circular, but also appears to have been bent outward on the buccal surface for attachment to the present mounting, resulting in the distance between the braces on the buccal surface being less than on the lingual surface. (All lengths in the table are from lingual surface.) The "circular" form suggests that this socket was meant to surround a living "peg"-shaped incisor, rather than a false tooth, which would have been made rectangular in cross section (cf. Copenhagen). The narrow width of the band of Bruschi III supports Deneffe's and Bliquez's conclusion that it was designed only to stabilize loose teeth.

The "ring" in the position of the I1 seems to be second smallest. This very small size, if it held a lateral incisor, is also consonant with a mandibular prosthesis. The socket formed for the left canine appears to be in the middle-range of sizes in this series of five. The I2 space within the band, however, has a M-D interior diameter of 7.2 mm. This distance seems distorted (elongated) through flattening of the band. This may explain why the tooth located in this socket was found, in 1991, to be rotated in its socket within the band.

The width of the "lingual" surface of the band, measured in five places, varies from 2.6 to 2.8mm (average 2.71 mm). Menconi and Fornaciari (1985: 94) give a range in width from 0.23 to 0.25 cm. The variations suggest that four individual units were joined by welding. Also, the buccal widths of the band appear much narrower than the lingual, but these could not be measured while the appliance was fixed to its display mount.

The three human teeth in Bruschi III

Although Becker believes that none of the associated teeth are original to this appliance, a history and description may be useful. Dunn (1894: 8) originally thought that this appliance encompassed five teeth or tooth spaces, believing that the three teeth were natural and served as anchors. Dunn's suggestion that there were two false teeth is indicated by the depiction of two rivets in his *drawing* of this appliance, although no rivets exist nor does Dunn indicate their presence in his text. At least one of the "false" teeth was said to be missing at an early date, but a later account states that one of the surviving false teeth was split. By the time that Menconi and Fornaciari (1985) examined this piece, at least one of the three human teeth that had been earlier in place appears to have been lost. This lost tooth had been replaced by another tooth before 1991, the premolar now seen in more recent illustrations.

This possible scenario, that lost teeth have been replaced, or did not survive with this appliance, brings us back to the problem of the location of the Bruschi III appliance in the jaws. It is doubtful whether *any* of the teeth now with the appliance were the owner's original teeth, serving as anchors for artificial teeth: we should infer that all have been replaced. All three teeth found with this appliance in 1991 appeared to be rotated in the sockets. The premolar appears rotated a full 90 degrees and an incisor is rotated about 45 degrees. We cannot even be certain which surface of the appliance is being viewed, but possibly what can be seen is the lingual surface, and the buccal is affixed to the plastic display panel. All observations and measurements were made with the supposition that we are examining the lingual surface.

No teeth were found in the sockets made for either left incisor; the tooth now found in the socket made to fit the I2 is actually a maxillary left canine. The tooth wear pattern on this I2 suggests that this person had an overbite, down in a left distal direction, indicating that this is a maxillary tooth. The extent of wear is considerable, suggesting that it comes from a mature individual who may have lost teeth or at least have had loose teeth. Some tartar remains on the tooth.

The left maxillary first premolar is so worn that both cusps are flattened almost to the level of the dividing groove, but not quite to a single flat surface. This premolar, which appears to be within the socket designed for a canine, appears to have had a great deal of tartar on it, but most of it has become detached, as indicated by the clean enamel showing through patches among the remaining tartar. The root has grooves on both surfaces but is not actually bifurcate, and also has some bumps at about one-third of its length up from its apical end. The articular surface of the tooth is worn down towards the lingual margins, again suggesting

Table 5.3 Dimensions of extant teeth in Bruschi III (believed to be modern inserts, of unknown sex)

Tooth	Height	A-P diameter	M-D diameter
Left canine	25.3	7.9	6.4
Left first PM	17.6	9.3	5.9
Right central I	?	6.9	7.2

an overbite such as is indicated by the canine, and suggesting that both derive from the same individual.

Critique of the literature relating to the Bruschi III appliance

Dunn (1894) describes Bruschi III as one of two examples that he saw in Count Bruschi's collection. This indicates that the third example owned by Count Bruschi (here identified as Bruschi I) came into his collection after 1894, but before 1899 when Deneffe indicated that Count Bruschi owned three examples.

Dunn suggests that the Bruschi III appliance was fashioned to replace the two front teeth (central incisors). His text does not mention rivets, but his illustration depicts rivets in both empty "central incisor" positions. The three "real" teeth shown by Dunn appear to be the maxillary left canine, a left lateral incisor (which in the drawing looks like a broad central incisor) and a right lateral incisor.

Deneffe (1899) describes this as one of three dental appliances then in Count Bruschi's collection. The accompanying illustration shows the left canine and both right incisors in place (differing from Dunn's illustration). Deneffe's description, however, is confused since he states that "*la canine droite*" is in place, while his fig. 5 suggests that it is the left canine in place. Casotti (1947) also says that three teeth are in place.

Deneffe (1899) describes the appliance as approx. 5 mm high, nearly twice the actual height (see also his evaluation of width for Bruschi II). His drawing, however, depicts a band much closer to the correct width. Deneffe's estimate of the band's length (40 mm) is reasonably accurate. Menconi and Fornaciari (1985) give the width of the band as 2.5 mm, but others tend to estimate the width as being much greater than it is, probably following Deneffe's published measurement. All descriptions supposed to be of Bruschi III, but including rivets, are probably of Corneto I, or derived from Dunn's (1894) early error. All the difficulties with the five examples supposed to be in Tarquinia (see Deneffe 1899: 59) appear to derive from these early contradictory descriptions.

11 Corneto I

Figure 5.11 Tarquinia appliance: Corneto I Appliance, drawing by Becker after Van Marter 1885a: figs 3–4.

Present location: missing (at least since *c.*1916–1925) from Museo Archeologico Nazionale Tarquiniense.

Type: braced band (?) for five spaces, one of which has a rivet (one space still had a replacement tooth; no other teeth remain). It is likely that the modern copies of this appliance are "braced," while the real example may have been formed by a series of welded rings.

Origin: excavated from a tomb in the necropolis of Corneto-Tarquinia, in contrada Montarozzi northwest of Secondi Archi, by Luigi Dasti *et al.* (season October 16, 1876 through Spring, 1877). The project was financed by the Comune and the *Arte agrariane* of Corneto-Tarquinia.

Jaw part: maxillary (?), left C–I2.

Date: sixth–fourth century BCE (on the basis of Helbig 1877: 64).

Sex: ?

Dimensions: L. 28, W.5–6 mm.

Description: following Deneffe's description, the five spaces of this "braced" oval band are believed to have surrounded all four maxillary incisors and the left canine. The construction appears remarkably like Bruschi III, but with a single rivet. This rivet would have passed through a replacement or cut-down central right incisor. Illustrations suggest a rivet 7.5 mm long, with a shaft length of approx. 6.7 mm. The peened heads of the rivet probably had dimensions similar to Bruschi II.

References

Bliquez 1996: 2651–2652, "M," figs 20 and 37 (no. 4).

Boissier 1927: 22, figs 3 and 4.

Brown 1934: fig. 4a.

Casotti 1947: pl. I (from Guerini 1894a, see below); and also Casotti's pl. II (from Platschick 1904–1905: fig. 6).

Dasti 1878: 17, 367–368.

Deneffe 1899: 77–78, fig. 4 (2.6 cm long, 0.5 cm wide) (Weinberger says p. 75, pl. II: fig. 4).

Dunn 1894: 8 (fig).

Emptoz 1987: 552, fig. 11? (no. XII?).

Farrar 1888: 33, figs 3–4.

Guerini 1894a: 394, figs 5–6; 1894b: figs 5, 6.

Guerini 1909: 73, fig. 18 ("very old Etruscan tomb").

Helbig 1877: 59–64 (see also Waarsenburg 1991a: 243, n. 11).

Koch 1909: 9, 16 figs 3–4.

Lufkin 1948: fig. 20.

Platschick 1904–1905: 241, fig. 6.

Ring 1985: 45, fig. 36 (from a copy? maxillary?).

Sudhoff 1926: 80–81, fig. 43.

Tabanelli 1962: 93.

Van Marter 1885a: 3, figs 3–4.

Waarsenburg 1991a: 243, n. 11.

Weinberger 1947: fig. 8 (supposedly from Sudhoff 1926: 90 [sic], but looks like a copy).

Weinberger 1948: 125, figs 41: 5 and 41: 9.

Woodforde 1967: fig. on p. 11 (inverted).

History/possible origins of Corneto I

From Helbig's early account (1877: 56–57) it appears that this piece was discovered during the 1876–1877 excavation season. Dasti (1878: 359) notes that the museum was inaugurated in 1878, on the ground and first floors of Palazzo Demaniale, Via dell'Ospedale, n. 15. This appliance was then displayed in room 3 on the ground floor. Van Marter (1885a: 2), who saw it in the Corneto Museum about 1885, says that he has a certificate from Dasti attesting to the dates during which this tomb and the tomb containing the Corneto II appliance were opened.

Dasti (1878: 367–368, Chapter IV, "*Oggetti d'Arte Etruschi di recente trovati*") notes that "this" appliance, along with smaller objects, was located in the "*3ª Stanza*" of the Museo Etrusco, Tarquiniese, suggesting that a piece in the Civic Museum is meant, very probably Corneto I.

> *Una dentiera formata di* [sic."da" in Helbig's version] *una lamina d'oro, lunga 0.03, con sei fori, uno dei quali, il quarto, contando dalla sinistra, contiene un dente. I due fori estremi, alquanto più larghi degli altri, erano destinati ad essere infissi in due denti effettivi della persona che doveva portare la dentiera.*
>
> A denture formed from a gold plate, 0.03 long, with six holes, one of which, the fourth counting from the left, contains a tooth. The two end holes, quite a bit wider than the others, were destined to be affixed to the two actual teeth of the person who was supposed to wear the denture.

This is the same description that appears, with slight orthographic variation, in Dasti's letter to Helbig (Helbig 1877: 64). Although no rivets are noted in this description, at least one appears to be present. Dasti may have counted the spaces on either side of the visible rivet (that actually would be halves of a single "tooth" location) as two separate "*fori*" ("holes," "openings") thus creating "*sei fori*" or six holes by his count.

Helbig's (1877: 59–64) publication of Dasti's letter contains the listing of the objects from all these chamber tombs combined, and distinguished only as having held Greek black- or red-figured vases (thus probably Attic imports of the sixth to fourth centuries BCE). There is no mention of finds of Etruscan bucchero pottery, often ignored in old excavations. Helbig (1877: 64; also Dasti) notes a sardonyx scarab and gold, granulation-decorated grape-cluster earrings, which sound typical of fourth-century Etruscan art, but there is no way to determine which burial produced them or the gold appliance.

Description, based on past publications

Van Marter (1885a) was the first to illustrate and describe this appliance in a clear and useful fashion, as an oval band with cross braces, an unlikely but not impossible construction. Usually it is described as made of five rings, as in Dunn's drawing (1894: 8; copied by Platschick 1904–1905), but elsewhere it appears to be a single band with four cross braces forming five sockets. Dunn's drawing and others showing five sockets appear to result from confusion with the Bruschi III appliance. Dunn (1894) illustrates in the central hole a single tooth with a portion of the root intact. This suggests a natural tooth and not an artificial or re-placed crown riveted into the appliance. In turn, the presence of a human tooth at this location implies that the appliance had but one rivet.

Van Marter (1885a: 3, figs 3–4) provides a description together with its most widely known illustrations, including what appears to be a hand-applied gilt overlay representing the appliance, approximately 5 mm broad. Van Marter says that the Corneto I appliance came from a "Roman" tomb, dated to 400 BCE: he gave no explanation for the statement, but many authors assumed that the more "complex" appliances are Roman rather than Etruscan in origin. This information, including Van Marter's illustration, was among the material copied by Koch (1909: 9, 16, figs 3–4).

Sudhoff (1926: 81) depicts a mandibular prosthesis (2I–C.), as indicated from its positioning and from the shape of the teeth, of which four are present, three being real tooth crowns and one apparently a replacement or false tooth. He shows a braced band with two rivets, stating (1926: 80) that the band is 5 mm wide on both the labial and lingual sides. By 1926 this piece may have been missing, so it would be useful to know if Sudhoff actually saw the appliance or instead derived his information from earlier sources or a copy. Other illustrations show but one tooth, the false tooth riveted in the central space in the band. Possibly Sudhoff's illustration was made before the loss of the natural tooth crowns that had been found with the appliance.

Deneffe describes this appliance, or a copy of it, as 26 mm long, 5 mm high, holding a well-preserved tooth crown riveted in the central opening, but lacking a root. The fourth hole from left also bears a rivet, but the false tooth is missing. Deneffe's description appears to have been taken from Guerini (1894a: figs 5 and 6). Deneffe (1899: 78) also credits Helbig with facilitating arrangements for making copies for the museum in Ghent of the two appliances then in the Corneto Civic Museum (see Appendix II.A).

Van Marter's figure illustrates this piece with what appears to be the crown of a small incisor in the central opening. Guerini (1894a: figs 5–6) also shows but one central incisor crown in place. However, Weinberger (1948: 125, figs 41: 5 and 41: 9) provides two interesting photographs. One, labeled 41: 5, appears to show this piece situated in a mandible, with all teeth present except for the top of the 1I. This is probably a photograph of a copy set in a mandible for display. Weinberger's illustration 41: 9 shows the appliance without a jaw, apparently the illustration used by Guerini (1894a) and Van Marter (1885a). Most interesting is Weinberger's failure to make any reference to his own fig. 41: 9 depicting this appliance.

Commonly published illustrations show but one remaining tooth and it is positioned as if it were a mandibular I1. If this tooth were a mandibular I1, then the chamber next to it (to the left when viewed from the rear; and the one with a rivet) would have held a replacement for the 1I. The openings or spaces in this appliance are relatively square in plan, and similar in shape to the central chamber in the Copenhagen appliance that was clearly meant to hold a false tooth. Possibly the I2 here was not false and we must conclude that the C and 2I served as anchor teeth. The exterior of the band appears perfectly flat.

Dunn's note on an appliance that has been confused with this prosthesis says that it is in the "*Stanza Ottava*" ("Eighth Room") of the museum. Platschick (1904–1905: 241) says that it is in the "*ottava sala*," and shows the false tooth as projecting below the appliance, but clearly most of the root is missing. Dunn suggests that only the fourth tooth was false, having a rivet located in that ring, but that when he saw it the tooth was missing. Clearly what he described is not the same piece as Corneto I, but which of the others (at Tarquinia or elsewhere) it might be is not certain.

12 Corneto II

Present location: missing (at least since *c.*1916–1925) from Museo Archeologico Nazionale Tarquiniense.

Type: compound: seven rings bridging eight spaces. Two of the five human teeth are in place as are "two" of the three false teeth. The "two" false teeth are fashioned from one piece of bone (possibly ivory). The false teeth were held in place by three rivets.

Origin: Necropolis of Tarquinia.

Jaw part: maxilla? Possibly 2PM–right canine.

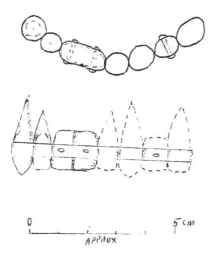

Figure 5.12 Tarquinia appliance: Corneto II, two sketch views. Becker's reconstruction, combining Clawson (1933: fig. 8a) and Van Marter (1885a: figs 1–2).

Date: 500 BCE (per Van Marter 1885a, citing Helbig).
Sex: Female??
Dimensions: L. 62.5, W. 4.0–4.3 mm.

Description: This impressive seven-ring appliance, spanning eight tooth spaces, is perhaps the most complex of Etruscan bridges. Three teeth are replaced, using three gold rivets. Both central incisors are replaced by the major feature, an elongate "ring" in which an animal tooth or piece of ivory was held in place by two rivets. The right lateral incisor and canine served as anchor teeth. This appliance also provided a replacement for the left first premolar, also riveted in place but not surviving. The second premolar served as the anchor tooth for this end of the bridge. Loss to decay of a first premolar prior to the loss of the molars and the second premolar is rare. The possibility that this tooth, like the incisors, was deliberately removed must be considered.

References

Bliquez 1996: 2653–2654, "Q," figs 26, 27 and 37 (no. 3).
Bobbio 1958: fig. 13 (figure credited to Van Marter 1885a, but actually from Rivault 1953: fig. 1, who took his illustration from a copy of the appliance in Paris).
Boissier 1927: fig. 8.
Brown 1934: fig. 5
Casotti 1947: 669, pl. 1 (from Guerini 1894a: figs 3 and 4).
Cavenago 1933: fig. 3.
Clawson 1933: fig. 8a; also 1934: 24, fig. 1.
Dunn 1894: 6–8, fig. p. 6.
Deneffe 1899: 73–76, fig. 3
Emptoz 1987: 556, fig. 17 (no. XIX). Dates it fourth century BCE.
Farrar 1888, I: 32–33, figs 1–2.
Guerini 1894a: 393–394, figs 3–4
Guerini 1894b: figs 3–4.
Guerini 1909: 71–73, figs 16, 17 (16 is printed in reverse).
Hoffmann-Axthelm 1985: 68, fig. 63 (also fig. 63 in 1981 edition). The "appliance" illustrated here is a copy.
Koch 1909: 9, 16, figs 1–2.
Lufkin 1948: figs 18, 19.
Platschick 1904–1905: 240, fig. 5.
Rivault 1953: fig. 1.
Sterpellone and Elsheikh 1990: 134, fig. 62 top (a drawing), 138–139.
Strömgren 1919: figs 2–3 (from Guerini 1909).
Sudhoff 1926: 82–83, fig. 46.
Tabanelli 1962: 93.
Van Marter 1885a: 3, figs 1–2 (best illustrations).
Weege 1913: 371.
Weinberger 1948: 126, fig. 41: 8 (error in transcribing date).
Woodforde 1967: fig. on p. 10.
Weiss 1989: fig. 28 (but mislabeled, with two views shown. Said to be in the "Civic Museum of Corneto," suggesting that his data comes from Guerini 1909).

History

This dental appliance appears to have been excavated around 1885, or during Van Marter's residence in Rome. First described by Van Marter (1885a: 2) when it was in the Museo Comunale di Corneto. He suggested a date based on Helbig's estimate of 500–400 BCE, presumably founded on the style of artifacts found with this appliance. Van Marter specifies that he received a certificate from Dasti attesting to the date on which the tomb was opened. While it is remotely possible that this unusual seven-ring appliance was excavated before 1885, the fact that it was located in the Museo Civico suggests that Corneto II was a local find.

Van Marter's report later (1909: fig. 16) indicates the "Civic Museum of Corneto," where it had been since at least 1885 (see Van Marter 1885a). Koch (1909) also copied Van Marter's data and illustrations. Platschick's reference (1904: 240) to "*otto anelli*" ("eight rings") probably indicates that this appliance extended over eight tooth spaces, bridged by an appliance of seven rings. Strömgren (1919: 24, figs 2–3) provides lower case letter designations for these rings (a–g), an extremely useful means of identification, a system unfortunately not followed by subsequent authors. Strömgren's letter "g" indicates the largest ring in this appliance, which may have circled the left 2PM.

Description, based on past publications

This appliance, if maxillary, appears to replace at least three teeth (1PM and 1I–I1). Deneffe gives the dimensions as 6 cm long, with a band 0.5 cm broad. Van Marter's illustration (1885a: fig. 1) suggests that the various rings are only 2.5 mm broad. Deneffe's illustration (also Platschick 1904–1905: fig. 5) shows one rivet for each of the three replaced teeth. The false incisor unit (the one-piece replacement for two teeth) has one rivet for each "tooth." The space for the 1PM has a rivet, but no false tooth remains. Details of construction techniques cannot be confirmed without direct inspection.

In place in this appliance are an intact, slender right canine and right lateral incisor. Next to them is a false tooth, replacing the central incisors, that appears to derive from an animal tooth with root filed down and otherwise sculpted. Platschick (1904–1905: 240) covered all possibilities when he noted that it might have been made "*di terra cotta o di pietra, oppure fatti da un pezzo di conchiglia*" ("of terracotta or of stone, or perhaps made of a piece of seashell") or from the tooth of a large animal. This "observation" clearly indicates that Platschick had not seen the appliance. Guerini (1909: 71–72) also suggests that one rooted anchor tooth was a canine. Guerini also suggested that either one of the owner's incisors never erupted (dental agenesis), or that shifting after the loss of a tooth may have allowed the teeth to close over this position, basing his inference on his belief that the large ring on one end was meant to fit over a molar (also Weinberger 1948: 126). In addition, Weinberger (1948: 126) believed that a "lug" (spacer bar?) was inserted between the last two empty rings, as suggested earlier by Guerini. No such "lug" existed, (a parallel is the fictional "spacer" often cited for the Bruschi I appliance).

The attachment of an Etruscan dental bridge to a molar is extremely unlikely. Van Marter is correct in indicating that the large empty ring probably fitted over a large left second premolar, which also reinforces the conclusion that this is a maxillary appliance. The cleverly carved replaced teeth make this is a sophisticated example of these appliances.

Guerini (1909: 72) also notes that "the large [false] tooth employed . . . does not show any signs of being worn by mastication" and suggests that it was made from an unerupted maxillary incisor taken from a calf (see also Deneffe 1899: 75, who cites Guerini). The replacement is cleverly carved with a vertical groove on the anterior surface to represent two incisors, complete with two rivets. Guerini, in English translation (Guerini 1909: 72) uses the British term "pivot" (in British dentistry the term used to describe a false tooth mounted on a pin set into a tooth root) rather than the term "rivet."

Guerini (1909: 72) states that when making copies of "all the ancient prosthetic pieces existing in the Italian museums, I met with special difficulty in the reproduction of . . ." this example. The copy of the Corneto II appliance illustrated by Hoffmann-Axthelm (1985: fig. 63) is not accurately made, having but one rivet securing the large, carved false tooth representing the original "pair" of incisors.

The two appliances in the Liverpool World Museum

In 1867 Joseph Mayer, a goldsmith of Liverpool, England, donated his entire collection of antiquities, including two Etruscan gold dental appliances, to the Public Museum of his city, then known as The William Brown Street Museum (Waite 1885a: 508). Mayer's Etruscan pieces had been purchased by or for him in Italy or in sales of collections formed in Italy. Many objects, especially bronzes and gold ornaments, can be traced to nineteenth-century collections gathered after what we today would consider the plundering of Vulci. Some items still bear labels linking them to finds sold by the estate of Prince Canino, one of the Bonapartes who had a country home in the vicinity of the city plain near the necropolis of ancient Vulci. Unfortunately, there is no documentation of the exact sources of the two dental appliances that were offered to Mayer because of his interest in gold-working. (None of Mayer's Etruscan gold jewels has a recognized provenance either.)

We know from Purland (1857–1858) that by 1857 Mayer already had "some examples" of Etruscan gold dental appliances in his collection (also Weinberger 1948: 79). Waite (1885a: 508) believes that Mayer had actually bought these pieces during the year 1857, but this is uncertain. Waite mistakenly states that Hockley (1858: 121) had published a note on at least one of these appliances in Mayer's collection (M 10334).

Perine (1883: 163) clearly knew of the existence of these two prostheses but his descriptions bear no relationship to the actual appliances. Quite possibly they derive from a verbal account provided to Perine by a third party. Arthur Weinberger (1948: 79) states that both of the Liverpool examples were reported in an article written by Henry H. Burchard, but this has not been confirmed. Emptoz (1987) includes in his inventory only one of the two examples from the Mayer Collection.

Both Liverpool dental appliances were studied (1980–1981) for incorporation in the catalogue of Etruscan objects being prepared by Turfa; they were then studied by Becker in 1988. After a theft occurred in 1989, the appliances were eventually recovered unscathed along with most other gold items. They were again examined by Turfa in 2011 with the assistance of Margarita Gleba and Cynthia Reed (goldsmith), and again examined by Turfa in May 2015 and May 2016. The descriptions that appear below are based on those direct observations, and the *Catalogue of the Etruscan and Italic Collection in the Liverpool World Museum* (Turfa, in press). What is most interesting about these two appliances, given that they became part of a single collection, is that both are bands enclosing four tooth spaces yet one has only what appear to be the natural lateral teeth in place and the other bears only the artificial central teeth (cf. Johnstone 1932b: 449). The gold bands are somewhat distorted, perhaps through post-excavation factors.

One of the copies of these Liverpool appliances in the Wellcome collection of the Science Museum, London (see Appendix II.B) came with the following note: "two pieces of Etruscan bridge work acquired Liverpool Museum 1915 ex Mayer collection there. WR 2/26/4 WR 2/25/28 (3)." Possible meanings of these numbers are discussed in Appendix II.B.

Bibliography for both Liverpool M 10334 and M 10335

These dental appliances have been cited in numerous general publications, with or (very often) without credit, often using the sketches published by Johnstone (1932b) or Macnamara (1973), or the photos of Tabanelli 1962: pl. 51. The main references are cited below:

Bonfante, L. 1986. "Daily Life and Afterlife," in L. Bonfante, ed., *Etruscan Life and Afterlife* [232–278] 251 fig. VIII–28. Detroit, IL: Wayne State University Press.

Cohen, R. A. 1959. "Methods and Materials Used for Artificial Teeth [Abridged]," *Proceedings of the Royal Society of Medicine* 52: 775–786, fig. 1. (Incorrect identification as Egyptian.)

Emptoz, F. 1987. "La Prothèse Dentaire dans la Civilisation Étrusque," in *Archéologie et Médecine: VII Rencontre Internationale d'Archéologie et d'Histoire (Antibes 1986)* [545–560] 554–555 no. XVII (inventory includes only one Liverpool appliance, M 10334). Juan-les-Pins: Editions A.P.D.C.A.

Grant, Michael, 1980. *The Etruscans*, 240–241, fig. London: Weidenfeld and Nicholson.

Hockley, A. 1858: 121 (M 10334 only). Waite (1885a: 508) gives this incorrect reference: "Mr. Hockley on Mechanical Dentistry." *Quarterly Journal of Dental Science* (April 1857–January 1858) I: 393–403.

Hoffmann-Axthelm, W. 1970. "The History of Tooth Replacement," *Dental Science and Research* 8 (9): 81–87, fig. 4.

Hoffmann-Axthelm, W. 1985. *Die Geschichte der Zahnheilkunde*, second edition, 78–79, fig. 64. Berlin: Quintessenz Verlags-GmbH.

Lloyd-Morgan, Glenys and S.P. Girardon, 1988. "The Etruscan Collection," in M. Gibson and S. M. Wright, eds, *Joseph Mayer of Liverpool, 1803–1886*, 77–85. London: Society of Antiquaries, Occasional Papers N.S. XI.

Macnamara, E. 1973. *Everyday Life of the* Etruscans, 170, fig. 104. London: Batsford.

Mayer, Joseph, 1852. *Egyptian Museum: No. VIII, Colquitt-Street, Liverpool.* 1852: 20, no. 222A (April 15). (Booklet/guide to Mayer's museum in Colquitt Street, Liverpool. Archival copy in the World Museum Liverpool is annotated with inventory numbers by Charles T. Gatty.)

Moorehead, T. F. 1983. "Chirurgia, Medicina, Dentifricium," *British Dental Journal* 154 (10): 340–342 (May 21): 341, fig.

Perine, G. H. 1883. "A History of Dentistry from the Earliest Period to the Present Time," *New England Journal of Dentistry* 2 (6): 161–166, 199–205, 269–273, 343–345 (descriptions inaccurate).

Purland, T. Jr., 1857–1858. "Dental Memoranda," *Quarterly Journal of Dental Science* I: 63–65, 201–204, 342–346, 460–463; II: 121–123, 242–243, 353–355, 490–493; see 1857: 63.

Waite, W. H. 1885."Association Intelligence, Western Counties' Branch" (Letter; Discussion), *Journal of the British Dental Association* (now *British Dental Journal*) 6: 316–317; 499–512, and 2 figures.

Weinberger, B. H. 1981 (1948). *An Introduction to the History of Dentistry*, Volume 1, 79. Saint Louis, MO: C. V. Mosby, 1948. Special edition by Gryphon Editions in Birmingham, Alabama, 1981.

Scarborough, J. 1969. *Roman Medicine*, pl. 8. Ithaca, NY: Cornell University Press.

Sterpellone, L. 2002. *La medicina etrusca. Demoiatria di un'antica Civiltà*, 139. Noceto: Edizioni Esembiemme.

Tabanelli, M. N. 1962. *La Medicina nel Mondo degli* Etruschi, pl. 51. Florence: Leo S. Olschki.

Numerous other popular and general publications mention or illustrate (often from the nineteenth-century drawing) one or both appliances (for instance, Recke and Wamser-Krasznai 2008: 139 fig. 58). The Wellcome Collection of the Science Museum, London, holds copies of these prostheses, said to have been acquired in 1915.

For additional discussion of Etruscan gold dental appliances, see:

Becker, M. J. 1999a. "Etruscan Gold Dental Appliances: Three Newly 'Discovered' Examples in America," *American Journal of Archaeology* 103: 103–111.

Becker, M. J. 1999b."The Valsiarosa Gold Dental Appliance: Etruscan Origins for Dental Prostheses," *Etruscan Studies* 6: 43–73.

Turfa, J. M. in press, 2016. *Catalogue of the Etruscan Collection in the World Museum Liverpool*, ed. Georgina Muskett, entries no. J29 and J30.

Turfa, J. M. and M. J. Becker 2013. "Chapter 47. Health and Medicine in Etruria," in J. M. Turfa, ed., *The Etruscan World*, 871 figs 47.8 and 47.9. London: Routledge.

13 Liverpool I (Cat. no. M. 10334)

Present location: World Museum Liverpool, Mayer Collection, inventory no. M 10334.

Type: band with two false teeth, which survive, each held in place with one rivet.

Origin: unknown, but surely from an excavation before or during 1857.

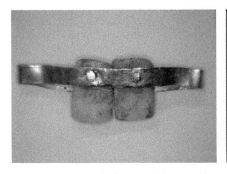
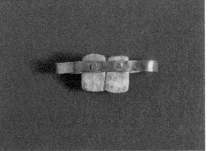

Figures 5.13a1–a2 Buccal views of appliance.

Source: courtesy of the National Museums Liverpool and Georgina Muskett, also by Margarita Gleba.

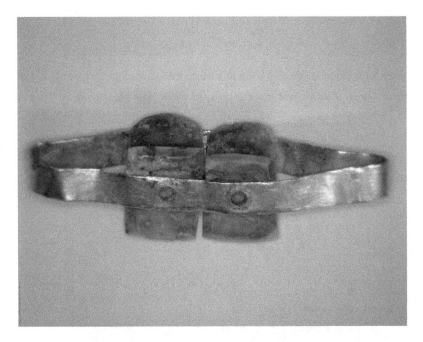

Figure 5.13b Lingual view.

Source: courtesy of the National Museums Liverpool and Georgina Muskett, also by Margarita Gleba.

Jaw part: maxillary 2I–I2.
Date: not known.
Sex: female?
Dimensions: L. 30.9, W. 3.0–3.1 mm. Rivets: L. 7.0 mm, diam. 1.1 mm.

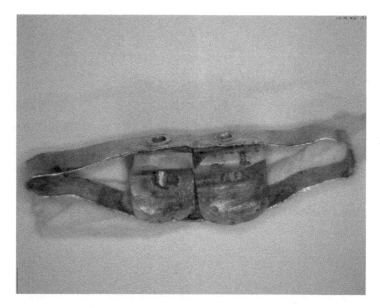

Figure 5.13c View of trimmed bases of inserted teeth.

Source: courtesy of the National Museums Liverpool and Georgina Muskett, also by Margarita Gleba.

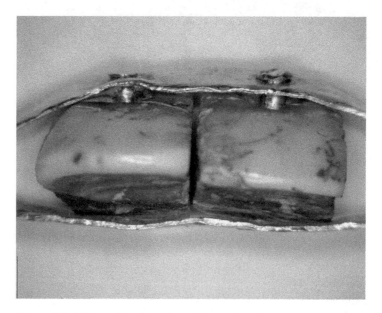

Figure 5.13d View of cutting edges of inserted teeth.

Source: courtesy of the National Museums Liverpool and Georgina Muskett, also by Margarita Gleba.

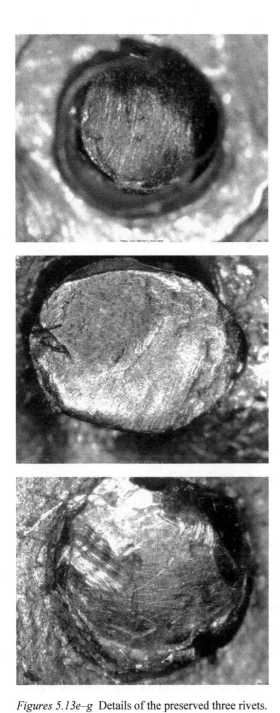

Figures 5.13e–g Details of the preserved three rivets.

Source: courtesy of the National Museums Liverpool and Georgina Muskett, also by Margarita Gleba.

Description: This single band that surrounded all four incisors is 0.3mm thick. Since the location of a weld cannot be visually identified it is possible that this seamless oval was formed from a piece of gold that was expanded to shape. The appliance has two cut-down human central incisors riveted into the center. These may have been the teeth removed from the owner. The open ends of the band were fitted over the owner's lateral incisors. The rivets holding the replaced teeth are 7.0 mm long and have heads peened so close to the surface of the band that in some locations they have pulled free.

References (main dental references for identification; see also preceding discussion)

See Turfa in press for additional nineteenth-century catalogues etc.

Bliquez 1996: 2650–2651, "K," fig. 17 upper.
Bonfante 1986: fig. VIII–28 (on p. 251: shown inverted).
Cohen 1959: fig. 1.
Emptoz 1987: 554–555, fig. 15 (no. XVII).
Hockley 1858: 121: a mistaken reference, see below.
Hoffmann-Axthelm 1970: 83, fig. 4 (upper).
Hoffmann-Axthelm 1985: 78–79, fig. 64 (upper).
Johnstone 1932a: 132–134, pl. 94 (17).
Johnstone 1932b: 448–449.
Macnamara 1973:170, fig. 104.
Mayer 1852: 20 no. 222A.
Moorehead 1983: 341, fig.
Naso 2011: 151 no. 12.
Purland 1857–1858: 63.
Scarborough 1969: pl. 8 (shown upside down).
Tabanelli 1962: pl. 51.
Waite 1885a: 316–317, 507–512, fig.

Description

Dental prosthesis made of gold sheet and rivets, covering the four upper incisors of a human jaw, preserves two central replacement teeth (the anchoring teeth are missing). The two "false teeth," held in place with one rivet each, are cut down from two human teeth, probably recycled teeth originally removed from this person (Johnstone 1932a: 448–449). They were heavy, robust teeth, with traces of large pulp cavities, and the back surfaces seem eroded or stained from burial (front surfaces are shiny white), making them resemble the teeth of a larger mammal. Recent examination (2012) by experts at the Liverpool Museum has affirmed that they are human. The replacement incisors are sharply trimmed with straight vertical edges, and are notched at the top to create a ledge that would have been seated against the gums. The band is a narrow strip of sheet gold worked to fit closely to the teeth, and band and rivets were carefully hammered and smoothed, to be worn comfortably. Small size of teeth implies a female owner.

Analysis

This band appears to have enclosed the spaces for the four maxillary incisors. The lateral incisors, on which this bridge was fixed, are not present. The space for the central incisors is occupied by two false "teeth" cut down from the incisors (almost certainly) of the human wearer, not from "some hard ivory" as Waite (1885a: 316) suggested. Both false teeth are notched at their uppermost surface (above the crown; see Figure 5.13c), suggesting that they were placed over the gums. The lateral edges appear to have been filed to ensure a close fit between the false teeth and the adjacent anchor teeth, (not extant). The pulp cavities of the crowns of these teeth are now exposed by the trimming, which created a ledge resting against the gum.

The length across the oval of the Liverpool I band is 3.09cm. The band has been effectively fashioned to form a seamless gold ribbon 0.3 mm thick, formed by expanding a single piece of gold. (No joint or alteration in the surface of the band could be detected in a series of examinations under magnification, confirmed by Turfa and staff at Liverpool Museums including Drs. Georgina Muskett and Chrissy Partheni, 5/31/2016. In May, 2016, on the lingual side of the proper right tooth there were visible several very short, shallow, parallel diagonal scratches that continue onto the gold band: it was not possible to determine if they resulted from ancient activity or nineteenth-century cleaning.) The band is 3.0 mm wide at the left side, as seen from the rear, and 3.1 mm wide at the right side, and molded to fit closely to both sides of the teeth. Each "tooth" has been drilled (B-L) and fixed within the band by a single rivet of gold, both of which are 7.0 mm long. Each rivet is estimated to be 1.1 mm in diameter, and passes through the tooth and band on each side. Both rivets have been hammered (peened) flush with the outer surfaces of the band. On the exterior or labial surface there is a slight bulge where the head of the rivet overlaps the band, the left being an oval 1.9 by 1.2 mm and the right almost circular, with diameters of 1.95 by 2.0 mm. On the lingual surface, where both rivets have been peened nearly flat, with less material overlapping the band, both have pulled free from the band. Dimensions of the cut-down replacement teeth are listed below.

Table 5.4 Dimensions of the false teeth in Liverpool I (in millimeters)

	Left	*Right*
B-L depth at the top	7.5	7.2
Height along buccal edge	11.4	11.0
M-D width at top	6.9	6.2
M-D width at cutting edge	6.5	7.0

14 Liverpool II

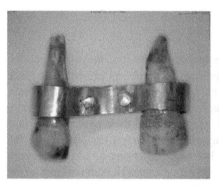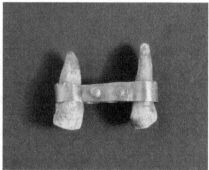

Figures 5.14a1–a2 Buccal views of appliance

Source: courtesy of the National Museums Liverpool and Georgina Muskett, also by Margarita Gleba.

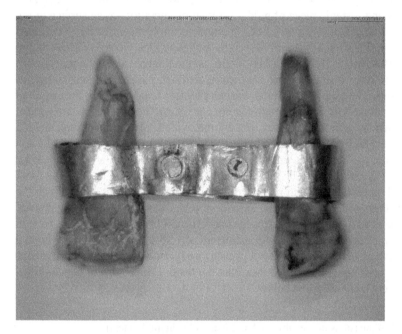

Figure 5.14b Lingual view.

Source: courtesy of the National Museums Liverpool and Georgina Muskett, also by Margarita Gleba.

Present location: World Museum Liverpool, Mayer Collection, inventory no. M 10335.

Type: band with 2 false teeth (now missing) riveted in place.

Origin: unknown, but surely from an excavation before or during 1857.

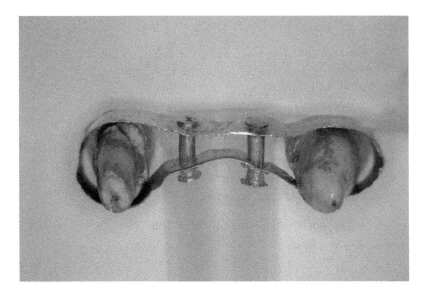

Figure 5.14c View of roots and rivets.

Source: courtesy of the National Museums Liverpool and Georgina Muskett, also by Margarita Gleba.

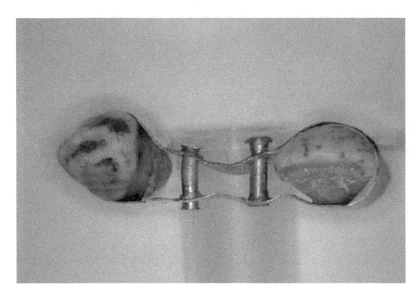

Figure 5.14d View of rivets.

Source: courtesy of the National Museums Liverpool and Georgina Muskett, also by Margarita Gleba.

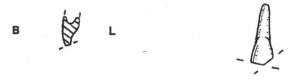

B   L

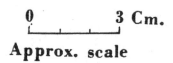

0   **3 Cm.**

Approx. scale

Figure 5.14e Diagram of cutting surface of rooted tooth.

Source: sketch by M. J. Becker.

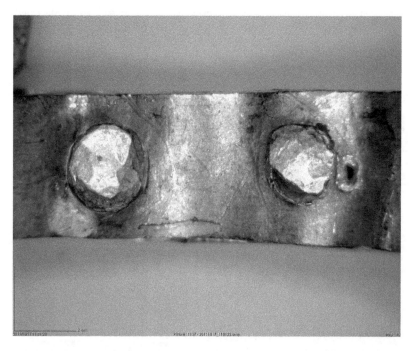

Figure 5.14f View of rivet surface.

Source: courtesy of the National Museums Liverpool and Georgina Muskett, also by Margarita Gleba.

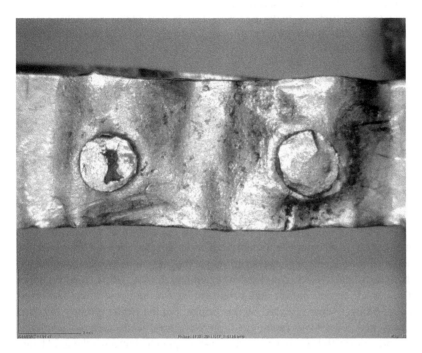

Figure 5.14g View of rivet surface.

Source: courtesy of the National Museums Liverpool and Georgina Muskett, also by Margarita Gleba.

Jaw part: maxilla, 2I–I2.
Date: not known.
Sex: female?, age 45+ years.
Dimensions: L. 28.2, W. 4.9–5.2 mm.

Description: this single band, once surrounding all four incisors, is ca 0.2 mm thick, considerably more gracile than the band of Liverpool I. Construction appears much the same, with two rivets where the centers of the central incisors would have been. The replacements, however, have not survived. Since we do not know the tomb conditions that would have influenced survival of artifacts, we cannot know if human teeth or some other organic materials had been used in forming the replacements. The rivets measured 6.0 and 6.2 mm long and have been peened nearly flat as with Liverpool I.

References

Bliquez 1996: 2650, "J," fig. 17 lower.
Bonfante 1986: fig. VIII–28 (p. 251, shown inverted).
Cohen 1959: fig. 1.

Hoffmann-Axthelm 1970: 83, fig. 4 (lower).
Hoffmann-Axthelm 1985: 78–79, fig. 64 (lower) (text in 1981 edition was unchanged).
Johnstone 1932a: 132–134, pl. 94 (18).
Johnstone 1932b: 448–449.
Macnamara 1973: 160, fig. 104.
Moorehead 1983: 341, fig.
Naso 2011: 151 no. 11.
Purland 1857: 63.
Scarborough 1969: fig. 8.
Tabanelli 1962: 94, pl. 51.
Waite 1885a: 316–317, 507–512, fig.

Description

Dental prosthesis made of gold sheet, surrounding four teeth of a human upper jaw, has spaces for two false teeth (missing) and currently preserves in the position at either end, two complete human teeth, although they may not have been the original anchoring teeth. With roots preserved, they resemble two canines but are actually, according to Becker and recent examination by Cynthia Reed (October 18, 2011), a left central incisor and a right canine (of the upper jaw). The original central incisors were replaced by this bridge, but the teeth currently installed are not original. Two rivets remain to show the central teeth were replacements. Becker and goldsmith Reed have noted a pin-hole punched through the gold band, with its rough edges smoothed, as if there had been a slight mistake in drilling and fitting the replacement tooth, or perhaps an adjustment to the appliance after it had been made and worn. Small size of teeth clearly implies a female owner. The rivets are slightly larger than those used in the other appliance. As with Liverpool I, there is no visible sign of the joining of two ends of the band: it seems possible that the band was worked from a pierced solid of gold into an oval ribbon-like band, using the techniques common in making gold and silver hollow wares.

Analysis

The Liverpool II dental appliance (examined by Becker when earlier on display in Case 44 at the Liverpool Public Museums, now Liverpool World Museum), is a band forming an elongate (3 cm long) oval 5 mm wide, which bridged four maxillary spaces. Most likely this example conforms to the general pattern of spanning the four maxillary incisors, with the present teeth placed within the appliance at a more recent date. The two false teeth, originally held in place by rivets, now are missing. Neither of the present human "anchor" teeth now in this appliance are securely fixed into the positions they occupy, at the extreme ends of the oval gold band. It is not at all certain that these are the original anchor teeth. Both appear to be from a female, as indicated by their size. The appliance originally may not have been well seated, and quite possibly, if these are indeed the original teeth, this was a removable cosmetic appliance, a possibility reinforced by the extremely high placement of the band on the teeth. The anchor teeth appear to be a left central incisor and a right canine, indicating that both right incisors were bridged.

The following comments assume that the teeth are the original ones (Figure 5.14e). The canine shows slight shoveling exhibited along the posterior mesial margin. Shovel shaped canines now have been found at several central Italian sites (e.g. Osteria del'Osa: Becker and Salvadei 1992) and this tooth is well within the expected range of configurations for canines. The right canine is 22.8 mm long, and has a maximum breadth of 7.2 mm. The wear pattern suggests the loss of one or more opposing teeth. The replacement central incisors would have a total M-D length of less than 12.5 mm. This suggests that the tooth now in place at the left is not original to this appliance.

The wide left central incisor is 20.9 mm long and 8.7 mm broad along the articular edge and is clearly shoveled. The degree of shoveling (2 on a 0–4 scale) is not great, which is also common with central incisors as compared with the more pronounced shoveling usually found on lateral incisors in central Italy (Becker and Salvadei 1992). Central incisor shape and width also are genetic characteristics.

This band, at approximately 5 mm wide (range 4.5 to 5.2), is wider than Liverpool I but has been made by the same technique, suggesting a related time and/or place of origin. The ribbon is particularly thin at *c.*0.2 mm and has been formed into a seamless band. The longest diameter of this oval band measured 28.2 mm. The width of the band varies from 4.9 mm in the center to 5.2 mm at the ends. Two holes were made (punched?) in the rear of the band and the rivets were driven through from that surface. The rivets were flattened at the rear, as in the other Liverpool example, and peened over on the anterior (buccal) surface. The left rivet is 6.2 mm long and has a head peened "flat" to form a circle some 2.9 mm in diameter. The right rivet is only 6.0 mm long and has a head peened into an oval some 2.2 by 2.0 mm.

An interesting, and unexpected, feature of this appliance is the presence of a small hole on the anterior surface of this band, lateral to the rivet on the right side and less than 0.5 mm from the edge, as seen from the inside of the band. This pin-size hole appears to have been punched from the rear (the interior) of the gold band, with the raised surface around the hole where it exits on the anterior surface then being peened over. If this was meant to add a small stabilizing pin to better secure the false tooth one would expect that it would have entered from the exterior. The origins and function of this very tiny hole remain unknown, but it appears to be a feature unique to this appliance.

15 Valsiarosa

The archaeological context from which the Valsiarosa appliance derives is the best documented of all the known examples. The specific tomb location has been identified and published. Only the Satricum appliance is nearly as well documented.

Present location: Museo Archeologico dell'Agro Falisco, in Forte Sangallo, Civita Castellana. (Formerly Museo Nazionale di Villa Giulia inv. no. 1515.)

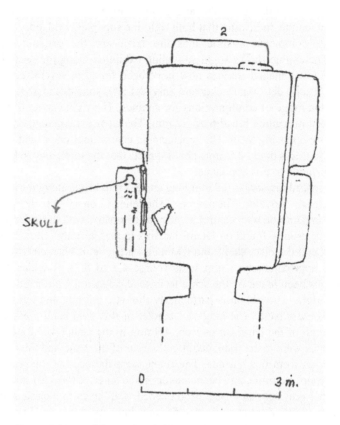

Figure 5.15a Valsiarosa Tomb 20 CIX (81). Plan, as rectified from Cozza and Pasqui (1981: 188, 201). They indicate that the chamber measures 2.50 m by 4.20 m. The arrow on the plan leading from the skull points to the text *"Teschio colla dentiera"*— "Skull with denture."

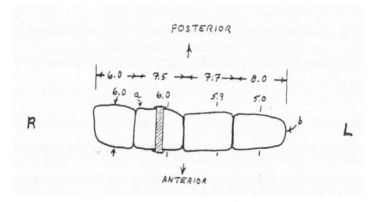

Figure 5.15b Drawing of the superior view, by Becker.

(c)

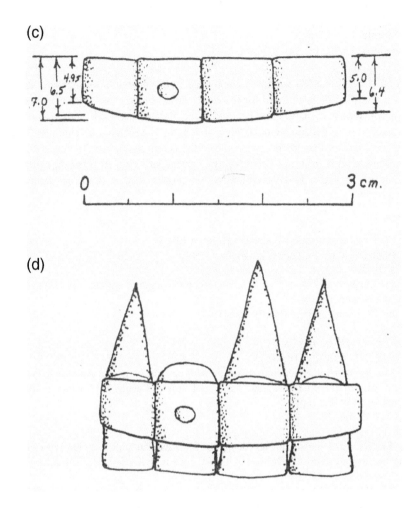

(d)

Figures 5.15c d (c) Drawing of the anterior view, by Becker; (d) view with teeth, roots in place, drawing by Becker.

Type: four chambers (for four maxillary teeth), which appear to be welded loops, with one rivet at 1I (cf. Copenhagen). No teeth survive. (Often confused with Populonia no. 6.)

Origin: Valsiarosa Necropolis about 0.5 km from modern Civita Castellana (ancient *Falerii Veteres*), "Tomba a camera CIX" = Tomb 20, a chamber tomb with *loculi* for bodies in the walls.

Jaw part: originally fitted to a maxillary 2I–I2 (spanning four spaces), although not so displayed today.

Date: fourth–third century BCE (based on Waarsenburg's evaluation of the grave goods).

Sex: female ?

Dimensions: L. 38, W. 5.0–7.0 mm.

Description: The Valsiarosa appliance sur rounded all four maxillary incisors, and provided a modified or false tooth for the right central incisor. No teeth survived, including any replacement tooth. The gold rivet, flattened at both ends, is now approximately 1 mm in diameter and 6.9 mm in length. The rectangular chamber for the left central incisor may reflect the shape of the actual tooth, but the buccal-lingual flattening of all four "rings" reflects post-mortem activities. At some time after its recovery this appliance had been mounted in a modern human skull for display.

References

Baggieri 1998: 68 (an error-filled prelude to Baggieri 1999).

Baggieri 1999: 39–40 (repeats errors in Baggieri 1998).

Baggieri 2001: 327–328, pl. XXXVIIC and E, graph 3.

Baggieri and Allegrezza 1994: 4–5. Includes a useful photograph of appliance as seen from below, but printed in reverse!

Baggieri and De Lucia 1993: 15 (briefly noted).

Becker 1994d.

Becker 1999b: 45, 49–59, figs 2A–2C, 4A-6.

Bliquez 1996: 2651, "L," figs 18 and 19.

Bobbio 1958: figs 9–10 (data taken from the modern copy in Paris (see Appendix II) as shown in Rivault 1953: figs 2–3), and fig. 12 (taken from Casotti 1947, who provides excellent views of this copy).

Boissier 1927: 27, fig. 2.

Cali 1901: 11.

Casotti 1927: 627, fig. 4 (illustrating an edentulous skull and mandible in a plate with the appliance on the left side (cf. Dall'Osso 1907), plus a stylized, but fairly accurate view (Casotti's Form B)).

Casotti 1947: 668, pl. I. Waarsenburg (1991a: n. 23) points out that five of Casotti's appliances (A, I, P, Q, R) are identical; see Bliquez 1996, and the text below.

Casotti 1957: 105 and fig. 6.

Cavenago 1933: fig. 2 (copy of Deneffe 1899).

Cozza and Pasqui 1981: 187–201 (archaeological data).

Dall'Osso 1907: fig. (illustrates this piece, incorrectly identified, in a skull resting on a plate).

De Lucia Brolli 1991: 35, 36 fig. 10.

Deneffe 1899: 59, 69–72, pl. 2 and 3. Plate 2 illustrates a copy of this appliance, mounted in a skull that has all of its teeth, also printed in reverse. Plate 3 shows what may be an original view of this appliance, seen as an unnumbered item in the upper left.

De Vecchis 1929: 18f.

Dunn 1894: 5 (Waarsenburg (1991a: 244) describes these drawings as "good").

Emptoz 1987: 553, figs 12, 14 (no. XIV, from "Falcini Veteres" [sic]; also XVI).

Guerini 1894b: figs 1–2.

Guerini 1909: 70–71, fig. 15 (probably a copy).

Laviosa *et al.* 1993: 130, figs V2 and V3 (these two color plates, from the Soprintendenza Archeologica per l'Etruria Meriodionale at the Villa Giulia Museum, are probably the two best now in print).

Menconi and Fornaciari 1985: 95–97, figs 5, 6.

Micheloni 1976 (illustrates the Praeneste appliance, but says it comes from Civita Castellana).

Naso 2011: 150 no. 2.

Platschick 1904–1905: 239, figs 3–4.

Quintarelli 1946: 104, fig. 2 (skull on plate plus view of appliance; cf Casotti 1927).

Rath 1958: fig. 4. (illustration provided by "Foto Anchora, Roma," shows only what appears to be a fragment of the mandible).

Rivault 1953: figs 2–3 (taken from modern copies in Paris).

Sterpellone and Elsheikh 1990: 138, fig. 67.

Strömgren 1919: fig. 4 (skull on plate).

Sudhoff 1926: 81–82, fig. 45.

Tabanelli 1962: 93 (from Dall'Osso 1907?).

Torino *et al.* 1997: 540–542.

Waarsenburg 1991a: figs 1–2.

Weege 1913: 371.

Weinberger 1948: 125, fig. 52. Text repeats Casotti (1947), but illustration, courtesy of Curt Proskauer, said to have been taken at the Villa Giulia in Rome, appears to be the Poggio Gaiella example in Florence.

History and date of the Valsiarosa appliance

The data published by Cozza and Pasqui (1981: 187) on excavations at Valsiarosa provide the most extensive archaeological record for the recovery of any ancient dental appliance. They include a map of the excavations with Tomb 20 noted. The grave goods (*corredo*) were identified by the number CIX, and the "Catalogo Pasqui" assigned number 81. The full series of numbers for this tomb at Valsiarosa often appears as 20CIX(81). The lack of human skeletal data from these tombs severely restricts our ability to interpret the details of their use.

Cozza and Pasqui (1981: 187) indicate that the "*Proprietario della tomba*" was "*Mancinelli (scavatore)*," the "year of excavation" 1888 (*anno di scavo 9/7/1888/a*). This information was not included elsewhere ("*Non e descritta in*" Notizie degli Scavi for 1887 "*ne dal catalogo Magliulo [10/3/1886– 10/7/1890]*"). Baggieri and De Lucia (1993) provide background on Francesco Mancinelli Scotti, who conducted numerous excavations for Italian and foreign sponsors in the territories (necropoleis) of Falerii and Narce—see Mancinelli Scotti 1917; for background on the Faliscan culture, see De Lucia Brolli and Tabolli 2013.

The site plan (Cozza and Pasqui 1981:188) locates Tomb 20: CIX(81) as the third in a line of eight large tombs running southwest to northeast along an ancient road, "*fra il terreno Brunelli e la strada comunale*" ("between the Brunelli land and the municipal road") (1981: 201). Entered from the southeast, it is trapezoidal in plan (2.50 by 4.20 m; see Figure 5.15a). *Loculi* (s. = *loculus*), body-length niches, were cut horizontally into the walls; two more *loculi* were set above one another in the back wall of the tomb. All were sealed with large pan tiles or flat stone slabs, a design common in the Faliscan region by the fourth century BCE.

The published Tomb 20 plan (Figure 5.15a) includes the *loculi*, but only one has the position of the skeleton sketched on it. A line drawn from the skull of this skeleton leads to the left where it ends in an arrow pointing to a text that reads "*Teschio colla dentiera*" ("skull with the denture"). In a note Cozza and Pasqui (1981: 201) state that this was the "*Teschio di scheletro che conserva nella mascella inferiore la legatura in lamina d'oro di quattro molari.*" ("Skull of skeleton that preserves in the lower jaw the binding in gold sheet of four molars.") They also cite page 75 of Della Seta's Villa Giulia Museum catalogue, which provides the catalogue number of "1515" for this appliance (see Guerini 1894b: figs 1–2).

A kylix (cup, probably Athenian) was mistakenly assigned to this tomb: "*Il Pasqui aggiunge una kylix che invece, secondo la sua Relazione, fa parte della tomba di Cella CIX bis*" (Cozza and Pasqui 1981: 143, 201). According to Waarsenburg (1991a), inv. no. 1516 was an Attic skyphos (cup) from "tomb CIX[bis]." A partial list of the goods recovered from Tomb 16: CXI(82) is in Cozza and Pasqui 1981: 199–200; see also Waarsenburg 1991a.

Tomb 20: contents and dating

Waarsenburg (1991a: n. 25) extracts an excellent description of the tomb from a document that he diligently sought out in Rome (*Archivio Centrale 1888*). It indicates that the tomb had been looted prior to the official excavation, but a large number of remaining items were recovered, including a "*dentiera a tre denti in oro, oggetto rarissimo*" ("dental appliance of three teeth in gold, a very rare object"). Waarsenburg (1991a) suggests that "*tre denti*" refers to the number of actual teeth then found in place in the prosthesis, not the number of spaces bridged, which clearly is four. Waarsenburg also points out that the appliance comes from Tomb 81, while the artifacts are noted as from Tomb 82. Why Cali (1901:11) says that item 1515 came from Tomb 84 of Faleri Veteres is unknown.

The date for the artifacts in Tomb 82 is based on their description, as reconstructed from the record by Waarsenburg (1991a: 245 with n. 25). He notes especially "a thymiaterion with lion's paws for stands and plastic doves along the plate, an Etrusco-Campanian jug and a bronze mirror with engraved Lasa." The first items might be fourth–third century in style, but the Lasa mirror is surely a third-century creation, although we cannot be sure that it belonged to the woman with the dental appliance rather than one of her relatives. Although the Valsiarosa appliance has one of the best archaeological records associated with it, the ability to date the tomb to any specific decade through ceramics was lost when the tomb was robbed. Tabanelli and Casotti both suggested a fourth-century date, also used by Bliquez (1996).

The association between the "*dentiera*" and the skull and mandible in which it is displayed is not known. We strongly doubt that the skull comes from any of the tombs noted by Cozza and Pasqui (1981). Very likely a convenient skull was selected in which to mount this appliance in order to create an attractive display.

This appliance was acquired by the Villa Giulia Museum soon after being exca- vated in 1888. Dennis (1888–1889: 164) notes that a gold dental appliance was present in a skull displayed among the Faliscan tomb groups at the Villa Giulia Museum when it opened in 1889 (see also Appendix I.B). Deneffe describes them there (1899: 69) when he says that a gentleman by the name of Barnabei (surely F. Barnabei), described as the conservator of the Villa Giulia Museum, gave him all possible help. Deneffe seems to have made a copy of the appliance. Platschick described it as at the Villa Giulia, as it was when Casotti (first?) saw it. The arti- facts from Tomb 82/CXI were returned from Rome to Civita Castellana in 1955 with other parts of the Faliscan collection (Waarsenburg 1991a: 245–246). The skull and appliance followed in 1967 and have been on display in the Museo Archeologico since 1977.

Waarsenburg, following Casotti (1947), reviews the early, confusing literature relating to the Valsiarosa piece and its "multiple identities." Citing Weege (1913: 371), Della Seta (1918: 75) and Leopold (1923: 208), Waarsenburg (1991a) attempts to clarify the history of the many "fabricated examples" (cf. Bliquez 1996). According to him, Cali (1901) also says these are the skull and mandible that he saw at the Villa Giulia Museum *"tra gli oggetti della tomba 84"* from *Falerii Veteres.*

Description of appliance and correction of past discrepancies

The Valsiarosa appliance, now in the Museo Archeologico dell'Agro Falisco in Civita Castellana, still retains the Villa Giulia inventory number "1515." Photographic negatives of the Valsiarosa appliance are on file at the Villa Giulia Museum, Rome (negative nos. 4044 and 4045, taken during the 1950s; see also 88-567 through 88-572). In August of 1993, with the aid of Dr. Maria Anna De Lucia Brolli (Director of the Museo Archeologico dell'Agro Falisco), Becker was granted permission to remove the skull from its display case and make a detailed study. Direct observation immediately resolved most of the confusion that exists in the literature, including the lack of any relationship between the Valsiarosa appliance and the skull in which it is displayed.

Examination of the shape of the individual rings of this appliance confirms that it had been designed to span the four maxillary incisors, with a rivet clearly demonstrating that a false tooth had replaced the 1I (upper left central incisor). The squared shape of the "loop" or "ring" that is pierced by this rivet further con- firms that a false tooth had occupied this space. The configuration of the loop for the living right central incisor (I1) of Valsiarosa reveals the delicate and careful shaping necessary to fit this gold band around a tooth that has a complex profile. The portion of the gold ring surrounding the crown of the I1 rapidly shifts from a nearly round shape near the gingival margin (gum line) to the chisel shape of the biting edge of this incisor. Although this natural tooth is now missing, as are all the natural teeth once surrounded by this appliance, the characteristic shape and size of a central incisor is retained in this loop, providing conclusive evidence for the original location in the owner's *upper* jaw. The relative size plus the precise incisor-shaped configurations of the four units in the appliance clearly indicate that it surrounded all four incisors. Furthermore, the shape of the "false" tooth so closely matches that of the right central incisor that we conclude that it *is* the original tooth, recycled after evulsion (see Becker 1995c). The absolute size of these teeth, as indicated by the size of the once tightly fitting loops, is not clearly diagnostic of the sex of this person. However, in each case where sex has been determined the wearers of such appliances have been female. In these examples, where high status individuals are most likely the owners, greater stature and general robusticity might be expected.

The Valsiarosa appliance is displayed in the skull of a person who had all of his teeth at death but had lost all of the dental crowns and most of the roots postmortem. Constructed to fit over the maxillary 2I–I2, the appliance as displayed rests in the left side of the face (area from 2M–2PM), and is attached to the mandible by wax or a similar material probably used in the conservation process in the 1880s. This display has led naive observers to assume that this was the original position of the bridge and assume that this is the skull for which it was intended. Menconi and Fornaciari (1985: 95, fig. 5) attribute a lesion in the *display* mandible as resulting from the wearing of this appliance during life.

The waxy material holding this appliance in place also fills several of the dental sockets, forming a coating that appears on superficial inspection to be like a second sheet of gold. This wax, or glue, reduced the opportunity to gather data from this appliance. Later in 1993 the Valsiarosa appliance was sent on loan to an exhibition in Rome (see Laviosa *et al.* 1993: 130). During its time away the material attaching it to the mandible was removed and both mandible and appliance were at least partially cleaned for photographing and study (Baggieri and Allegrezza 1994: 5; Baggieri 1998: 68; Baggieri 1999: 39). Baggieri (2001: 327) states that the weight of the appliance is 1.96 grams, apparently after cleaning.

The actual construction technique used in making this piece continues to be uncertain. The four units were fashioned as individual loops that then were welded to each other (not as a single long loop or braced band). Each ring now is roughly rectangular when viewed from "above" (looking at the superior margin, or into the appliance from the alveolus). The loop for the false tooth (the 1I) clearly has the most rectangular configuration. Thus the rectangularity of the superior margins of each of these loops reflects the configuration of the appliance when it was made, and affixed into the owner's mouth.

The original superior margin of the Valsiarosa appliance, which would have been close to the gums when worn, has been subjected to considerable bending and distortion by being battered by the maxilla of the display skull. The actual edges on both sides of each loop are distorted, bent and torn. The total length of the Valsiarosa appliance was approximately 29.2 mm, although it now has a somewhat greater maximum length (particularly along the exposed edge) due to distortion at the right lingual corner by the I2 and a flattening of the ring for the 2I.

Table 5.5 Tooth measurements (socket diameters, at centers), in millimeters

Tooth	A-P	M-D
2I	6.0	6.0
1I	6.0	7.5
I1	5.9	7.7
I2	5.0	8.0 (greatest distortion)

The peculiar "dihedral" form of the anterior view of this appliance appears to be unique. This shape is not evident in Waarsenburg's illustrations (1991a), but it can be detected in the color plates provided by Laviosa *et al.* (1993). From an anterior view (see Figure 5.15d) one may note the differing heights of the appliance where it passes between the teeth. Thus at the far right margin of the appliance, where it separated the I2 and the right canine, the band is only a bit more than 4.9 mm high. Where the ring surrounding the I2 is attached to the I1, the height of the band is 6.5 mm. In the very center of the appliance, between the loops for the two central incisors, the height of the band is greatest (7.0 mm). The band narrows from the center down to 6.4 mm at a point between the 1I and the 2I, and ends at the distal side of the 2I with a height of only 5.0 mm. The thickness of the ribbon of the loop for the I2 is the only one that could be measured at that time due to a coating of glue, but it appears to be 0.2 mm thick.

The rivet pierces the anterior and posterior walls of the ring or chamber for the 1I, but the diameter of this pin could not be determined. Becker estimates a diameter of approximately 1.0 mm (cf. Menconi and Fornaciari 1985: 95). The loop pierced by this rivet has an anterior-posterior diameter of 5.9 mm at its inferior and superior margin. Since the rivet itself has been peened to a length of 6.9 mm, where it passes through the center of the ring, the false tooth must have been closer to 6.0 to 6.1 mm in diameter. Even accounting for the thickness of the heads on both ends of the rivet, plus the thickness of the loop on both sides, the false tooth at the point where the rivet passes through it clearly has a greater diameter than is seen at the inferior opening of the chamber, similar to Copenhagen. The rivet head on the lingual side has been peened to a rough oval about 1.9 by 2.1 mm in diameter. On the anterior surface the configuration of the head is nearly the same, with diameters of 2.0 by 1.8 mm.

Although we do not know what material was used for the false tooth in this appliance, only minimal functional use could be inferred. The soft gold used could bear only limited stress. The positioning of the appliance across all four incisors balances the decorative design, as seen in the Liverpool appliances, and was not an attempt to provide additional support by adding a loop around another tooth, as suggested by Baggieri and Alegrezza (1994: 5).

Analysis: the skull now associated with the "Valsiarosa" appliance

Two important publications contribute to our understanding of the archaeology and recent history of the Valsiarosa appliance. Francesco Mancinelli Scotti's nineteenth-century excavation data has been published by Cozza and Pasqui (1981). Waarsenburg (1991a) adds the archival records, but does not refer to Cozza and Pasqui (1981).

All of the photographs of the Valsiarosa appliance published prior to that of Baggieri and Allegrezza (1994: 4) show an edentulous skull and mandible, with the appliance resting between the left jaws, approximately in the location of 1M–C (see Waarsenburg 1991a; Laviosa *et al.* 1993). These illustrations plus all of the earlier descriptions suggest that Valsiarosa had been mounted in this skull soon after it was discovered, probably when it was first displayed at the Villa Giulia. The skull in which the appliance has been displayed is that of a male who died at about 40 years of age (Becker 1994d). All of his incisors were in place at the time of his death. Since none of these teeth had been lost, there would have been no need for this person to be fitted with a false incisor. As Baggieri and Allegrezza (1994) point out, the mandibular right second molar appears to be the only tooth lost before death; yet this observation does not prevent them from reaching the incongruous conclusion that this is the skull of the owner of the appliance.

In the skull now displayed, from a source yet to be determined, 29 of the 30 original teeth (two molars never erupted) were in place at death. The margins are in good condition, reflecting relatively good dental health. At least 13 fragmentary roots of these teeth remain in place (Baggieri and Allegrezza 1994). The partial survival of these dental roots reflects normal conditions within Etruscan tombs where the variably moist environments are conducive to hydration (water bonding) of bone. The boney portions of the skull in question have survived quite well, but the teeth have splintered (see Becker 1999d). Becker's age evaluation derives from the configurations of the cranial sutures as well as by the pattern of tooth loss. The Etruscan population from Tarquinia appears to have enjoyed generally good dental health, but molar loss due to developing dental caries commonly begins at about age 40–50 in that population (Becker 1993a). We infer that soon after its discovery this appliance was mounted in a skull from another context at Valsiarosa. Baggieri and Allegrezza (1994: 4) offer notes on pathologies associated with the skull, and recognize that the Valsiarosa prosthesis is a maxillary appliance, but Baggieri (1998: 68, 69) failed to recognize that this skull was not the one for which it was made.

Much of the confusion regarding the Valsiarosa prosthesis derives from earlier observers making fanciful evaluations from the original or from a number of poorly constructed replicas. The extent of confusion among these authors is addressed elsewhere (Becker 1994d; Becker 1999b: 45, 49–59, figs 2A–2C, 4A-6). These problems were exaggerated by reversing negatives or printing them upside down. One illustration commonly associated with the Valsiarosa appliance, the source of which remains unclear, depicts this skull resting in what looks like a dinner plate. Sudhoff (1926) shows the skull in this plate, but his print is probably a copy. This also is what Casotti (1927: fig. 4) illustrates. Casotti (1947: 674–675) says that this piece is about 30 mm long and 6 mm high, figures repeated by Weinberger (1948: 125) and Waarsenburg

(1991a: 243). In many respects the piece that Sudhoff and others depict resembles a model from which copies appear to have been *cast*, rather than fabricated using techniques like those employed in making the original. Casotti (1947: figs 4–6 and pl. II) provides illustrations of five "different" appliances, all of which appear to be created from the Valsiarosa example. Casotti realizes, from photographs, that at least five different identities had been created from this prosthesis, but then he creates at least two new examples in his own text (see Appendix I.B). Casotti's problems multiplied over the years, as noted by Becker (1999b).

16 Teano

Present location: Institut für Geschichte der Medizin, Universitätsklinikum Charité, Humboldt-Universität zu Berlin.

Type: six "rings" plus an outer "jacket," no rivets. No roots survive but two relatively intact tooth crowns plus portions of two other tooth crowns were in place in 1909 (Hoffmann-Axthelm 1970: fig. 5).

Origin: Hellenistic necropolis (Tomb 18) at the Fondo Gradavola (on the property of Signore Luigi Nobile) at Teano dei Sidicini (*c.*32 km northwest of Caserta), Province of Caserta in the Campagna. (Excavated February 1907.)

Jaw part: maxillary C–C (although generally said to be mandibular).

Date: fourth–third century BCE (Guerini 1909: 79, via C. Dall'Osso). Waarsenburg (1991a: n. 8) suggests *c.*300 BCE.

Sex: female (via tomb contents; confirmed by tooth size).

Dimensions: total dimensions: L. 47; W. 12; H. 4.5 mm (tapering at distal ends).

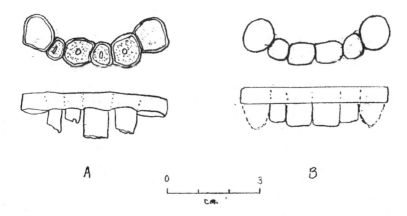

Figure 5.16 The Teano appliance, Becker's reconstruction (inferred from Hoffmann-Axthelm 1970: fig. 5), four views. Photographs as illustrated by Rath (1958: fig. 2) are probably from the FEHR copy rather than the original find.

Description: constructed of six attached rings, no rivets, originally retaining portions of four teeth. Presumably fashioned to stabilize four loose incisors. The two end rings, empty when collected, presumably were looped over canines as anchors. The extant teeth, almost certainly those of the original wearer, have become much more fragmentary since 1910–1911. The unusual construction is unlike any other example. The six-ring welded construction is surrounded by a single gold-band "jacket." The double layer measures approx. 0.2 mm thick. Later photographs reveal a premolar inserted into the left lateral incisor position.

References

Bliquez 1996: 2653, "P," figs 22–25.
Casotti 1927: 628 (typographical error in pagination), fig. 5 (blurred front and top views).
Dieck 1911: no. 114.
Dieck 1934: VIII.
Gàbrici 1910: cols. 44–45, 70, fig. 25.
Guerini 1909: 78–79, figs 25–26 (figures reveal only three dental crowns in place).
Hoffmann-Axthelm 1970: 83, fig. 5.
Hoffmann-Axthelm 1985: 78–79, fig. 66 (two views); (Hoffmann-Axthelm 1981: fig. 66; shown as maxillary in all cases).
Marz 2010.
Naso 2011: 152, no. 15: cited as *"collocazione attuale sconosciuta."*
Rath 1958: 11, fig. 2 (photograph of a copy in Cologne).
Schweitzer 1936 (catalogue, March).
Sterpellone and Elsheikh 1990: 137, fig. 65.
Strömgren 1919: 26, figs 5–6 (from Guerini 1909).
Sudhoff 1926: 93, figs 53a and b.
Waarsenburg 1991a: n. 5: no. 15, and n. 8.
Weinberger 1948: 146–147, fig. 51.

History and context

"Teanum of the Sidicini" (an Oscan/Italic tribe of central Italy) is situated north-northwest of Naples and 32 km northwest of the town of Caserta in the ancient region of Campania. Teanum, situated on the fertile slopes of an extinct volcano, was a waypoint on the Via Latina. As the influence of Etruscan culture, strong in Campania through the Archaic period (c.650–480 BCE), waned, the Oscan-speaking Sidicini came under Roman domination c.334 BCE.

Portions of a "Greek-Roman" necropolis near Teano were excavated in February of 1907 from the land of Signor Luigi Nobile. Guerini's (1909: 78) earliest published description states that this prosthesis was found in the jaw of a woman's skeleton in one of six *loculi* (niches) cut into the walls of a tomb constructed and roofed with stone slabs. The tomb held many vases and a gold necklace that went missing soon after discovery. Only the skull with this appliance and one "shin-bone" were recovered. At the time of excavation, a stylistic date of c.400–200 BCE was assigned based on the grave goods.

Signor Nobile retained this appliance until 1910 when it was acquired by Professor W. Dieck for his private collection of objects relating to the history of dentistry (cf. Becker 1999a). In 1911 the Teano appliance, identified as man-dibular, made an impression on visitors to the International Hygiene Exposition in Dresden (exhibit no. 114). By then someone had replaced (?) a lateral incisor (the left, if identified as a maxillary appliance; see Marz 2010: 45), or perhaps inserted a tooth into that space that previously had been empty. The origins of the two apparently intact dental crowns (if maxillary, the left incisors) now seem questionable, and perhaps represent recent insertions.

In 1934 Dieck arranged to transfer by sale, perhaps through his will, his entire collection of dental antiquities to the Zahnärztlichen Universitätsinstitut, Berlin. Dr. I. Marz (2010) provides the historical sequence of events (also Dieck 1934: VIII):

Bemerkenswert ist, dass sich unter den Objekten auch ein aus einem kam-panischen Grabe bei Teano herrührendes antikes aus Gold mit natürlichen Zähnen gefertigtes Zahnersatzstück befindet, welches vor c.20 Jahren für 1700 Mk. angekauft worden ist.

It is worthy of note that among the objects there was included, originating from an ancient Campanian tomb, a denture made of gold with natural teeth, which was bought for 1700 Marks around 20 years ago.

The purchase price is that paid by Dieck; transfer of his collection was completed about 1935, a year after his death. A catalogue of the "*Dieck Sammlung,*" dated March of the following year (Schweitzer 1936), suggests that at least one copy of this appliance had been made by 1936 (see Appendix II). The text of that cata-logue describes a *copy* of the Teano appliance as follows (via Dr. I. Marz):

Antikes Ersatzstück, 2400 Jahre alt (Original im Geldschrank) Nachbildung Ancient prosthesis, 2,400 years old (Original in the Coin cabinet) Reproduction.

Dieck, who dates the original prosthesis to the third century BCE, notes that:

Da neben diesem Ersatzstück sich auch Schmucksachen befanden, unter ihnen ein Diadem aus gepunzten Goldblättern, so ist anzunehmen, dass die Trägerin sehr vornehmen oder zumindest reichen Standes war.

Since near this denture pieces of jewelry were also found, among which was a diadem of beaten gold leaves, it is likely that the woman who wore them was of noble birth or at least of an affluent class.

Gàbrici (1910) dates the necropolis at Teano dei Sidicini to the Hellenistic period. He describes Tomb 18 (27) [sic] (1910: cols. 69–70), noting that the two associ-ated teeth included a rootless lateral incisor that now appears lost (see Bernhard Weinberger's illustration 1948: 146–147, fig. 51). The dental appliance, he says, was "*fatta mediante due fascette d'oro, che cingono di dentro e di fuori quattro denti del cadavere"* ("made using two strips of gold, which bind on inside and out four teeth of the cadaver").

Gàbrici's 1910 description is the first to note that construction involved "*due fascette d'oro.*" His description and illustration (fig. 25) indicate that this series of rings enclosed six spaces, with four central incisors still in place, stabilized and anchored using the canines. At least some portions of the four incisor (?) crowns, and bits of root are shown. Guerini's 1909 photograph reveals only three crowns still in place. One of the crowns (left lateral I) shown in prints made from glass plate negatives appears to be a replacement tooth without a root, probably not original to this appliance. Both the color and type of deterioration of the root suggest a different origin, although differential decay within the tomb is entirely possible. Data kept with the Wellcome copy in London (see Appendix II.B) is quite erroneous, but suggests that the fourth tooth had been lost by the time this copy was made, probably by Guerini. Possibly Guerini's copies were fitted with complete teeth while largely rootless examples were found with the original. Marz notes (personal communication) that a copy of this appliance is in the same institute in Berlin where the original is held, and that a second copy was then, in 1988–1996, in Köln (see Appendix II.C). Possibly both copies were made by, or at the time of Guerini's work in reproducing all the known examples.

Guerini indicates that the appliance was meant to support the left central to right lateral incisors, reflecting the loss of one of these teeth by the time that he saw and copied it. Gàbrici also notes (1910: col. 45) that

> *[s]imili dentiere si rinvennero in tombe di Conca, dell Agro Falisco, di Corneto, e se ne conservano nella raccolta Barberini del Museo di Villa Giulia e nei depositi del Museo Archaeologico di Firenze.*
>
> [s]imilar dentures were found in tombs at Conca [ancient Satricum], in the *Ager Faliscus*, and at Corneto [Tarquinia] and they now are preserved in the Barberini collection of the Villa Giulia Museum and in the storage collections of the Florence Museo Archeologico.

His listing provides an indication of which appliances were well known in 1910 (cf. Guerini 1909).

The six dental spaces involved cannot be identified with certainty from the illustrations, but the large rings at the ends suggest maxillary canines and a maxillary placement. Detailed measurements and examination clarify some of these problems.

Micheloni (1976: 284) says that the copy of Teano that he saw in Berlin was damaged. Rath (1958: 11, fig. 2) also refers to a copy in Berlin (cf. Waarsenburg 1991a: n. 5, no.15), then in the collection of Professor Carl-Ulrich Fehr. Earlier Rath also notes that he saw various copies at the Forschungsinstitut für Geschichte der Zahnheilkunde, Köln. Rath's illustration depicts an appliance in which parts or all of four dental crowns are present, two of which appear severely decayed. No roots are evident.

Techniques of construction

The Teano appliance is made of six separate rings, welded in a series to form a slight arc, similar to the Valsiarosa example. Weinberger (following Guerini 1909) provides an entirely fanciful description of the way in which the Teano piece was made, suggesting that he never examined the Teano example, and was unfamiliar with gold-working or construction techniques used for the other gold-band appliances. The most recent laboratory study of this appliance (Marz 2010) appears based as much on the recent literature as on first-hand observation. Marz's observation of what appear to be the two layers of gold, first described by Gàbrici (1910) led Becker to scrutinize the available illustrations assumed to be of the original appliance (Marz 2010: figs 2.6 and 2.7). Becker suggests that six individual rings were formed separately each to fit the specific teeth intended to be surrounded. Then they were "tacked" together in a series using a punch. Then the entire set of rings was outlined by another gold band, which was fitted to the exterior of what became the internal ring-set. This technique seems odd, despite adding strength to a simple set of rings. The over-engineering might be due to a naïve goldsmith following verbal orders from a new client in an attempt to create a particularly stabile appliance. Since there are no rivets and no indication, even in this latest study, of false teeth, a device to stabilize loose teeth could be strengthened by such a design.

The Marz (2010) illustrations, like Hoffmann-Axthelm's photographs, confirm that no rivets were used in this appliance. The "roots" of the four original teeth (2I–I2) clearly have largely rotted off, although the I2 appears to have some traces. This suggests that the four "central" teeth were merely loose, and that this appliance was intended to hold them in place. Quite possibly the "anchor" teeth were also present when this appliance was found, and the discoverer pulled the appliance, and any teeth therein, from the jaw, where the more firmly rooted "anchor" teeth remained.

Unfortunately, during Becker's 1988 and 1989 visits to (East) Berlin, the appliance was not available for study. The story of that visit, and the search for this appliance, reads like a Cold War parody that is, sadly, too true. While an informative lesson in life behind the Iron Curtain led Becker to within 10 meters of the safe in which the appliance was held, permission to see the piece was denied. Some years later, with the encouragement of Dr. Ernst Künzl, Becker contacted Professor J.-F. Roulet (Freie Universität Berlin), who kindly indicated (Roulet to Becker, personal communication February 7, 1994) that this appliance is in the Charité clinic. Professor Roulet requested that Professor Zuhrt at the Charité clinic oversee the request, and later in 1994 Professor Zuhrt asked Dr. Ilona Marz to provide a set of prints of the Teano appliance, taken from glass negatives dating from *c.*1912. Although these prints are extremely good, a description derived from photographic prints is far inferior to one taken through careful direct observation. Attempts to clean this appliance appear not have involved preservation of all of the fragmentary elements of the surviving dentition.

The size and shape of the central four "rings" are not as would be expected: e.g. a pair of spaces for the central incisors flanked by slightly smaller spaces for the lateral incisors. Instead, we find the next largest opening after the canines appears to be that meant for the 2I, with the space for the I1 appearing nearly as large. The space for the 1I appears to be the third largest, and that for the I2 appears to be the smallest in the series. However, the shapes of all of these elements may have been distorted; only direct examination will provide crucial information regarding its construction.

"The dentition"

The position of the left lateral incisor (2I) is shown as occupied by a tooth crown lacking the color, wear pattern, in-tomb decomposition pattern, and residue apparent on the other teeth. In addition, this crown occupies a space that probably once held the 2I, but the crown (in the photograph) may be a first premolar. It is likely that this relatively unworn crown was added to the appliance from another source. This tooth retains its entire crown, and the dentine within, completely intact, with just the root missing. From the photograph it seems likely that this root was attached whenever this tooth was found (certainly not in its present location), but that it was dislodged by a blow, and not by natural decomposition within a tomb.

The left central incisor (1I) is represented by just the enamel shell of a crown, together with what appear to be remnants of the dentine within. None of the root appears to have survived, but some portion of the neck may be obscured within the appliance. The labial surface of this 1I appears intact, but what may be a pattern of wear is evident on the lingual aspect, suggesting an overbite that led to wearing down into the dentine. This suggests that a relatively old individual (well over 50 years at death) is represented. The extensive wear on the 1I may explain why so little of the right incisors now remain. Both these teeth retain only "shredded" aspects of the base of the enamel crowns, all only evident above the level of the appliance as illustrated. Hidden within the appliance, and extending to a slight degree "above" it are the nearly equal surviving portions of both roots, probably not original to these spaces in the appliance.

Dr. Marz (personal communication, July 25, 1994) had hoped that the organic material surviving in association with the Teano appliance would enable a precise date to be determined. Marz notes that experts involved in the study or evaluation of this piece over the years included C.-U. Fehr and a colleague identified only as Dr. Blum. The two copies now known may have been made by or for either of these scholars. Professor C. U. Fehr, of Berlin, is listed as the source of the excellent illustrations used by Sterpellone and Elsheikh (1990: 37, fig. 65).

17 Praeneste (modern Palestrina)

Present location: Villa Giulia Museum, Rome (inv. no. 13213).
Type: band surrounding four tooth spaces, central pair riveted.
Origin: Praeneste (ancient Palestrina).
Jaw part: maxilla; 2I–I2 (only three teeth are present).

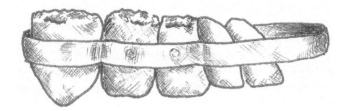

Figure 5.17 Praeneste appliance.

Source: drawing by Tim Downs.

Date: not known.

Sex: female.

Dimensions: measured by Becker, June 1988 and June 1999. See Table 5.7 for rivets. L. 31; W. varies from 2.7 to 2.9 mm.

Description: simple band surrounding all four maxillary incisors, with two rivets fastening replaced or replacement central incisors. Central incisors probably were teeth removed from the owner and filed down. The canine displayed with this appliance may derive from the same person, but this tooth did not originally serve as an anchor tooth for the band. See Table 5.6.

References

Baggieri 1998: 67 (this prelude to Baggieri 1999 depicts the appliance in an inverted position; erroneously suggests that five spaces are bridged).

Baggieri 1999: 37, fig. 6.

Baggieri 2001: 323–324, pl. XXXVIIf, g (repeats Baggieri 1999).

Bliquez 1996: 2655, "T," fig. 31.

Bonfante 1986: 250, n. 63 (noting Helbig 1969: 827, no. 2957).

Della Seta 1918: 444.

Emptoz 1987: 553 (no. XV).

Helbig 1969: 827

Henzen 1855: 75.

Menconi and Fornaciari 1985: 94, 97 fig. 9 (excellent photograph).

Micheloni 1976 (illustrates Praeneste, but text describes Valsiarosa).

Naso 2011: 151 no. 13.

Pot 1985: 37–38, fig. 2.

Sterpellone and Elsheikh 1990: 125, fig. 61; 142, fig. 70 (illustrations are quite good).

Tabanelli 1962: 93.

Torino *et al.* 1996: 121–122.

Torino *et al.* 1997: 538–539.

Van Marter 1886: 57.

Waarsenburg 1991a: n. 15.

Weege 1913: 354–355 lists "Garg E 5758"); 371 notes "n. 1768d."

History and chronology

The excavations of Giorgi and Mattia in the Colombelle necropolis west of the city of Palestrina (Henzen 1855: 75; see also Braun 1855), were just outside the city wall. The necropolis of Latin Praeneste yielded rich finds including "Princely Tombs" (*Tombe principesche*) of the mid-seventh century BCE and others the Archaic through Hellenistic periods. Pot (1985: 36) cautions that the fourth-century BCE date sometimes associated with this appliance is not supported by any known evidence.

The Praeneste appliance was seen by Van Marter in 1885 in the library of the Barberini Palace in Rome. In 1908 it was acquired, with the Barberini collection, by the Villa Giulia Museum (Waarsenburg 1991a: n. 15). Waarsenburg transcribed from the Villa Giulia inventory book: "*acquistata dal Prof. Elia Volpi, Agosto 1908. Buono no. 49.*" Waarsenburg includes Villa Giulia inventory numbers for items 12755 to 13658, including pieces that may relate to the tomb group within which this appliance was found. The Praeneste appliance, inv. no. 13213, is described as "*Quattro denti con fascia d'oro, Lire 120*" ("four teeth with gold band, 120 *Lire*"). This suggests that four teeth were then with this appliance, although they may have been added after being recovered from its tomb. For data on the history of the Villa Giulia Museum see Pelagatti (1985), Rizzo (1985), and Sforzini (1985).

Della Seta (1918: 444) includes this example in his description of the items in the Collezioni Barberini at the Villa Giulia Museum:

> *Dentiera. Una fascetta d'oro unisce l'incisivo centrale superiore di desta col canino di sinistra. In mezzo vi sono i due denti rimpiazzati che sono tenuti fermi da due bullettine.*
>
> Denture. A small band of gold joins the upper right central incisor with the left canine.
>
> In the middle there are two substituted teeth that are held tight by two little tacks [i.e. rivets].

Quoting Della Seta (1918: 444), Tobias Dohrn ("Kunstliches Gebiss," in Helbig 1969: 827) lists the Praeneste piece as no. 2957 (cf. Bonfante 1986: 250, n. 63), with its "Helbig number" in the third edition "1768d."

Description

In 1999 the Praeneste appliance, a maxillary pontic in the Museum of the Villa Giulia was on display in Room 34, as item no. 10 in a case featuring sporadic finds from the Praeneste necropolis, the gold band mounted vertically, with the now empty space for the actual I2 at the superior position.

The configuration of this appliance and the evaluation of the three teeth now held in, but not necessarily original to it suggest that it was worn by a female at least 35 to 45 years old at the time of death (see Becker 2002a). The evaluation of age, however, is based solely on dental wear and the presumption that these teeth belonged to the original owner. Since foods such as white bread, lacking in the coarse husk materials, cause lower rates of dental wear than bread made from less finely sifted flours, we might assume that these high-status individuals show somewhat lower rates of tooth wear—but in the absence of a skeleton, caution is indicated.

This is a simple band that surrounded four maxillary teeth, with the central pair, possibly the owner's, riveted into place. The presence of a canine when the appliance was on display led some to believe that this band enclosed the maxillary left canine, the left lateral incisor and both central incisors, using the canine and right central incisor as anchor teeth. In fact, almost certainly this appliance spanned the four maxillary incisors (compare the Liverpool appliances).

The "apparent" I1 (certainly the actual I2 position) now is empty, the tooth missing and presumed lost. However, Becker found that part of the tooth on display (perhaps all of its crown) had been in the actual 1I position, but then was shifted to the actual I2 socket. The two riveted central incisors are human and match the surviving anchor tooth in general size, color, and even degree of wear. The canine might have come from this person, although it was not originally displayed with the appliance. At least one tooth displayed in the slot for the I1 was actually the original I2 anchor tooth that, when split, could be placed in the I1 position. The other tooth used in making this display version of the appliance may be a natural canine, but was not originally within the band, but put into the bridge when it was recovered. This conclusion was independently reached by Menconi and Fornaciari (1985).

A canine now within the appliance, represented by the crown only, has a mesial-distal length of 7.5 mm and a buccal-lingual diameter estimated at 8.8 mm. Most of the dentine within the enamel of this crown has decayed away, probably during burial. The lateral incisors that served as anchor teeth are not evident among the teeth displayed with this appliance.

The teeth used in the spaces of the 2I and I1 are represented only by crowns, with much of their interior dentine lost, as in the case of the canine. This precludes determining if the roots of the central incisors had been filed or cut down before being riveted into the band. The I1 is quite narrow for a central incisor, with a mesial-distal breadth of 6.3 mm. The buccal-lingual diameter is suggested by the length of the rivet, about 5.2 mm or less. Incisor shoveling is quite evident on the I1, about level 2 to 3 (0–4 scale; cf. Becker and Salvadei 1992). The tooth fragments in the position of the 1I are problematical since they seem to be a single tooth split in two. Although the 1I appears wider than I1, Becker suspects that the two halves of this

Table 5.6 Configuration of teeth in appliance no. 17 (Praeneste)

Apparent	Actual	Tooth in place
Left C	2I	Canine, in 1999
2I	1I	Fragments
1I	I1	Split tooth
I1	I2	Empty

Table 5.7 Rivet dimensions of the Praeneste appliance

Tooth (replacement)	Rivet length	Rivet head diameter (as peened) labial	Rivet head diameter (as peened) buccal
2I	5.8	2.5/2.0	2.3/1.8*
1I	6.0	2.4/2.2	2.5/2.3

* Peened into the depressed area of the shoveled surface.

"crown" may not belong to the same tooth, or may be all or part of the "missing" 1I noted above. Slight shoveling appears in the margin of the distal portion, which is now firmly set in the bridge. The mesial margin of this broken tooth, however, is loose within the band. Either this half has been poorly glued to its other half, or it is not the mesial half at all. Becker suspects that what is set in the mesial position within the location of the 1I is actually a portion of the I1 (right central incisor), which has been restored in the band incorrectly.[5]

The gold ribbon forming the band is quite thin (0.3 mm or less) and very narrow, ranging unevenly from 2.7 mm wide along the anterior surface of the incisors to 2.9 mm at the left lateral incisor. Many of the irregular bends may be a result of modern forces adjusting the gold to these tooth surfaces. The original band need not have been so curved to adjust from the narrow buccal-lingual (B-L) diameter of the 2I to the very wide B-L diameter of the left lateral incisor. As Pot (1985: 37) points out, this band passes across the teeth close to the centers of the crowns, or much higher than is the case with the Satricum appliance, which had a different construction and function.

The replacement teeth were held in place on the band with gold rivets (rivet diameters not visible). The lengths of the rivets, their heads carefully and delicately peened (see Table 5.7), are just sufficient to hold the band tightly to the teeth. The process of affixing the rivet in the band was one of the more delicate aspects of the production of these appliances.

18 Satricum

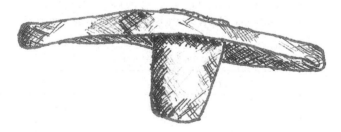

Figure 5.18a Satricum appliance, without natural tooth.

Source: drawing by Tim Downs.

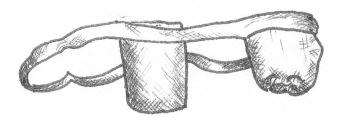

Figure 5.18b Satricum appliance, as published.

Source: drawing by Tim Downs.

Present location: Villa Giulia Museum, Rome (inv. no. 12206).

Type: band spanning five spaces with an artificial hollow gold tooth attached at the center.

Origin: Conca (Borgo Le Ferriere, ancient Satricum), northwest Necropolis, Tumulus C, 'Tomb' XVIII, Grave C 11, the "*tomba dell'oro.*"

Jaw part: maxillary, 2I–C. (false "tooth" at I1).

Date: seventh century BCE. Waarsenburg (1991a: 320; 1995: 366) suggests 700–650 BCE.

Sex: female (Mengarelli 1898; Becker 1994a).

Dimensions: measured in Villa Giulia Museum by Becker June 1988 and June 1999. L. 29, W. 1.8 (mesial)–2.2 mm (distal). Gold tooth height 10.2 mm (2.9 x 0.2 x 0.02 cm; Waarsenburg 1995: 372 no. 18.50). Baggieri (2001: 325) gives the total weight of the appliance as 1.2 grams.

Description: This gold dental appliance is the only example in which the replacement tooth also was fashioned from gold and then fastened to a very thin band surrounding five dental spaces, almost certainly all four incisors and one canine. This also is the earliest example known, probably made between 700 and 650 BCE.

References

Ampolo 1980: 177, 185–187 (regarding the date).
Baggieri 1998: 67 (prelude to Baggieri 1999 includes an inverted (?) illustration).
Baggieri 1999: 36–37, fig. 5.
Baggieri 2001: 325–326, pl. XXXVIIb, graph 2.
Baggieri and De Lucia 1993: 16–17, fig. 1 (from Della Seta 1918).
Becker 1994a.
Bliquez 1996: 2655–2556, "U," figs 32–35.
Boissier 1927: figs 6 and 7 (well drawn).
Brown 1934: figs 6a and 6b.
Casotti 1947: fig. 7 (fig. from Dall'Osso 1907).
Casotti 1957: 675–676 (data derives from Piperno (?))

Colonna 1974: 315; 1988: 308.
Dall'Osso 1907.
Della Seta 1918: 250–251 (see n. 20).
Della Seta 1928: 304f.
Emptoz 1987: 556 (no. XX).
Ginge 1996: 21, 39–40.
Gnade 1986: 125, fig. 214.
Guerini 1904: 280.
Guerini 1909: 101, figs 31, 32.
Menconi and Fornaciari 1985: 94–95, 96 figs 7 and 8 (excellent illustrations).
Mengarelli 1898: 169–170, figs.
Naso 2011: 151 no. 14.
Piergili 1906–1907 (incorrectly attributed to lower jaw).
Piperno 1913: 4, fig. (via Della Seta).
Pot 1985: 36, fig. 1.
Proskaur 1979 (2): 13 (mentioned only).
Sterpellone and Elsheikh 1990: 137–138, fig. 66.
Strömgren 1919: figs 7–8 (from Guerini 1909).
Sudhoff 1926: 93, fig. 54 (clearly a copy, shown in a mandible)
Torino *et al.* 1996: 121–122.
Torino *et al.* 1997: 539–540.
Waarsenburg 1994: 319–321.
Waarsenburg 1995: 360–372; 365–367; catalogue entry p. 372 no. 18.50, pl. 72.
Weege 1913, Vol. II: 354–355.
Weinberger 1948: 147, fig. 54.

History of the Satricum appliance

The present crossroads hamlet, Borgo Le Ferriere, within the region south of Rome once called *Latium Vetus* ("Old Latium") includes a necropolis of the city of Satricum (for archaeological history of the area see Waarsenburg (1994: 314–329; 1995: 10–30). Waarsenburg also provides a complete description of the archaeological context from which this prosthesis was recovered. R. Mengarelli identified the person in this tomb as a woman according to diary entries he made in 1940, more than 40 years after he excavated a burial (Tomba XVIII) from the center of Tumulus C in 1898 (Mengarelli 1898: 169–171; Waarsenburg 1994: 319–329; 1995: 374–377; Gnade 1986: 125; Ginge 1996: 21). His evaluation of gender based on associated artifacts now is independently supported through examination of the teeth associated with the appliance (Becker 1994a).[6] The monumental tomb type and grave goods indicate a family of aristocratic status.

Carefully combing excavation records (daybooks, *Giornale di Scavo*), Waarsenburg was able to identify the original burial of this appliance as "Tomb" XVIII. This was not a single tomb, but a group of several tombs with varying numbers of burials, all found beneath the large Tumulus C at Satricum. Della Seta (1918: 249) had identified this context, overlooked by later authors (Waarsenburg 1995: 360, n. 947). The burial complex held grave goods ranging from the second half of the eighth to the later seventh century BCE (Waarsenburg 1995: 361). The appliance was found on a skeleton buried in Grave C 11, the only burial containing gold (although looting may account for this). Grave C 11 held two inhumations and one cremation burial, with one body apparently dressed in a costume decorated with gold appliqués and amber ornaments, and still wearing this gold dental appliance. The various offerings from these three funerals were not differentiated spatially when the tomb was excavated. They included three Etrusco-Corinthian kylikes (painted wine cups) and another painted vase, as well as impasto cups of earlier style (inv. C 11.8f.) Metal goods included a sheet-bronze vessel, a bronze fibula, and various ornaments, including some of amber. The impasto vases are fine quality seventh-century ceramics; the latest objects are the painted vases, all now lost. Etrusco-Corinthian wares began in the late seventh century and flourished in the sixth.

Mengarelli's approximate date for this tomb, at *c.*600 BCE, has been accepted by many scholars (cf. Della Seta 1918: 250–251; Della Seta 1928: 304; Colonna 1977; 1988: 308). Ampolo (1980: 177) dates the tomb specifically to 620–610 BCE, but Waarsenburg (1994) suggests an even earlier date, between 700 and 650 BCE, based upon painstaking review of the inventories and extant finds. The deposition of the woman with gold-ornamented robe (*roba di parata*) is characteristic of Latial period IVA, or the first half of the seventh century BCE (Waarsenburg 1995: 349, n. 914; 366). The Satricum appliance clearly is the earliest as well as the most securely dated of any of the known Etruscan pontics, and of course, it would have been made and worn *before* the time of death and burial.

Waarsenburg (1991a) determined that many authors such as Casotti (1957: 676) identify all gold dental appliances considered to be of "better quality" as Roman in origin. On that very subjective basis alone they suggest a later date. We point out that this example appears to be prototypic, and a precursor to Etruscan riveted and other examples, and therefore support Waarsenburg's evaluation of an early date.

Detailed description of the Satricum appliance

The possibility that this appliance was worn in the mandible is suggested by the small size, but it could have been intended for the maxilla of a small woman.

The Satricum pontic is a unique example of a variant form of gold dental appliance. It was constructed in two parts. First, a thin gold band (ribbon) was fashioned, 29 mm long, 0.2 to 0.25 mm thick, varying in width from 1.8 mm at the mesial end to 2.2 near the distal end.

This looped around five dental spaces. Attached at the center of the band is a hollow false tooth fashioned to replicate a dental 'crown' (the portion of a tooth that projects above the gum) 10.2 mm high. The mesial-distal breadth of this false tooth is 6.1 mm, the buccal-lingual breadth is 5.0 mm. Both maxima appear slightly above the relatively constricted lower margin of this "crown." The base measures 5.8 × 4.8 mm, replicating the constricted neck of a natural tooth. The false tooth is made from two thin swaged (molded by hammering into a form) gold plates (labial and buccal) welded together to form a hollow false tooth that is neither a dental "cap," nor a true crown as in modern dental terminology.

While the shape of this false tooth resembles a mandibular incisor, it may have replaced a canine. The form may be a result of the manufacturing process rather than a skillful representation of the missing tooth. The bends now in the band suggest that it originally surrounded the two teeth on either side of the gold "capsule." The band also fits low on the teeth, or at the neck, much lower, for instance, than the band in the appliance that secures the Praeneste teeth (cf. Pot 1985: 37).

Mengarelli correctly notes that this hollow false tooth was made of two thin parts, but suggests that it was designed to imitate the left lateral maxillary incisor, an evaluation with which Becker originally concurred, but since has come to question. Guerini (1909: 101) believes that the piece is made from two plates of gold stamped out and then soldered together. More likely, the pure gold band and false tooth were assembled by welding. This shell of the false tooth may have covered a relatively hard material, now lost or dissolved in the tomb, as suggested by Pot (1985). No evidence indicates that anything more than a single false tooth had been secured to this band.

The Satricum false tooth is welded, at its base, between the labial and buccal (lingual) surfaces of the gold strip. The weld between the tooth and the band on the buccal surface has separated and the band itself has come apart where it had been joined at the midpoint of the labial surface of the false tooth. This separation suggests that the bonding point of the band and the weld that attached the false tooth to the band were at the same location, and may have been achieved in a single step. Guerini (1904: 280) notes that he had made "an exact reproduction" of this appliance (see "Copies" in Appendix II). What has become of Guerini's copy remains unknown.

Discoloration evident at various junctures along the band appliance probably relates to the manufacturing process, which at this early period may have involved true soldering rather than welding. The dark color patches may be metals or fluxes used in such a process rather than impurities in the gold. The suggestion that a silver-rich solder was used to join various aspects of this appliance (Baggieri 2001: 326) has not been tested. No modern attempts to repair this appliance are known, but such attempts could be another possible source of these discolorations.

The "real" tooth associated with the appliance

No skeletal material is known to have been preserved from the excavations that yielded this appliance (Becker 1994a). The crown of a single tooth, a mandibular first premolar, appears in some early photographs of the Satricum appliance, at the left distal end of the band (Weinberger 1948: fig. 54; Baggieri and De Lucia 1993: fig. 1) appears in some of the early photographs of this appliance (Mengarelli 1898: 169). Guerini's (1909: figs 31, 32) photographs show the appliance without a human tooth, suggesting that the human tooth now there was only later glued into the band. Whether it is the same tooth has not been demonstrated. Guerini also notes that he saw this piece only a few months after its excavation, at the

"Museum of Pope Julius in Rome" (then the new Museum of the Villa Giulia), but the date of his photograph is unknown.

On the basis of close examination of this premolar crown, and comparison with numerous other dental series in central Italy, Becker suggests that this is a mandibular first premolar of a mature adult female (see also Pot 1985: 36). Only a small portion of the root of this premolar remains, but most of the root appears to have dissolved while still in a tomb. The area around this tooth remnant, at the base of the crown, appears to be covered with modern glue or some agent that may have been used to conserve the bit of root still present, or to hold the tooth within the band for display or conservation. Even if this fragment of tooth is original to the Satricum appliance, belonging to the person who wore this device, it may not be in the correct place within the band. More probably it never was within any of the four spaces of the band, but was recovered from elsewhere. Even less probable is that this tooth has been relocated from the place in the band in which it was found to another space.

The gold replacement tooth

The band has slight undulations that appear to bracket spaces for four healthy teeth, two flanking each side of the false tooth. If the human premolar is a 1PM and is in its correct position within the band, then the appliance would have enclosed the spaces from 1PM to I1. Baggieri and De Lucia (1993) suggest that the false tooth would have replaced the mandibular 2I, since it has the morphology of a small incisor. Although the two mesial spaces within the band are small, or about the size of mandibular incisors, the distal spaces are of the same size. Furthermore, the false tooth is as large as any of the empty spaces, and there is no reason to believe that this unique false tooth was accurately modeled on the tooth it replaces.

Clearly this false tooth was *not* meant as a tight fitting cover or "crown" to a worked or filed tooth since the neck of the "tooth" is constricted and thus could not be seated properly over a decaying tooth, as Waarsenburg (1994) and some others suggest (cf. Pot 1985: 36). Mengarelli (1898) wrongly believed that this hollow false tooth was meant to be a "crown" to cover a carious incisor, an idea that Guerini (1909: 101) seems to have accepted. This idea may derive from Talmudic references, which simply err in their translation, or otherwise distort any possible relationship between false and rotted teeth and are not founded on actual dental possibilities.

The gold used to form the hollow false tooth must be relatively pure, and therefore relatively soft. If such a thin shell had been used as a "crown" over a decayed tooth, it would have collapsed as the tooth below it decayed. Thus this hollow gold "tooth" must have been intended to fill a vacant space. Clearly this gold "tooth" was meant only as a decorative spacer. The use of two pairs of "anchor" or "post" teeth, one pair on *either* side of the gold tooth, may reflect early technological caution and inexperience. Another possibility is that the adjacent teeth had been loosened due to periodontal disease. Most likely the appliance was made as an ornamental replacement for a tooth that had been deliberately removed.

Summary, interpretation

Excavated from a tomb within Tumulus C of the Satricum necropolis, this unique gold appliance is the earliest known, probably made between 700 and 650 BCE and buried no later than *c.*630 BCE. It is the only example in which the entire replacement tooth was fashioned from gold and welded to a very thin band that surrounded five dental spaces. All four maxillary incisors and one canine were enclosed by this band, but which canine cannot be determined. It was worn by an adult female of 50 years of age or older (Becker 1994a), of elevated social status in her community.

This appliance, unique in technique and early date, presents two scenarios. One is an evolutionary pattern, with this appliance using a tooth made from gold, while later versions re-used the owner's cut-down teeth or teeth from other humans, animals or other substances. The second views this early piece as one of a kind, commissioned especially by the wearer. Great variety in approaches to design and manufacturing technique may be expected, due to the individuality of goldsmiths and wearers. Our sample, with a maximum of 21 examples, is too small to permit generalizations about techniques of manufacture or evolution of the tradition.

Several authors have inferred that the Satricum appliance, perceived as more "complex" than the simple bands, is therefore of later date and Roman manufacture (Sudhoff 1926: 93; Weinburger 1948: 148). Casotti (1947) even fabricated a false origin for this piece to confirm his "conclusion" that it is Roman. Tabanelli's (1963) omission of this example from his "Etruscan" series suggests that he, too, may have believed it to be Roman (see Waarsenburg 1991a: n. 12). The archaeological context tells us that exactly the reverse is true. As the oldest dated dental appliance, the Satricum piece provides possible insights into the development of dental appliances. Later Etruscan appliances tend to anchor a false tooth only to the immediately adjacent teeth. This "prototype" may have been "overdesigned" simply because the makers were as yet uncertain as to how much support would be needed to steady a replacement tooth. Using a long band also provides more margin for errors in calculating the length needed.

Della Seta (1918: 250–251) errs in presenting both the archaeological and descriptive data, citing Weege (1913, II: 355) and Piperno (1913: 4, fig.). Baggieri (1998: 67; 1999) echos Della Seta by illustrating the Satricum appliance upside down, identifying the false tooth as a left (mandibular?) premolar, and using imprecise terms such as *capsula*, commonly translated as "dental crown," for the false tooth. His use of *saldata* for the join has been incorrectly translated as "soldered" or "welded" in the English version (Baggieri 1999).

The date of the Satricum appliance, as the earliest known dental bridge, certainly reflects the evolving social structure of the urbanizing peoples of central Italy during the era of the *Tombe principesche* (see Ampolo 1980: 185–187, and his n. 96 referring to CLP: 34).

19 Bracciano

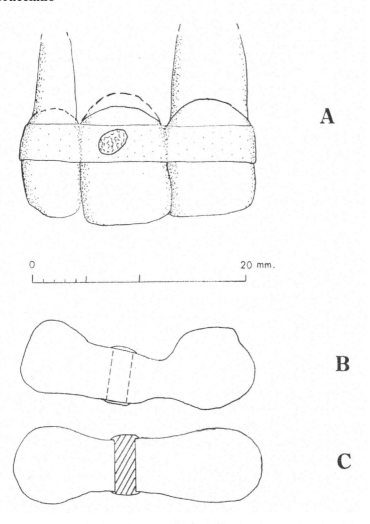

Figures 5.19a–c Bracciano appliance, drawings by Becker: (a) anterior view (adapted from Teschler-Nicola *et al.* 1994a); (b) superior aspect of the Bracciano appliance (without the teeth), adjusted from Teschler-Nicola *et al.* (1994a) using their dimensions; (c) the Bracciano appliance as it may have been originally constructed (without the teeth in place). (Note: Naso 2011: 147 fig. 65 provides a color frontal photo.)

Present location: Department of Anthropology, Museum of Natural History, Vienna (Wiener Naturhistorisches Museum), inventory no. 24.286.
Type: simple band, with one rivet holding a false tooth.
Origin : "Etruscan tomb" near Lake Bracciano.

Jaw Part: maxillary 1I–I2 (three spaces).

Date: seventh century BCE (?).

Sex: female (?) aged 35–40 years (Becker); 25 to 40 years (according to wear patterns, per Teshler-Nicola *et al.* 1998: 61).

Dimensions: L. 24 (est.), W. 3.5–3.8 (depicted as *c.*3.0) mm. Becker: gold band at least 3.5 to 3.8 mm in width, and 0.24 to 0.30 mm thick; Teschler-Nicola *et al.* (1998: 61) suggest a band width of 2.4 to 3.0 mm (3.9 mm at overlap); diameter of rivet approx. 2.55 mm.

Description: simple gold-band appliance, of somewhat mysterious provenance, spans three dental spaces and holds a surviving cut-down right central incisor. Most unusually, both anchor teeth survive. The gold of the band is 0.24 to 0.30 mm thick, much thicker than in most bands. The diameter of the gold pin is indicated as 2.0 to 2.5 mm; either measurement appears large, prompting questions of authenticity.

References

Naso 2011: 147 fig. 65; 151 no. 5.
Teschler-Nicola *et al.* 1994a.
Teschler-Nicola *et al.* 1994b.
Teschler-Nicola *et al.* 1998.

History, provenance

If the seventh-century BCE date of this Etruscan dental bridge, suggested by Teschler-Nicola and colleagues (1998), is accurate, it would be among the earliest known, comparable in date to the Satricum example. The date, like the sex of the wearer, is said to be based on "some accompanying archaeological artifacts" of 700–600 BCE found in "an Etruscan tomb near Lake Bracciano north of Rome" preserved in the Department of Prehistory of the Vienna Natural History Museum (Teschler-Nicola *et al.* 1998: 57). In 1998 it was said to have been "found a few years ago," or prior to 1994, but no details of excavation or finds have been published. Teschler-Nicola *et al.* stated in 1998 "We have incomplete information as to the arrangement of the grave goods in the tomb" (1998: 61). If the finds were obtained and transported to Vienna prior to 1970 they may have been studied in accordance with international laws. We include some of the published data here in the interests of a complete catalogue of Etruscan appliances, but we have not seen any of this tomb material. Study of the documents of the previous owner of these materials may enable scholars to determine a more precise location for the tomb from which they came and the excavations that brought it to light.

The Bracciano appliance may provide new information that confirms earlier inferences regarding the technology employed in the fabrication of Etruscan prostheses. In addition to macroscopic examination of this appliance, Teschler-Nicola and colleagues (1994b) used "radiological and light-microscopical [analytical] techniques." The tooth structure was examined with a scanning electron microscope (DSM 962 ZEISS, Germany). Scanning electron microscopy (SEM) was used in conjunction with a Link eXL microanalysis system (Oxford Instruments Ltd., UK) to determine precise metallic composition (at 20kV, with X-ray signal collected for 500 seconds; Teschler-Nicola 1994b). The X-ray provided by Teschler-Nicola *et al.* (1998: 62, fig. 6) indicates that the rivet used is approximately 2.5 mm in diameter, or much larger than other examples.

Description of the teeth

The Vienna team estimated age and sex by size and wear on the teeth, determining the female wearer of the appliance was between 25 and 40 years at time of death. This bridge had the unusual feature, when found, of retaining both anchor teeth as well as the "false" tooth. The "false" tooth riveted into this appliance is the right central incisor, believed by Teschler-Nicola *et al.* (1994b: 28) to be the person's own tooth with a filed root. The anchor teeth are the right lateral and left central incisors, the entire crowns of which survive intact, but with only small portions of the neck areas. The roots are entirely deteriorated, a common condition in the dentition of individuals buried in Etruscan chamber tombs (Becker 2004). Damage to the roots has not resulted from postmortem removal of this device, as Teschler-Nicola and her colleagues suggest (1994b). More likely little if any of the skull remained intact in this tomb.

Both anchor teeth show "moderate shoveling" (cf. Becker and Salvadei 1992), and the left central incisor also has a lingual tuberosity. None of the observations make reference to this clear example of a typically Etruscan lateral incisor trait (see Pinto-Cisternas *et al.* 1995).

Teschler-Nicola *et al.* (1994b: 28) noted that the right central incisor (the "false" tooth) was similar to the anchor teeth in "form, size, color and degree of dental abrasion." Color, however, can be derived from staining in the tomb context, and is not as useful a diagnostic trait as would be metric or morphological data. If the false tooth is actually a tooth from this person, shoveling might be expected, however, the lingual surface of this false tooth "is partly ground off . . . to achieve a flat surface for the fixation of the gold band" (Teschler-Nicola *et al.* 1994a: 132). Their study of the false tooth by "light and scanning-electron microscopic investigations" indicates that "all parts seem to be artificially treated" (Teschler-Nicola *et al.* 1992: 57, 55) including the lingual surface. Unclear is whether the articular surface of the crown also had been ground down, as the authors later suggest that both central incisors share the same degree of "dental abrasion." This information contradicts the statement regarding "all parts" being artificially treated. In any case, such extensive treatment of "all parts" of this tooth would seriously reduce its identifiability, and reduce our ability to compare the two central incisors.

Most of the "false" tooth root had been removed, with the remnant rounded and smoothed. The degree of dental abrasion on the natural teeth suggests to Teschler-Nicola and colleagues an age at death greater than 25 years. Based on

Becker's observations of high status Etruscans from this area we suggest an age at death of 35 to 45 years. Teschler-Nicola *et al.* (1994a) infer that the dental metrics (Teschler-Nicola *et al.* 1998: 61, table 1) indicate that a female is represented, using for their comparative sample an Early Bronze Age population (Teschler-Nicola 1992). Becker (1994b) concurs with her conclusion (Teschler-Nicola *et al.* 1994a) regarding the wearer's sex (Becker 1992a).

Technical aspects, construction

The appliance is formed from a simple gold band varying from 3.5 to 3.8 mm in width, and 0.24 to 0.30 mm thick. These dimensions suggest a coarser example (wider and thicker) than the Poggio Gaiella appliance (no. 5). The band was made into a long oval by overlapping the ends of a long strip for some 8 mm and welding along this overlap (cf. Teschler-Nicola *et al.* 1994a). These authors indicate that the welded section of the appliance is "between the right medial and lateral incisor," but whether placed on the labial or lingual (buccal) surface is not stated, nor is it evident from the drawings. Where this overlap has been welded, it ranges up to 0.39 mm in thickness. Important in the Teschler-Nicola observations is that "[O]ne of the broader scratches shows signs of repair, obviously done by the goldsmith," a point to which we shall return (Teschler-Nicola *et al.* 1994a: 132). Note that these authors depict the superior margin of this maxillary appliance as shorter than the inferior margin. Unless post-excavation damage has occurred this could only be achieved if there was post-insertion molding of the appliance around the anchor teeth.

The rivet holding the false tooth is depicted (Teschler-Nicola *et al.* 1994a) as just under 2 mm in diameter or approximately the same width as the diameter of its peened ends. This is highly unlikely, and the diameter is far greater than the approximately 1.0 mm of the pins used in other appliances. Drawings of the Bracciano appliance showing the placement of the rivet are not in agreement, leaving the exact pattern of riveting uncertain. Also, despite the high technology applied in the study of the Bracciano appliance, no attempt appears to have been made to verify the rivet diameter. Larger holes are not only more difficult to drill, but in this case they would leave both the artificial tooth and the band to which they are affixed more fragile.

The most significant contribution of the study by Teschler-Nicola and her colleagues (1994a, reprised 1998) is in the analysis of the gold used to make the Bracciano appliance (cf. Becker 2003). The authors made "10 examinations from different regions of the gold band and the rivet" but do not indicate the loci of these tests (1994a: 132). The gold component was found to be from 92.2 to 98.6 percent (by weight; mode *c.*97 percent), with silver varying from 0.74 to 7.0 percent (mode *c.*2.2 percent) and copper varying from 0.00 to 0.8 percent (mode *c.*0.7 percent). These figures reveal that the gold employed in making this appliance was exceptionally pure (Becker 2003); compare the results of analyses of Liverpool I and II (nos. 13–14).

Discussion and conclusions

Teschler-Nicola (*et al.* 1994b: 28) conclude that "the functionality" of this appliance

> is indicated by lesions, such as tiny chips, situated on the occlusal margin along the gold band and the presence of very small scratches (–0.5 m [sic]) on the labial as well as on the lingual surface of the band.

They infer "that this prosthesis was in use for at least several years." While this inference is reasonable, it is not at all likely that this "seems to be primarily a functional device." The soft quality of the gold led to the scratches and distortions, including the large one that supposedly required repair. An appliance fashioned from this quality of pure gold would be easily bent out of shape by very slight pressure. Thus the possible use of this person's own incisor as a false tooth might *require* that the occlusal edge be filed down to *prevent* it from being in alignment with the other teeth, where it would be torn apart by normal use! The kinds of damage evident on this appliance suggest that it was kept in place during mastication, but the purity of the gold could *not* tolerate even the simplest masticatory functions—in other words, the wearer had to chew very carefully around the cosmetic appliance!

20 Tanagra (Greece)

Present location: National Archaeological Museum, Athens. Lambros Collection, no. 358.
Type: compound band made of two joined loops (no rivets).
Origin: Tanagra (Boeotia) Greece.
Jaw part: maxillary, C–C (6 spaces)
Date: fourth–third century BCE (?)

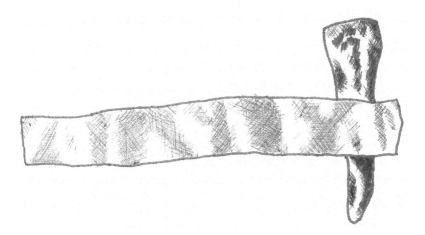

Figure 5.20 Tanagra appliance, drawing after Weinberger 1948: fig. 39.

Sex: female?
Dimensions: L. 43.3, W. 4.3–5.6 mm.

Description: gold band appliance designed to surround six maxillary (?) teeth; almost certainly the four incisors and both canines. The two long gold loops that were welded at the "center" were formed from two strips each nearly 25 mm long and 0.2 mm thick. The ends for each strip may have overlapped for about 6 mm before being welded to form an elongated oval. Then the bands were welded to form a single appliance (cf. Poggio Gaiella). Given the apparently unusual flexibility of the alloy used for this example, the fitting must have been extremely delicate. The possibility that this had been a mandibular appliance cannot be ruled out.

References

Becker 1997: 87–88, figs (written prior to direct observation).
Bliquez 1996: 2648, "G," fig.12.
Deneffe 1899: 26–27, 59 (no illustrations).
Emptoz 1987, no. IX.
Guerini 1909: 60, fig. 9 upper.
Koch 1909: 6.
Lufkin 1948: 56.
Micheloni 1976: 264.
Sudhoff 1926: 63, figs 39b and c.
Weinberger 1948: 119, fig. 39 upper.

History

The Tanagra dental appliance is one of only two of this type known from outside Italy. It may have been worn by an Etruscan immigrant or made to Etruscan specifications. Very little is known of the tomb goods and other conditions of this find. One hundred years ago Platschick (1904–1905: 241), although apparently unaware of the Tanagra example, predicted that Etruscan dental appliances would be found in Greece.

Deneffe (1899: 26–27) published the first reference to this appliance, believing that it had been recovered from excavations at ancient Tanagra, near Greek Thebes (*Thēbai*), a site 55 km northwest of Athens. Deneffe's description had been provided to him, we presume, verbally, by Dr. Lambros, who told Deneffe that this piece was bought from a private collector in Boeotian Thêbes, where it had been deteriorating. Deneffe notes that but one incisor was left, and later illustrations show one intact tooth (with root) within the appliance. The intact state of the tooth suggests a later substitution. Illustrations depict a narrow band, which has been crushed flat (pinched together) except for one end, where it encloses a tooth (see Sudhoff 1926; Lufkin 1948; Weinberger 1948). From the illustrations the tooth appears to be a maxillary 2I, but Becker does not believe this tooth to have been in the appliance when it was found. It had probably been inserted after excavation to indicate the inferred function of this band.

Deneffe (1899) describes an oval band 5 mm wide, but illustrations suggest slightly *less*. Deneffe, noting an absence of rivets, believes that it was affixed around four incisors to hold the loose centrals in position. Micheloni (1976), stating that the band measures 70 mm long (referring to the total length of the gold ribbon before forming the oval?), gives the width as varying from 5 to 6 mm.

Description

Direct observations of the Tanagra appliance were made by Becker at the National Archaeological Museum in Athens in June, 2002 through a permit issued by the Ministry of Culture. The kind co-operation of Dr. Rosa Proskynitopoulou greatly facilitated this research. Unfortunately, arrangements to secure an XRF analysis of its metallurgical content were blocked by Museum officials. The appliance was apparently recovered in its present flattened condition, but what taphonomic processes or conditions led to this crushing (distortion) remain speculative. At present a single human tooth is encircled within the gold band at one extreme end of the appliance.

Published illustrations give the impression that this appliance was a simple, one-loop band that bounded the upper four central incisors. It actually has a compound or two-loop construction, formed by fashioning two units or "long gold rings" that together encircled six (maxillary?) teeth, the canines as well as the incisors. Each of the two units of the appliance extended from the distal surface of the canine to the medial point in the dental arch, between the central incisors. This two-loop configuration would provide a much tighter fit around these six teeth than could be achieved by fashioning a single loop band.

The tooth now found in the band is tightly pinched into place, but rotated some 90° from any likely original orientation. In fact, the buccal (labial) surface of the tooth now faces the "right" end of the band rather than either the "front" or the "back" of the appliance. For the purposes of this description the end of the appliance with tooth will be considered as the right end, and the "front" of the appliance is thus arbitrarily determined. With the appliance in this position, the catalogue number ("Λ. 358"), carefully written in black ink, appears inverted at the lower left corner of the band.

Two lines of evidence strongly imply that the association of the incisor now in the Tanagra appliance occurred after the excavation and recovery of this artifact. First, this is the only tooth now in association with the appliance and this tooth shows no signs of the deterioration that commonly occurs in the environment of ancient chamber tombs. Since all six teeth encircled by this appliance, both canines and four incisors, must have been present in the owner's mouth at the time of death, the recovery of only one perfectly intact tooth would be unlikely. Additional evidence relates to the present configuration of the band. Becker found the band to be highly resilient and not easily distorted, as might be expected in a pure gold strip. The tooth, somewhat obscured by the gold band, is missing a portion (approximately one-third) of the crown, but appears to be a left central maxillary incisor with slight shoveling (1 on a scale of 0–4). At present the tooth measures 21.5 mm long; the apical (root) tip is slightly damaged. An original length of *c.*23.0 mm is suggested here. The crown of the tooth has a vertical fracture and a portion of the "right" side (when looking at the labial surface of the tooth) has been lost (cf. Copenhagen, no. 4). The breadth of the surviving piece of crown is 3.9 mm, and the maximum probable breadth of the dental enamel of the crown may have been *c.*5.8 mm, that point falling just below the level of the encircling band. A lateral measurement made from the left side of the crown to the exterior surface of the band on the right side (rear surface of the "encircling" part of the band) is approx. 5.8 mm. The breadth of the dental crown where it now emerges from the band appears to be about 5.4 mm, from which point a slight expansion of the crown takes us to its widest point.

Age and sex

The degree of wear seen on the articular surface of the incisor is slight to medium, implying an age of perhaps 45 ±10 years at death. Without a comparative population of appropriate social class, though, this estimation of age must be considered as tentative. The estimated breadth of the incisor, *if Etruscan*, indicates a female. The estimated length of the tooth is less diagnostic of sex. As noted, it is not likely that this tooth is original to the appliance. In the selection of a "random" tooth to be part of a "display" or even to indicate function of this artifact, there is an approximately 50 percent chance that it came from someone of the same sex as the original owner.

The appliance: a band formed from a pair of long loops

The color of the surface of the appliance is largely a pure yellow commonly associated with gold, but several irregular blotches of reddish- or "copper"-colored "highlights" are easily observed. Whether these reflect metallurgical variations in composition remains to be investigated. Quite possibly the surface hammering of the gold to form the basic band led to differential surface enrichment of the gold (Becker 2003).

The composite appliance, formed by two relatively long loops, is now largely flattened. The "right" loop retains some slight degree of physical separation over its entire length. The other, or "left" loop, has a portion of its length so tightly "crushed" together that Becker could not visually detect the two thicknesses of the band. At present the greatest length of this "crushed" appliance, at point "N" on the "lower" margin of the band, is 43.3 mm. The length at "M" on the "upper" part of the band, at the present tooth root direction, is only 0.1 mm less, or a length of 43.2 mm.

The width of the gold strip varies from 4.3 to 5.6 mm, narrowest on the left end. Seven points (A through G) have been located along the "upper" margin of the "anterior" part of the band, with widths listed in mm at these locations.

A   4.3

B   4.8

C   5.4

D   "6.0" (represents the total width of the two overlapping portions of one band)

E   5.3 (only the anterior width; total width at this point including overlap is 5.8 mm)

F   5.6

G   5.4

In the anterior view of this appliance there appear two faintly visible "lines" evident between the points D and E. While both lines appear to be scratch-like in origin, the "line" at point E, which crosses the entire band, almost certainly represents the point of overlap in the band. This overlap remains evident despite the hammering or welding that was used to form the original loop. The line that appears closer to point D does not cross the entire band and is angled in such a way as to further suggest that this line may be only a surface scratch.

The thickness of the gold strip or strips used to form this appliance could not be measured, as there is no location at which a precision instrument of the types available could bracket both surfaces. At point W, where two parts of the appliance have been crushed or beaten together, the metal in the two parts of the band has a total thickness of *c.*0.4 mm, suggesting that at this point the individual dimensions are approximately 0.2 mm thick. These figures may be compared with the details of band thickness from other appliances.

Bilateral variations in mesial-distal tooth lengths are normal in any population (cf. Becker 2002a). Thus the lengths of each of the two loops in a well-fitted appliance such as this would be expected to reflect these slight differences. A simple band appliance surrounding six teeth would best be fitted with a two-loop system. While more difficult to fit among the teeth in a healthy maxilla, a two-loop system could provide a tighter and more stable appliance while an "open" or single-loop band around six teeth would be relatively unstable.

21 Sardis (Ancient Lydia)

Present location: Private collection, Ankara, Turkey. Present owner Dr. Ilter Uzel.
Type: band encircling four teeth; the two central incisors are replacements each held by one rivet; second incisors serve as anchor teeth.
Origin: said to have been discovered by a Turkish farmer in a tomb at Salihli, the area of ancient Sardis (Lydia, Anatolia), shortly before 1986 when it was first published. Details of the tomb context are cast into doubt because of the apparently illegal excavation/collection of the burial.
Jaw part: securely attached to original mandible—anchored to mandibular lateral incisors.
Date: earring and wreath said to match grave goods of Teano appliance, dated by Terzioğlu and Uzel to third century BCE (unsubstantiated).
Sex: female? Currently in what is said to be the original female skull; small tooth size (apparently).
Dimensions: gold band L. 48; W. 4 mm.

Description: an unusual mandibular prosthesis formed from a single strip of gold that Terzioglu and Uzel measured at 48 mm long; hammered into a loop. The central incisor tooth sockets appear to have been fully resorbed (healed), perhaps after the appliance was made. If correct, this would provide important evidence for evulsion and replacement of these teeth with an Etruscan-style pontic. Only the buccal ends of the rivets are illustrated, revealing irregular peening.

References

Terzioğlu and Uzel 1986.
Terzioğlu and Uzel 1987.

(Incorrectly cited as from an Etruscan tomb, by Teschler-Nicola *et al.* 1998: 64.)

Circumstances and description

The prosthesis, along with a skull and mandible in which it is said to have been found, is presented only in two brief articles by dentistry professors from the University of Istanbul and the Gülhane Military Medical Academy in Ankara. The appliance has not been made available for scholarly study. Such restriction of access has been known to occur in cases in which scrutiny of the evidence would reveal that this is a modern attempt to create an "archaeologically significant" object.

The complete skull (missing many teeth) was said to have been found in a tomb, with one gold earring and one small gold wreath, which led the authors to identify the deceased as female. They imply that it is similar to the appliance from Teano (third century BCE), stating that radiographic and other analyses show the skull to have an asymmetrical nasal bone (as do many/most persons today).

Five natural teeth are preserved with the skull; the owner later "found" the upper front teeth (Terzioğlu, and Uzel, 1987: 112, fig. 10). According to Terzioğlu and Uzel, tartar deposits on the replacement teeth show that the appliance was worn constantly. They maintain that the design and technical features of the appliance are of Etruscan manufacture.

Gold band 4 mm wide, 48 mm in length. As illustrated, two replacement teeth, carved from human teeth (or possibly bovine teeth, according to the authors) are each set with a rivet within a gold band; they are anchored by the two second incisors, wrapped with the gold band. The replacement teeth project slightly below the gold band, and their irregular, convex edges must have abutted the gum uncomfortably—or else the gum had already receded. The publications imply that the band held the false teeth above the gum so that it did not press on the tender gums, and thus was helpful for appearance and speech but not for biting or chewing. Given the evident loss (postmortem) of most of the other teeth, it seems odd that this appliance should have remained in place.

The authors cite Herodotus' claim of Lydian origins for the Etruscans to explain the presence of a person wearing this prosthesis in the Lydian capital of Sardis. While the tale of Lydian migration to Italy has been debunked (Briquel 2013), there certainly were intensive commercial interactions and travel between Etruria and Lydia during the Archaic period (seventh–sixth centuries BCE) (Demetriou 2012: 82–83). By the third century BCE, though, conditions were very different.

PART II: CATALOGUE OF ANCIENT WIRE DENTAL APPLIANCES

The history of dentistry and oral medicine in the Near East is a subject only recently addressed by diligent scholars. Musitelli (1996: 213–217, n. 12–22) provides an excellent summary of the general topic with suggestions regarding future directions of research. Relevant to Etruscan ornamental dental appliances is the evidence from the Eastern Mediterranean and Levant of a completely different use of gold and silver wire as ligatures to retain loose teeth in place. This important aspect of dental medicine appears to have developed in the Eastern Mediterranean and Levant, passing into Western dental medicine. Unlike much medical knowledge in the Arabic world that derived from Greek and Roman traditions, the use of wire dental appliances may have had beginnings in the area of the Levantine coast and Egypt, to judge from archaeological evidence. Relationships with early Hebrew medical knowledge remain to be explored in greater depth, but wire ligatures were found to be so useful that the technology survived well into the twentieth century.

This tradition of fashioning dental appliances from gold or silver wire is documented from only seven examples, identified as W-1 through W-7 below. Six examples were retrieved from archaeological contexts along a small part of the eastern Mediterannean, two from Phoenicia, three from Egypt and one from Greece (Becker 1997). Carroll's (1972) comprehensive study of the process by which wire was manufactured in antiquity is of considerable value in understanding the technology involved in fabricating the wire used in these appliances (also Formigli 1979). (See description in Chapter 2).

Origins

In an attempt to demonstrate what they believed to be an Egyptian origin for all of these pieces Iskander, Harris and Farid (1978: 107) noted that the Phoenician Sidon I example was found with an impressive array of "Egyptian" artifacts. The Sidon II appliance also had Egyptian faience figurines with it. In fact, by the later first millennium BCE, much faience of Egyptian appearance (scarabs, amulets, beads) was actually produced in Phoenician factories in the Nile delta, Levant, and/or Phoenician colonies. Such amulets and faience vessels were avidly sought across the entire Mediterranean, so their presence cannot be construed as diagnostic of ethnicity. There is no evidence for an Egyptian origin for these appliances. Wiring to support loose teeth was mentioned in Greek medical texts (a fifth–fourth-century BCE Hippocratic work, reiterated in the first century CE by Celsus). Greek and Roman doctors knew about the treatment, yet most of the meager evidence has been found in the Levant and Egypt, with one example in Greece, and one in Rome.

While a case can be made that wire appliances were "Phoenician" in origin, the extant specimens are dated from the end of the fifth century through the

Hellenistic period or later—none approach in date the Etruscan example(s) of the second half of the seventh century BCE. Although some authors believe that all seven known examples may have been influenced from the Western tradition of dentistry, namely, the Etruscan gold-band appliances, no prototypes exist. The distribution and manufacturing techniques of the wire appliances suggest a Levantine origin for this distinctly medical procedure, apparently also informed by Greek medical traditions. More is involved in their design and installation than would be necessary for Etruscan band appliances.

No dental prosthesis of any type was known in Egypt until the Hellenistic (Ptolemaic) period. The literature on Egyptian examples is summarized by Bardinet (1990), who provides references to his own thesis (1977) and the paper by Rombauts and Monier concerning Egyptian dentistry (Bardinet 1990: n. 10).

W-1 Sidon I (sometimes referred to as "Gaillardot")

Present location: Musée du Louvre, Paris, inv. no. AO 5777.
Type: gold wire, holding two (?) replacement teeth together with four others.
Origin: Sidon (Saïda), Lebanon. Tomb XI, Room 1, fosse b (1861) (Phoenician).
Jaw part: mandibular (???), C–C, holding replaced incisors I1 and I2.
Date: fourth century BCE or later (intruded into an earlier tomb? See Clawson 1933: 155).
Sex: female.
Dimensions: L. 34 mm (est.), W. variable, but generally three widths of wire.

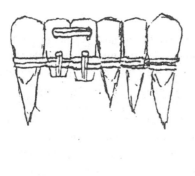

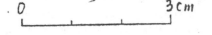

Figure 5.21a Wire appliance W-1 (Sidon I), drawing after Hoffmann-Axthelm 1970: fig. 2. Drawing by Becker.

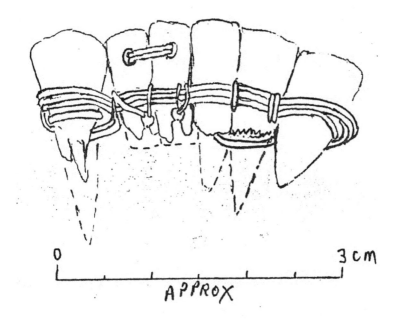

Figure 5.21b Schematic view of the buccal surface (?) of appliance Sidon I, after
Clawson (1933: 156, fig. 8c). Drawing by Becker.

Description: gold wire pontic, used to replace both mandibular right incisors that
had been lost or deliberately removed. These incisors were re-placed in position
using wires that pass through two holes drilled front to back (buccal-lingual) in
each tooth. Two horizontal ligatures pass through the crowns of these drilled
teeth, and two vertical sets of wires pass through the neck hole and around the
cut-down base of each replacement tooth. These lower vertical bindings pass
over the three wires that pass horizontally around six teeth, including both
canines. The wires that surround all six teeth were tightened by running wires
between the teeth, and then pulling the external horizontal wires in towards the
center. Where and how the ends of the gold wire were tied off is not indicated
by any illustration.

References

Asbell 1948: figs 1 and 2.
Becker 1997: 79–80, figs.
Bertolin 1955: figs 1–2.
Bliquez 1996: 2645, "A," figs 1 and 37 (no. 8), using data via A. Caubet (Louvre).
Bobbio 1958: figs 2–4.
Brown 1934: figs 3a and 3b.

Casotti 1927: 625, fig. 1 (drawing and photograph).
Clawson 1933: 155–157, figs 8c, 8d; 1934: 25–26, fig. 3 (the usually careful Clawson could provide only a poor schematic sketch of this appliance).
Deneffe 1899: 52, 59, 83–88, fig. 8.
Emptoz 1987: 546, 548–549, figs 4 and 5 (no. VII). (fig. 3 is incorrectly labeled).
Farrar 1888: fig. 9.
Filderman 1931 (with 5 figs).
Guerini 1894a: 396 and fig. 9.
Guerini 1894b: fig. 9.
Guerini 1909: 29–31, figs 3–4.
Fontan 2004: 293 no. 92, catalogue entry by Elisabeth Fontan, with recent color photos. Gives Louvre inv. no. AO 5977.
Hoffmann-Axthelm 1970: 81, fig. 2 (superior).
Hoffmann-Axthelm 1985: 38–39, fig. 22.
Iskander *et al.* 1978: 106–107, pl. V, B (from Weinberger 1946).
Koch 1909: 8–9, fig. 6.
Lufkin 1948: 49, fig. 15.
Quintarelli 1946: 36, fig. 5.
Rath 1958: fig. 1 (photograph of a copy in Köln).
Renan 1864: 462–463, 472–473 with poor sketch of appliance, 484 (updated inventory of finds).
Ring 1985: 28, fig. 19, and on p. 6 (excellent photographs).
Sterpellone and Elsheikh 1990: 124, fig. 60. Depicts a plaster reproduction said to be in a Roman museum (see Appendix II). On p. 134, fig. 62 center reproduces two different drawings of this same appliance.
Sudhoff 1926: 34, fig. 26 (drawing and photograph).
Van Marter 1886: 60, fig. 4
Weinberger 1946: fig. 4; 1947: fig. 5; 1948:100–103, fig. 32.
Weiss 1989: fig. 30 (from Renan 1864).
Woodforde 1967: fig. on p. 10.

History and context

The Sidon I appliance is one of two wire prostheses recovered from the Phoenician necropoleis at Sidon (modern Saïda), in southern Lebanon. Sidon was, since the Bronze Age, a major Canaanite and Phoenician city, prospering again through the Hellenistic and Roman Imperial periods. Some Phoenician-period tombs (sixth–fourth centuries BCE) appear to have been re-used in the Roman era.

(Joseph) Ernest Renan (1823–1892) was with the invasion team sent by Napoleon III into the Lebanon, ca 1860. His monumental *Mission de Phénicie* (1864) published exciting discoveries at several Phoenician cities, including the first account of the discovery of the Sidon I appliance, based on Gaillardot's journal (daybook) of the excavations in 1861. Finds were consigned to the Louvre and Gaillardot updated the inventory once they were received in Paris (Renan 1864: 484). Elisabeth Fontan (2004: 293, no. 92) gives the name of the necropolis location as Magharat Tablun.

Working in the southeast necropolis on the outskirts of Sidon, on April 14, 1861 Gaillardot began excavating the pit (*grande caveau* XV) in which on May

14–24 workmen cleared several linked, rectangular chambers. The tomb at issue, 8 meters below the surface, was labeled Tomb XI, Room 1, fosse b. (In 1901, Charles C. Torrey of the American School of Oriental Research (Jerusalem) would excavate a nearby tomb and discover the Sidon II appliance (no. W-2). Gaillardot suggested that the ceiling had collapsed before the tomb could be looted, preserving somewhat sparse finds and fragmentary skeletons. The room held two trenches (*fosses*), one on each long side, which may have held disintegrated wooden coffins.

"*Fosse b*" held several grave goods mixed in the sand filling along with the portion of what was thought to be a woman's upper jaw with the wire appliance in place. Also recovered were: 1 "teardrop" (vase) in white glass; 1 blue glass bead; 2 copper coins (bronze?) illegible; 1 small copper disc with suspension hole (not cited in updated inventory); 12 small figurines/amulets in faience depicting Egyptian gods, all pierced to be strung as a necklace; 4 small faience amulets in the form of fantastic animals; 1 scarab, pierced for suspension; 1 small pierced ornament, described as "(phallus?)"—perhaps a *djed*-pillar amulet; 1 heavy iron finger ring "*forme chevalière*"; and 1 ceramic vase (variously described as small or large).

Gaillardot's final inventory also cites four mirrors, but this might be a confusion with mirrors found in adjacent burials. No images of the objects were published, and the descriptions are not very useful: the glass beads and faience amulets are types favored from the eighth century BCE through the Ptolemaic period. A very likely date, given the proximity of similar tombs and finds would be the fourth or third century BCE. Since the tomb was near that in which the other wire appliance was found, within a well-dated marble sarcophagus (of the fourth quarter of the fifth century BCE), it is tempting to assume a date around 400–350 BCE, but this could be improved if the associated offerings can be more closely dated. Elizabeth Fontan (2004: 293, no. 92) dates the appliance *c.*400 BCE. She states that an X-ray study showed that an abscess had infected the bone of the lower jaw.)

Description

Renan's published description (1864) of this wire dental appliance was provided by Dr. Gaillardot, who actually discovered the piece and acted as Renan's medical assistant. The fragmentary "upper jaw" (actually mandible) that Renan found (there is no mention of a sarcophagus or complete skeleton) held a gold-wire appliance holding two canines and four incisors. The two right incisors were held tightly in place with wire wound through holes drilled in them. Clearly the roots of the owner's live teeth encircled by this appliance had deteriorated while in the tomb, having almost completely rotted away. The surviving teeth as well as the cut-down and re-placed incisors in this pontic appeared quite similar when excavated.

The canines and incisors bound by the gold wire are said to derive from "*une portion de mâchoire supérieure de femme*," but the teeth as illustrated appear to be mandibular. Since none of the roots are intact, the bound set of teeth may have been in a position that was ambiguous to an archaeologist—no mention was made of the rest of the skull or skeleton, and other burials had only fragmentary bones found in the sandy fill. The specific configuration of the crowns of these teeth, however, leaves no doubt as to their original location in the jaws of this person. Two human incisors are held in place as false teeth. Clawson suggests that they derive from another individual, but they may be the owner's own teeth, lost through a blow, if not deliberately removed.

Filderman (1931: 336) provides the best and most complete description of the Sidon I appliance itself, including detailed measurements of the teeth and (correctly?) suggests that this is mandibular (Clawson 1933, 1934). Gaillardot (in Renan 1864: 423–473) had (incorrectly?) identified this piece as maxillary (Deneffe 1899: fig. 8; Hoffmann-Axthelm 1970: fig. 2), but correctly identified the wearer as a female. Although Clawson (1934: 26) is correct in noting that no gender-related morphological variations can be detected, absolute size may be used to identify gender in some populations (Becker and Salvadei 1992).

One or more complexly wound wires are used to suspend two "replacement" teeth in position. The replaced, or artificial teeth each have two holes drilled through them (buccal-labial) to allow the gold wires to attach these to the sound teeth. The roots of the replacement teeth have been cut off.

The I1 and I2 (probably the natural teeth) are suspended above the area from which they were lost, possibly due to periodontal disease. In some illustrations the 1I also appears to be replaced. Weinberger (1948) reviews related data with copies of the early drawings and two new photographs, but possibly errs in believing these to be maxillary. Weinberger suggests that the wire had been taken off these teeth and later replaced, with the teeth not returned to their proper order. Weinberger (1948: 102) also believes that at least one of the replacement teeth comes from another individual. Hoffmann-Axthelm's (1970: fig. 2) illustration appears to show a left canine in the appliance, which may derive from another person. Van Marter (1886, repeated by Lufkin 1948: 50) suggests that both "replacement" teeth come from another person. Ring (1985) erroneously believes the replacement teeth are ivory. Fontan (2004) presumably follows this in stating the material is ivory. She states that X-ray studies revealed an abscess affecting the bone, but without references.

The wire binding these teeth passes around the anchor teeth at the base of the crowns. A hole for the wire is drilled B-L through the center of the crown of each "replaced" tooth. This wire also appears to pass through a second hole drilled in each tooth, near the base of the crown. Two turns of wire are visible on the buccal surface, passing between the holes near the centers of the crowns, and this wire (or wires) must be evident on the lingual surfaces of these two replacement teeth. How they were "tied off," whether they were connected to wire holding all six teeth, and if there are two or three wires involved in this prosthesis would require further detailed study of the actual appliance.

W-2 Sidon II (sometimes called "Ford" or "Torrey")

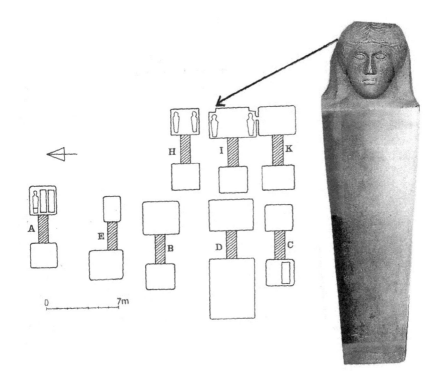

Figure 5.22a Plan of the tomb in which the appliance was found, within the Sidon
necropolis (near the tomb of Sidon I), after Clawson 1933: 142; inset:
approximation of the sarcophagus in which the appliance was found.

Present location: Archaeological Museum of the American University in Beirut,
Lebanon. Catalogue no. 5998. (Sarcophagus that contained the skeleton is in
Beirut, National Museum no. 4366).
Type: gold-wire brace.
Origin: Sidon (modern Saïda), Lebanon, 'Ain Ḥilweh necropolis, Tomb I, East
room.
Jaw part: mandible, C–C.
Date: fifth century BCE.
Sex: male.
Dimensions: L. 35 (est.), W. 3–4 (?) mm.

Description: This gold-wire retention device was woven around and between six
teeth, probably the mandibular canines and incisors. The detailed pattern of this
wiring, made from a single gold strand over 100 mm long, and technique of manufacture are well illustrated by Clawson (1933).

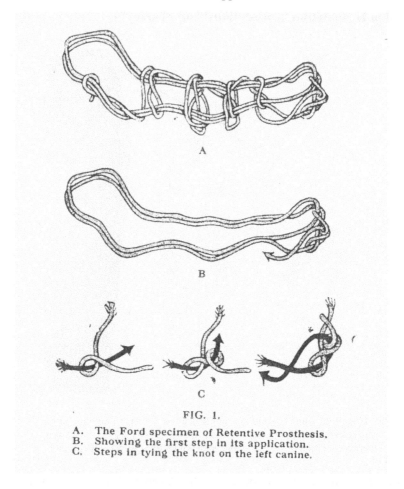

FIG. 1.

A. The Ford specimen of Retentive Prosthesis.
B. Showing the first step in its application.
C. Steps in tying the knot on the left canine.

Figure 5.22b Sidon II appliance, after Clawson (1933: 147, fig. 1), showing it as it was
         removed from the teeth, plus drawings showing details of the ligation.

References

Asbell 1948: 816, figs 5 and 6.
Badre 1986.
Badre 2004: with recent color photograph of appliance in mandible.
Becker 1997: 80–81, figs.
Bertolino 1955: figs 4, 5.
Bliquez 1996 (noted under his "A").
Bobbio 1958: figs 5–7 (from Bertolino 1955).
Clawson 1933: 142–143, 147, 150–153, 159; figs 1 and 8e (very detailed account with
     archaeological drawings of excavation area and appliance, as well as photographs;
     figs 1–3).
Clawson 1934: 27–31, figs 5–6c.

Deneffe 1899: 52, 59, 83–88, fig. 8.

Emptoz 1987: no. VIII.

Ginestet 1927: figs 1, 2 (poor illustrations).

Guerini 1909: 29 (mentions it, only).

Fontan 2004: 292–293 no. 91

Hoffmann-Axthelm 1970: fig. 3 (the lower illustration, the appliance removed from mandible, is either the reverse or the underside of Clawson's illustration (1933: 147, fig 1a).

Hoffmann-Axthelm 1985: 38–39, fig. 23 (from Torrey 1920: figs 14, 15).

Iskander *et al.* 1978: 107–108, pl. VI A.

Ring 1985: fig. 18, and page 28.

Tabourian 1932 (cited by Clawson 1933: 160, n. 10, but not located for this project).

Torrey 1920, vol. I: 14–15, figs 14–15.

Weinberger 1946: fig. 5.

Weinberger 1947: fig. 6; 1948: 103–106, figs 33–34.

History and context

The Sidon II appliance was discovered in January, 1901 during excavations by the American School of Oriental Research in Jerusalem in the 'Ain Ḥilweh necropolis, which lay about one mile southeast of the boundary of the ancient Phoenician city of Sidon. Tomb I containing this gold-wire appliance (plan and section in Clawson 1933: 142; reproduced by Lembke 2001: 14 fig. 6) lay immediately east of Tomb XI, where another wire dental appliance (Sidon I) was found by the French expedition of 1860. Tomb I (reused and joined to adjacent Tomb H in antiquity) was a rock-cut chamber tomb accessed by a deep plastered shaft; the larger of two rooms, on the east, had a niche on each side to accommodate a marble anthropoid sarcophagus. The tomb later held bodies in wooden sarcophagi, when the necropolis was reused during the Roman Empire, but the pair of Phoenician-era marble sarcophagi remained undisturbed. One sarcophagus portrayed a youthful male, the other was interpreted as his wife, but Lembke (2001: 15, 131–133, no. 41) has noted the rather short hair, suggesting that this sarcophagus also depicted a male (see Clawson 1934: pl. VII; and Torrey 1920: 3, fig. 2; 14–15, figs 14–15; 20, fig. 18).

"Anthropoid no. 8," the male sarcophagus, held a well-preserved skeleton that had been wrapped in linen (presumably many of the occupants of these sarcophagi had been mummified). (See Lembke 2001: 129, no. 29 for full analysis and additional references on the sarcophagus and its style.) With successive cycles of flooding of the tomb, the linen had disintegrated except for some tatters adhering to the sides of the sarcophagus (Torrey 1920: 13, fig. 12, upper right corner illustrates a fragment of the textile). The two sarcophagi seem never to have been disturbed and no. 8 was said to have contained a gold seal ring "of excellent Greek workmanship" (Torrey 1920: 21, not illustrated). The sarcophagus (2.15 m. long) is smooth with only the head carefully carved, with classical Greek features and short, wavy hair, and bosses for handling on shoulders and foot. On the foot was incised the Greek letter Δ, a mason's mark indicating East Greek, or Ionian, workmanship (Lembke 2001: 107–109), and traces of red paint remained in the man's hair. Stylistically, the sarcophagus shows the influence of Greek art on the Egyptianizing, mummiform format favored by the Phoenicians.

Marble sarcophagi are not common, but have been found in other Phoenician cities and in the colonies of Cadiz and Soloeis/Solunto (Sicily), where they may denote high-born personages. Similar sarcophagi in terracotta or wood imitated these forms for less expense. Certainly, the extremely costly (in terms of manpower and time) tomb and rare sarcophagi attest to their occupants' importance in Persian-occupied Phoenicia. Only the very affluent could have availed themselves of such gold prostheses. The necropolis area that held this tomb and that of the Sidon I appliance probably was used by members of related families, and may represent the earliest context for wire appliances: Katja Lembke, in a survey of all Phoenician anthropoid sarcophagi, has dated the one which held the dental appliance to the fourth quarter of the fifth century BCE, and placed the companion sarcophagus just slightly later, in the first quarter of the fourth century (Lembke 2001: 129 no. 29; 131–132, no. 41; 98–99, figs 20–21, pls. 16a–d and 22d—she does not mention the dental appliance).

This dental prosthesis was found on the jaw of the skeleton identified as a middle-aged adult male (Clawson 1934: 27; Asbell 1948: fig. 7). For this information Clawson (1933: 160, n. 4) cites T. Reinach ("Necropole" pp. 145–178, presumably Hamdî and Reinach 1892, describing finds in this necropolis). Leila Badre (catalogue entry for Fontan 2004: 293) notes that the skeleton was that of a man of uncommon body size, whose lower front teeth were affected by periodontal disease, occasioning the need for bracing with wire. Clawson (1933: 160; 1934: 27) identifies this appliance as the "Ford" specimen, naming it for an American physician who had lived in Sidon for over 20 years, but who had died by 1933. Ford's will left this appliance to the Museum of the American University in Beirut. We do not know the details of the apportionment of the finds from this excavation. Clawson (1933) provides the best description. Dr. C. F. Torrey, first Director of the American School of Oriental Research (ASOR) in Jerusalem (established 1901) often has his name associated with this appliance, because ASOR was the agency directing the excavation of these tombs (Torrey 1920). Along with W-1, this prosthesis (in a mandible) was shown in 2004 in the exhibition *"Hannibal ad Portas. Macht und Reichtum Karthagos"* held in Karlsruhe, Germany, at the Badisches Landesmuseum.

Description

Clawson (1933: 143, photographs and fig. 1) shows two views of this appliance as it had been removed from the jaw. Theses views indicate that the Sidon II appliance had enclosed six teeth, with the wire completely encircling each of the four teeth on the left (?), but with the two teeth on the right (?) bound as a single unit with no wire passing between them. The appliance is fashioned from a single strand of pure gold wire, 24 gauge, and weighs just over two grams (Clawson 1933: 146; 1934). Clearly this was meant to hold loose teeth in place;

teeth that Clawson believes had been loosened by extensive pyorrhea. Gold wire was looped around six teeth (C–C). The mandibular 1PM had been lost before death, and Clawson (1933: 149; 160, n. 10) suggests that Tabourian believes that the lost tooth was the result of an accident. Interestingly, the only decay noted in the other teeth appears in the right (first?) premolar (Clawson 1933: 149). Serious periodontal resorption, most strongly noted around the central incisors, shows a bilateral symmetry in its degree around the lateral incisors and declines past the area surrounding the canines, to a trace around the molars. All of the bones are well preserved and said to be tinted with a greenish color, possibly from proximity to copper salts (Clawson 1933: 151). Clawson also provides a summary of the associated grave goods (from Torrey 1920).

Clawson (1933: fig. 1) illustrates the pattern used to weave the gold wire around the teeth, describing the weaving in some detail (Clawson 1933: 146–147), noting, "salivary [calcareous] deposits had overlain the appliance at this point and had to be scaled away before the splint [appliance] could be taken from the teeth." Clawson (1934: 24) notes that Ginestet (1927: 17) errs in describing this piece as composed of two separate wires. Asbell (1948: 816) provides fine illustrations of the teeth and sarcophagus.

W-3. Alexandria

Present location: Greco-Roman Museum, Alexandria, Egypt (appliance now lost?).
Type: gold wire.
Origin: Ibrahimia (Ibrahimieh), near Alexandria, Egypt.

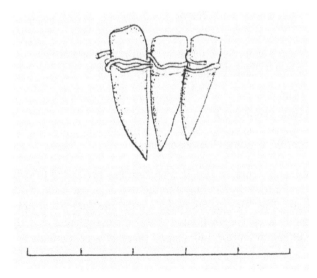

Figure 5.23a Wire appliance, W-3 (Alexandria), showing buccal surface of the right canine and incisors (after Weinberger 1948: fig. 40). Drawing by Becker.

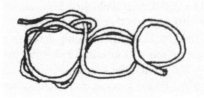

Figure 5.23b Alexandria appliance, a superior view, adjusted from Weinberger (1948). Drawing by Becker.

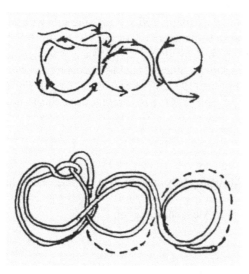

Figure 5.23c Alexandria appliance, diagram and sketch, showing Becker's suggested method of ligation. Drawing by Becker.

Jaw part: mandible, I1–C.
Date: Roman period (first century CE).
Sex: ?
Dimensions: L. 25 mm, W. variable (loosened wire).

Description: thin gold wire, 1 mm or less in diameter, has been used to stabilize a mandibular left lateral incisor by binding it to the two adjacent teeth. No holes are drilled in any tooth. The wire passes twice around the canine but now not completely around the incisors. Originally it probably did complete a second loop around the central and lateral incisor, but a small piece of wire, perhaps 21 mm long, has broken off.

References

Bardinet 1990: 2554, fig. 3 (after Weinberger).
Becker 1997: 82–83, figs.

Brown 1933: 584; 1934: 829.
Iskander *et al.* 1978: 105–106, pl. V, A (drawing from Weinberger 1946).
Lufkin 1948: 41 (citing Ruffer 1921: 314).
Ruffer 1921: 314 (but, see below).
Weinberger 1946: fig. 7.
Weinberger 1948: 119, fig. 40.

History and provenance

The origins of the Alexandria appliance remain vague. Ruffer (1921: 314, cited in Lufkin 1948: 41) appears to refer to this appliance as a series of teeth bound with a gold wire, found in a Roman tomb in Egypt by a Professor Breccia (obviously about or before 1921).[7] Earlier, Ruffer (1920) appears to have referred to the same appliance, as a set of artificial teeth, suggesting a denture. Since the Greco-Roman Museum was founded in 1892, this appliance probably was acquired by the Museum between that date and 1920.

Brown (1933: 584) was given some information about the Alexandria piece by a Mr. Aloriani of the Greco-Roman Museum in Alexandria (below), so it may have been there in 1933. Weinberger (1946: fig. 7) stated that it was found in a Roman grave of the third century CE at Ibrahimia. Some years later Iskander and colleagues (1978: 106) could not find it. More recently Bardinet (1990) tried to locate it, but also was unsuccessful. An attempt by Becker to clarify its location with the Director of the Greco-Roman Museum, Dr. Doreya Said (Becker to Said, personal communication, July 1, 1994) was unsuccessful.

In reply to Brown's (1933: 584) enquiry, Mr. Aloriani of the Greco-Roman Museum indicated that this mandibular appliance included three natural teeth (designated as 3, 2/1) connected with gold wire. Weinberger's drawing (1948: fig. 40) seems to indicate that the teeth are a mandibular right central incisor to right canine. He notes that a single piece of gold wire around their gingeval margins binds these three teeth, the middle one of the three, or the I2, most probably being supported by the appliance. Weinberger says that "signs of abrasion" are present on the teeth, suggesting that this is "due undoubtedly to the mechanical action of the gold wire." He states that "The teeth are considerably worn and over calcified, with tartar extending halfway down the roots." Dr. L. Avrouskini of Alexandria had sent photographs to Weinberger, who stated stated that the photographs "show the accompanying drawing to be correct" (Weinberger 1948: fig. 40).

Description

In Becker's redrawing of Weinberger's illustration of the Alexandria appliance it became evident that no means of providing tension or a secure bond is evident between the incisors. However, if the end of the gold wire at the lingual-distal aspect of the canine, as shown by Weinberger, is turned in the *opposite* direction and passed in front (buccal) of the lateral incisor and then behind (lingual) to the central incisor, it would meet the other end of the wire. At that location the ends could be twisted together to lock the appliance in place and provide the needed tension to retain a loose lateral incisor in place. The present wire may be sufficiently long to achieve this closure if all the slack now seen were removed by pulling. It seems likely that a small section of the wire may have been lost.

W-4 El-Qatta

(a)

(b)

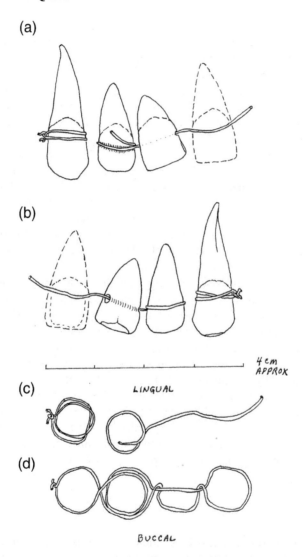

(c)

(d)

Figures 5.24a–d Wire appliance W-4 (El-Qatta): (a) labial surface, with teeth; (b) lingual (buccal) surface, with teeth; (c) configuration of the wire, as inferred by Becker from Harris *et al.* (1975); (d) a possible arrangement of the wire appliance, as suggested by Becker. Drawings by Becker.

Present location: believed to be at the "Cairo Museum," inv. no. 8/75:2/1 (or 82/751).

Type: gold wire support for a re-placed maxillary central incisor.

Origin: a mastaba of the Old Kingdom, reused in Roman period, in the cemetery of El-Qatta (near Imbaba, according to Harris *et al.* 1975: 401) about 40 km northwest of Cairo.

Jaw part: maxilla, 1I–C?? (but only I1, I2, and C survive).

Date: Ptolemaic? (32–31 BCE) or Roman era

Sex: uncertain.

Dimensions: L. 43 mm (broken), W. variable (loosened and broken wire).

Description: The two pieces of gold wire assumed to have been part of a single original length of wire now are associated with three maxillary teeth. A right canine is surrounded by two loops of gold wire, twisted closed at the distal side. A right lateral incisor is surrounded by a single loop of wire, which then passes through a hole drilled laterally through a right central incisor that has been cut down for replacement in this jaw. On the mesial exit from the drilled hole the wire now extends 17 or 18 mm. No other tooth was recovered but Becker reconstructs this appliance as having encircled the now-missing left central incisor for use as an anchor tooth. The fact that the root of the drilled tooth has been filed down suggests that this appliance was intended to re-place a central incisor in the Etruscan fashion.

References

Bardinet 1990: 2554, fig. 2 (a poor sketch).
Becker 1997: 83–84, fig.
Harris *et al.* 1975 (includes four figures and an extensive but imprecise description).
Harris and Ponitz 1980: 50, fig. 3.5 (an error-filled summary).
Hoffmann-Axthelm 1985: 29, figs 15–16.
Iskander *et al.* 1978: 108–112, pl. VI, B and also pl. VII through X.
Ring 1985: 36, fig. 28 (an enlarged, but indistinct photograph.)

History and provenance

The archaeological location known as El-Qatta is located on the edge of Egypt's Western Desert. The site is primarily known for a series of "mastaba" tombs ("bench"-shaped burial structures) of the Old Kingdom, probably Fourth Dynasty. Iskander and colleagues, including the excavator (1978: 109) indicate that the superstructure of Tomb no. 90, the mastaba from which the appliance derives, had been re-used for burials during the Roman period.

The appliance was found in 1952 by Dr. Shafik Farid (Exc. Reg. 58), but was overlooked until 1974. Details of the archaeological context have never been published (but see Iskander *et al.* 1978: 109). The wired series of three teeth are said to be from the crushed skull of a burial in Shaft 5 (of 6). Harris (*et al.* 1975; also Iskander *et al.* 1978) seem to imply that this appliance has an Old Kingdom date because it was associated with a mastaba (see Iskander *et al.* 1978: pl. I) of that period, but re-use of such funerary structures was quite common. Ring (1985) suggests an Old Kingdom mortuary prosthesis, made to be fitted to a mummy. No Egyptian "mortuary prostheses" of any date are known, however (see Chapter 2).

Bardinet (1990: 2554) carefully points out that the burial chamber from which the El-Qatta appliance was recovered had been reused in the Roman period. This appears to be a true dental prosthesis, but it most certainly dates to the Roman period. Leek (1967, also 1981) provides the best evaluations of the dates of these artifacts. The errors made by Harris and his colleagues are similar to those made in their evaluation of the Junker amulet.[8] The quality of the archaeological record for El-Qatta leaves a great deal to be desired. The lack of any scale in the published illustrations, and the absence of measurements of any of the associated teeth renders impossible an evaluation of gender.

Both Quenouille (1975) and Emptoz (1987) refer to a gold-wire appliance that they believe to be located in Cairo, but their commentaries are not sufficiently specific to enable us to identify it. Both of these authors probably refer to the El-Qatta piece, which Emptoz dates to the fourth–third centuries BCE; the basis for the date is not explained. Becker's attempts to locate it in Cairo in 1993, through the efforts of Professor Krishna Kumar (West Chester University), were not successful. Attempts to trace the history of this appliance, through a program of letter writing, have been equally unrewarding.

Description

The evaluation of the El-Qatta appliance as a dental prosthesis is based on the teeth involved as well as on the apparent technique of fastening. Direct descriptions are available from Harris *et al.* (1975) and are repeated by Iskander *et al.* (1978). The latter account provides a somewhat more clear evaluation and much better illustrations, but the overall presentation is still wanting.

Iskander *et al.* (1978: 111) believe that the presence of "calculus" (tartar) "on the cuspid and the substituted lateral incisor demonstrate that the bridge was worn by the patient for [a] relatively long period of time." Whether this "calculus" is true dental detritus or actually a coating that formed on all the objects in the tomb need not be considered here.

The teeth recovered appear to be a right central incisor, a right lateral incisor, plus a "cuspid" (canine). This worn canine, "around which has been placed a double strand of gold wire twisted into a knot on the distal surface" (Iskander *et al.* 1978: 110), is generally believed to be an abutment (anchor) for a bridge. Only the photograph (Iskander *et al.* 1978: pl. IX) provides evidence that this is a *single* wire, in the form of a crossing-over of the wire that is evident on the buccal surface of the canine. Iskander and colleagues (1978: 110) believe that the canine "has a gold loop in the wire that was twisted around it on its distal surface. To this loop was attached by a hook the gold wire on which were placed the two teeth just described." The other anchor tooth, the left central incisor, is said to have "been lost with the broken parts of the skull" (Iskander *et al.* 1978: 404).

In fact, no hook and loop arrangement is evident around the canine in the illustrations provided by Iskander *et al.* (1979). A hook and loop arrangement would not be a possible attachment method for a dental appliance using soft gold. Furthermore, why the "loop" would be on the "distal" surface of the tooth when the replaced teeth abut this canine's mesial surface cannot be explained. Clearly what we have here, called a "loop," is a typical twist of the wire ends used to "tie off" the wire appliance (see Harris *et al.* 1975: 402, fig. 4).

What is evident from both of these texts is that the two components were not described *in situ*, and that the arrangement or order of the teeth is a matter of some speculation. Iskander *et al.* (1978: 111) clearly states that "this prosthesis was originally an anterior bridge. The arrangement of the three teeth as presented to us must have been, therefore, changed since its discovery or *post mortem*." They then conclude that this appliance included two false teeth bound to two living teeth, a pattern that may be possible. However, if this appliance held two replacement incisors, then we must ask why only one of the two "replacement" incisors has been drilled (see below)? Considering the nature of this find and the early "descriptions," another scenario may be suggested. The drilled central incisor may be the only replacement tooth, but it was anchored to the lateral incisor as well as to the canine and left central incisor.

One illustration of the El-Qatta appliance (Iskander *et al.* 1978: pl. VI, B) clearly indicates that someone has linked these teeth by bending, as well as straightening, various parts of the gold wire, a procedure that has destroyed the evidence for the way in which the wire originally related to these teeth. It depicts a length of gold wire that might have been sufficiently long to encircle two replacement teeth. Our understanding of the specific construction arrangement of the El-Qatta appliance may be distorted because the original author failed to provide a careful description of the appliance before someone tampered with it. We have no idea how the "appliance" was "constructed" before it was "assembled" in the pattern generally seen in various illustrations. The label for fig. 2 of Harris *et al.* (1975: 403) states that: "The lingual view of the bridge *assembled according to the author's* [sic] *contention* that the cuspid was a right maxillary abutment tooth" (emphasis added).

The other "two teeth placed on a long gold wire completed the specimen" (Harris *et al.* 1975: 402). One of these

> two teeth appears to be a central Incisor [sic] where a hole has been drilled in a mesial distal direction through the crown. The root of the tooth is said to have been scraped to give the root a smooth and artificial appearance. Also, a buccal groove is said to have been prepared parallel to the hole to accommodate the gold wire from outside.
>
> (Harris *et al.* 1975: 402)

Harris (*et al.* 1975: 402, figs 2, 4) indicate that the central incisor has had extensive wear, and is extremely "shoveled" (about which more below). In fact, the groove is on the labial surface, as they correctly note in fig. 3 (caption) and again on p. 404. However, the wire is *not* shown encircling this incisor, but only passing through it. The "groove" on this central incisor (I1) is described by Iskander and colleagues (1978: 110) as located on the buccal surface, but on the following page (p. 111) it is said to be "a labial groove." The photographs provided do not help solve this problem as no "groove" is evident on any of these teeth. *Drawings* of the right central incisor, however, do seem to indicate a groove on the labial surface of the crown.

The possible lateral incisor is not likely to be a second "false" tooth secured by this appliance. Iskander *et al.* (1978: 110) state that "The other tooth has the gold wire wrapped around it with a labial groove prepared to accommodate this wire" (see also Harris *et al.* 1975: 402, 404). This tooth would appear to be a lateral incisor, and these authors state that the root has been scraped giving it an artificial morphology. This supposed reconfiguration of the I2 is less certain. Iskander *et al.* (1978: 110) also note that "[I]n addition, considerable tartar is found on the gingeval two thirds of the root."

Bardinet (1990) points out that the technique of mesial-distal drilling, assumed to hold one tooth in place (the I1) for the El-Qatta appliance, is like that found with the Tura El-Asmant silver wire appliance (no. 15), another example where only one tooth has been replaced. Bardinet suggests that El-Qatta has a similar date, probably during the Ptolemaic period, or during the Roman period in Egypt. Bardinet's fig. 2 shows the three teeth of this El-Qatta appliance (I1–C.), so well illustrated by Harris and his colleagues. No mention is made by Harris *et al.* (1975) of how this appliance functioned.

Regarding the shoveling observed on this tooth, this non-metric dental feature is relatively common in central Italy and probably elsewhere, but the trait is rarely mentioned in dental studies in the Mediterranean region. While noted as common in central Italic populations, the exact incidence is not known for other regions. Professor Joel Irish (2006) provides a review of up to 36 morphological dental variants in 15 Egyptian samples, Neolithic through Roman, revealing shoveling incidence greater than 40 percent in some groups, while others have none. The high incidence groups suggest that the person at El-Qatta with this appliance was most likely a local resident.

W-5 Tura El-Asmant

Present location: Iskander *et al.* (1978: 105) state that this appliance is at the Centre of Research and Conservation of Antiquities, General Organization of Egyptian Antiquities, Cairo, "but it will be shortly exhibited in the Cairo Museum."

Type: silver wire.

Origin: Tura El-Asmant, Egypt.

Jaw part: maxilla (I1–I2)

Date: Ptolemaic (323–31 BCE)

Sex: male??

Dimensions: L. 27 mm, W. two lengths of silver wire, each less than 1 mm diameter.

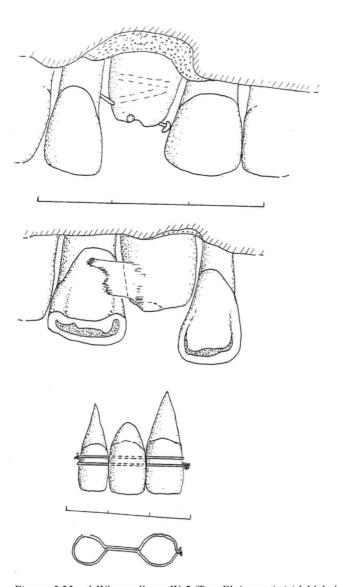

Figures 5.25a–d Wire appliance W-5 (Tura El-Asmant): (a) labial view, after
photographs by Quenouille (in Iskander *et al.* 1978: pl. III, IV);
(b) lingual view (cf. Figure 5.25a); (c) and (d) a possible technique
for affixing the Tura El-Asmant wire appliance. Drawings by
Becker.

Description: This bridge supports between its natural adjacent teeth a re-placed
maxillary right central incisor, with root filed down. The re-placed tooth has had
two holes, one above the other, drilled through the mesial-distal aspects. A single
silver wire, about 75 mm long, passed around one anchor tooth, with both ends

then passing through a single hole in the re-placed tooth and dividing again to surround the opposite anchor tooth where it was then twisted closed. The second silver wire, of about the same length, passed in the opposite direction at the level of the second drilled hole and parallel to the first wire, similarly passing around the opposite anchor tooth and tied off with a twist. These two wires at no point were in contact.

References

Bardinet 1990.
Becker 1997: 84–86, figs 5a and 5b.
Iskander and Harris 1977: 85–90, pl. I–III.
Iskander *et al.* 1978: 104–105, pl. III and IV.

History and provenance

During archaeological rescue excavations of a burial area at Tura El-Asmant during the 1952/3 season, Mr. Mohammed abd El-Tawab El-Hetta recovered over 100 mummies from 182 tombs of the Ptolemaic period. Tura el-Asmant, in the region/state of Al Qahirah, is today a small town near the eastern bank of the Nile, south of Cairo and Giza, and east of Saqqara. The exact location of the archaeological site is not specified; salvage excavation was initiated in response to the expansion of "the Portland Cement Company." At the time Mr. El-Hetta was a co-excavator with Zaky Youssef Saad at nearby Helwan, which lies only a few kilometers south of Cairo.

Simple graves (T-1 through T-182) held mummies described (Iskander and Harris 1977: 86) as exemplifying an embalming technique noted by Herodotus (2.88) as the third, and least expensive, method of mummification. This implies that the tombs at Tura El-Asmant were not those of families of the highest status. This is an important observation, since it is the only case where there is a possible indication of a dental appliance being available to other than the elite members of society.

Tomb T-121 (Iskander and Harris 1977: 86; but Iskander *et al.* 1978: 104 identify the tomb as T-127) held a mummy whose skull was associated with traces of what has been interpreted to be silver wire. The skull was sent to the Department of Antiquities in Cairo for conservation and study. The subsequent location of the skeleton and/or the "dental appliance" is not provided by Iskander and Harris (1977), and has not been determined by Professor Krishna Kumar's attempt on behalf of Becker to locate the skull or the appliance in Cairo in 1993.

Description

Testing revealed that silver, with slight copper impurities, had been used in some form of "wire," but that this metal, or perhaps alloy, had corroded into something like silver chloride. Iskander and Harris identify the metal as "horn silver," which is a heavy halide mineral composed of silver chloride (AgCl). This is an extremely important observation. If this material reflects the use of a silver wire dental appliance, this would suggest that inexpensive silver appliances (see Iskander and Harris 1977: 88–89 for ancient values of silver) may have been used by affluent but non-aristocratic Egyptians of the Ptolemaic period. This would also confirm those texts of Ptolemaic and later date, which discuss silver dental appliances in contexts that would suggest that they were commonly available. Quite probably the silver in such prostheses has deteriorated and therefore gone unrecognized in most cases.

The illustrations provided by Iskander and Harris (1977) suggest that this is the skeleton of an adult (young?) with all teeth present, except for a "false" or replacement tooth wired in place. Iskander *et al.* (1978: pl. III, IV) include two excellent photographs taken by Dr. Jean-Jacques Quenouille (cf. Quenouille 1975). These plates offer detailed views of only the three teeth involved plus the adjacent alveolus. The photographs clearly indicate that the I2 and I1 are shoveled, which on a scale of 0–4 could be noted as 2 and 1 respectively. This non-metric dental trait is discussed above (no. W-4). The considerable wear on the lingual surface of these teeth also reflects a severe malocclusion (overbite).

What appears in the photographs to be a rotted stump of the right central incisor (I1) is situated in a severely abcessed area of the alveolus, or has a necrotic depression surrounding the root area. The illustrations provided by Iskander and his colleagues (1978) are not sufficiently clear to permit a secure evaluation, but the photograph appears to indicate a male. A detailed examination of the teeth and of this skeleton is needed.

A maxillary right central incisor (I1), which may have been lost due to trauma or to deliberate ablation, appears to have been placed back in the mouth (or replaced with another human incisor). The replacement may have taken place after some interval of time, while the injury (?) healed from the loss. Two holes ("or a bifurcate hole": Iskander *et al.* 1978: 105) are said to have been drilled through "the lower half of the crown" of the replaced or replacement incisor, through which silver wire was passed and then tied. The relationship of these two drilled holes and the pattern of wiring and tying the replacement tooth to the flanking incisors is unclear from even Quenouille's excellent photographs (in Iskander *et al.* 1978: pl. III, IV).

The dental health of this individual, as represented by surviving dentition, is good. If the traces of metal discovered represent a wire dental appliance, one possible method by which this tooth may have been suspended in place would have been to use two wires and to place the two drilled holes one above the other. Each wire would pass from one flanking or support tooth, through a drilled hole and around the opposite "post" or support tooth, then back through the same drilled hole. When the wire emerges it would pass around the opposite side of the first flanking tooth, and the ends would be "tied off" or twisted together near the distal margin of the post tooth.

Iskander and Harris (1977: 87) note that the root of the replacement or replaced right central incisor "is considerably shorter than that of the left" central incisor.

We concur in suggesting that this tooth could be the owner's original tooth with a root modified after loss for replacement in the space. The pattern of construction of the Tura El-Asmant dental appliance appears similar to that used in the El-Qatta appliance.

W-6 Eretria

Present location: National Archaeological Museum, Athens, inventory no. 733.
Type: gold wire.
Origin: Eretria, on the island of Euboea, Greece.
Jaw part: mandibular I1–PM1 (?).
Date: fourth century BCE (Clawson 1934: 25).

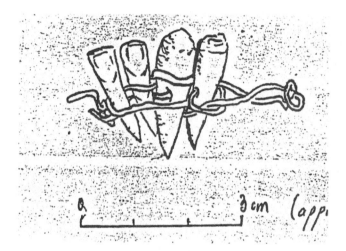

Figure 5.26a Wire appliance W-6 (Eretria). View of the lingual surface suggesting that teeth had been drilled (after Clawson 1933: 156, fig. 8b; also Weinberger 1948: fig. 39, lower). Drawing by Becker.

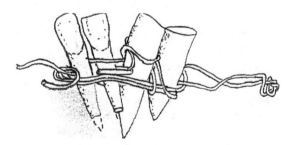

Figure 5.26b Becker's reconstruction of Eretria as a wire appliance with no drilled teeth. Drawing by Becker.

Sex: female ??? Becker (1997: 86) originally suggested that this was a male, but now questions that evaluation.

Dimensions: L. 49 mm (est.); W. variable (2–4 widths of wire).

Description: The poor original drawing and subsequent unavailability of this gold-wire appliance render difficult any efforts at description. This appears to have been a classic use of wire to stabilize loose teeth, but whether the four teeth apparently depicted were original to this artifact is another of the many unknowns. Clawson's (1934) effort to depict this appliance and the teeth associated with it reveals a confusing tangle that appears to represent a single strand. Our efforts to decode the path of that strand around the teeth do not result in a coherent or reasonable appliance such as would have been the effort of any practitioner. We can only assume that the appliance is incomplete as is.

References

Becker 1997: 86–87, fig. 6.

Bliquez 1996: 2645, "B," fig. 2

Clawson 1933: 158, fig. 8b; 1934: 25, fig. 2. This illustration, possibly taken from Guerini (1909) seems to depict two drilled teeth, emphasized by the lack of surviving roots on them.

Emptoz 1987: 551, fig. 9 (illustration depicts an extremely poor *copy* of the Eretria appliance, possibly a copy in Paris; see Appendix II).

Guerini 1909: fig. 9, lower.

Lufkin 1948: fig. 16.

Papabasileiou 1903: 65.

Sudhoff 1926: 63, fig. 39a (this is *probably* Eretria).

Weinberger 1946: fig. 6 (this figure appears to be the Eretria appliance, but may depict the Alexandria example; see Weinberger 1946: fig. 7).

Weinberger 1947: fig. 7 (same as 1946: fig. 6).

Weinberger 1948: 118, fig. 39 lower (this illustration derives either from Clawson (1933) or Guerini (1909)).

History and context

The Eretria prosthesis, apparently discovered in 1902 (Papabasileiou 1903: 64–65), is said to have come from a necropolis excavated at Eretria, where at least one burial (not that with the appliance) was found with a gold coin (stater) of Alexander the Great placed in the mouth. No details were published on the tomb in which the appliance was found, however. Clawson (1934: fig. 2) derives his depiction of this example from Guerini (1909: 60). Emptoz (1987) repeats the belief that it came from the skull of a woman, probably deriving his evaluation from the Papabasileiou text. The present disposition of related skeletal material, if any was recovered, is unknown. Micheloni (1976: 264) suggests a similarity between this example and the Sidon pieces (nos. W-1, W-2), and now we can link this form of appliance with others known from the Eastern Mediterranean and Rome.

Description

Four teeth appear entwined (bound?) by this wire, which extends off at either end of the appliance as if other teeth may have been involved. The four teeth involved might be the right central incisor through the right first premolar, but only if these are the original teeth that are depicted and if they are shown in proper order. Becker has redrawn them with an estimate of their relative size, as derived from published drawings. The presence of four teeth appears to be the only detail on which there is general agreement among those early authors describing this appliance, but all this information may have been copied from a single original source. As in many other cases, earlier descriptions were so uniformly poor that readers cannot be certain of anything. We cannot determine from the literature if the teeth are all natural, or were bound in place, or if one or two are "artificial," or at least lost and replaced in correct position by drilling through them and suspending them with wires, as is the case with the Sidon I appliance. Although Clawson's rough drawing (1934: fig. 2) may appear to represent one or more holes drilled through the canine, this is an unlikely tooth to be replaced after loss. Our reconstruction (Figure 5.27b) suggests that no drilling had been used to put in place this gold-wire appliance. The two visits made by Becker to the National Archaeological Museum in Athens (see no. 20) failed to locate this example.

Without detailed direct examination, no conclusions can be drawn at this time, but it would be very unlikely that holes would have been drilled in any teeth still in position, and these teeth appear to have intact roots. In some illustrations at least the canine appears to be pierced, but the total number of teeth originally involved is not evident. The original appliance probably spanned six teeth, but the anchor teeth are no longer associated with the fourth teeth illustrated. These four teeth usually appear to be gracile when depicted, thus might derive from a woman. However, dentition among Greek populations appears uniformly gracile, and gender variation has not been specifically demonstrated for Greek populations, so it remains possible that the individual wearing this appliance was male.

The Eretria prosthesis was formed through a complex pattern of wiring, but whether the wires pass through holes drilled mesial-distally through the teeth at the base of the crown, or only pass around the teeth remains unclear. Whether the two teeth in the middle (I2 and C.) may be the only ones drilled also is not clear. Quite possibly all four teeth are not even original to the appliance, but are replacements used for display, or in the process of making a copy of this appliance. If these are original teeth, the anchor teeth to which they might have been tied would have been the 1I and the PM2, which are not present.

Interpretation

Perhaps the presence of this appliance reflects some technological/dental connection between Greece and the eastern/Levantine practice of using wire dental appliances. The Hippocratic texts of the Classical era (fifth–fourth centuries BCE) mention wiring to stabilize loose teeth. It is also late enough in date (early Hellenistic, if we may date it by the gold stater placed as Charon's coin in the mouth of someone in the same necropolis) that many traders, diplomats, slaves, mercenaries and their families, were circulating across the Mediterranean. It is true that Etruria was intimately associated with Euboea since the Iron Age (eighth century BCE) through the settlers of the colony of Pithekoussai in the Bay of Naples. Ancient literary sources (Strabo 5.247C) note that gold was being purveyed there (processed, probably into diadems for the burials of native Italian wives of the original Greek and Levantine colonists (although there are no gold sources on or near the island itself). Archaeology has opened new vistas on these early, shared efforts at trade and colonization, with the excavation of burials of families of mixed ethnic background: Greeks from Eretria, Chalkis, and Corinth, men and women from Phoenicia and North Syria, Italic persons (Daunian, Latin, Campanian, etc.) and Etruscans who all all married and raised (and often buried) numerous children. (See Ridgway 1992: 111–118; Buchner 1979; Buchner and Ridgway 1993; Becker and Donadio 1992; Becker 1995b.) The grand cooperative enterprise of Etruscans and Euboean Greeks occurred in the Iron Age-Archaic periods, the era of Etruscan band-type appliances.

Professor Larry Bliquez (personal communication 2002) wisely urges caution in identifying any dental appliance found outside of Etruria or Phoenicia as deriving from one source or another. He suggests that Greeks may have derived such technology from their Levantine trading partners, and employed the technology at home. This might be consistent with Lucian's Roman-era testimony, which certainly notes the existence of these devices, probably in the Greek world. Becker emphasises, however, that there would have been cultural inhibitors on the use of such appliances in Greek society. Certainly the Greeks would not wish their wives to bedeck themselves with the kinds of ornamentation to be seen on those Etruscan women present during dining sessions, who made the visiting Greeks so uncomfortable by their presence.

W-7 Collatina (Rome)

Present location: Soprintendenza Archeologica di Roma, Palazzo Altemps, Rome.
Type: wire.
Origin: Rome, Collatina Necropolis, Viale della Serenissima (Municipio V di Roma).
Jaw part: mandible, spanning five teeth.
Date: Imperial Era (first–second century CE?).
Sex: female.
Dimensions: L 39; Extant W. 10 mm.

Description: This simple gold-wire dental prosthesis from the Collatina Necropolis holds one re-placed tooth, a right central incisor in an otherwise normal mandible. It is fashioned from a single length of gold wire, less than

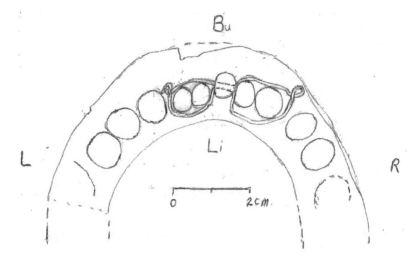

Figure 5.27 Roman wire appliance from Collatina necropolis, Rome. Drawing of placement in jaw as found, by M. J. Becker.

1 mm in diameter, with an estimated length of perhaps 100 mm. The appliance as wound in place measures 39 mm long and now approximately 10 mm across the lingual-buccal plane, probably due to post-mortem distortion. Originally this appliance probably measured only 8 mm across, the distance needed to surround the right canine. The wire passes around two teeth on each side of the single "replacement" or re-placed tooth, held in place by wire passing through a mesial-distal hole.

References

Catalano *et al.* 2007.
Minozzi *et al.* 2007.

Context

The complete reports on the excavations from the Collatina Necropolis remain in production, but Simona Minozzi kindly provides us with an important glimpse of an object of great interest. Excavations in a necropolis near the Viale della Serenissima (Municipio V di Roma, the southeast sector of Rome) during the year 2000 brought to light the only archaeologically documented gold-wire appliance found in Rome, or anywhere on the Italian peninsula. The necropolis of the Viale delle Serenissima is now identified as the Collatina Necropolis, relating it to the ancient Via Collatina, which passes nearby. An impressive stretch of the original surface of this ancient road has been found nearly intact in the area of Rome's Serenissima train station (Buccellato *et al.* (2008).

The full extent of the Collatina necropolis, as with most of Rome's sprawling ancient burial areas, remains unknown; it is now the largest known necropolis of the Imperial Age (31/27 BCE–476 CE) within the area of modern Rome. Excavations were directed by Dr. Stefano Musso, then an Inspector for the Archaeological Superintendence of Rome, and its director in 2014.

The specific archaeological context of this cremation burial is provided only in Catalano *et al.* (2007), who describe a "Tomba Monumentale" identified as "M1 T.1." The cremation with this appliance is said to have been at the center of the tomb, where the cremation itself took place. This suggests that the tomb was built around the pyre. In addition to mausoleums, most of the "tombs" from the Collatina Necropolis are said to be inhumations. Over 2,200 burials have been recovered (Minozzi *et al.* 2012: 269), but among them the cremations encountered are said to be few (Buccellato *et al.* 2008: 63). Specific numbers have not been tabulated, but the three cinerary urns that are mentioned appear to be only a small percentage. The burned bones from these various cremations are to be studied by Elena Santandrea (Buccellato *et al.* 2008: 86, n. 42).

Recognition of the importance of the find of a gold-wire dental appliance in peninsular Italy led to the rapid publication of this object by a team of scholars (Minozzi *et al.* 2007). The archaeological context has been roughly dated first–second centuries CE, or early in the Imperial Age. Specific details regarding this individual burial have not yet been published more precisely. The bones are described as representing "the partially cremated remains of an adult woman" (Minozzi *et al.* 2007: e1). The focus of the poster presentation and article is on the gold appliance and the mandibular corpus that holds the teeth found bound with gold wire. This is the only cremated bone from this burial yet described. A photograph of the complete surviving *corpus mandibularis* appears in Catalano *et al.* (2007: fig. 1). The publications and their illustrations provided the primary sources for the evaluation that follows.

The use of photographs to evaluate the age and sex of an individual is a notoriously risky business. Given that only the body of the mandible is illustrated, any statement made here regarding age and sex must be considered with caution. The apparent presence of robust third molars might be an indication that this person might be a high status female, but the evaluation of sex of a single individual without others from that population is extremely difficult (Huntsman and Becker 2013). The absence of apparent dental decay should be compared with others in this population, but the extent of periodontal deterioration suggests an adult of perhaps 50 years of age (± 10 years) at death.

Becker interprets the illustrated evidence associated with this appliance as indicating the product of a complete and perfectly normal cremation, probably at a temperature of 900–950°C. The presence of an un-crushed mandibular corpus within this cremation burial presents one of two possibilities. First, that the cremated remains had been buried in a large container (sarcophagus, large chest, wooden coffin, etc.) or; second, that only selected portions of the *ossilegium* (the bones that normally survive cremation) had been chosen for deposit in this grave. The second alternative is less likely than that the burned bones lay where they were burned as indicated by the authors.

Minozzi *et al.* (2007) carefully note that the typical cremation damage to the crowns of teeth that were in place at death applies to this individual. All the missing crowns were lost due to fire damage in a process that Becker has described as "exploding." They add that, "the jaw was largely preserved from the third left molar to the second right premolar. The single tooth held in place by this gold "bridge" does not manifest the type of fire damage common to teeth that were living at the time of death. This seems as if the "replaced" tooth was a dry (non-living) inclusion, supported by gold wire, and not subject to the kinds of spalling or explosive damage to the crown as the living teeth. Whether this "replacement" was the owner's original tooth re-placed in this position is uncertain.

The melting point of pure (24 ct) gold is 1063°C. Silver melts at 961°C. The pyre temperatures of most cremations in antiquity did not exceed 950° C. It is not surprising that the gold dental appliance survived the process; we might expect more of them to be found, if they had been popular.

The detailed illustrations in these publications focus on the appliance and omit some important evidence concerning the surviving mandibular corpus and the condition of the individual teeth therein. The descriptions below derive from the published photographic evidence (Minozzi *et al.* 2007: page e2, figs a–c).

The dentition

Some evidence of periodontal deterioration is evident, suggesting an age of perhaps 30 to 35 years. Roots of the left third and second molars are in place (Catalano *et al.* 2007: fig. 1). The root and neck of the first molar appear firmly anchored. Aside from the missing ("exploded") crowns, the left premolars appear to have been healthy at death. The authors' observation of a "peculiar abrasion of the buccal surface of the left first premolar" warrants further study. The socket for the left canine reveals a relatively healthy tooth, aside from the periodontal inflammation. The root itself is not present, having been lost post-mortem, and almost certainly post-cremation.

The left lateral incisor served as an "anchor" for the dental appliance. Despite its precarious position, next to an extremely loose central incisor, it maintained this small pontic during life and even after cremation and burial. A root canal, as suggested by the authors, is not visible. The "left central incisor is not preserved." Becker strongly disagrees with the authors' belief that it "is certainly 'artificial,' as suggested by the space apparent in the gold wire" (Minozzi et al. 2007). If it were "artificial" or the original tooth held in place by the wire, the tooth would have been drilled and the wire would have been pinched to pass through the hole, not simply passed around the tooth. The space for the left central incisor is evident in the wire of the prosthesis. However, the area of the socket of the left central incisor reveals extensive periodontal deterioration. The same deterioration certainly caused the right central incisor to fall out, probably providing the "replacement" tooth, as the authors also believe. Becker believes that the left central incisor was extremely loose in a deteriorating and shrinking socket, but that it had not yet fallen out. In that loosened condition it would not have served as an anchor tooth, requiring that the wire appliance incorporate the left lateral incisor to support the pontic.

The right central incisor is the dental space for which this pontic was constructed using the person's own lost tooth to create this appliance. The re-placed tooth has been drilled at the base of the enamel with a mesial-distal hole, approx. 2 mm in diameter, to pass both the lingual and buccal aspects of the appliance wire through it. Minozzi *et al.* (2007) suggest that the root of this tooth has been filed down to allow it to fit above the gingival tissue without causing further irritation. Note that this tooth is the best preserved of the series in that it retains its crown. This suggests that this dry (dead) tooth was not subject to the same effects of the fire as the others.

The right lateral incisor and canine appear to be angled toward the medial area, probably in response to the periodontal conditions that were causing dental loss of the central incisors. Not mentioned in the publication is a flake of burned bone shown lodged within the gold prosthesis against the lingual surface of the right lateral incisor. The right premolars were present at death, but the roots probably became dislodged from their sockets after cremation. The second premolar socket has what appears to be an abscess at its base. The socket for the right first molar is so extensively damaged as to preclude any evaluation. The extent of the post-cremation bone loss suggests that a tooth had been in place at death. Had that tooth been lost, bone formation at the site probably would have survived combustion. The Minozzi *et al.* (2007) text suggests that the region of the corpus below the second and third molars does not survive, but the illustration in Catalano *et al.* (2007) reveals that the area below both teeth is present, although extensively damaged.

The loss of anterior teeth, or general looseness of the anterior teeth in the elderly is seen here to be associated with extensive periodontal disease, as noted by the authors. Becker's experience with Italic pre-Imperial populations is that dental loss most often begins with caries among the molars. Anterior teeth tend to remain in place to very old age.

The need to use two teeth on either side to anchor this tooth reflects the extent of periodontal loss that caused this right first incisor to fall out. The immediately adjacent teeth were so compromised as to be incapable of

(continued on p.299)

Table 5.8 Etruscan and related dental appliances

#	Name	Provenance	Date	Sex	Jaw region	Type	*	Comments, location
1	Barrett I	Etruria	? 5th c.	F?	Maxilla I1 plus	Simple band, 3 spaces Stabilizing	NA	Formerly private collection of Dr. Wm. C. Barrett, Buffalo, NY—location unknown, believed to be in Buffalo area
2	Barrett II	Bisenzio, tomb on Capodimonte	500–480	F	Maxilla (2PM–I1?)	Simple band, 5 spaces Stabilizing	NA	Formerly private collection of Dr. Wm. C. Barrett, Buffalo, NY—location unknown, believed to be in Buffalo area
3	Van Marter	"Lake of Valseno" (Bolsena?)	600??	F??	Maxilla?	Ring series 3 spaces, with central false tooth	NA	Formerly private collection of Dr. Wm. C. Barrett, Buffalo, NY—location unknown, believed to be in Buffalo area Obtained by Dr. James Gilbert Van Marter in Italy
4	Copenhagen	Orvieto?	500–490	F	Maxilla I1–I2	3 welded loops, no rivet	*	National Museum, Copenhagen inv. no. 8319
5	Poggio Gaiella	Chiusine necropolis Poggio Gaiella	?4th–3rd c.	F 25–40 yrs	Maxilla 1PM to PM1	Single, complex band Now in 2 pieces	*	Florence, Museo Archeologico, inv. no. 11782 Now in wrong skull and mandible
6	Populonia	Populonia, San Cerbone necropolis (tomb destroyed)	4th c.	?	Maxilla (2I–I2)?	4-ring series, 4 spaces, 1 rivet	NA	Florence, Museo Archeologico, inv. no. 84467—lost in Florence Flood 1966, Minto, Populonia 1943: pl. 48,1 (mandible)

7	Ghent	"Near Orvieto"	6th c. or later?	?	Maxilla (2I–I2?)	Complex band 3 loops, 4 spaces	NA	(Ghent University Museum, 1899—looted by German invasion forces WWII) attached to skull fragment by canine tooth
8	Bruschi I	Probably territory of Tarquinia	5th c.?	F	Maxilla 4 spaces (incisors)	Narrow band, 4 spaces Stabilizing	*	Museo Nazionale Archeologico, Tarquinia, Ex collection, Count Bruschi-Falgari, Corneto Displayed with two teeth
9	Bruschi II	Territory of Tarquinia?	?	F???	Maxilla (2I–I2?)	4 rings, 1 rivet (1 false tooth, 3 spaces)	NA	Collection, Count Bruschi-Falgari, Corneto Missing since 1916–1925 transfer to Museo Nazionale Archeologico, Tarquinia
10	Bruschi III	Territory of Tarquinia?	2nd c.??	F	Maxilla?	4 braces, 5 spaces, No rivets Stabilizing	*	Museo Nazionale Archeologico, Tarquinia Ex collection, Count Bruschi-Falgari, Corneto Often confused with Corneto I Teeth now associated are recent replacement
11	Corneto I	Tarquinia	530–510?	??	Maxilla? Left C–I2	Braced? band, 5 spaces, 2 rivets, 1 false tooth	NA	Museo Nazionale Archeologico, Tarquinia. Probably excavated 1876–1877 Missing since 1916–1925 (or earlier)
12	Corneto II	Tarquinia	500?	F??	Maxilla? (2PM–right C?)	Compound: 7 rings, 8 spaces, 3 rivets, ivory	NA	Museo Nazionale Archeologico, Tarquinia. Possibly excavated c.1875 Missing since 1916–1925 (or earlier)

(continued)

Table 5.8 (continued)

#	Name	Provenance	Date	Sex	Jaw region	Type	*	Comments, location
13	Liverpool I	Unknown	?	F?	Maxilla 2I–I2	Band with 2 false teeth, 2 rivets, 4 spaces	*	Liverpool World History Museum inv. no. 10334 Ex collection of Joseph Mayer Collected before 1857
14	Liverpool II	Unknown	?	F? 45+ yrs	Maxilla 2I–I2	Band for 2 false teeth, 2 rivets, 4 spaces	*	Liverpool World History Museum inv. no. 10335 Ex collection of Joseph Mayer Collected before 1857 Anchor teeth may be replacements
15	Valsiarosa	Valsiarosa necropolis of Falerii Veteres, Tomb 20	4th c.?	F?	Maxilla 2I–I2	4 welded loops, 4 spaces, 1 rivet	*	Museo Archeologico del Agro Falisco, Civita Castellana, previously Villa Giulia inv. no. 1515 Displayed since 1880s on ancient skull that is not original owner
16	Teano	Teano, Tomb 18, Fondo Gradavola necropolis, Campania	4th– 3rd c.	F	Maxilla C–C	6 rings, no rivets Stabilizing?	NA	Institut für Geschichte der Medizin, Universitätsklinikum Charité, Humboldt-Universität, Berlin; Excavated 1907 Ex collection Professor W. Dieck
17	Praeneste	Praeneste, Sporadic find in necropolis	?	F 35–45 yrs**	Maxilla 2I–I2 3 teeth	Band, 4 spaces Central pair riveted	*	Villa Giulia inv. no. 13213, on display In 1885 was in Palazzo Barberini, Rome

No.	Site	Provenance	Date	Sex/Age	Location	Appliance		Museum
18	Satricum	Satricum, Borgo Le Ferriere, Tumulus C	7th c. c.630	F 50 yrs	Maxilla 21-C	Band, 5 spaces Gold tooth (I1)	*	Villa Giulia inv. no. 12206
19	Bracciano	Near Lake Bracciano	7th c.?	F?	Maxilla I1-I2	Band, 3 spaces, 1 rivet holds false tooth	NA	Vienna, Museum of Natural History inv. no. 24.296 (acquired or catalogued c.1990), apparently part of a tomb group in museum
20	Tanagra	Tanagra, Boeotia	4th–3rd c.?	F? 45±10 yrs**	Maxilla C–C	Compound band of 2 joined loops, no rivets	NA	Athens National Museum: Lambros Collection inv. no. 358
21	Sardis	Salihli "ancient Sardis" found by farmer in a tomb	3rd c.??	F 25–40 yrs	skull + mandible 2 central incisors false; anchors 2 second incisors	Stabilizing band, 4 loops, 2 rivets (in 2 false teeth)	NA	Private collection, Ankara, Turkey. Present owner Dr. Ilter Uzel

Note: where noted, sex has been assigned based on (small) tooth size, determined by the spaces in appliances.
  * Autopsied by M. Becker.
NA Not available for examination or lost.
 ** Age estimate based on dental wear or extant teeth.

Table 5.9 Typological details of Etruscan gold-band appliances

#	Name	Provenance	Date	Sex/age	Gold design	# Rivets	False: material	Living teeth present	Type/design
1	Barrett I	Etruria	5th c.	F?	Simple band				3 spaces Stabilizing
2	Barrett II	Bisenzio	500	F	Simple band				5 spaces Stabilizing
3	Van Marter	Bolsena?	600	F??	Ring series		?		3 rings Replacement
4	Copenhagen	Orvieto?	500	F	Welded loops				3 rings Stabilizing
5	Poggio Gaiella	Chiusi	4th–3rd c.	F, 25–40	Complex band			Wrong skull	4 rings, 8 teeth Stabilizing
6	Populonia	Populonia	4th c.	?	Ring series	1	1		4 rings Replacement
7	Ghent	Orvieto	6th c.??	?	Complex band				3 rings, one double-size Lost
8	Bruschi I	Tarquinia	5th c.?	F	Narrow band				4 spaces Stabilizing
9	Bruschi II	Tarquinia	?	F??	Ring series	1	1		4 rings Replacement
10	Bruschi III	Tarquinia	2nd c.?	F	Braces?	No			5 spaces, braced Stabilizing band
11	Corneto I	Tarquinia	530?	??	Braced band?	2	2		5 spaces, band Replacement

12	Corneto II	Tarquinia	500?	F??	Compound rings	3	Ivory		7 rings Replacement
13	Liverpool I	??	?	F?	Band	2	Human		Band, 4 spaces Replacement
14	Liverpool II	??	?	F? 45+	Band	2	2		Band, 4 spaces Replacement
15	Valsiarosa	Falerii	4th c.	F?	Welded loops	1	1 at 1I	Wrong skull	4 rings? Replacement
16	Teano	Teano	4th–3rd c.	F	Ring series				6 rings Stabilizing?
17	Praeneste	Praeneste	?	F, 35–45	Band	2	2		Band, 4 spaces Replacement
18	Satricum	Satricum	630	F, 50	Band		Gold		Band, 5 spaces Replacement
19	Bracciano	Bracciano	7th c.?	F?	Band	1	1		Band, 3 spaces Replacement
20	Tanagra	Boeotia	4th–3rd c.?	F? 45	Compound band				Band, 2 loops Stabilizing
21	Sardis	Sardis, Turkey	3rd c.?	F 25–40	Band	2	2		Mandibular, band Replacement

Note: where material is not noted, false teeth are missing but attested by presence of rivet(s). Shading denotes appliances missing or not available for study.

Table 5.10 Technical details of Etruscan gold-band appliances

Appliance	Band type	# Rings	Total # teeth/ replacements	Replacement Teeth	# Rivets	Purpose/ conditions
Barrett I	Simple, narrow	—	3 spaces maxillary	No	None	Stabilize (poor info)
Barrett II	Simple, narrow	—	5 spaces maxillary	No	None	Stabilize
Van Marter	—	3 rings	2 + 1 replace maxillary	R central incisor	None	Replacement human tooth
Copenhagen/ Orvieto?	—	3 rings	2 + 1 replace maxillary	R central incisor lost	None	Replacement; anchors worn
Gaiella (Chiusi)	Complex band	4 "rings"	8 teeth maxillary	No	None	Stabilize; skull substituted
Populonia	—	4 rings	4 maxillary incisors	Central incisor lost	1 rivet	Replacement; fragments of the maxilla remain
Ghent (Orvieto?)	—	3 ring— one double	4 incisors	No	None	Stabilize; a tooth substituted
Bruschi I Caere/Tarquinia	Simple, narrow band	—	4 maxillary teeth	No	None	Stabilize loose teeth
Bruschi II Tarquinia	—	4 rings	3 + 1 replace	Central incisor lost	1 rivet	Replacement
Bruschi III Tarquinia	Braced band	—	5 teeth—L canine to R lateral incisor	No	None	Stabilize; teeth recent inserts
Corneto I Tarquinia	Braced band	—	3 + 2 replace	Central lateral incisors—1 lost	2 rivets	Replacement unknown material

	Band type	Rings	Spaces	Teeth lost	Rivets	Function/Replacement
Corneto II Tarquinia	—	7 rings compound rings	8 spaces = 5 + 3 replace maxillary	1PM; II and II one lost	3 rivets	Replacement 2 "teeth" carved in one piece (animal tooth)
Liverpool I	Band	—	2 + 2 replace maxillary	2 central incisors	2 rivets	Replacement; human teeth
Liverpool II	Band	—	2 + 2 replace	2 R incisors lost	2 rivets	Replacement; only anchors remain
Valsiarosa Falerii	—	4 rings welded loops	3 + 1 replace maxillary	Central incisor lost	1 rivet	Replacement; skull substituted
Teano	—	6 rings	4 + 2 spaces maxillary	No	None	Stabilize; probably original teeth overbite, worn
Praeneste	Band	—	2 + 2 replace maxillary	2 central incisors	2 rivets	Replacement human teeth
Satricum	Band	—	4 + 1 replace maxillary	Central incisor	None	Replacement; hollow gold tooth
Bracciano	Band, compound	—	2 + 1 replace maxillary	R central incisor	1 rivet	Replacement; owner's tooth, filed down?
Tanagra	Compound band	—	6 spaces, canines, incisors	No	None	Stabilize, 2 loops
Sardis	Band	—	2 + 2 replace mandible	2 central incisors	2 rivets	Owner's teeth filed down; tartar on both replacements

Note: shading denotes appliances now missing or unavailable.

Table 5.11 Wire-appliances (Hellenistic and Roman periods: not Etruscan)*

Item	Provenance, location	Date	Sex/age	Gold design	False: material	Living teeth present	Type/ design
W1. Gaillardot	Sidon, Tomb XI, Room 1, fosse b (1861 excavations) Louvre	1st 1/4 4th c. BCE	F	Wire	2 human incisors—I1, I2 2 holes drilled in each	4 C to C roots not intact	Mandibular?? Wire binding 6 teeth
W2. Ford	Sidon, Tomb I, 'Ain H ilweh necropolis, East sarcophagus American University Museum Beirut	5th–4th c. BCE	M? middle aged	Wire brace	No	6, with decay etc. C to C	Mandible
W3. Alexandria	Ibrahimieh, Tomb Greco-Roman Museum, Alexandria	Roman 1st c. CE	?	Wire	No	3: I1 to C?. Poor condition	Mandible
W4. El-Qatta	El-Qatta Tomb no. 90 reused mastaba, shaft 5 Cairo Museum?	Roman	?	Wire	1 tooth drilled	3 teeth wired series 1I to C? anchor on R canine and C incisor	Maxilla

W5. Tura el-Asmant	Tomb T-121 in Ptolemaic necropolis Cairo/Museum etc.?	Ptolemaic	M?? young adult?	Silver wire	R central incisor returned to mouth (drilled) root modified	I1 to I2 necrotic abscess R central incisor	maxilla severe malocclusion 2 teeth drilled—or caries?
W6. Eretria	Tomb at Eretria Athens Nat.Arch. Museum	4th c. BCE	F???	Wire	Human teeth, drilled	4 teeth—I1 to PM1? originally spanned 6 teeth I2 and C are drilled	Mandibular complex pattern wiring—originally binding 6 teeth, 2 of them replacements (drilled, wired)
W7. Rome	Tomb in Collatina necropolis, partially cremated skeleton	Imperial Roman	F 50?	Wire	Original tooth: R central incisor, root missing (drilled, wired)	R canine thru L lateral incisor:	Mandibular: adjacent teeth damaged by periodontal disease, so anchored to next teeth

* All gold wire except where otherwise noted.

Table 5.12 Measurements of ancient appliances

Item	Length	Width	Thickness	Length of strip	Buccal-lingual	Rivets	Type	# Teeth spanned	Details
Barrett I	20	6	0.2 to 0.3?	53	6	—	S	3	Lost?
Barrett II	25	2.0 to 2.5	0.2 to 0.3?	60	6 to 7	—	S	4	Lost?
Van Marter	25	4	—	—	5	—	R + 1	3	Lost?
Copenhagen	21.6	5.5 to 6.2	—	NA	5.1 to 6.7	—	R + 1	3	NA
Poggio Gaiella	42	2.82 to 3.3	0.12 to 0.17	*90 and	—	—	S	8	*2 strips
Populonia	(25 to −30)	—	—	—	—	1	R + 1	4	Lost
Ghent	27	2.8	—	—	—	—	S	4	Lost
Bruschi I	32	1.9 to 2.1	0.20	74	—	—	S	4	
Bruschi II	29	2.1	—	—	—	1	R + 1	4	NA
Bruschi III	36.8	2.6 to 2.8	—	83	—	—	S	5	
Corneto I	28	5 to 6	—	—	—	2	R + 2	5	NA
Corneto II	62.5	4.0 to 4.3	—	—	—	3	R + 3	8	NA
									Most complex
Liverpool I	30.9	3.0 to 3.1	0.3	?	?	2	R + 2	4	NA
Liverpool II	28.2	4.9 to 5.2	0.2	?	?	2	R + 2	4	Unique 2-layer construction
Valsiarosa	38	5.0 to 7.0	?	?	?	1	R + 1	4	
Teano	47	4.5	—	—	—	—	S	6	
Praeneste	31	2.7 to 2.9	?	?	?	2	R + 2	4	
Satricum	29	1.8 to 2.2	?	?	?	—	R + 1	5	Gold tooth
Bracciano	24	3.5 to 3.8	0.24 to 0.30	?	?	1	R + 1	3	
Tanagra	43.3	4.3 to 5.6	0.2	*2 × 25	?	—	S	6	* 2 strips
(Sardis)	18	4.0	—	—	—	2	R + 2	4	NA

Note: all measurements in millimeters; many approximated or estimated from illustrations (see catalogue).
NA = not available.
Function: S = Stabilize; R = Replacement (R + # teeth replaced); ? = Some doubt as to exact identification.

Table 5.13 Wire appliances*

Item	Length	Width	Thickness	Length of wire	Type	# Teeth spanned	
Sidon I	34	Varies			R + 2	6	
Sidon II	35	3 to 4?		over 100	S	(6)	
Alexandria	25	Varies	1 or less		S	(3)	
El Qatta	(43)	Varies			R + 1	3 or more	
Tura el-Asmant	27	Varies			R + 1	3?	2 silver wires
Eretria		Varies			R + 2	6	
Rome		Varies			R + 1	5	

* Measurements in millimeters, mainly from published illustrations.

Function: S = Stabilize; R = Replacement (R + # teeth replaced); ? = Some doubt as to exact identification.

providing supports for this simple pontic. The single wire passes in a single loop around the right canine and then the right lateral incisor before being pinched together to pass through the hole drilled through the re-placed tooth. Upon exiting from this hole (or holes), the two ends of the wire extend around the left central incisor (now lost) and the left lateral incisor that serves as the anchor tooth. The left central incisor must have been quite loose at the time that this appliance was fashioned. The ends of the wire are then twisted, at the distal-buccal position, in a clockwise direction for two and one-half turns, and then end. Not noted in the publications is the extremely loose fit of the right distal aspect of the wire and what seems to be a small loop at the right distal end, at the distal-buccal surface of the canine. This is not clearly revealed in the illustrations but appears to be a tiny loop, of less than 3 mm diameter that was made in the wire at the end near where it begins to pass around the right canine, and then the right lateral incisor. This loop might have served to take up slack in the appliance by allowing the wire to be tightened by twisting it with a small pair of pliers.

Summary

This use of gold wire to fit a replacement tooth is the only example yet known from Rome (or Italy), and was excavated under controlled conditions from a tomb of the first–second century CE in the Collatina necropolis of Rome. A woman who died around 50 years of age was wearing the appliance to replace a mandibular central incisor probably lost to periodontal disease. If such appliances had been common, more examples should have survived. This Roman example of the Early Imperial Age falls within the same medical tradition known from the Hippocratic corpus, and also reflects specimens buried in the eastern Mediterranean, Levant and Egypt.

Table 5.14 Appliances ordered by type and number of replaced teeth, number of teeth spanned

Item	Length	Width	Thickness	Length of strip	Buccal-lingual	Rivets	Type	# Teeth spanned	Details
Barrett I	20	6	0.2 to 0.3?	53	6	—	S	3	Lost?
Barrett II	25	2.0 to 2.5	0.2 to 0.3?	60	6 to 7	—	S	4	Lost?
Ghent	27	2.8	—	—	—	—	S	4	Lost
Bruschi I	32	1.9 to 2.1	0.20	74		—	S	4	
Bruschi III	36.8	2.6 to 2.8	—	83		—	S	5	
Teano	47	4.5	—	—	—	—	S	6	NA unique 2-layer construction
Tanagra	43.3	4.3 to 5.6	0.2	*2 × 25	?	—	S	6	*2 strips
Poggio Gaiella	42	2.82 to 3.3	0.12 to 0.17	*90 and 42		—	S	8	*2 strips
Van Marter	25	4	—	—	5	—	R + 1	3	Lost?
Copenhagen	21.6	5.5 to 6.2	—	NA	5.1 to 6.7	—	R + 1	3	
Bracciano	24	3.5 to 3.8	0.24 to 0.30	?	?	1	R + 1	3	
Populonia	(25 to −30)	—	—	—	—	1	R + 1	4	Lost
Bruschi II	29	2.1	—	—	—	1	R + 1	4	NA
Valsiarosa	38	5.0 to 7.0	?	?	?	—	R + 1	4	
Satricum	29	1.8 to 2.2	?	?	?	—	R + 1	5	Gold tooth
Liverpool I	30.9	3.0 to 3.1	0.3	?	?	2	R + 2	4	
Liverpool II	28.2	4.9 to 5.2	0.2	?	?	2	R + 2	4	
Praeneste	31	2.7 to 2.9	?	?	?	2	R + 2	4	
(Sardis)	18	4.0	—	—	—	2	R + 2	4	NA
Corneto I	28	5 to 6	—	—	—	2	R + 2	5	NA
Corneto II	62.5	4.0 to 4.3	—	—	—	3	R + 3	8	NA Most complex

NA = not available; ? = indicates imperfection of data.

Function: S = Stabilize; R = Replacement (R + # teeth replaced); ? = Some doubt as to exact identification.

Notes

1 A note in *The Dental Record* (Waite 1885b) erroneously suggests that these prostheses had been described by Waite in the April (1885) issue of the *Independent Practitioner*. The text reveals that Waite actually refers to Van Marter's (1885a) publication.

2 Shoveling here indicates the condition of the incisors being "shovel-shaped," dish-shaped in profile so that the back face is concave, the front face flat or convex. The condition is a harmless genetic variation providing a greater articular surface for chewing or use of teeth as tools. Given a large enough sample this trait might indicate familial, regional or ethnic affiliations.

3 Post-mortem tooth loss occurs as the skull and its tissues dry during burial. It can be recognized, with some experience, by the clearly defined edges of the tooth sockets: the gums have disappeared, the jaw is dry and teeth with straight roots can easily drop out (often they are shoved back into the wrong sockets for a better display!).

4 For background on the Bruschi archaeological collection, see Fabrizio Santi, 2002. "La famiglia Bruschi-Falgari e la sua collezione di antichità etrusche," *Bollettino della Società Tarquiniese d'Arte e Storia* 31: 159–188. The Attic Black Figure vases in the collection, surely imports found in Etruscan tombs, are catalogued by Danilo Nati (2012). *La collezione Bruschi Falgari. Materiali del Museo Archeologico Nazionale di Tarquinia*, 20 (Archeologia 168), Rome: G. Bretschneider.

5 Pot, who fails to recognize that that the replaced teeth in the Praeneste appliance are held with rivets with peened heads, also presents an inaccurate drawing of the appliance (1985: fig. 2), as well as an incorrect interpretation of the method of its manufacture. Van Marter (1886: 57) also failed to note the rivets that held the two false teeth in place. Van Marter notes that he saw "four natural teeth" in 1885 or early 1886, but his general description is too poor to determine if one of the anchor teeth was lost only after 1886.

6 This Tomba XVIII, sometimes noted as "Tomb 18," is distinct from the Tomb 18 that was recovered during the 1907–1910 excavations at Satricum (Ginge 1996: 171).

7 Presumably Evaristo Breccia (1876–1967) who published extensively on Alexandrian archaeology and the Greco-Roman Museum.

8 Those scholars who ignored Euler's report, submitted to Junker in 1928 (Junker 1929: 256–257), fail to understand the function of that amulet as well as its date. Euler's report on the Junker amulet, written long before the discovery of the El-Qatta appliance, reflects many of the same problems of interpreting archaeological context and providing an accurate date.

6 Concluding remarks

Our research has shown that no culture prior to the Etruscans of the first millennium BCE ever attempted any sort of dental interventions, even when simple extraction of an infected tooth might have saved a life. Certainly there were no dental prostheses before the first gold-band appliances were constructed and fitted by goldsmiths working in the Etruscan tradition, during the seventh century BCE (Satricum, no. 18, is the oldest proven example). People in Neolithic Italy, and in many other regions of the world, from prehistoric times to the modern day, certainly did remove or reconfigure their living front teeth for aesthetic, social and cultic purposes. This seemingly basic human trait may relate to the demand for replacement teeth in Etruria, where women of the affluent families occasionally lost—or had removed—one or two front teeth. The corpus of surviving gold-band dental appliances is too small to justify sweeping theories. It may be that, like modern immigrants who have moved from Sub-Saharan Africa to Europe and America, that a woman of the neighboring Italic regions came to Etruria in a dynastic marriage and wished to alter her appearance, which had been marred by a deliberate tooth evulsion. (It would have been appropriate, and looked right, in her own culture, but was seriously out of place in the Etruscan cities.) Or it may be that the ruling families of Etruria occasionally demanded of a daughter a small sacrifice to commemorate a rite of passage, a death or other landmark in the great family. In contrast to the situation in dozens of other cultures of antiquity, these women were permitted to correct the deficit with golden-band prostheses, leading several others to commission similar dental appliances to brace loose teeth and help them to look normal in their public roles as leaders' wives, heads of households or of cults.

It may seem odd that the long-standing Etruscan tradition—although confined to the very affluent or ruling classes—did not continue under the Roman rule of Italy. We cannot be sure of the latest date for the gold-band appliances, but none are known from any first-century CE or early Imperial-era burials. The wiring tradition seems to have begun slightly later and developed in parallel to band appliances, if the fifth–fourth century BCE dates are correct for the Sidon examples; the single recent find from Rome (the Collatina burial) is dated to the second century CE. The wire appliances appear to be following the dictates of the Greek and Roman medical authors, and some seem to have been worn by men. They were also mainly worn in the lower jaw, in contrast to the Etruscan type, which was almost always fitted to the upper dentition. The Etruscan bands may all be associated with women. One wonders if the prejudice expressed by Martial against Roman women wearing dentures expressed a deeper disapproval than might be occasioned by women's vanity and the social faux pas of revealing an imperfection. Could it be prejudice against Etruscan mores? If the reasons for frontal tooth loss were still known in Martial's day, they might explain his reaction, particularly if some alien custom of tooth evulsion to honor dead ancestors or to mark a special threshold event were the reason.

It is interesting to note that, for funerary ideology, the Etruscans at the dawn of urban society, the seventh century BCE, had adopted a number of Egyptian-influenced customs, such as the use of golden coverings for bodies in burials. The famous Regolini-Galassi Tomb of Cerveteri held the body of Larthia, wife (or daughter) of Velthur, adorned with massive gold jewelry including a bib-like pectoral over her chest. This was not an especially native accessory, but does closely resemble the pectoral plates or mask extensions found in pharaonic Egyptian burials (like that of Tutankhamun). Maurizio Sannibale (2006, 2008) points out that Egyptian funerary ideology maintained that, when the pharaoh died and became the Osiris, like the gods, his bones were silver, his flesh gold, and it appears that Larthia's family, of the ruling class of Caere-Cerveteri, intended that she receive the utmost respect, with a gold ornament made especially for her burial. And over several centuries, very many Etruscan women were buried with some amount of gold jewelry, even if, in some cases, it was actually clay jewelry covered in thin gold foil. While religion shows most strongly in funerary traditions, we may imagine that the exhibition of gold as an intrinsic part of the body of an empowered woman (an aristocrat) was considered representative of the importance of her family as well as an expression of her beauty and well-being.

Even today, some individuals will go to great lengths in permanently altering personal appearance to express identity or status, as we have seen in twenty-first-century America. *Vice Magazine* reporter Lauren Schwartzberg (2014) gives a comprehensive and carefully researched (she interviewed Turfa and a number of scholars and read Becker's articles as well) survey of the background of the modern gold phenomenon. Schwartzberg points out that ancient mythology in the Philippines described the creator god Melu as having gold teeth, and by 1300 CE some people had begun to decorate their teeth with gold or to file or inlay them, apparently for ideological purposes. The Tagalog and Bikol languages include words for gold pegs or coverings inserted into living teeth, apparently as status symbols for those in control of chiefdoms. With the advent of Spanish colonists, just as had happened with the Maya, this form of adornment was banned as being barbarous. Modern immigrants to the USA from Central America, descendants of the Maya, and emigrating Tajiks from Central Asia have preferred to have their gold inlays or fillings removed so that they may blend in better in their new homelands.

But gold will always dazzle. William Faulkner's novel *The Reivers* (1962/1999: 114) has a cameo description of a minor but strong character, Minnie, the black servant who works in a brothel. She saved up her money until she could have a front tooth pulled and replaced with a gold one. The little boy narrator, on his first trip away from home, stands in awe of the little woman and her tooth:

> Ned was still looking at Minnie's tooth. I mean, he was waiting for it again. Maybe Miss Reba had said something to her or maybe Minnie had spoken herself. What I do remember is the rich instantaneous glint of gold out of the middle of whatever Minnie said, in the electric light of the kitchen, as if the tooth itself had gained a new luster, lambence from the softer light of the lamp in the outside darkness, like the horse's eyes had—this, and its effect on Ned. It had stopped him cold for that moment, instant, like basilisk. So had it stopped me when I first saw it, so I knew what Ned was experiencing. Only his was more so. . . . Here, in the ancient battle of the sexes, was a foeman worthy of his steel; in the ancient, mystic solidarity of race, here was a high priestess worth dying for.

Ned invites Minnie out to dinner, saying (Faulkner 1962/1999: 116) "let that tooth do its shining amongst something good enough to match it, like a dish of catfish or maybe hog-meat if it likes hog-meat better"—we see that society (Minnie's would-be male suitor) admires the extravagance of gold and expects it to be displayed in public dining . . . Later a bad character steals the tooth while Minnie sleeps, but a quiet hero regains it for her: when without it, she feels lost.

During the 1980s gold inlays and removable tooth covers began to come into fashion in the entertainment world, and then spread among the teenage emulators of rock, hip-hop and rap stars. Johnny Depp and Madonna are among the Hollywood types who have popularized gold teeth. Katy Perry, in an Ungaro designer dress, showed off her grillz at the MTV Video Music Awards in 2013: rock stars may be the new aristocracy, filling the ecological niche of those Etruscan noblewomen of millennia ago. In 2005, the artist known as Nelly released his rap single "Grillz" and the trend expanded, with Californian high-school students acquiring expensive, removable grills, especially young women who wore them for the school prom (see May 2005). And those who craft the gold teeth and grills are goldsmiths—as Meredith May (2005) noted: "While most dentists shudder at the thought of all that bacteria growing behind the bling, jewelers who make the teeth are counting their gold." The variety of ornamental expression of identity is great, thanks to modern technology and easy access to gold: some grills have diamonds, or are etched with the wearer's choice of words, symbols, initials, phone numbers or gang names. The ability to remove the grills easily has probably contributed to their popularity: originally a symbol of edgy, male characters from stage and ghetto, they are now widely displayed among affluent teenage females . . . so while this modern group need not have their teeth pulled for beauty or belonging, the golden smile shines on.

Appendix I

Uncertain examples of Etruscan dental appliances

This list includes several possible examples of ancient gold dental appliances not analyzed in the corpus. Most of the other supposed appliances listed below are, in fact, erroneous duplications created in the literature as commentators relied upon written descriptions and did not autopsy actual objects; others are modern copies of one or more of the examples catalogued above (see Appendix II). Other of the false appliances may be votive plaques, such as the terracotta example from Veii illustrated by Hoffmann-Axthelm (1985: 68, fig. 62; see Appendix IV.A below).

In particular, the Hamilton appliance (no. I.A) certainly was an actual Etruscan-type dental appliance, but it is believed to have been lost for nearly two centuries. Its description, by Böttiger (1797: 63–65, quoted below) makes it seem very similar to the Corneto II appliance, once in the Museo Civico di Corneto and now said to be lost. Corneto II (see Corpus no. 12, and fig. 5.12) was a complex appliance with seven rings, a configuration remarkably similar to that of the Hamilton appliance. Becker had earlier suspected that these were one and the same piece, but now we suggest that they may be two distinct examples.

I.A Hamilton

Present location: unknown.
Type: "*Golddrahte*" ("gold wire") binding seven teeth.
Origin: "Southern Italy" (?)
Jaw Part: ?
Date: contemporary with "Attic vases" (which were probably sixth or fifth century BCE)
Sex: ?
Description: see below, no illustrations exist.

References

Böttiger 1797: 63.
Waarsenburg 1991a: n. 5 (no. 19).
See also: Castorina 1998: *passim*.

The earliest documented "modern" discovery of an actual Etruscan gold dental appliance appears to have been in the late eighteenth century. This find verified the existence of ancient dental appliances, a category of artifacts that previously had only been known from the ancient texts, which were familiar to most educated Europeans. This first archaeological find was known to be in the collections of Sir William Hamilton during the late eighteenth century, but is believed to have been lost during the Napoleonic wars.

The original description of the Hamilton dental appliance and of the context in which it was found (Böttiger 1797: 63) is transcribed below for readers who may not have access to this rare publication. Böttiger's text suggests that this appliance was one of the more complicated examples, possibly spanning five or more dental spaces. A recent review of notebooks relating to seventeenth- and eighteenth-century excavations (*c.* 1725–1830), including some relating to the recovery of items that entered Sir William Hamilton's collection, may offer circumstantial clues to the archaeological context of that appliance (Castorina 1998). A study of the Pompeii excavation records of about that period (Pagano 1997, see also 1996) also might be productive. Since we infer that the Hamilton appliance derived from a high-status tomb, probably in the vicinity of the Bay of Naples/Campania, searches of these early documents may yet reveal important information regarding a specific context.

The Hamilton appliance does not appear to have been discovered during the excavations in the year 1789 or 1790 in the Kingdom of the Two Sicilies, or in some part of Magna Graecia (Böttiger 1797: viii, 1). Böttiger (1797: 62) notes that this piece was among the objects included with a collection of vases bought by Sir William Hamilton for 30,000 *Thaler* at some time prior to 1797, and probably after the sale of Sir William's first collection to the British Museum in 1772 (see Ramage 1989, 1990). Thus this dental appliance was probably among the items in the second Hamilton Collection in Naples, and had probably been found or bought by the person whose collection Hamilton had purchased for 30,000 *Thaler*. (The "*thaler*" was then a silver German coin, worth about $US5 in 1990). Unfortunately, no small items are illustrated among the magnificent drawings of vases published by Hamilton (1791, the famous Tischbein drawings). Campania had strong Etruscan ties during the Iron Age and Archaic periods, and it is quite plausible that a person wearing an Etruscan gold appliance was buried in one of the necropoleis, for instance, at Capua, where much Etruscan material, including inscriptions, has been found (see discussion under no. 16, and Cuozzo 2013 for background.)

Waarsenburg (1991a) believes that this dental appliance was among the items from Hamilton's collection later lost at sea. Approximately one-third of Hamilton's second vase collection was lost when the *H.M.S. Colossus*, a 74-gun Royal Navy *Courageux*-class ship of the line carrying eight crates of vases as well as men wounded in the Battle of the Nile, sank in storm on December 10, 1798 off the Scilly Isles en route to England. However, the list of Hamilton's property recently published (Ramage 1989, 1990) includes no small items such as jewelry, among which a curiosity such as this dental appliance might have been noted.

These long submerged vases were salvaged in the 1980s, and after exhibition in the British Museum some were placed in academic museums for teaching and study (the painted vases had been ravaged by the North Sea currents: see Ramage 1989: 704, n. 2 and 1990: 479, n. 65). In 2001 more of the wreck was exposed and an ongoing program of underwater excavation began, with relics displayed in the Isles of Scilly Museum. (For background and Hamilton's collections, see Jenkins and Sloan 1996; on Colossus materials, see 1996: 58–59, 89, 186.)

Appliances that bridge or include five or more teeth are not common. Only one example, Corneto II (missing since at least 1925 from the Tarquinia Museum), is depicted as having seven rings (see fig. 5.12).

Dunn (1894) mentions that five appliances had already been lost by the time that he studied these Etruscan examples, perhaps in reference to pieces which by then had passed into private or unknown hands, such as Barrett I and quite possibly both Barrett II and Van Marter. We also do not know if he included the Hamilton appliance among the five pieces he then described as lost.

I.A Supplemental material: Passages from Böttiger (1797: 63–65) relating to the gold dental appliance once in the Hamilton collection

Scholars may have difficulty in locating Böttiger's volume, warranting transcription of those portions of his text of interest in this research. The following transcription is taken from the copy in the Rare Books Collection of the University of Pennsylvania (Cat. no. NK/4645/G84/1797).

Böttiger, Carl August, 1797. *Griechische Vasengemälde. Mit archäologischen und artistischen Erläuterungen der Originalkupfer.* Ersten Bandes, Erster Heft. Weimar: Industrie-comptoir. (IV Nachrichten über die griechischen Vasen aus Briefen von Tischbein und Meyer [January 3, 1796: Naples].)

(Page 63, bottom)

> *In eben den Gräbern, wo die Vasen gefunden werden, sind auch noch manche andere Sachen ausgegraben worden. In dem einem fand man sieben Zähne, welche mit einem Golddrathe zusammen gefügt waren. Diese Zähne befinden sich noch jetzt im Museum des Ritters Hamilton *. Die Vasen sind gewöhnlich ganz leer, so dass die ehemalige Vorstellung, sie für Aschenkrüge zu halten, durchaus unstatt-*

(Page 64)

> *-haft ist. Findet sich ja zuweilen etwas darinn, so sind es Dinge, die auf Todtenopfer Beziehung haben. So fand man einmal ein paar Eier in einem Vase. Dessgleichen fand man in einer andern eine Materie, die viele Aehnlichkeit mit weissen Wachse hat, wovon ich selbst etwas besitze. Fände sich also doch zuweilen eine Vase mit Knochen und Asche, so müsste man annehmen, dass*

zie aus einem geöffneten Grabe genommen, und in spätern Zeiten erst von den Römern als Aschen krug gebraucht worden sey. Diese Muthmassung findet durch folgende Begebenheit noch mehr Bestätigung. Vivenzio fand einst ohnweit Nola eine sehr schöne Vase, auf welcher der Tod und die Vertilgung der Familie des Priamus abgebildet ist. Sie war mit Asche und Menschenknocken, auch mit kleinen Gefässen, die man gewöhnlich Thränen krüglein nennt, angefällt, und in eine andere Vase van grober Erde gestellt, die ihr gleichsam zum Futterale dienst. Hieraus

(Page 65)

lässt sich vermuthen, dass die Römer diese Vase von den Griechen an sich gebracht, oder sonst ausgegraben hatten, undem sie solche schon damals als eine kostbare Seltenheit ansahen, und einem vornehmen Mann oder geliebten Freund nicht besser ehren konnten, als wenn sie ihm diese Vase zur Begräbniss urne gabe.

Im vorigen Jahre hat Vivenzio wieder im römischen Gräbern . . .

* Es ist merk würdig, dass von dergleichen mit Gold eingesetzten Zähnen (odontes chrysio endedemenoi [original in Greek script] *in der Beschreibung eines 70 jährigen Mütterchens beim Lucian in Rhet. Praec. C. 24. T.III. p. 26.) schon in den Gesetzen der 12 Tafeln die Rede war, wo alle Verschwendung des Goldes an die Leichen untersagt wurde, die mit Gold eingesetzten Zähne ausgennomen: quoi auro dentes vincti sient, im cum ollo sepelire—se fraude esto. Cic. de Legg. II, 24. s. 60.*

Section relevant to the Hamilton appliance:

In the tombs where the vases were found, many other things also have been excavated. In one were found seven teeth which were bound together with a golden wire (wire = *Draht* in modern German). These teeth are now in the Museum of Lord Hamilton.* The vases are usually quite empty, so that the original display, showing them as cinerary urns, is not at all correct.

* It is noteworthy that those very teeth that are worked with gold (*odontes chrysio endedemenoi* [original in Greek script = "teeth worked with gold"] in the description of a 70-year-old little old lady in Lucian's *Rhet. Praec. C. 24. T.III. p. 26*) were already spoken of in the Laws of the Twelve Tables, where all disposal of gold on corpses is forbidden with the exception of gold-bound teeth: *quoi auro dentes vincti sient, im cum ollo sepelire—se fraude esto.* Cic. *de Legg. II, 24. s. 60.*

The remainder of the passage notes discoveries in the excavations of waxy substances in some vases, eggs and other food, and human bones (surely cremation burials) in other vases. The ancient literary sources he quotes, Cicero/The Twelve Tables and Lucian, are discussed in Chapter 1.

I.B Castellani collection: an alleged example

Present location: unknown. (Possibly this is the same as that which is part of the
  Villa Giulia's Castellani Collection, Rome, Praeneste no. 17.)
Type: ?
Origin: a tomb near Cerveteri in 1865 (Guerini 1909: figs 23–24).
Jaw part: ?
Date: Etruscan.
Sex: ?

References

Bliquez 1996: "S," figs 29 and 30.
Casotti 1957: 105 and fig. B.
Guerini 1909: 76.
Sudhoff 1926.
Waarsenburg 1991a: n. 5, no. 17, *passim*.
Weinberger 1948: 124–126, fig. 41.

This "example," so frequently described in the literature, actually may be the Praeneste (no. 17) appliance, now in Rome, but references to it may also have been derived from Bruschi I (no. 8) or one of the phantom variations of the Valsiarosa piece (no. 15). Bliquez gathered the limited data relating to this appliance from Guerini (1909), whose brief description is useless.Guerini notes that this appliance was in the Castellani Collection in Rome, but the collections of the two Castellani brothers each went to a different Roman museum (one to the Capitoline and the other to the Villa Giulia). No one has identified a gold dental appliance as being in either of the Castellani collections. Quite probably Guerini saw the example now at Civita Castellana (Valsiarosa) while it was at the Villa Giulia Museum, and later erroneously attributed it to the Castellani collection at the Villa Giulia Museum. Alternately, Guerini, in his notes, may have confused the Civita Castellana museum with the Castellani Collection, or collections, in Rome.

  Sudhoff (1926) also describes a piece from the "Castellani Collection" (cf. Valsiarosa, now in the Museo del Agro Falisco), but probably takes his data from Guerini (1909). The Sudhoff description appears divergent from any known example, and probably is simply erroneous in nature. Casotti (1957) recognizes the various problems in the multiple identities of this piece, noting at least five. However, Casotti himself provides two separate descriptions, one that clearly is Valsiarosa (1957: 674–675) and another that is less clear (1957: 105 and fig. 6). This latter refers to a supposed skull and mandible at the Villa Giulia Museum from which all teeth were lost post-mortem except for eight teeth in the right mandible:

che risulta non completamente erotto. Si nota, appoggiata, una protesi inferiore di quattro elemente (sostegni compresi). É visibile la copiglia che fissava il primo molare. La provenienza é ignota. La fotografia é stata cortesemente trasmessa.

which was not completely disintegrated. One notes, propped up, a lower prosthesis of four elements (supports included). The cotter pin (*copiglia)* that attached the first molar is visible. The provenance is unknown. The photograph was kindly provided.

In this photograph we see no lower teeth, and the apparent gold appliance seems to extend from the canine to the first molar, but is not surrounding any teeth. Emptoz also lists an appliance of unknown provenience (his no. XVI), which replaces a right lower molar, as being in the Villa Giulia Museum in Rome. This "example" apparently derives from the information presented in this paragraph.

Bliquez (1996) also cites Hoffmann-Axthelm (1981: 68, fig. 65) as providing relevant information regarding the "Castellani Collection." Waarsenburg (1994) follows Weinberger (1948) in suggesting that this prosthesis is a mandibular band, extending from C–M1, 30 mm long and 6 mm high, and divided into four chambers by three "soldered cross divisions." This error-filled description, nevertheless, also appears to be that of the appliance in the Museo dell'Agro Falisco (Valsiarosa, no. 15).

I.C Rath example (dubious)

Rath (1958: 11, fig. 2) describes a gold dental appliance supposedly in private hands. Waarsenburg (1991a) suspects that this may be the Teano example. Becker believes that Rath may be describing a *copy* of the Teano piece (see below under "copies"). There is no other evidence for such a piece apart from the Teano appliance (no. 16).

I.D Dresden: "old German" cremations (prostheses of bone?)

Linderer (1848: 406) notes that before 1848 there was in a collection of antiquities that he saw in Dresden, in glass cases, two osseous (?) pieces along with others that derived from ancient German urns. His observation is as follows:

die dortige Antikenkammer . . . kammartige Stücke Knocken, welche in altgermanischen Urnen gefunden wären. Beim ersten Anblick sah ich aber, dass es künstliche Zähne sind, doch vermochte ich nicht, da ich sie nicht ganz nah betrachten konnte, zu entscheiden, aus welcher Substanz sie auffallend weiss. Jedes Stück besteht, wenn ich mich recht besinne, aus fünf Zähnen, nämlich ein Augenzahn und vier Schneidezänen.

the antiquities gallery there . . . comb-like pieces of bone, which had been found in Old German [Iron Age? or Dark Age?] urns. At first glance I saw, however, that they were synthetic teeth, but I was not able to determine, since I could not look at them close up, of what material they [were made]. Each piece consisted, if I recall correctly, of five teeth, namely one eye-tooth [canine] and four incisors.

Guerini (1909: 162) elaborates on Linderer's "comb-like pieces of bone" with the statement that each had five teeth, a canine and four incisors. Guerini goes on to "translate" Linderer to the effect that the major difference distinguishing

these pieces from the prosthetic pieces in ivory still in use [1848] consists in this, that the pieces of which I speak have not at all a broad base, designed to rest on the gums, the base having instead the same thickness as the rest. The five teeth are well separated from one another. Besides, the canine makes the proper angle with the incisors, and . . . a hole seems to have been drilled at each end.

(Guerini 1909: 162)

Linderer noted that he could not get a close enough look to determine the exact material of the teeth/appliances. Quite possibly whatever Linderer saw may have been a bit of cremated bone, possibly of the sutural area of the skull, which he mistook for an ancient dental appliance.

Brown (1934: 835) suggests that these cremations may have belonged to the collections of the Archaeological Society of Saxony, in Dresden. All of their collections were acquired in 1887 "by the Museum of Antiquities in the Zwinger" in Dresden. Brown was unable to locate such items in the Zwinger (*c.*1930?), and Becker was unable to identify these cremations in 1989.

I.E Metz Museum pivot tooth (from Merovingian France)

Brown (1934: 834–835, figs 7a, 7b) describes what he believes to be the earliest known pivot tooth. This upper left lateral incisor, illustrated by a labial and palatal view) is believed to be Merovingian in date (420–737 CE). Brown, who provides several useful references, describes it as having a natural crown affixed by "a gold post or 'pivot' which is inserted in the retained natural root and secured there with resin; the pivot tooth also being ligated to the proximal cuspid with gold wire" (1934: 834–835). However, note should be made that the gold rivets or pins used in many Etruscan dental appliances have been translated as "pivots" in many English language texts. There is no other source for this item.

I.F Emptoz's votives

Several "examples" of dental appliances are listed by Emptoz (1987: 546, fig. 2), all four of which are probably votive models. At least one of these appliances is certainly a copy of a votive (see Appendix IV under "Votives").

Appendix II

Modern copies of Etruscan dental appliances

Modern interest in all things Etruscan can be traced back to the Renaissance (see, for instance, Rowland 2013 and De Angelis 2013). Interest in several aspects of Etruscan culture reached new highs during the late nineteenth and early twentieth centuries (see Haack 2013). Architectural and other artistic developments in Europe and North America generated a vogue for reproducing the best of Etruscan art, much of which was then being recovered from the necropoleis of Tarquinia and other cities. These tombs were then being mined in search of their treasures. Between 1895 and 1913 the indefatigable Wolfgang Helbig, among his many activities (see Molteson 1987), made complete copies of the paintings in 28 tombs and facsimiles of some 90 other elements (Molteson and Weber-Lehmann 1991). The production of copies of specific objects from these tombs was proving even more profitable.

This renewed interest in Etruscan art coincided with a period of important developments in modern dental technology, and the spread of ideas regarding modern dental care. Looking back over the history of dentistry led historians to recognize the impressive talents of the ancient Etruscans in fashioning dental appliances. The few true pieces being recovered in Italy were eagerly sought. Dental museums were then being created, and individual scholars also·generated a demand for copies of the appliances that had been fashioned more than 2,000 years earlier. Numerous copies, often in what were described as complete sets, as well as specific and single examples, were being created c.1900 and have come to add confusion to the extensive literature on Etruscan gold dental appliances.

Most of these copies were made during the period from 1895 to c.1913. To some extent these copies now may be used to determine the configurations of some dental appliances that are now lost or missing. However, at this point it appears that most of these copies were poorly made. Their study is another area of research yet to be pursued.

Copies of ancient dental appliances frequently appear in popular as well as scientific publications, both as illustrations and as references. In many cases the referencing does little to clarify their origins as copies (see Waarsenburg 1991a: n. 19). In others the authors actually believe the copies to be real examples (e.g. Sterpellone and Elsheikh 1990: 124, fig. 60). Guerini, identified by Deneffe (1899: 66) as a dental surgeon, provides us with some of the few contemporary references to the actual creation of these copies. Guerini (1904: 280) discussed the reproduction of the Satricum appliance, and also (1909: 72) says that he himself made copies of all the Italian pieces, noting that he had special difficulty in making a copy of Corneto II.

Guerini (1909) and Lufkin (1948: fig. 23) each provide a photograph of the *copy* of the thin band from Tarquinia (Bruschi I, above), but they do not note the location of this copy or the source of the illustration. Brothwell and Carr (1962: fig. 3) clearly indicate that this is one of the copies of dental appliances in the Wellcome Historical Medical Museum in London. Other references to copies of these prostheses often emerge, but at this time it is not completely clear how many examples have been copied, how many copies were made and by whom, how accurate the copies are, and where these copies may be found.

Bliquez (1996: fig. 37) provides an illustration of one such copy, and his observation is important because some of the "duplicate" pieces identified by later authors may simply be modern (c. 1899) reproductions. Photographs of these copies are generally published without indicating where the objects can be found, and often no hint is provided regarding the original appliance that is being represented (e.g. Proskaur 1979 (3): 13). A listing of the known copies, therefore, is important to this study of ancient appliances.

The appliance from the Museum in Florence (Populonia, no. 6, inv. 84467), excavated in the Populonia necropolis and lost in the Florence flood of 1963, is commonly confused with the skull and jaw in which there is now displayed an appliance: Valsiarosa (no. 15). This confusion is evident in Weinberger (1948), who illustrates (p. 124, fig. 41: 7) what we believe to be a copy of the appliance from Populonia, and two views of what we believe is the original piece (Weinberger 1948 148: fig. 53). The location and source of the piece in the photograph of what we believe to be the copy are not noted.

II.A The Ghent copies

Deneffe (1899: 59–61) indicates that copies had been made of eight gold dental appliances for the University of Ghent, Belgium. The University of Ghent had purchased one original about that time, the Ghent appliance still attached to its maxilla (no. 7). Deneffe (1899) described the Ghent original as well as copies of eight other appliances in his study of ancient prostheses. The eight copies presented by Deneffe (1899: 59) are as follows:

1 Tanagra band (not illustrated).
2 Sidon II (fig. 8).
3 Valsiarosa (fig. 2).
4–8 Tarquinia (all five: Bruschi I–III, Corneto I–II; figs 3–7).
Plus: Ghent (the original (?); Deneffe 1899: fig. 1)

Presumably Deneffe used the eight copies, plus the Ghent original, for all of his published descriptions, including those of the five pieces from Tarquinia (of which only two are known to survive today) and the two examples now at the Villa Giulia Museum in Rome (see Bliquez 1996). Presumably the Ghent piece is an original (see Ghent, above), but even this might be questioned. Thus the accuracy of the Ghent copies of the two surviving appliances in Tarquinia can be used to evaluate the accuracy of the form of the other three Ghent copies of pieces now missing from the Museo Nazionale in Tarquinia. Since the simple band of Bruschi I (no. 8) would be the easiest of these appliances to reproduce, and thus to evaluate, inspection of the Ghent copy of this appliance would provide a good indication of how accurately the series had been duplicated. The copy of Bruschi I, which is shown by Guerini (1909: fig. 20), and possibly made by or for him, erroneously depicts two rings separated by a bar. If the Ghent copy were similarly inaccurate, all of the other Ghent copies as well as Deneffe's observations based on them could be considered as useless.

Dr. A. Boddaert, the secretary of an early (before 1899) Medical Congress in Rome, collected a series of copies for exhibition in Ghent. Possibly the person who actually made the copies was V. Guerini. However, Deneffe's (1899: 66) discussion of Guerini's works makes no mention of any involvement by Guerini in the fabrication of the Ghent copies. Quite possibly Boddaert had a goldsmith fashion the Ghent copies. In 1904 Guerini (p. 280) states that "an exact reproduction" of the Satricum appliance "may be seen in my archaeological collection," but does not indicate details regarding the origins of this copy. However, at a later date Guerini (1909: 72) indicates that he made copies "of all the ancient prosthetic pieces existing in the Italian Museums." Unfortunately, it is unclear just how many pieces Guerini copied (or had copied), which museum collections were involved, or how many copies were made. What has become of these reproductions in Guerini's collections or elsewhere remains largely unknown (but, see Teano, no. 16).

II.B The Wellcome copies, now in the Science Museum in London

There are 12, or possibly 13, copies of ancient gold dental appliances now in the collections of the Science Museum in London where they were transferred in the late 1970s as a part of the collections from the Wellcome Historical Medical Museum of the Wellcome Institute. Some may date from the period around 1900 when the Ghent copies were made. A listing of the Wellcome copies appears below in Table AII.1. The Science Museum catalogue entry states only "1901–1930." This information implies that these items had been acquired over a 30-year period, an idea reinforced by the "date" appearing on the Brothwell and Carr illustration (1962: fig. 3) derived from this series.

The Wellcome Collection item catalogued as "8556," a copy of Teano (cf. no. 16), provides no clue to the origins of these copies. The two copies (1047 and 1048) of the Liverpool pieces (cf. nos. 13–14) are noted in the Wellcome catalogue as acquired from the "Liverpool University Museum" in exchange for four Congo drums. They were registered at the Wellcome Museum on February 15, 1915 (S. Emmens, personal communication July 29, 1991). One of these two bears the note: "two pieces of Etruscan bridge work acquired Liverpool Museum 1915 ex Mayer collection there. WR 2/26/4 WR 2/25/28 (3)." The fact that these "two pieces" were copies of the two appliances held in Liverpool is nowhere noted.

Table AII.1 The copies in the Wellcome Collection

Wellcome#	Science Museum#	Width/height/ thickness	Original model/present location
R8547*	?	—	Corneto II (missing)
1047	A622193	29 — —	Liverpool II (Liverpool Museum)
1048	A622194	35 12 10	Liverpool I (Liverpool Museum)
8549	A634910	46 11 19	Sidon II (Paris, Louvre)
8550	A646729	65 25 10	Tanagra (Athens, National Museum)
8551	A646732 +	51 27 67	Brushci III? (missing)
8553*	A622191 +	28 — —	Bruschi I (Tarquinia, Museo Nazionale)
8554	A622195 +	31 10 8	Corneto I (missing)
8555	A622196 +	26 — —	Ghent (missing)
8556	646 731 +	45 18 10	Teano (Berlin, Humboldt University)
8557	A622192 +	35 — —	Bruschi II (missing)
8558**	A622197 +	28 — —	(To be determined)
8559	A622198	29 13 8	Satricum (Rome, Villa Giulia)

* Important in the history of these copies is the presentation by Brothwell and Carr (1962: fig. 4) of a copy of the appliance that they identify as "Wellcome R 8547." They clearly state that this is a copy of an "original in the Corneto Tarquinio [sic] Museum," and the piece illustrated by Brothwell and Carr is indeed a copy of Corneto II. This copy is shown mounted in the maxilla of a skull, bridging at least eight spaces from approximately 2PM to PM1. Both central incisors are made from one piece (ox tooth?), and this piece is held in the band by two rivets. However, this appliance does not appear on the list of copies in the Science Museum provided by Mr. Emmens, nor was he able to identify any object with this number by a computer search (October 1992).

Brothwell and Carr (1962: fig. 3) also indicate that the second appliance they illustrate is a copy of an example that had been in the collections of Conte Bruschi of Corneto (Tarquinia). This copy was in the Wellcome Historical Medical Museum in 1962, with a catalogue number of "R 8553." This is clearly the copy of Bruschi I listed above, but the illustration shows a number that appears to be "1930" printed on one of the two teeth. This appears to relate to the date of acquisition by the Wellcome Museum.

** The typed label for 8558 identifies this as a "roman denture from Near Teano," and also has "Etruscan." printed by hand. It seems likely that the original labels while at the Wellcome Museum were jumbled. This is suggested because the item with label 8553 is said to be a copy of a Liverpool appliance, but is actually Bruschi I. Thus the piece said to be from "Near Teano" may not be from that area, but at least one of the others may be.

+ The four-number registration system (e.g. 8551), no longer in use by the Wellcome Institute, enables these pieces to be linked to catalogue cards, but the cards for these seven examples provide no information on their origins other than that all were registered December 18, 1918. However, the catalogue card for 8553 mentions the Liverpool Museum, but the role of that museum in the acquisition of this piece is unknown.

Heurgon (1964: fig. 5) depicts a gold bridge using a photograph depicting an appliance that in 1964 was at the Wellcome Institute for the History of Medicine, with the catalogue number 8553. Heurgon's photograph appears to depict a very narrow band in which two apparently false teeth flank an empty space, possibly a copy of Bruschi I (cf. no. 8).

The Science Museum piece A646732 may be a copy of Bruschi III (cf. no. 10), the original of which (a very confusing piece) now is missing. The Wellcome copies, or those copies at Ghent, may enable us to resolve the difficult problem of the 3 missing pieces from Tarquinia. The Wellcome copy has a (false?) human tooth in place at the right end of the band; and the band is broken, or open, at the left end. The tooth is described as being 27 mm "high," indicating that the band is a bit wider than 6 mm. The possibility that this copy was made from an original that is not yet known to us, cannot be discounted. One further note should be made regarding the copies in the Wellcome Collection. A photograph in the "Bettmann Archive," a vast collection of high-quality photographs, depicts a copy of the Corneto II appliance (cf. no. 12), and is believed to derive from one of the Wellcome copies.

II.C Copies in Berlin and other German cities

In addition to the original Teano prosthesis (no. 16), several copies of Etruscan dental appliances are to be found in various German collections. Rath (1958: 11, fig. 2), Hoffmann-Axthelm (1970), and Micheloni (1976: 284) all refer to the copy of the Teano appliance also in Berlin. Ilona Marz (personal communication) had informed Becker that a copy of the Teano piece was in a separate safe in the same institute where the original was held. This copy appears to have been made before 1936 (Schweitzer 1936) for Professor Dieck, and may have gone with his private collection to the University of Berlin *c.* 1935 (see Teano, above). Subsequently, Dr. Marz (personal communication to Becker July 25, 1994) says that "the copy in Berlin is made of a non-metallic material and is plated with gold."

Rath (1958: 10) suggests that a collection of copies is in Köln at the Forschungsinstitut für Geschichte der Zahnheilkunde, possibly (in 1994) to be found in the care of Dr. F. H. Witt (see also Waarsenburg 1991a: n. 5, no. 15, and n. 19). This Köln group may be part of the collection that was produced by Guerini in the 1890s. The copy of the Teano appliance noted by Marz as having been in Köln also may be there (see below). Since Rath (1958: 10, fig. 1) illustrates a copy of the Sidon II appliance, said to be in Köln, as well as a copy of the Teano piece, one may infer that both examples are in the same collection. The other two pieces illustrated by Rath (1958: figs 3 and 4) are from photographs, but the text implies that copies exist in Köln (of Bruschi I and Valsiarosa, cf. nos. 8 and 15).

Hoffmann-Axthelm (1970: fig. 2, lower) provides a clear illustration of the copy of "Sidon II" (cf. no. W1) in Köln, and indicates that it was to be found in the research Institute for the History of Dentistry. This copy is poorly made and lacks necessary construction features found on the original.

The copy of the Teano piece (No. 16, above) that Marz has noted as being in Berlin may be the same copy noted by Micheloni (1976: 284) as the property of the wife of Professor Carl Ulrich Fehr, in Berlin. A second copy of Teano appears to be in Köln. Rath (1958: 11, fig. 2) appears to illustrate the copy of the Teano piece owned by Professor Fehr. Marz (personal communication 1994) says that the Köln copy, in metal, also may have been made by Professor Fehr, but when is not known. Marz further states that Fehr was at the Dental Institute in Berlin during two separate periods. The first was from *c.*1912–1914, about the period when Dieck bought the Teano appliance, and he was again there from 1946 to 1948. Fehr's skills at sculpting and copying are well known to Dr. Marz and others, but no clear record of his having made these copies can be produced.

At the 1988 Berlin conference, "Die Welt Der Etrusker" (see Becker 1990) Dr. Ernest Stirnad gave Becker basic and important information regarding the Teano appliance, and also said that he believed that a copy of an Etruscan dental appliance might be in Leipzig. Dr. Stirnad did not then know where the original might be. This "Leipzig" copy may be one of the Teano duplicates noted by Marz.

II.D Musée Pierre Fauchard copies (*Musée de L'École Dentaire de Paris*)

The various copies of Etruscan dental appliances in the Pierre Fauchard Museum were "made by Guerini and offered to our museum" (Dr. Claude Rousseau: personal communication to Becker March 23, 1991). Details as well as the total number of pieces remain unknown, but Rivault (1953) publishes Corneto II (fig. 1), Valsiarosa (figs 2 and 3), and what may be Bruschi II (fig. 4). At least one votive piece is among these copies (see Appendix IV). Rousseau's letter states that "The ex-voto published by Dr. Emptoz [1987: 559, fig. 21] came from our copies." This votive piece may be the Junker specimen (see Appendix IV, below), but a clear confirmation is in order.

Boissier (1927) illustrates a large number of appliances (as well as the Vetulonia "crowns": see Appendix III, no. 5, below). The date of his publication and place where he appears to have conducted his work are consonant with his having used the copies in Paris for his study. Dechaume and Huard (1977: fig. 4) illustrate seven "prostheses," but this is the least clear illustration in this book. All of these examples may be copies now in Paris. The labeling here is so poor that one cannot be certain which pieces are being shown, but their fig. 4a appears to be Sidon II and 4b2 depicts Tanagra and Eretria. Also, in fig. 4b1, is an appliance with a rivet said to be from Greece, but this must be an error in labeling.

Ring (1985: 45, fig. 36) illustrates a dental appliance that appears to be a copy of Corneto I. The photograph is copyrighted by W.O. Funk of Cologne. This braced band, shown as a maxillary appliance, has 5 spaces (C-I2). What may be real teeth appear in the spaces for the canine as well as 2I and I2 (N = 3). Rivets are at both central incisor spaces, but the right space is empty. The short replacement "tooth" in the left central incisor socket appears to be a human tooth from which the root has been filed.

The photograph of the Valsiarosa piece illustrated by Bobbio (1958: figs 9 and 10; taken from Rivault 1953) appears to have been made from a copy that is in the *Musée Pierre Fauchard*. A copy that may be of the complex Bruschi II piece (?) also is in this collection (max. 1I-C), and is illustrated by Bobbio (1958: fig. 11; also from Rivault 1953).

II.E Dr. Samuel D. Harris National Museum of Dentistry: Baltimore, Maryland, USA

This museum opened in Baltimore, Maryland in 1996 in a building originally built in 1904 for the Dental Department of the University of Maryland (31 South Greene Street). The University of Maryland in Baltimore claims to having opened the world's first dental school, as the Baltimore College of Dental Surgery (1840). The collections in the Museum of that College began to be assembled in the 1850s, and recently were merged into the holdings of the National Museum of Dentistry (Sutter 1996).

Along with some supposed native Ecuadorian gold dental inlays, said to have been donated by an archaeologist at the University of New Mexico *c.*1996, and several different dentures attributed to George Washington, two replicas of ancient gold appliances may be seen in this museum's collections. These are as follow, illustrated on the museum's website:

1   Copy of a Near Eastern wire appliance. This would appear to be a very loose copy of Sidon I, set in a trimmed down human mandible. Photo at: www3. nd.edu/~sheridan/Baltimore%202006/Baltimore%202006-Pages/Image17. html, consulted July 18, 2014.
2   Copy of an Etruscan appliance with gold band spanning all four upper incisors, set into a fragmentary human maxilla. Photo at: www3. nd.edu/~sheridan/Baltimore%202006/Baltimore%202006-Pages/Image18. html, consulted June 29, 2016.

While details concerning the shapes and origins of these exhibits remain unknown, their presence in this collection indicates the extent to which the discovery of Etruscan and other dental appliances has influenced the story of dental medicine.

Note: the Dr. John Harris Dental Museum, Ohio

In the context of the National Dental Museum mention also should be made of a small museum at 207 Main Street in Bainbridge, Ohio (see Dalton 1946). This Museum claims descent from the first dental school in America, dating their origins to 1827. During the autumn of 1827 Dr. John Harris, a medical doctor from Cincinnati, offered instruction to those supposedly interested in entering a medical college. Whether medical schools were operating at that time remains subject to debate. By the following year Harris's "advertisements emphasized his interest in dentistry" (Museum brochure). By 1830 Harris had moved to nearby Chillicothe, leaving a total of nine known students behind, among them his younger brother Chapin A. Harris. Chapin Harris is said to have been one of the founders of the Baltimore College of Dental Surgery and became an extremely important figure in pioneering dental research and education in America.

II.F Ward's copies, Edinburgh Dental School, and clues to other copies

G. Ward (1962) illustrates a series of Etruscan dental appliances (his figs 1–4) that all appear to be copies of the better-known examples reviewed here. At least two appear to have been made by Ward himself, and at least two of these copies may be in Edinburgh. The four copies, with corresponding figure numbers, appear to be as follow:

1   A copy of the Sidon I example (cf. no. W-1) appears in a photograph that Ward credits to the courtesy of the Edinburgh Dental School. The copy shown in this illustration may be in Edinburgh, but it appears very similar to a copy in Germany (see above).

2   Copy of the Sidon II appliance (cf. no. W-2), made by (for?) the Oral Pathology Department of the Edinburgh Dental School, to whom the illustration is credited.

3   Frontal and inferior views of a copy of the Ghent appliance (cf. no. 7), made by Ward. The appliance is shown mounted on a pair of maxillae (possibly a cast of these bones?), with the latter view showing the appliance anchored to a right canine. The appliance appears to span at least the right incisors. The copy seems poorly made, and appears to be a 3-ring (or 4-ring) appliance.

4   A copy of Corneto I (?, cf. no. 11). The appliance is an oval with 4 braces (5 spaces), which appears to duplicate a 5-ring example. Spaces 2 and 3 have rivets in them, and an incisor is riveted into the central location. The photograph is credited courtesy of the Baltimore College of Dental Surgery, suggesting a possible location for this copy.

II.G Copies now held in Italy

Although one might expect that many copies of these ancient dental appliances might exist in Italy, the opposite appears to be the case. Perhaps with so many originals available, Italian scholars were less concerned with making copies for display.

Rome Exhibition, 1993–1994

Becker has seen only two of the three known copies of ancient dental appliances in Italy, and both of these had been on display in an exhibition organized by

Professor Luigi Capasso in Rome (December 1993–January 1994). Both are assumed to have been borrowed from Italian collections, and both include plaster duplicates of jaws into which they are set for display. The appliance copies appear to have been fashioned from metal, and to be duplicates of the Sidon II and the Valsiarosa appliances (cf. nos. W-1 and 15). Unfortunately, these two pieces are not included in the extensive and well-illustrated catalogue of this exhibition (Capasso 1993). However, the publication of Sterpellone and Elsheikh (1990: fig. 60) does illustrate these copies (*Museo dell'Istituto de Storia della Medicina, Roma*; see below). In that exhibition, the actual Valsiarosa and Poggio Gaiella appliances (see nos. 15 and 5) were also displayed (Laviosa *et al.* 1993).

Museo dell'Istituto de Storia della Medicina, Roma

An illustration in Sterpellone and Elsheikh's paper (1990: 124, fig. 60) depicts three plaster replicas of dental appliances presented together in a single display, but presented as if all three are real examples of Etruscan dentistry. These three, identified by their location in the illustration, must be as follow:

1   *Upper left.* A plaster mandible with a reproduction of the Sidon II wire appliance (cf. no. W1).
2   *Upper right.* A plaster mandible with a reproduction of the Poggio Gaiella appliance (cf. no. 5).
3   *Lower.* A plaster skull and mandible with a reproduction of the Valsiarosa appliance (cf. no. 15), shown mounted in the same position as the original had been prior to *c.*1995.

II.H Other copies?

Sudhoff (1926) illustrates his dental publications with a number of photographs depicting copies of dental appliances (e.g. his fig. 52 depicts a poor copy of Barrett II, and his fig. 54 shows a copy of Satricum mounted in a mandible). Sudhoff's fig. 55 (1926: 93) depicts two views of a bizarre creation that is presented as an appliance dating to the "Römische Kaiserzeit" (Roman Empire). Shown in plan is the gold appliance alone, with a rectangular box for the false tooth, made of bone, in the upper right central incisor position. A "bar" links this to the ring for the right canine. The frontal view shows the false incisor in place within the band. There is no other indication of what real appliance (if any) this creation is intended to depict, nor where this supposed replica was made or where it now may be.

Appendix III

Spurious examples of dental implants or appliances

The literature on dentistry, dental history, and the history of medicine is filled with references to "examples of ancient dentistry" that have no basis in fact (see Becker 1994c). These erroneously evaluated situations, like the many copies of ancient dental appliances and the various examples of appliances that remain uncertain, do a great deal to confuse the casual reader. The considerable numbers of spurious reports relating to dental bridges, or the manufacture of ancient crowns, inlays, or fillings, constitute a significant body of supposed evidence waiting to ensnare the unwary observer. Also creating difficulties in understanding the published literature is an inability to recognize dental abnormalities. Kocsis (*et al.* 1994) provide an excellent description of some abnormal, or atypical, characteristics in a sixth-century BC Etruscan individual. Others who are less familiar with these dental anomalies might reach different conclusions.

Most of the publications relating to these spurious examples, such as a "dental implant" made of stone that was found in Turkey (Atilla 1993, see III.11 below), appear only in secondary journals. A few, however, have been accepted by scholars supposedly well versed in the literature (e.g. Guerini 1909: 68, n.1, including a comment on one such piece). In most cases these spurious examples are the result of wishful thinking combined with poor referencing of earlier secondary sources (see Becker 1994c). Simple ignorance of the technology involved, plus a lack of scholarly communication, appears to have led to the fabrication of several such "examples of ancient dentistry."

Classical literature yields a few definite references to ancient gold dental appliances, as noted in Chapter 1. The first documented discovery of an Etruscan gold dental appliance, the lost piece once in the collection of Lord William Hamilton, dates from the end of the eighteenth century (Böttiger 1797). This archaeological verification of the ancient texts appears to have spawned numerous reports, which cannot be confirmed. Spurious reports of ancient dental appliances were so common that Van Marter (1886: 57–58) was led to spend considerable time attempting to trace supposed Egyptian examples. Van Marter searched for these spurious gold appliances in Naples and elsewhere, but always without success. Mummery (1870) had already discounted claims of early Egyptian examples of ancient dental appliances, but the poor scholarship and gullibility of authors over the decades continues to fill the literature with fanciful accounts. Weinberger's

(1948: 77–81) excellent review dismisses most of these tales, but in the process he appears to generate still other mythical examples (cf. Waarsenburg 1991a: 243, n. 13 and 20). A listing of the more commonly noted, but entirely spurious, dental "appliances, crowns, or implants" appears below.

III.A The "dental bridge" in the "skull of Pliny"

A skull with non-matching mandible, together with "Pliny's sword," is now on display in the Museo Storico dell'Arte Sanitaria of the Accademia di Storia dell'Arte Sanitaria in Rome (see Waarsenburg 1991b: 41, plates). Excavations believed to have been conducted during the nineteenth century at Boscotrecase, near Pompei, revealed many skeletons/bodies of victims of the 79 CE eruption of Vesuvius of which the bones subsequently may have been reburied. Matrone (1909:7–12) provides a section entitled "Le squelette de Pline l'ancien" in which (1909: 10, fig. 2a) appears a skull, lacking the face, and a mandible.

Waarsenburg (1991b) believes that at some point subsequent to these excavations the excavator at Boscotrecase was asked if the body of Pliny had been found among the bodies uncovered. According to Waarsenburg a skull and a mandible were then produced and identified as belonging to Pliny the Elder (Cannizzaro 1901), who died in the eruption of Vesuvius in 79 CE (see also Micheloni 1976: 311). Waarsenburg (personal communication to Becker) also suggests that a 1903 edition of Matrone (1909) had been issued by publishers at Castellamare di Stabia.

Many years after this identification of the skull of Pliny, S. Baglioni (1952) fantasized the presence of evidence suggesting that the mandible of this skull had been fitted with a dental bridge (see Becker 1994c: 5–6). Fortunately, this fable has rarely been repeated (but, see Sgarbi 1984: 582, fig.). Waarsenburg (1991b) traces the origins of the legend that this skull belonged to Pliny. In an attempt to clarify the record Dr. Waarsenburg escorted Becker, in January of 1991, to the Museo Storico dell'Arte Sanitaria in Rome to examine the mandible for evidence of the bridge allegedly seen by Baglioni (1952). At that time Becker determined that no evidence for any dental appliance, artificial drilling, or filing can be found in association with this mandible, and that the mandible does not even match the skull (Becker n.d. b). Waarsenburg had hoped to correct his manuscript (1991b), in which the myth of the "skull of Pliny" unfortunately had been repeated, but the manuscript had already gone to press.

Evidence for "oral surgery" was also detected on this mandible by Baglioni. Such fantasies are neither new nor uncommon, and even appear in the works of E. A. Hooton (1917). Weinberger (1948: 69–73) reviews several of these studies of oral surgery in an historical survey, which Baglioni does not appear to have consulted. While tooth extraction and rudimentary dental surgery may have been performed prior to 1,000 BCE, there is no evidence that dental prostheses were made prior to the seventh century BCE, nor that they were fashioned in Egypt, or even present in Egypt, until after 400 BCE.

Recently Musitelli (1996: 232, n. 24) claimed that a gold wire (*filo d'oro*) appliance of Roman origin was in Rome at the "Museo dell'Istituto di Storia della Medicina." Musitelli appears to derive his data from one of Sterpellone's publications (supposedly 1990), but it has not been possible to identify the citation. Elsewhere in his text Musitelli (1996: 217) refers to *laminette d'oro* (bands of gold) as distinct from a *filo d'oro*, but does not define the differences. This confusion probably derives from erroneous citations relating to the false skull of Pliny.

III.B Baglioni's "bridge"

In addition to the "dental work" (Baglioni 1952: 14–20) imagined in the "skull of Pliny" (see above), Baglioni also claims great antiquity for a gold dental plate with a set of 12 sockets purported to hold teeth. This mysterious "dental plate," coming from "*la campagna etrusco-laziale*" ("the Etruscan-Latial countryside") was said to have been in private hands, and now is missing or unknown (see De Vecchis 1939: fig. on p. 85). Bobbio (1958: 370, fig. 16) illustrates this piece, noting that the object (or the photograph) actually was in the collection of Professor S. Baglioni in Rome. Bobbio gives a supposed date for this piece as the Roman Imperial Period, but this clearly appears to be in error (Becker 1994c: 6).

Given the fabulation involved in the "skull of Pliny" episode one may also discount this reference to ancient dentistry. Waarsenburg (1991a: n. 5, no. 16) initially accepted Baglioni's statement and included this spurious "denture" in his inventory. Thus two appliances have been added to the literature (Waarsenburg 1991a: n. 5 and 8) through a process similar to those that Waarsenburg (1991a: n. 13) himself describes. Baglioni's "dental plate" may be an example of dentistry dating from after 1700 AD, the golden age of dental bridges.

III.C Cali's various creations

In a single publication by Giuseppe Cali (1901) three spurious examples of ancient dentistry are created or listed. Fortunately, only one author has incorporated any of Cali's dental creations in a subsequent inventory. All three are listed here together, with brief comments on their validity.

A   Thebes (a mummy?): supposedly found *c.*1880 by a Professor Sanders (Cali 1901: 5).
B   "Meyer Museum, London": the maxilla from a mummy (Cali 1901:10). Even the museum cannot be identified. Cali may be confusing the Mayer prostheses in Liverpool.
C   The Vatican Museum piece (Cali 1901:11): this may be a reference to an object associated with an Egyptian mummy.
D   Villa Giulia confusion: Cali's specimen from the "Museo di Papa Luigi" is one and the same as his piece from the Museo di Antichità nella Villa di Papa Giulio III. Cali believes they are two separate pieces, as does Weinberger (1948: 125, 145), who attributes one to the Etruscans and the other to the Romans (see Waarsenburg 1991a: n. 20; Becker 1994c: 6).

III.D Platschick's piece supposedly from Populonia

Waarsenburg (1991a: n.1) points out that Ghinst (1930) took the Valsiarosa appliance, moved it to a maxillary position, and claimed that it came from a context of the fourth-century BCE at Populonia (Becker 1994c: 6).

III.E Marzabotto (near Bologna, Italy)

Platschick (1904–1905: 239) notes that Count Pompeio Aria had in his collection a supposed dental appliance from Marzabotto, an Etruscan colonial town of the fifth century BCE excavated in the countryside south of Bologna. The Count apparently had in his possession a gold pendant in the form of, or incorporating, a human incisor and furnished this information to Dunn (Dunn 1894: 4–5). Platschick (1904–1905: 239) describes this as a deciduous tooth exquisitely mounted in gold, with a ring to place it on a "*cordicella*" for suspension as an ornament. Platschick, unfortunately, was given to unwarranted speculations not necessarily based on any particular evidence (see Becker 1994c: 6–7).

Count Pompeio Aria alleged that he had at one time owned a skull in which there was an artificial tooth attached with a gold wire (band?). "This skull was sent with other Etruscan objects to a foreign scientific society, but it was never returned to Count Aria" (Dunn 1894: 5). Although the year 1894 is remarkably close to the time when Guerini is believed to have made copies of the Italian dental appliances, the probability that such an artifact, or collection of artifacts, would not be recovered by the owner is seen as quite low. Note also that Dunn (1894: 4) indicates that he himself owned the skull and mandible with complex gold band (Poggio Gaiella, no. 5), which he subsequently donated to the Museo Archeologico Etrusco in Florence (their Inv. no. 11782).

III.F Vetulonia "crowns" (in the Museo Nazionale, Firenze)

Some of the early references to these teeth as being artificial dental crowns include Dunn (1894: 3) and Falchi (1885, 1891, 1908). In fact, they are natural and unworked human teeth now in the Museo Archeologico Etrusco, Florence, Inventory nos. 7820–7824. In 1957 they were displayed in Room XXVI; by 1994 most of the archaeological material from Vetulonia, which had been in Sala XXVII, had been placed in storage. This stored material also may include these stained teeth formerly in Sala XXVI. Becker was unable to locate them in storage in 1994 (Becker 1994c: 7).

This series of 11 natural human dental crowns derives from four different tomb contexts, and thus at least four different people may be represented. As Bliquez (1996: 2656, 2659, 2660, n. 19–20, item "V") points out, the metallic appearance of these teeth may have confused Guerini (1909). The teeth are stained to a green color from contact with copper salts derived from a corroding bronze coin placed in the mouth or from a bronze artifact that was part of the tomb offerings (see Capasso 1985: 52). Such stains on bones and teeth are common features in ancient tombs (see, e.g., Becker 1985: 221, 223, 1990; also Clawson 1934), and the process of roots and dentine becoming dissolved leaving the natural dental enamel crowns intact also is common at archaeological sites. Another example is a set of now-green natural enamel crowns from a middle-aged woman collected in Etruria in the nineteenth century (probably at Chiusi or Orvieto) and sent to the University of Pennsylvania Museum (see Becker *et al.* 2009: 98). Brown (1934: 958) suggests that cast gold tooth caps are not documented before *c.*1593 CE.

These teeth, from which the roots have deteriorated while in the tombs, were recovered by Isidoro Falchi from the Vetulonia necropolis area, northeast of Monte di Colonna (see Levi 1931 for site location, and Casotti 1957, fig. 1 for details). Falchi (1885: 98–114, 398–417) describes the general context and offers a plan of the excavated area (pl. VI), as well as a detailed plan of the specific location (tav. XII) from which some of these human teeth were recovered. Objects from the excavation also are illustrated (tav. VII–IX).

Falchi's illustration of teeth from Vetulonia

Falchi's Vetulonia report (1891: tav. XIV, 15) illustrates, at full scale, two teeth that look like those of a small dog. They almost certainly are the fragments of human teeth, but drawn to indicate a metallic appearance, so that they could even be mistaken as having a band around their outer surfaces. If that were so, it might indicate teeth worn as amulets, but this is unlikely. The crowns of four teeth are shown in Falchi's tav. VII, with the roots reconstructed (see also tav. XV, 2 and XVII, 20; these depict two teeth each). The graves (Falchi 1891: 67) from which three "human" teeth derive (p. 68) may actually have produced material from a necklace: "*e attorno ad essi, e accomodate con molto cura, sono: una collana di pallottole di vetro e di ambra, un' altra di anelli di bronzo infilati 4 a 4, insieme a tubetti piccoli*" ("and along with these, mended with great care, are: a necklace of spherical beads of glass and amber, another of interwoven rings of bronze in 4 x 4 pattern together with little tubes"). Several fine necklaces are known with fossil or other animal teeth set in gold mounts: see four examples from the Metropolitan Museum in New York published by Richard De Puma (2013: 260 nos. 7.16a–d).

Casotti (1957: 105–111, fig. 7, citing Falchi 1885 and 1891: 67) reviews the archaeological data regarding these 11 crowns from at least 4 different contexts at Vetulonia. Casotti's discussion and illustration (1957: fig. 7) are of importance, and provide many references to others who have published information about or related to these human teeth. Bobbio (1958: 368, fig. 15, from Casotti 1957) discusses these stained teeth, noting the various interpretations of them as either natural human crowns or, incorrectly, as early artificial dental crowns.

Platschick (1904–1905: 239, fig. 1) clearly notes that the roots and dentine had rotted out of these human teeth, and that the color is the result of being in contact with bronze artifacts that were also in the tombs. Brown (1934: 958–959) and Weinberger (1941: 1853) also clearly recognized that these teeth are not gold castings, but simply the stained crowns of human teeth (see also Casotti 1957: 105–106). Others were not so observant and erroneously identified these human teeth as cast gold "crowns" or as parts of a dental appliance. Dunn (1894: 3–4) ambiguously refers to these green stained enamel crowns of human teeth from Vetulonia only as "crowns," but the implication in his text is that they were fabricated and meant to serve a purpose like that of modern dental crowns (see also Guerini (1909: 70, figs 13, 14).

Despite the many good observations made of these stained teeth, the existence of this "appliance" remains imbedded in the popular literature. Boissier (1927: 25, fig. 1) is among the early authors mistaking these teeth for artificial crowns. Tabanelli (1962: 92, pl. 49), erroneously citing Platschick's imperfect description, repeats the error of calling these teeth a dental appliance, and Emptoz (1987: 546) unfortunately applies this information to one of his "examples." Ghinst (1930: 406) seems to cite these teeth in suggesting an appliance from Chiusi. Waarsenburg (personal communication) provides useful data on appliance no. 6, described above, as well as these "green" teeth that are so often confused with it.

III.G The Purland "Egyptian" example (1857–1858)

References

Becker 1994c: 7.
Brown 1934: 830–831.
Purland 1857 (1857–1858), Vol. I: 63.

Purland claimed to have (inherited?) a "pivot" tooth from the "head of a mummy [that had been?] in the collection of a lamented friend." A "pivot" tooth is a false crown affixed to a natural root by means of "a gold post or 'pivot'." The date and origin of such an example must be considered unreliable, as Brown (1934) clearly indicates. What it was that Purland was identifying as a false tooth remains unknown.

Purland (1857–1858) also repeats the myth that Giovanni Belzoni had found false teeth and teeth stopped (filled) with gold in Egyptian mummies (see Chapter 2, above). Purland does note that examples of dental prostheses are in the collection of Joseph Mayer (Liverpool I and II), and that others are in collections in Berlin and Paris. Aside from the true appliances in Mayer's collection in Liverpool these other "examples" may refer to gold items associated with mummies. However, the possibility that they are correct evaluations of actual appliances, as in the Liverpool case, cannot be determined.

Purland's claims to ancient Egyptian examples of dental prostheses are unfortunately cited as if they were valid by Perine (1883: 163) and Casotti (1947), and still later are repeated by Micheloni (1976: 159).

III.H Other spurious ancient Egyptian examples supposedly dating from before the Hellenistic period

As noted above, there is a vast literature stating that the ancient Egyptians had fabricated and used dental prostheses (Becker 1994c: 8). Textual evidence does suggest that the Egyptians were practicing complex oral *medicine* as early as 2,900 BCE (Jonckheere 1958), and probably earlier. However, no evidence for the presence of dental appliances before *c.*400 BCE can be documented, and even dental extractions are not clearly described in the early Egyptian texts (Ruffer 1920: 377). Most commonly mistaken for appliances are votive objects, a few examples of which are listed below (Appendix IV).

No sooner than Quenouille (1975) had efficiently discounted the possibility that these votives were anything else, with a well-reasoned discussion, then Trillou (1976) assembled the spurious and indirect "evidence" in an attempt to prove that early examples of dental prostheses actually did exist in Egypt. Another recent repetition of the popular fantasies involving several of these votives appears in a paper by Puech *et al.* (1970: 2006). Although it is quite clear that no dental prostheses were fabricated in ancient Egypt prior to the fourth century BC, readers should consult Bardinot's (1990) extremely useful summary of the direct evidence discounting these many spurious claims.

Sir Armand Ruffer (1920: 377), whose careful observations are extremely important, suggested that the "artificial teeth" that were in the Alexandria Museum came from a Roman grave. Ruffer describes them as like the "set of teeth" from Sidon, a clear reference to a known Near Eastern dental appliance. But many other commentators ignored genuine pieces to continue the myth of early Egyptian dentistry.

III.I Saint Benedict's dentures

The founder of the Benedictine Order, who died in 543, is often claimed to have worn dentures or a dental appliance. Brown (1934: 835, n. 6) examined the skull said to be that of St. Benedict and found no evidence that would support this myth (cf. The skull of Pliny, no. 1, above; Becker 1994c: 8).

III.J The Nabatean "wire implant" described by Zias

A skull of a male found in a mass grave from the northern Negev, dated to 200 BCE, was found to have "a bronze wire approximately 2.5 mm in length firmly implanted in the canal" of a maxillary right lateral incisor (Zias and Numeroff 1986a, 1986b, 1987). Zias and Numeroff suggest that the "pin" had been deliberately inserted after artificially expanding the chamber; in effect "a primitive 'root canal' operation, or an attempt to "prevent 'tooth worms'." They also suggest that this may have been a pin to hold an "artificial tooth" in place, or that something had been done (drilling?) to provide a drain for a large palatal cyst which they identify as being at the root of the tooth. More recently, Zias (1993) has become interested in the medical aspects of *Cannabis*.

All of these inferences are equally unlikely, given what is known about the state of dental medicine and technology at that time. None of the suggestions put forth by Zias has been demonstrated through scanning electron microscopy or other techniques that might confirm these speculations. Equally unlikely is the insertion of a bronze pin, or even a gold pin, for any of the purposes suggested by Zias.

The possibility that a false crown might have been mounted on this tooth is also unlikely (Becker 1994c: 8).

Not suggested by Zias and Numeroff is the possibility that the tip of a bronze tool may have accidentally broken off in this tooth while it was being probed in relationship to the cyst noted. Vicissitudes of burial or excavation could have caused a foreign object to become lodged in a space where tissues had decomposed and disappeared. Powers (1988) clearly points out the errors associated with the idea that this example represents a deliberate dental insert (see also Zias and Powers 1989). Powers (1988) also notes another similar example of an apparently filled tooth from the Levantine site of Lachish (see the following, example no.11).

III.K The "filled tooth" from Lachish in Palestine

Under the heading "apparent adventitious filling of a tooth" D. L. Risdon (1938: 120–121) reports on findings in the maxilla of a female cranium (no. 518) excavated at the site of Biblical Lachish in central Israel, a city of importance in the Bronze and Iron Ages. Risdon concludes that the piece of metal embedded in the worn second right molar has an "appearance [that] was precisely similar to that of an artificial stopping." This "stopping," or what in American English would be termed a "dental filling" is well illustrated in Risdon's Plate XIX. When removed by Risdon this metal piece, with a 1 x 3 mm exposure, was found to be only 1 mm in height. The pit in the tooth in which it was found was not a prepared cavity, and similar pitting was seen in the teeth from other skulls in this large collection. These details led Risdon to conclude that this was not a result of dental intervention but an accidental embedding of a bit of metal into the articular surface of the molar. This example is in the British Museum collection (BM 1944. 10. 20. 518: Lachish Series, Iron Age), as noted by Powers (1988).

III.L The Danish "bead" insert

Another case of an accidental insertion of a foreign object into a tooth has been reported from Denmark. There a "bead" (or "pearl" in some languages, but meaning a bead, not necessarily the product of an oyster) has been found "fixed into a caries cavity," reported to derive from a medieval context (Møller-Christensen 1958, in Bennike 1985: 176). Subsequently, Bennike (1985: 81) quotes Møller-Christensen (1969) as reporting this medieval "implant" from the Aebelholt monastery as being a deliberately placed "pearl." One may infer that this bead, like the "bronze wire" noted above, found its way into this context by accident, or possibly through post-mortem placement (Becker 1994c: 8).

III.M The "stone implant" from the Kalabah Necropolis, Klazomenai, Turkey

Gul Atilla (1993) reports the discovery of a piece of stone, that he believed to be the same size and general shape as a tooth, in a limestone sarcophagus with a limestone lid (Tomb Nr. 81/6). The tomb is located in the Kalabak Necropolis, situated to the east of the ancient Ionian city of Klazomenai on the Aegean coast (now "located in the Urla Iskelesi suburb of Izmir province," or to the west of modern Izmir/Smyrna). The report, and the comparanda noted, are not always clearly presented. In addition, Atilla uses data from the more obscure literature to support his interpretation of this object as an implant. The evidence is summarized here (see also Becker 1994c: 8–9) in order to evaluate these data in the light of documented examples of dental appliances.

This stone object was discovered in 1981 inside a looted limestone sarcophagus (Tomb Nr. 81/6) of the Kalabak Necropolis. The date of the sarcophagus is given as 550 BCE, based on its placement over a cremation burial (Tomb Nr. 81/3), which had associated offerings dated "to the first half of the sixth century BC [*c.*600–550 BCE]. In the Kalabak Necropolis nothing has been found later than mid-sixth century BC." "The southern half of the tomb had been found partly opened and the contents stolen." Recovered from inside were "some bones, teeth, and a tooth-like structure carved out of stone . . . with a gold hair-spiral as a burial offering." Later Atilla notes that this "object, which was found among broken bones, did not resemble a piece of an ornament." No specific location of any of the artifacts within this tomb has been provided.

Atilla suggests that the plundering of the tomb is the reason why the "tooth" was not found in place, which he suggests was in the "upper right canine" position. No list of human teeth found in the tomb is given, nor evidence for what portions of the face survived. The mandible is noted as present, with a pattern of molar eruption suggesting an age of 14 to 16 years at death. The presence of the hair spiral leads them to suggest that the deceased was a woman.

The material and the object from Turkey

Atilla notes that the size (length) of the object that he believes to be a dental implant is "the same" as is generally noted for upper canines, believed to be 27 mm. The actual dimensions listed later in the article suggest that this object is 29 mm long. The shape, and the "inclination" (bevel of the area believed to be the crown?) led Atilla to suggest that this is an upper right canine. The shape of the stone, which Atilla claims does not exist in nature, has led him to postulate that "the implant was attached to the adjacent tooth [sic] with special wires or devices." That is the way it is depicted in an artist's drawing (Atilla 1993: fig. 3), as wired to the upper right lateral incisor and first premolar.

Geological study requested by Atilla demonstrates that this stone seems to be composed of a hematite travertine portion, and a calcite section, the latter probably representing the pseudo-crown. Calcite is noted as having a hardness of three on Moh's scale, which is quite soft. The "crown" measures 6 × 5 × 11 mm, and fractures seen on it under a stereomicroscope are said to have led to "the theory that this object had functioned as a tooth." The neck area of the stone is believed to have "erosion lines resulting from the gold wire or band," and a polarizing light microscope is said to have revealed "gold pieces a few microns in diameter," supposedly traces of a gold fastening.

A new analysis of the Atilla (1993) report

Although this piece of stone is said by Atilla to have been "carved," he later says it "did not resemble a piece of an ornament." In fact, such pieces are found by amateur archaeologists and interested geologists with great frequency. Such randomly formed stones, produced by chance in nature, are commonly collected and mounted as charms or amulets. This clearly is a natural stone, differentially eroded (not worked), which has a slight resemblance to a tooth (or a phallus).

The traces of gold at the neck of this object may indicate that it was bound in a gold device, but they may be part of the mineralogical composition of the stone. Alternately, a gold mounting for an amulet might have held this stone. None of the adjacent teeth (if such existed) have been tested to support the theory that this stone was bound in place by a gold ligature.

At 29 mm in length this stone piece clearly is too long to have served as a false tooth in a bridgework unit. Artificial teeth are always limited to the crown portion alone, being suspended in a pontic device by bands (as in the Etruscan designs) or wires, as in Eastern Mediterranean examples. The "crown" part of the stone also is far too soft to have functioned as an artificial tooth. The preferred materials have always been ivory, human or animal teeth, and very dense woods. The single example of an artificial gold tooth, from Satricum, is also the earliest known dental appliance. (Quite probably problems involved with the soft gold shell rapidly led to the use of more durable replacement materials.) Despite Atilla's claim that stone has been used for other dental pontics, no example of this has been verified.

Most likely this piece of stone was a random inclusion within the opened sarcophagus, either entering when the tomb was looted or at any other point when the box was open. It also seems possible that some ancient person, such as a young girl, found this interesting stone and carried it as a charm. Amulets and decorations, on gold or silver wires, were commonly made in antiquity from all sorts of natural formations, including fossils and also "fairy darts," the term given to chipped stone arrow points and other tools of the European Mesolithic. Far from being a dental implant, the stone artifact noted by Atilla appears to be one of the large number of spurious objects wishfully suggested as representing these fascinating examples of ancient dental technology. (Note also that none of the known examples of dental appliances derive from the burial of an adolescent.)

III.N Bulgarian boasting: "brass" teeth of the fourth century CE

In 1997 a report was circulated (United Press International, January 13) that Nikolai Panaiotov, described as a Bulgarian archaeologist, planned to wear a pair of "brass" teeth that he discovered during excavations supposedly conducted near the port city of Varna on the Black Sea. His goal is said to be a listing in the Guinness Book of Records as the person wearing the oldest teeth. At the time of this report the archaeologist's dentist was said to have removed two healthy teeth from Panaiotov's upper jaw, and to be searching for a means by which the supposedly Roman teeth could be implanted using "ancient Roman" methods.

Aside from the questionable curation of archaeological findings, the toxicity of any uncovered brass (copper alloy) implant would lead to a severe shortening of the user's life. This artifact, quite possibly an amulet, merits further study, perhaps along with its excavator.

III.O An Hungarian ring found "surrounding" a tooth

A traditional Mordvin (western Hungarian) folk tale involves the story of a young girl who had a silver tooth (Dr. T. Grynaeus, personal communication, citing the Hungarian translations from the German as "*Az ezüstfogu lány. Mordvin népmesek*," Budapest, 1990: p. 163). This tale came to mind during the discovery of the bones of a young woman of the tenth–twelfth-century period who had what some believed to be a silver ring binding a tooth. Other aspects of this cemetery reflect the presence of numerous local, and non-Christian, funerary customs.

Trogmeyer (1960–1962: 11, 14, 36) reports that Grave 34 of the Békés-Povádzug cemetery (tenth–twelfth centuries) in southeast Hungary is that of a young woman. She died while pregnant or in childbirth, since the bones of the infant were identified within the mother's pelvis. Her mandibular right first molar was found to be extensively decayed, with but a small part of the crown left attached to the root. "Molded" into and around this surviving portion of crown, possibly by chewing or tooth clenching, was a silver hair ring of the type identified as "S-shape" (Trogmeyer 1960–1962: pl. II, no. 13; see Eogan 1997). The ring has a diameter of some 14 mm, with the loop made from a tube only 1 to 1.4 mm in diameter. Three other rings of the same type (Trogmeyer 1960–1962: pl. II, nos. 10–12) were in normal positions within the grave.

The archaeologist suggested to Dr. Thomas Grynaeus that she may have been chewing on her own braid, or the ring binding it, at the time of her death—perhaps in a painful and unsuccessful delivery. Although the published information might lead naive readers to conclude that this ornament was somehow involved in a dental context, none of the scholars associated with the excavation see any possibility that the ring was in the mouth of this woman during the course of her life.

III.P The drilled adult tooth from an Upper Paleolithic context

Note is made in a report on hominid remains from the Upper Paleolithic Period in France of a drilled adult tooth from Saint-Germain-la-Rivière, Pille-Bourse (Gambier and Houet 1991a: xix, 112–116, fig. 11). This tooth (STG 13) has indeed been drilled, but this occurred during a post-mortem event in order to pierce it through the root near the apex to allow the tooth to be suspended as a pendant.

This tooth and three others derive from a Magdalenian context (Upper Pleistocene, recent Würm). This tooth, found in July of 1966, and the 3 others found 2 years later are among the 15 hominid specimens described by Gambier and Lenoir (1991). The caption for Gambier and Houet's (1993: fig. 11) illustration may err in noting perforated "teeth." Clearly this tooth is not an example of ancient dentistry, although the fact that it has been drilled may confuse readers.

III.Q The "filling" in a pig's tooth

An interesting case of misidentification of a dental filling in a tooth, believed to be an amalgam restoration, led to the belief that the remains of a human being had been discovered.

Like examples 10 and 11 above, the "filling" in this case was entirely accidental. The dentition of pigs does resemble that of humans, reflecting to some extent the omnivorous behaviors of both species. Thus when a tooth with an apparent restoration was found in a case where a possible crime may have been involved, the initial observers focused on the metal "filling" rather than the morphology of the tooth.

Careful examination (Ubelaker 1996: 234–235, fig. 3) revealed that this is the mandibular molar of a pig. The crenulation between the tooth cusps had become packed with aluminum foil that some believed was an amalgam filling (silver and mercury dental restoration). Becker suggests that the surface of the aluminum was kept polished by continued use, a feature that may have been involved in the two supposed human cases (10 and 11) noted above.

III.R A French fantasy in Algeria

In 1954 an isolated skull of the Upper Capsian period (ninth–fifth millennia BCE) was recovered in Algeria (Vallois 1971: 206–208, figs 3–5). Six incisors, including all of the maxillary, had been deliberately removed (dental evulsion). According to Verger-Pratoucy (Personal communication, February 1996) a human(?) "phalange" was found wedged between the molar teeth identified as 14 and 16 (upper right molars). The apparently rough shaping of this bone led Vallois to claim that this piece of bone was meant to be a "*Prothèse dentaire*" (dental replacement) for the maxillary right second molar.

Appendix IV

Amulets and votives resembling or incorporating teeth

Factors contributing considerably to the confusion in tracing the history of dental prostheses are the many references to ancient votives and amulets involving human teeth or depictions of teeth (see Fenelli 1992; also Weinberger 1948: 128–129). Many descriptions of this type of votive or amulet erroneously suggest that they had been used as dental prostheses. The limitations of ancient Egyptian medicine and "dentistry" that were noted earlier help us to understand why charms or amulets were used by these people to deal with dental problems.

Among the amulets used by the ancient Egyptians were several that were very important, and thus popular, for the living as well as the dead (Andrews 1994). Flinders Petrie (1914) had recognized five specific categories of amulets, of which three are relevant to various aspects of medicine (homopoeic, phylactic and theophoric; see also Nunn 1996: 110). The "phylactic" category (from Greek *phylax*, "guard") is that which provides protection to the living, and thus must have included those amulets that were used to protect against tooth ailments. However, amulets involved in oral contexts are nowhere clearly described, nor is a clear association demonstrated between any specific amulet and the concerns of either dentists or patients (see Dawson 1953). An outstanding classification of amulets from ancient Egypt, based on the British Museum collections, is provided by Andrews (1994; see also Pinch 1995).

Dental votives were rarely used in Etruria (see Turfa 1994, and Chapter 2 for models of jaw or mouth). Guerini (1909: figs 10–11) illustrates two votives in terracotta, and one (fig. 12) that he believes to be a denture. Quite clearly this is simply another anatomical votive. Some Egyptian models generally appear to have been magical items (Nataf 1988, 1989). Magical amulets of all types have been surveyed by Bonner (1950), who provides information on a useful range of basic types. In many situations where confusion can be noted in the literature, this generally is the result of the description of an amulet as if it were a dental appliance. The source of the confusion for most, if not all of the following examples can be traced to such basic errors (see Leek 1967b).

IV.A Veio

Two terracotta examples of votive lips and teeth, supposedly from a votive deposit at the Etruscan city of Veii, are illustrated by Weinberger (1948: 129, fig. 42). One of Weinberger's examples is taken from Sudhoff (1921: 75; also 1926: 78, fig. 42), and the other from Guerini (1909: 68). Sudhoff (1926: 78) clearly identifies this item as a votive offering. (For properly documented "oral" votives, see Cederna 1951: 218; Baggieri 1996–1999: 40–41, 93.) Hoffmann-Axthelm (1985: 77, fig. 62; also 1981: fig. 62) illustrates an example also believed to be from Veii. All of these items may be various views of the same two terracotta votive pieces. Compare Figure 3.4, a votive in the Wellcome Collection.

IV.B Junker

The object most commonly imagined to be a dental appliance is a linked pair of teeth, attached by a gold wire, recovered from excavations at Gizeh, Egypt. Puech (1995: 5–6) provides the best illustrations now available as well as important data about comparative dental wear (cf. Puech 1987, Puech *et al.* 1983).

The Junker piece is identified by Iskander *et al.* (1978: pl. II) as Inv. 2453 at the Pelizäus Museum (once Römer-Pelizäus) in Hildesheim, Germany (see Eggebrecht 1994). These two linked teeth had been excavated by Junker from the shaft fill, of mixed date, from a tomb in a mastaba-like structure believed to date *c*.2,500 BCE (Tomb shaft 984: see Puech 1995; Leek 1972: 405). This amulet has come to be promoted as an Egyptian example of an early gold-wire appliance.

In fact, the Junker teeth derive not from an early tomb but from a fill deposit of late date (probably Hellenistic/Ptolemaic). They cannot be demonstrated to have been wired into the mouth of a living person to stabilize a loose tooth by joining it to a rooted one, nor to have a date before 500 BCE. Most likely this arti-fact actually is an amulet or charm of some type, although it might have been a post-mortem attempt to replace teeth in a mummy of the Hellenistic period. Gizeh has been the source of numerous mummies for centuries, and several supposedly have been of interest to dental historians (see Weinberger 1948: 70–73), but no dental appliances have ever been found there. Numerous scholars (e.g. Sigerist 1955: 347) wondered why no ancient Egyptian dental appliances had been found in the more than 20,000 well-preserved skulls of high-status individuals that were known! The two Egyptian wire amulets in the Egyptian Museum in Torino, Italy (E. Rabino Massa, personal communication, May 1996; see IV.J below) should be examined for possible similarities with the Junker piece.

References

Bardinet 1990: 2554–2555.
Eggebrecht 1994.
Emptoz 1987: 546 (also p. 559), no. I, fig. 21.

Euler 1928 (published in Junker 1929; also by Sallou 1975).
Hoffmann-Axthelm 1970: 81, fig. 1; 1985: 28–30, figs 13, 14.
Iskander and Harris 1977: 88.
Iskander *et al.* 1978: 104, pl. II, A and B. The illustrations were provided via the German
  Institute of Archaeology in Cairo and the Pelizäus Museum in Hildesheim, Germany.
Junker 1914: 169.
Junker 1927.
Junker 1929: 256–257, pl. LX, c.
Leek 1967a.
Leek 1972.
Micheloni 1976: 158.
Nataf 1989: fig. 2.
Puech 1995.
Peuch *et al.* 1983.
Proskaur 1979, Pt. 1: 9–10 (illustration on p. 8).
Ring 1985: 36, fig. 28.
Sallou 1975.
Euler 1928.
Weinberger 1946: fig. 3; 1947: 180–181, fig. 4.
Weinberger 1948: 73–75, fig 29 (from Euler 1928, Junker 1929: pl. 50a, and unpublished
  records).

Junker recovered these two teeth, which are at opposite ends of what appear to be
two or more strands of gold wire, from debris in the shaft of Tomb 984 at Gizeh.
The tomb itself is believed to date from the late Fourth or early Fifth Dynasty, or
about 2,500—2,000 B.C. The shaft debris, however, appears to be much later in
date. Bardinet (1990) correctly concludes that the debris in the shaft of Junker's
tomb cannot be dated. Strouhal and Perizonius (1993: 7) note that shaft contents
in Egyptian tombs are generally mixed and messy, and require special care in their
excavation as well as in their interpretation. These teeth were not in association
with any known human skeletal material.

Junker, in his first report on the teeth (1914) assumed that the gold wire was
used to link these two teeth only after death, as part of the mummification process.
This idea appears to have altered through time, but not necessarily as a result of
Euler's report, as Leek (1972: 405) suggests. Euler (in Junker 1929: 256–257,
fig. XL, c) describes and illustrates the Junker "piece" (see Junker 1929: i, 53–54;
vii, 113–117; viii, 26–27). Euler saw the teeth at the Römer-Pelizäus Museum in
Hildesheim, out of any archaeological context. Euler, believing that the "distal"
molar had lost its roots through pathological absorption, concluded that the wire
had been applied during the life of the patient in an attempt to retain the more
distal tooth in place. We believe instead that root loss reflects the deciduous origin
of this tooth.

F. F. Leek, whose impressive observations of dental appliances have contributed enormously to clarifying the record, offers several important observations on
these two teeth and the associated wire. Leek made his own direct examination of
the teeth and associated wire *c.*1970 and provides the most accurate description

of them. He notes that the wire is bound around the gingival margins, which is the narrowest point on these molars. Leek (1972: 405–406) says that the wire had been twisted into a figure 8, with further twists thereafter. Leek believed that the junction of the two loops of the figure 8 had been broken at some time after it came to the museum. He notes double loops of the gold wire around each tooth, and indicates that the wire is 0.35 mm in diameter. Leek says that several of the twists of wire around the junction of the two loops could not have been made during the life of this person since access to that part of the mouth would have prevented this type of maneuver.

Strangely, Leek describes what he thought was a "tubular construction" of this wire, revealed by a seam along the length of the wire, or wires. This is probably an extrusion imperfection (much ancient wire was spirally twisted and hammered rather than drawn), but Leek believes that he could detect a central bore when he used an 8x lens in his examination. This unlikely construction is so remarkable that we must question this otherwise generally accurate observer.

Leek (1972: 405) found the tooth with "completely absorbed roots" to have such "pronounced attrition on the occlusal surface of the tooth" as to make it impossible to assign a place in the dentition. This is the tooth that Becker believes to be deciduous. Leek (1972: 405) says that the "dark gray color of the enamel of this tooth indicates that the irritation caused by attrition created an inflammation of the dental pulp which resulted in its necrosis." He infers that associated pain would lead to the desire to have the tooth removed. Removal of a deciduous tooth with a root that had been largely absorbed would have been a simple problem. More likely Leek is describing a deciduous tooth that simply fell out and was probably saved by the owner or her/his family as a charm. Sallou (1975; see also Puech 1995) reports that the wire is 0.4 mm in diameter and is actually not a single strand but rather six short lengths that have been knotted together.

Junker came to believe that "tartar" found on both the teeth and the gold wire was evidence that the wire was placed into the mouth of a living person. Leek (1967b: 55) questions the evaluation of this material as tartar, suggesting that more probably this coating was a concretion of mineral salts that formed after this amulet was placed in a tomb, in fact a common phenomenon and not an organic deposit derived from the saliva. By the time that Leek (1972: 405) came to examine this piece he found "no accretions whatsoever around the gold wire."

Junker (1927: 68–70) states that this piece indicates that ancient Egyptian medicine was comparable to ancient Greek medicine, but his argument is far from convincing. No photographs, nor accurate description of where this piece was located when it was in the fill of the tomb shaft, appear in Junker 1914 and 1927, but an illustration of the teeth appears in 1929 (see also Hoffmann-Axthelm 1970: fig. 1; 1985: fig. 13). Leek (1967a) also suggests that it is an amulet, a conclusion that Bardinet (1990: 2553–2555) reaffirms, saying "*L'ensemble est isolé de tout contexte osseux*" [The group is isolated from all contexts with bones]. Hoffmann-Axthelm (1970: 81) sums it up by saying "This was in no way [an example of] restorative dentistry."

Bardinet (1990) notes the magical possibilities that may have been associated with this piece. The fact that the involved teeth are clearly molars appears to rule out any possibility that this material reflects the presence of a wire dental appliance. More likely this item is an amulet, such as described by Roldan *et al.* (1992; see IV.J below). Leek (1967b: 54) provides an excellent summary of relevant data from the stela of 'Iry", from Gizeh and of Junker's comments (1927) about this stela.

The molars of the Junker piece are generally said to be the right mandibular M2 and M3 with wire wound around them at their gingeval margins (possibly two turns). In fact, these teeth are far from being "bound together," nor are they even closely linked by the gold wire (see also Leek 1967b: 54). Weinberger (1948: 73, 75) and Leek (1967b: 55) describe this amulet as including a worn third molar with absorbed roots. Hoffmann-Axthelm (1970: 81) says that the item consists of a worn second molar, which is bound to a third molar, suggesting that both are permanent teeth.

Significantly, the supposed second molar clearly appears to be an extremely worn molar with what appears to be resorbed roots, but it is possible that they are fractured. The illustrations are generally good, but are insufficiently clear to permit a conclusion to be drawn about these teeth. I believe that this is a deciduous molar that had been lost by natural processes, which would include the resorption of the roots. The wear on this molar is deep into the dentine, and its surface is nearly flat (see Becker n.d. c), while the other molar is much less worn, a point also independently noted by Leek (1967b: 56). This makes considerable sense if the more worn example is a deciduous tooth that as a child's molar may have been saved as a charm. This may be especially true if loss of this tooth had been delayed. Leek suggests that one was lost due to an infection, noting (1967b: 56) that there is no mention of a skull or of other teeth from the archaeological context in which it was found. The absence of other skeletal evidence strongly suggests that this amulet was not connected to a specific burial when discovered.

While Emptoz (1987) provides a good review of the Junker amulet, Sallou (1975) offers an excruciatingly detailed and well-illustrated study of this specimen, which was first illustrated in 1929. Sallou (1975: 524), who examined this amulet in 1973, also provides Euler's report, signed at Breslau on October 15, 1928 and included in Junker's publication (1929). The report states that tartar appears on both teeth as well as the gold wire. Sallou (1975: 531) states that "*nous refusons la thèse d'une insertion post mortem religieuse sur le cadavre.*" Note is made that the (supposed) third molar is small and much more worn than the other molar, believed to be a lower left second molar. Careful measurements are provided. Hoffmann-Axthelm (1985: fig. 14) provides a good review of the relevant literature as well as his own photograph taken in 1972.

Despite a series of very good photographs, Sallou (1975) offers no lower view of the smaller tooth, which would conclusively indicate that what is said to be decay is actually the normal resorption process of deciduous tooth roots. Perhaps both the child's tooth and the adult tooth were retained to be used as an amulet.

One of the copies in Paris may represent this piece. Claude Rousseau (personal communication March 23, 1991) states that "The ex-voto published by Dr. Emptoz [1987: 559, fig. 21] came from our copies." This copy of a votive piece in the *Musée Pierre Fauchard* (Paris) may be a copy of the Junker specimen, and may explain why several published descriptions of the Junker piece are problematical. If these descriptions rely on a faulty copy, or one clearly taken out of context, the resulting evaluations would also be suspect.

IV.C Cairo, fourth–third centuries BCE

Various votive (?) pieces said to be dental appliances are vaguely noted as being "in Cairo." One of these specimens may be the same as that silver appliance listed above (Tura El-Asmant, no. W-5) noted by Iskander and Harris (1977) as taken to Cairo for conservation and study. Other of these vague references may relate to finds made in association with various mummies. Such references include Emptoz (1987: 546, no. II) and Quenelle (1975).

IV.D Vienna Museum

Egyptian mummy(?) dated to 200 BCE (Emptoz 1987: 546, no. III). While Professor Dr. Szilvassy in Vienna may be able to identify this item, at present we have only the vague note by Emptoz to account for this possible votive.

IV.E National Museum of Hungary in Budapest

Via X-ray, 1959 (Emptoz 1987:5 46, no. IV).

This piece may be a nasal "prosthesis" that had been described by Mérei and Nemeskéri (1959, as taken from Trillou 1976: 60).

IV.F Rijksmuseum van Oudheden, Leiden, amulets supposedly detected via X-ray in Egyptian mummies

References

Dawson and Gray 1968: xii, n. 2.
Emptoz 1987: 546, no. V.
Gray 1966; 1967: 41, fig. 6
Trillou 1976: 59.

The large sample (more than 25) of mummies in Leiden provides evidence for numerous Egyptian amulets of all periods, but no dental appliances have been found associated with these people.

IV.J Turin Egyptian collections

Dr. Emma Rubino Massa (*Università degli Studi, Torino*) reported to Becker (personal communication May 1996) that Egyptian "wire" amulets associated with mummies now in Turin resemble the Eastern Mediterranean-style dental appliances. These should be examined for possible relationships with the Junker amulet ("B" above).

IV.K Roman molar

A human molar set in a silver mount (ring), and dated to the Roman period, is described by Roldan *et al.* (1992). This worn human tooth, apparently a left maxillary second molar, had been rounded off (at the root?). The use of teeth as charms and amulets is a widely distributed custom, and this piece could date from the Roman period, but could have been made at almost any time in history.

Appendix V
Pliny on cures for oral pathologies

Although much of the pharmacopoeia of the ancient Greeks may appear somewhat peculiar to modern minds, the efficacy of many ancient drugs was, and remains, quite easily demonstrated. The therapeutic philosophers documenting the details of Greek medicine indicate that it derived from principals of sympathy (ink mixes with water, resinous gums dissolve in vinegars) and antipathy (water puts out fire), yet the results often were quite good (Scarborough 1987; Riddle 1985, 1987).

Toothache remedies were particularly sought after, as the pain induced is considerable and the incidence of dental decay tended to increase with age. Pliny (*Natural History*) is often cited as listing a series of toothache remedies, but in fact his repertoire involved treatments for a wide range of oral pathologies within which were a number specifically for the teeth. Some remedies prescribed by Pliny were meant to be poured into the ear located on the same side of the head as the tooth that was painful. Others are put into the ear on the opposite side of the head. Jones (in Pliny 1963: 564) notes that many of Pliny's remedies are not "rational" (e.g. the use of a hyena's tooth to dispel the pain in a decayed tooth), and suggests that the bases of such cures must have been derived from magic and from folk medicine, like much of Pliny's information. What was magic and what was science (both then and now) is often a matter of opinion. A more complete understanding of the sources of the ingredients would be needed before one could determine the place of such remedies in the world of pharmacy or magic, as it then was known (cf. Scarborough 1986). Many ingredients can be shown to have been available or collected in central Italy, and thus of relevance to Etruscan practices as well (for herbal ingredients, see Harrison and Bartels 2006; Scarborough 2006; Jannot 2009; Harrison and Turfa 2010; Turfa and Becker 2013: 869–870).

The preponderance of the Greek pharmaceutical agents that originate in plants, as listed in the various pharmacopoeias, renders all the more interesting our discussion of the remedies that Pliny listed for toothaches. Plant-derived pharmaceuticals appear to have outnumbered animal sources by a great margin, as general categories of palliatives among the ancient Greeks. The ancient uses of plants are documented by surveys of specific plants used in remedies, and their use continued right down to early nineteenth-century pharmaceutical inventories. A survey of the inventory lists of a Philadelphia druggist from 1812–1820 indicate that he carried some 300 items in his stock (Buerki 1988). The most common category, involving some 116 (38.9 percent) items, was drugs or drug products derived from plants. In stark contrast to this number are the seven drugs of animal origin. In fact, despite 2,000 years of accumulating knowledge, only 66 of the drugs in stock had chemical or mineral origins. Other categories, such as dyestuffs, patent medicines, medical equipment, and "sundries" (castile soap, glue and sealing wax) also reveal a great deal about what may have been in ancient "drugstores."

Plants and herbs "*d'antica tradizione etrusca*" are reviewed by Russo (1992: 265), who notes various examples [of plants and herbs] used during the extraction or treatment of a diseased tooth. The proportions of the agents used for dental pain by Pliny, almost invariably derived from animals, are all the more striking when seen in light of ancient as well as more recent pharmacopoeias. Animal sources dominate the ingredients found in the "dental" part of Pliny's *pharmocopoeia* (see Bonet 1995), but all kinds of variations may have been practiced by different medical specialists. For example, Marcellus Empiricus (*c.*400 AD) presents numerous remedies that actually may include pharmacologically useful ingredients (see Scarborough 1987). The Pseudo-Apuleius, in the fifth century CE, focused on herbal remedies, but his contemporary Sextus Placitus made recipes exclusively from birds and terrestrial animals. While the traditional medicine of ancient Rome was developing a complex pharmocopoiea there certainly was sufficient room in this complex society to allow a tremendous range of "treatments" to flourish, just as they do today.

The listing below derives only from just two books of Pliny's *Natural History* (Books 28 and 30; see Pliny 1963: 66–67, 290–295, 566). Many other remedies are scattered through the other 35 books, most of which illustrate Pliny's efforts to collect and record folk remedies (see Pliny 1870–1898, edited by Jan and Mayhoff). The information presented here is ordered simply by grouping the remedies according to their principal ingredient, which is always derived from a formerly "living" thing. The observation that these recipes require an animate (animal) agent to effect a cure may be of importance in understanding the philosophy of medicine as then practiced. Secondary ingredients, such as frankincense, or transport agents such as rose oil or pitch-pine resin, appear throughout the list and clearly reflect the pharmaceutical nature of these potions.

The contexts in which these medications were used and associated treatments noted by Pliny as useful in effecting the same cure (end result) may be important in understanding exactly how these remedies were understood at that time. The ingredients in the prescriptions listed below suggest just how much of Pliny's information derived from folk medicine, and may explain why these particular prescriptions are clustered in these two books while other formulae are scattered throughout the collected works. Some of the remedies listed are clearly attributed to the Magi, as is one of the preventatives listed (*Natural History* 30.8.23): "There are among them those who order that a mouse be chewed twice monthly to avoid [tooth]aches."

We are certain that the distraction of chewing up a mouse might work wonders in altering perceptions of pain, but also point out that mice are common ingredients in folk remedies throughout the world. (Consuming a live mouse was a remedy in Egyptian papyri, and remains of a mouse are said to have been found lodged in some mummies—where it obviously failed to cure.) Lady Eveline Gurdon's survey of folk remedies that were common throughout the Suffolk countryside at the end of the nineteenth century includes several that call for mice. As a cure for whooping cough "let the patient eat a roasted mouse" (Gurdon 1893: 14; see also Billson 1895: 55). "Fried mice are relied on as a specific for the small-pox" but "it is considered necessary that they should be fried *alive*" (emphasis in the original, Gurdon 1893: 18). And Lady Eveline Gurdon also notes (1893: 20) that, "*For Rheumatism*—ashes of a mouse baked alive." Hartland's parallel survey from Gloucestershire (1892: 51) lists the cure for whooping cough simply as "eat a roasted mouse." Billson (1895) surveyed printed sources of remedies from Leicestershire and Rutland, from as early as 1768. He notes Gurdon's data, as well as information from Henderson's folklore of the northern counties. Fried mice seem to be commonly prescribed for whooping cough, but also for quinsy (Billson 1895: 55). Shrew mice are used in entirely different remedies, or charms (Billson 1895: 29). This small sampling of remedies from various parts of England dating from only a bit more than a century ago suggests that the folk remedies listed by Pliny were ancient even in his time, and survived into the age of modern, largely science-based medicine. Presumably Pliny's remedies survived in Italy well past the Renaissance.

Pliny: Natural History, Book 30

Toothache remedies (relief). Gum therapies and agents that cause aching teeth to fall out with ease (*Natural History* 30.21–27; Jones translations, in Pliny 1963: 290–297):

Dog head and/or teeth

a)   The ash of the fleshless burned heads of dogs that have died of madness [rabies], [dissolved in] cyprus oil and dropped into the ear on the side of the pain [Magi].
b)   Left eye-tooth (canine) of a dog, use to scrape around aching tooth [Magi?].
c)   An amulet made of the two upper teeth [of a dog?; central incisors or canines?], if the pain is in the upper jaw; teeth from the lower jaw are used for lower jaw pain.
d)   The magi rinse the mouth with a decoction of dogs' teeth in wine, boiled down to one-half. The ash of these teeth, with honey, helps children who are slow in teething, and also is made into a dentifrice.

Earthworms

a)   Boiled down in oil and poured into the ear on the side with the pain.
b)   Reduced to ash (burned in an earthen pot) and plugged into decayed teeth cause them to fall out easily, and applied to sound teeth relieves any pain in them.
c)   Boiled down in squill[1] vinegar with the root of a mulberry tree, makes a wash for the teeth.

Hens

Touching the afflicted tooth or scraping the gum with the "*ossiculi gallinarum*," little bones of hens [that] "have been kept hanging on the wall of a room, with the gullet intact," and then throwing the bone away . . . "they assure us that the pain at once disappears."

Hyenas' teeth

a) The touch of the corresponding tooth.
b) Use [of the corresponding tooth?] as an amulet.

Insects

Bugs from the mallow are poured into the ears with rose oil [to make teeth fall out or to relieve pain]. Scarborough points out that Pliny elsewhere (*Natural History* 29.62–63) notes that these insects (*cinices*, not *cimices*) are to be burnt.[2]

Lizard

a) Scrape the teeth with bones extracted, at a full moon, from the forehead of a lizard, without their [the bones] touching the earth.

Maggots

a) The maggot found on the plant called Venus' Bath,[3] plugged into teeth [cavities], is wonderfully good.
b) At the touch of the cabbage caterpillar [*Urucae brassicae*?] [teeth] fall out.

Mice

a) Ash of mouse dung, or dried lizard's liver, stuffed into the cavity of a decayed tooth (relieves pain).
b) The ash of burned mice mixed with honey (with some fennel root added) when rubbed on the teeth makes the taste in the mouth agreeable. [probably as a "remedy" for sour stomach rather than bad breath].

Moles' teeth

Pliny notes that the Magi place great faith in the mole, implying that this remedy is one recommended by them: a tooth extracted from a living mole worn as an amulet.

Ravens' dung

Kills dental pain when wrapped in wool and worn as an amulet.

Snails

a)   The little grains of sand found in the horns of snails, if put into hollow teeth, free them at once from pain.
b)   Empty snail shells, reduced to ash and with myrrh added, is good for gums.

Snakes

a)   Heart of a snake, eaten or worn as an amulet.
b)   Ash of a serpent burned with salt in an earthen pot, poured with rose oil into the opposite ear, is good for gums [pain].
c)   The slough (shed skin) of a snake, with oil and pitch-pine resin, warmed and poured into either ear, is good for the gums (some add frankincense and rose oil). If put [the slough?] into hollow teeth it also makes them fall out without trouble.[4]
d)   Snake's tooth [fang?] worn as an amulet.
e)   One of the vertebrae of the "draco" (a snake, usually non-poisonous; cf. Pliny *Natural History* 24.180) or of an "*enhydris*" (a water snake), the serpent being a white male [scraped around the aching tooth? See Dog "b"].

Sparrows

a)   Sparrow dung, wrapped in wool and worn as an amulet, causes dental pain to disappear. But this causes unbearable itching [so Pliny suggests that the following is preferable].
b)   Take the ash of a sparrow's nestlings, which have been burned on twigs and mix it with vinegar. Rub this on the part [near the pain?].[5]

Spider

"Some think a spider is beneficial." To be effective the spider must be caught with the left hand, beaten up in rose oil, and poured into the ear on the side of the pain.[6]

Notes

1 Squill is the bulb or the root of the sea-onion, or related plants: *Silla* or *Urginea maritima*. The squill has been used in pharmaceuticals from ancient Greek to modern times (see Stannard 1974; Riddle 1987: 52). Sternberg (1998) offers a more recent identification for squill as *Drimia maritime*, a member of the family *Liliaeae*, noting that this plant contains a number of cardioactive glycosides, such as *Proscillaridin*, which now is an important cardiotonic pharmaceutical. Any effects on the teeth or gums remains undocumented, but indirect benefits may be present.
2 Professor John Scarborough (personal communication to Becker) points out that the original text reads "*a malva cimices infunduntur auribus cum rosaceo*," and that "*cimices*" (sing. *cimex*) usually translates as "bed bugs" (*Cimex lectularius L.*). Professor Scarborough notes that in the text of Dioscorides (II, 34) the term clearly means "bugs from a bed." In the context of the mallow (*Malva sylvestris L.*), however, Professor Scarborough translates "*cinices*" as "aphids."

For data on the medicinal and other uses of insects, as well as other invertebrates, in Classical antiquity (drugs, poisons, etc.) see Beavis (1988). Also of interest is the work of Davies and Kathirithamby (1986). For specific references to medical uses of insects see Scarborough (1988).

3 Venus' Bath, also called Venus' Basin, is the wild teasel, *Dipsacus sylvestris*.

4 Elsewhere Pliny (1963: 294) notes that it is an idle tale that white snakes shed about at the time of the rising of the Dog Star, since in Italy he notes that such castings are seen before the rising. Pliny suggests that in warmer regions it is even less probable that the sloughing would be so late. "But they say this slough *even when dry* [emphasis added] combined with wax" causes teeth to come out quickly. Obviously fresh and still soft shed skins are preferred for this remedy. The mixture most probably was to be inserted into the carious hole in one's tooth.

5 Whether this is a specific treatment for dental pain or a general painkiller is not clear.

6 Almost all spiders are venomous, but very few have biting mechanisms capable of penetrating human skin. Quite probably the toxins in the poison sacs of many spiders may have an anesthetic effect of pharmacological value, with possible chemical variations in how a preparation would operate to achieve this end. Some venom might be best applied to the surface of the skin, while others might be effective if taken internally. Scarborough (1979: 7–14) provides useful information on this subject in addition to considerable folklore regarding noxious biting creatures.

Appendix VI

Evidence for dental extractions in ancient Rome

A summary of the analysis of teeth excavated at the Temple of Castor and Pollux in the Roman Forum

Modern European and North American dental practice involving tooth loss generally involves disposal of removed teeth as a waste product. Only in the case of children's rituals (the "tooth fairy"), and the cash value of deciduous teeth, do we find any transient interest in these "body parts." Even among Catholics we know of no cases where teeth are ritually conserved to be rejoined with the remainder of the body for the afterlife. There may be modern societies in which the teeth and perhaps other elements of the human body are not casually discarded. J. Oyamada (personal communication 2003) affirms that in eighteenth- and nineteenth-century Japan a person would save teeth lost during life with the expectation that they would be buried with the body. One grave from an extensive cemetery adjacent to Prague Castle in the Czech Republic contained an individual identified as an edentulous woman buried c. 850–880 CE. Near her left hand, possibly in a pouch, were 15 teeth said to derive from at least four individuals (Smetáka 1988). While some may have been her own teeth, this has not been confirmed. Since this is a unique example within this region (cf. Becker 2000b) no cultural norm can be inferred.

The teeth from the excavations of one of the *tabernae* in the massive base of the Castor and Pollux Temple (Becker 2014) are overwhelmingly characterized by extensive decay. The uniformly carious condition of these teeth and their concentration in a limited area of this shop strongly indicate that they derive from a location where dental extractions had been performed. Not only does the vast majority have caries, but these decayed portions of the teeth are invariably of large size and almost all penetrate well into the pulp chambers. The considerable pain generated clearly would lead a sufferer to seek aid in the form of extraction, as any use of painkillers would have been of only limited and temporary value.

The Temple of Castor and Pollux, a landmark in the ancient Roman Forum recognized today by its three standing columns (Szegedy-Maszak 1988: 20), had numerous important functions. Housed within its massive base were a series of *tabernae*; small shops in which an enormous variety of trades were plied. We may be sure that one of these trades involved money changing. That a dentist or "cosmetologist" occupied one of these shops should not be surprising (see also Russo 1992: 266–267). The juxtaposition of small shops within or among temples has been known throughout ancient Rome (see Reynolds 1997). Continuity in this Italian tradition of placing shops and offices within the platforms or at the ground level of buildings is evident in the base of the massive fourteenth-century town hall in the center of modern Tarquinia (formerly Corneto). The small niches beneath the imposing entry stairs are now occupied by a simple electrical repair shop and by a store selling inexpensive toys.

The complex cosmology of the ancient Romans permits numerous relationships to be worked out between the deities and the lives of the worshippers. Does the god Castor, one of the Greek Dioscuri, in any way relate to dentistry? The European beaver (genus *Castor*) is identified as *castor* in both Greek and Latin. The secretion from the perineal glands of the beaver, as well as the dried glands themselves, is also called "castor." This material has traditionally been used in medicine and in perfumes. The medicines may have been important adjuncts to dental extractions. *Castoria*, or castor oil, is a plant-derived product completely unrelated to the beaver. However, *castoria* has been prescribed for the pain of childbirth and may have been used in ancient dentistry. (The mythical association of the Twins with boxing might have implications for oral/dental health as well.)

In the study of the teeth from this *taberna* no X-rays were considered as necessary as the large dental caries are easily described by naked eye examination. The enamel surfaces of the teeth, however, were examined with a 10x lens to search for evidence of tool marks or any indications of treatment that might have left detectable signs on any tooth surface. No such markings were found, which is consistent with the literary evidence that indicates that teeth were firmly grasped and wiggled loose before extraction (see Figures 1.2a and b). The person, or persons, who removed these teeth must have been quite skilled in the procedure, employing techniques of wiggling and otherwise loosening, which permitted the successful extraction of the afflicted (or designated) tooth. All cases of broken roots in this sample were examined to determine when the breaks occurred—either during extraction or subsequently as the result of being trodden underfoot (see Figures 1.2a and b). The examples of broken teeth from this collection, with either fractured crowns or snapped roots, all appear to have resulted from being trod underfoot in the establishment prior to finding their way into the drain from which they were recovered. The drain was filled with these extracted teeth and with fragments of materials that appear related to the trade in ointments and cosmetics. The floor drain passes under the door sill and joins a larger drain that passed along the side of the temple. This drain in turn connects with the *cloaca maxima*, the central sewer of Rome that drained the Forum and emptied into the Tiber.

Sex evaluation was made on the basis of tooth size. Individual teeth were identified as to position in the jaws, and then measurements were taken of each tooth (see Becker, 2016, in press: tables). Sex evaluation can be made by the study of tooth size, a process that has been well documented as noted in the above text. This procedure has been employed with success in Italy at the site of Osteria dell'Osa, the Iron Age cemetery of ancient Gabii, which was the settlement nearest to ancient Rome on the east (Becker and Salvadei 1992). Although the period covered at Gabii is somewhat earlier (ninth–eighth century BCE) than that with which we are concerned in this study, the geographic area is nearly identical.

Dental pathology, as it is generally studied within archaeological contexts, focuses in most cases on disease as it is found in cemetery populations. This kind of information, an historical summary of which is provided by Emery (1963), offers a "normal" cross section of dental disorders. The unusual case that we have here provides us with a pre-selected sample of a limited range of pathological types.

1   These teeth clearly represent a sample of diseased teeth, which appear to have been extracted in a *taberna* in the center of the Roman Forum. The tooth categories represented and the patterns of decay clearly rule out any possibility that these teeth came from a relatively small number of people. They appear to be extractions from a great number of individuals, possibly as many as represented by the entire number of teeth.

2   The variety in this series reflects the fact that these are the decayed teeth of a large number of people, and not the dental remains from a few skulls from which the teeth had been lost.

3   The success of the method of extraction used is attested by the absence of tooth fragments broken across or through the decayed area. In no case did the tooth crown break as a result of poor procedures employed. No lead fillings, to prevent breakage during extraction, were found. Quite possibly lint stuffing was used to stabilize the teeth and thus to prevent breaking during removal. More probably no effort was made to prevent crown damage and the teeth were simply loosened through cutting of the gums and nearby boney tissue.

4   These teeth primarily derive from adults, although two deciduous teeth indicate that extractions from children's mouths also were practiced here. Dental wear patterns suggest that most of these adults were from 30 to 60 years of age at the time of extraction. The degrees of wear on the surfaces of the teeth suggest that the age of the persons from whom they came was generally between 30 to 40 years, but this estimate of age from dental wear may be low since it is without a complete comparative population. The age distribution, however, is consistent with data that we have from the Iron Age population in the area of Rome (Gabii) (Becker and Salvadei 1992), which suggest that caries rates increased with age, and tended to be strongly concentrated in the molar teeth. This pattern, which might seem logical, is actually very different from that found in contemporary America where caries rates are very high in children, but tend to decelerate with increasing age. In modern America, by age 25 dental caries generally are superseded as a problem by periodontal disorders. The causes for this pattern, whether diet or food consumption pattern, are not known.

5   In the Castor and Pollux sample, decay appears to have been concentrated in the interdental areas of the premolars and molars rather than on articular surfaces. Eating coarse foods may have "polished" the working surfaces of teeth and reduced decay in those areas.

6   Periodontal problems also afflicted these ancient Romans. The loss of bone surrounding the roots of teeth, due to ineffective or absent periodontal care, was rarely a severe problem for these people, but certainly did exist. For the practicing dentist of this period such periodontal difficulties were an aid to extraction of the teeth since the loss of supporting hard tissue surrounding the roots facilitated the removal of a diseased tooth.

7   The presence of only one possible abscess is suggested from the study of these teeth.

In association with these teeth from the Roman Forum were a number of tools, both fragmentary and intact, which completely support the conclusion that this shop plied a trade in pharmaceuticals as well as providing dental extractions (Guldager and Slej 1986: 33). Künzl (1982: 5–6), on the basis of extensive studies of medical instruments, concludes that medicine and pharmacy together with cosmetics and painting were closely linked in the Roman world (see also Miller 1981: 48 for cosmetics in a Late Antique grave). Many of Künzl's finds (1982) were intact sets of instruments, which had been contained in "physicians'" tool kits. On rare occasion, such as in shipwrecks, the actual box and normally perishable contents could survive. However, one of the few examples suggested as a tool or pharmaceutical kit appears to be a jewelry case (Mas 1985). Another yielded cumin and coriander among the organic remains that could be visually identified (D'Atri and Gianfrotta 1986: 206). Whether this was a spice box or medicine case remains unclear.

Mas (1985: 219) specifically examined the objects from the House of the Surgeon at Pompeii and now in the National Museum at Naples. Mas concludes that a surgical kit is not among these objects. Bliquez (1994: 79–80) notes that only two instruments associated with the House of the Surgeon can be identified. The small cylindrical box containing a bone needle, which Mas (1985: 212, n. 15 and16) also recovered appears to be a sewing kit. The small or miniature wooden box from the Crimea now in Berlin (Cat. no. 11863; Richter 1966: fig. 402) has been termed a "pharmaceutical box," but no evidence exists to make such an association.

Künzl's publication of numerous items related to the trade in pharmaceuticals provides outstanding comparative data for the assemblage found in the Temple of Castor and Pollux. Of particular note is the appearance, in a third-century BCE context, of a barber's shears in association with a round- bellied ointment jar (Künzl 1982: 94–95) identical to those jars found with the teeth from the Temple of Castor and Pollux. These are characterized by a small base and mouth of nearly the same size, with a bulbous center. Other medical equipment illustrated by Künzl (1982) that parallels the material from the Temple of Castor and Pollux are numbers of pins and rods (pp. 96–97), a bone spatula (pp. 114–116), and small scoops from Syria (p. 123, fig. 97).

The information from the teeth and the associated artifacts recovered from this *taberna* in the Temple of Castor and Pollux provide conclusive evidence for the practice of dentistry at this location. Analysis of the contents of the jars may offer

Table AVI.1   Taberna in Roman Forum, findspots of extracted teeth

Excavation unit #	1	2	5	6	8	9	10	11	12	19	31	32	34	36	37
# of teeth	11	13	4	1	8	2	1	5	1	1	2	2	2	30	3
(Total number of teeth = 86)															

further clues to specific ointments, potions, or drugs being offered for sale or used in the course of extracting teeth from the many customers who were living active lives in the center of ancient Rome.

Contexts and evaluation of the teeth, Castor and Pollux Trench "T"

All of the teeth recovered in this excavation derive from a single small test area, designated as "Trench T," located beneath the northernmost aspect of the Temple stairway. The excavation location within Trench "T" is given here as a "unit" number, and this location is also noted after the identification of the position in the mouth that has been evaluated for each tooth.

The specific data regarding the dentition, both adult and sub-adult, appear in a series of tables (Becker 2016, in press) (see Table VI.1).

Observations

1   Almost every tooth in this sample has extensive caries.
2   Only two of these teeth are deciduous, thus representing children.
3   Five of the "teeth" are large fragments that show vertical fractures, certainly as a result of post-extraction damage.
4   A large number of these teeth have lost at least a small portion of the enamel that was still intact at the time of extraction, again probably as a result of post-extraction exfoliation due to being trampled, etc.
5   Sex has been evaluated on the basis of crown dimensions, as well as from an evaluation of root size and root configuration. Errors in these evaluations could be significant. Even the evaluation of the jaw location for individual teeth has a degree of uncertainty.
6   Wear cannot be used as an effective indicator of age in individual teeth (cf. Molnar 1971), since no evidence for presence or absence of the opposing tooth is available.
7   Very few of these teeth are free from decay. While no X-rays have been taken to determine possible disease in these apparently disease-free examples, the assumption is that they were healthy teeth removed for reasons not readily evident. A worn mandibular third molar (from Trench 2, Unit 2) is among these caries-free examples.

Possibly these healthy teeth were extracted in error, but more probably they were pulled in conjunction with therapies for disorders other than dental disease (e.g. chronic headaches, Bell's Palsy, etc., but see observation no. 9, below). All the ancient authors as well as modern dental scholars agree that preservation of one's natural teeth is to be preferred.

8   Based on relative tooth size, fewer females than males appear to be represented. Did many Roman women suffer in silence, or did they have better teeth, or were they less likely to seek external treatment (either suffering the pain or being treated informally, perhaps by other women)?

9   Of the healthy (decay free) teeth, females appear to be overrepresented. Were the teeth of women removed when symptoms other than decay-generated toothache were present? Were teeth removed in antiquity the way other portions of the female anatomy have been removed in more recent times, for symptoms (some would say "as punishment for") of ills perceived as "female complaints"? (This could be relevant to the reasons for Etruscan tooth evulsion that resulted in gold appliances, but in the absence of literature, we cannot know.)

Appendix VII

Report on analysis of gold bands in Liverpool appliances (nos. 13 and 14)

*Matthew J. Ponting and Pablo Fernandez-Reyes,
Department of Archaeology, Classics and
Egyptology, University of Liverpool (May 2015)*

**Report on the analysis by scanning electron
microscope with energy-dispersive spectrometry
(SEM-EDS) of two Etruscan gold denture fittings**

Introduction

Two Etruscan dental fittings (M10334 and M10335) were submitted for SEM-EDS analysis with the aim of establishing the chemical composition of the yellow-metal strips and attaching rivets.

Analytical method

The SEM used is a JEOL JSM-5300 scanning microscope fitted with both secondary electron (SE) and backscattered electron (BE) detectors together with an ultra-thin window EDS detector controlled by a Princeton Gamma Tech Spirit EDS and imaging system. The analysis was conducted at an accelerating voltage of 20 kV, counting for 100 seconds with an approximate count rate of 2,000 cps on pure copper. The system was calibrated on pure metal standards and periodically checked against a gold-alloy standard prepared and certified by the Edinburgh Assay Office. The level of agreement with the certified reference sample is tabulated below:

The level of agreement is acceptable given that the surface of the standard had not been polished or otherwise prepared prior to analysis. This was intentional so as to match as closely as possible the surface morphology of the Etruscan

Table AVII.1 The level of agreement with the certified sample.

	Gold (wt. %)	*Silver (wt. %)*	*Copper (wt. %)*
Certified	80.5	9.6	9.9
At start	81.1	10.0	8.8
At finish	79.9	9.2	10.9

objects. Unprepared surfaces with less than perfect geometry to the incident electron beam is known to adversely affect EDS analysis, in analysing the gold-alloy standard under similar circumstances to those expected of the samples, we are able to better gauge the level of error caused by the unprepared surfaces and poor geometry. It can be seen that the errors are relatively minor; around ±1 percent or less.

In analysing the Etruscan objects, both rivets and the main sheet were measured independently. Two areas were selected for each rivet and three areas were selected across the sheet to provide as representative an analysis as possible.

Results

In all cases the gold alloy used in these objects is high in gold with relatively little silver and copper present. In no case was more than 2 percent of either silver or copper detected, usually rather less.

M10334: rivet A

This has an average composition of 97.3 percent gold, 1.5 percent silver and 1.2 percent copper.

M10334: Rivet B

This has an average composition of 98.5 percent gold, 0.39 percent silver and 1.1 percent copper.

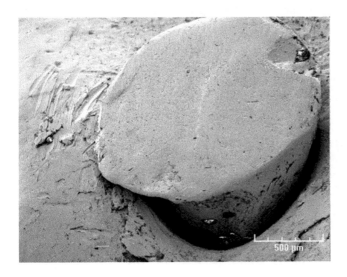

Figure AVII.1 SEI image of rivet A in M10334.

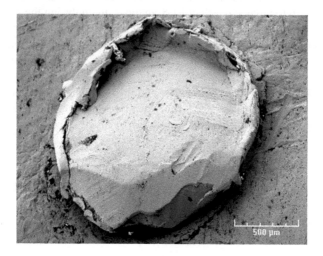

Figure AVII.2 SEI image of rivet B in M10334.

M10334: Main sheet (band)

This has an average composition of 98.2 percent gold, 0.24 percent silver and 1.6 percent copper. The three points were equidistantly spaced across the rivets, with one area located between the rivets and one on each side of the pair.

M10335: Rivet A

This has an average composition of 99.3 percent gold, no detectable silver and 0.7 percent copper.

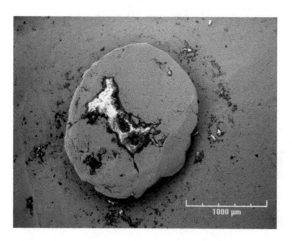

Figure AVII.3. SEI image of rivet A in M10335.

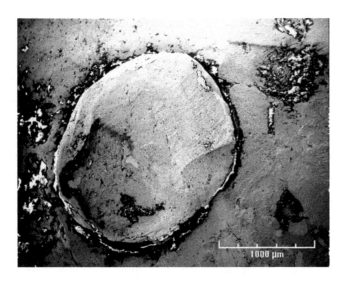

Figure AVII.4 SEI image of rivet B in M10335.

M10335: Rivet B

The average composition of this is 99.4 percent gold, 0.1 percent silver and 0.6 percent copper.

M10335: Main sheet (band)

The areas analysed were spaced in the same fashion as on the previous object. The average composition is 96.8 percent gold, 1.8 percent silver and 1.4 percent copper.

Discussion

Both pieces are made of relatively pure gold containing less than 2 percent of silver or copper. The rivets are of broadly the same alloy type as the sheet, although the rivets in M10335 are of slightly purer gold than the sheet containing only around 0.5 percent of alloying metals. The rivets used in M10334, however, are of essentially the same purity as the sheet, with rivet A containing slightly higher levels of silver and copper than rivet B. It does not appear that softer, purer gold was intentionally used for the rivets.

No platinum group metal inclusions (PGEs) were identified during the study and so the gold alloy from which these objects were made is unlikely to be alluvial. Primary vein gold would be the probably source.

Table AVII.2 Gold, silver, and copper content of all areas analyzed, with average for each item (rivet or band).

	Gold	Silver	Copper
M10334 RA1	97.36	1.43	1.21
M10334 RA2	97.26	1.59	1.15
M10334 rivet A	97.31	1.51	1.18
M10334 RB1	98.99	0.00	1.01
M10334 RB2	98.41	0.37	1.22
M10334 RB3	98.64	0.42	0.94
M10334 rivet B	98.53	0.39	1.08
M10334 SH1	98.75	0.00	1.25
M10334 SH2	98.41	0.36	1.22
M10334 SH3	98.00	0.11	1.89
M10334 sheet	98.21	0.24	1.56
M10335 RA1	99.26	0.00	0.74
M10335 RA2	99.43	0.00	0.57
M10335 rivet A	99.34	0.00	0.66
M10335 RB1	99.48	0.12	0.40
M10335 RB2	99.26	0.00	0.74
M10335 rivet B	99.37	0.06	0.57
M10335 SH1	97.36	1.43	1.21
M10335 SH2	97.00	1.55	1.46
M10335 SH3	96.62	2.04	1.35
M10335 sheet	96.81	1.79	1.40

Note: shaded entries denote the average of elements in each item (rivet or band), for comparison with the exact values for each area sampled.

Bibliography

Abenguefit, 1533. *De uirtutibus Ciborum, & Medicinarum*, trans. Gerardo Cremonesi. In *Sex Rervm non naturalium, cum earum naturis, operationibus, & rectificationibus* (see Tacuinus, Domus Sextadecima), 119–139. Cum praerogatiua Caef. Maiestatis ad sexeñium. (Volume located in the Biblioteca Statale Cremona, Italy, bound with other works of Tacuinus).

Accorsi, S., M. Fabiani, N. Ferrarese, R. Iriso, M. Lukwiya, and S. Declich, 2003. "The burden of traditional practices, ebino and tea-tea, on child health in Northern Uganda," *Social Science and Medicine* 57 (11): 2183–2191.

Adams, Francis, 1844. *The Seven Books of Paulus Aegineta, Translated by Francis Adams* (3 volumes). London: For the Sydenham Society.

Adams, Francis, 1849. *Genuine Works of Hippocrates, Translated by Francis Adams* (2 volumes). London: For the Sydenham Society.

Aetius of Amida, 1935. *Aetii Amideni. Libri Medicinales I–IV*, ed. Alexander Olivieri. Corpus Medicorum Graecorum VIII, 1. Leipzig: B. G. Teubner.

Agbor, Ashu M., Sudeshni Naidoo, and Awono M. Mbia, 2011. "The role of traditional healers in tooth extractions in Lekie Division, Cameroon," *Journal of Ethnobiology and Ethnomedicine* 7: 15. Online: www.ethnobiomed.com/content/7/1/15 (consulted November 15, 2016).

Albrektsson, T. and G. A. Zarb, 1993. "Current interpretations of the osseointegrated response: clinical significance," *International Journal of Prosthodontics* 6 (2): 203–208.

Albrektsson, T., G. A. Zarb, P. Worthington, and A. R. Eriksson, 1986. "The long-term efficacy of currently used dental implants: a review and proposed criteria of success," *International Journal of Oral and Maxillofacial Implants* 1 (1): 11–25.

Alexeyev, Andrey, 2012. *The Gold of the Scythian Kings in the Hermitage Collection.* St. Petersburg: The State Hermitage Publishers.

Alimen, Henriette, 1957. *The Prehistory of Africa*, trans. Alan H. Brodrica. London: Hutchinson.

Allbutt, T. Clifford, 1921. *Greek Medicine in Rome*. London: Macmillan.

Allen, Charles, 1969 (1685). *The Operator for the Teeth, Shewing How to Preserve the Teeth and Gums*, with a new introduction by R. A. Cohen. London: Dawsons.

Allison, Penelope M., 1997a. "Artefact distribution and spacial function in Pompeian houses." In Beryl Rawson and Paul Weaver, eds, *The Roman Family III: Status, Sentiment, Space*, 321–354. Oxford: Clarendon Press.

Allison, Penelope M., 1997b. "Roman households: an archaeological perspective." In Helen M. Parkinson, ed., *Roman City*, 112–146. New York: Routledge.

Alt, Kurt W., 1989. "Odontologische Befunde aus Archäologie und Anthropologie," *Zahnärztliche Mitteilungen* 79 (7/89): 785–796.

Alt, Kurt W., 1993. "Praktische Zahnmedizin im 18. Jahrhundert. Historische Grabfunde aus Saint-Hippolyte, Grand Saconnex, Genf, Schweiz," *Monatsschrifte Zahnmedizin* 103: 1146–1154 (followed by a French translation, pp. 1155–1157).

Alt, Kurt W., 1994. "Prosthetics, periodontal therapy and conservative dentistry in the eighteenth century: archaeological findings from Grand Sacconex [sic], Geneva, Switzerland," *Bulletin of the History of Dentistry* 42 (2): 67–70.

Alt, Kurt W., 1997. *Odontologische Verwandtschaftsanalyse*. Stuttgart: Gustav Fischer.

Alt, Kurt W. and H. Newesely, 1994. "Ein Anfangskapitel der modernen Prosthetik," *Zahnärztliche Mitteilungen* 84: 66–68 [518–520].

Alt, Kurt W., Wolfgang M. Pahl, Gerfried Ziegelmayer and Franz Parsche, 1990. "Gebissdeformation als 'Körperschmuck'—Verbreitung, Motive und Hintergründe." *Zahnärztliche Mitteilungen* 80 (22): 2448–2456.

Alt, Kurt W., F. Parsche, W. M. Pahl, and G. Ziegelmayer, 1989. "Gebissdeformation als 'Körperschmuck'—Verbreitung, Motive und Hintergründe," *Zahnärztliche Mitteilungen* 80 (22/90): 2448–2456.

Alt, Kurt W. and Sandra L. Pichler, 1998. "Artifical modifications on human teeth." In Kurt W. Alt, Friedrich W. Rösing, and Maria Teschler-Nicola, eds, *Dental Anthropology: Fundamentals, Limits, and Prospects*, 387–415. Vienna: Springer.

Alt, Kurt W., S. Rieger, W. Vach, and G. Krekeler, 1995. "Odontometrische Geschlechtsbestimmung. Evaluierung frümittelalterlicher Bestattungen," *Rechtsmedizin* 5: 82–87.

Alt, Kurt W., Friedrich W. Rösing, and Maria Teschler-Nicola (eds), 1998. *Dental Anthropology: Fundamentals, Limits, and Prospects*. Vienna: Springer.

Alt, Kurt W. and Werner Vach, 1998. "Kinship studies in skeletal remains: concepts and examples." In Kurt W. Alt, Friedrich W. Rösing, and Maria Teschler-Nicola, eds, *Dental Anthropology: Fundamentals, Limits, and Prospects*, 537–554. Vienna: Springer.

Amann, Petra, 2001. *Die Etruskerin. Geschlechterverhältnis und Stellung der Frau im frühen Etrurien (9.–5. Jr.v.Ch.)*. (Denkschriften der philologie-historisches Klasse, 289.) Archäologische Forshungen, 5. Rome: Giorgio Bretschneider.

Ampolo, Carmine, 1980. "Periodo IV B (con un contributo di Gilda Bartoloni)," *La Formazione della Città nel Lazio = Dialoghi di Archeologia* (New Series) 2: 165–192.

Ampolo, Carmine, 1984. "Il lusso funerario e la città antica," *Annali del Istituto Orientale— Napoli, Arch.* 6: 71–102.

Anderson, John G. and Keith Manchester, 1992. "The rhino-maxillary syndrome in leprosy: a clinical, radiological and paleopathological study," *International Journal of Osteoarchaeology* 2: 121–129.

Anderson, John G., Keith Manchester, and Charlotte Roberts, 1994. "Septic bone changes in leprosy: a clinical, radiological and paleopathological review," *International Journal of Osteoarchaeology* 4: 21–30.

André, Jacques, 1987. *Être médecin à Rome*. Paris: Société d'Edition "Les Belles Lettres".

André-Bonnet, J.-L., 1910. *Histoire générale de la chirurgie dentaire depuis les temps primitifs jusqu'à l'époque moderne*. First edition. Paris, Lyon and Marseille: Société des Auteurs Modernes and P.-C. Ash.

André-Bonnet, J.-L., 1955. *Histoire générale de la chirurgie dentaire depuis les temps primitifs jusqu'à l'époque moderne*. Second edition. Lyon: Fleuve.

Andrews, A. R., 1994. *Amulets of Ancient Egypt*. Austin, TX: University of Texas Press (London: British Museum Press).

Angeletti, L. R., R. Mariani-Costantini, U. Agrimi, and L. Frati, 1993. "Serpenti sacri e medicina teurgica nel mondo antico." In Luigi Capasso, ed., *Le Origini della Chirurgia Italiana*, 9–14. S. Atto Teramo: Officine Grafiche Edigrafital, for the Ministero dei Beni Culturali e Ambientali, Rome.

Anonymous (P. F.), 1987. "La médecine de la préhistoire au moyen-age," *Archeologia* 224 (May): 13–14.

Anonymous, 1994. "It's a black male thing," *New Yorker* May 16: 41.

Anonymous, 1997. "Breakthroughs in science, technology and medicine: archeology: a pre-Columbian cavity," *Discover* 18 (12): 24.

Anonymous, 1998a. "Beauty file: how do I look?" Style (section), *The Sunday Times* (London) March 8: 38.

Anonymous, 1998b. "Golden boy," *New Yorker* March 30: 108–109.

Apse, P., G. A. Zarb, A. Schmitt, and D. W. Lewis, 1991. "The longitudinal effectiveness of osseointegrated dental implants. The Toronto study: peri-implant muscosal response," *International Journal of Periodontics and Restorative Dentistry* 11 (2): 94–111.

Archivio Centrale, 1888. Min. P. I., AA.BB.AA., II. vers., I sezione, b. 231: Museo di Villa Giulia. Acquisiti 1888, fasc. 4000, documento sin numero. Archivio Centrale dello Stato a EUR (Roma).

Arcolani, Giovanni (Arculanus, Joannis), 1480. *Practica. Expositio noni libri Almansoris edita a clarissimo viro Joanne Arculano cive Veronensi*. Venice: Bernardium Stagninum de Tridino Monteferrato.

Arsuaga, J. L., J. M. Carretero, C. Lorenzo, A. Garcia, L. Martinez, J. M. Bermúdez de Castro, and E. Carbonell, 1997. "Size variation in Middle Pleistocene humans," *Science* 277: 1086–1088.

Arthur, Robert, 1854. *A Treatise on the Use of Adhesive Gold Foil*. Philadelphia, PA: Jones, White and McCurdy.

Asbell, Milton B., 1941. "The practice of dentistry among the ancient Hebrew: a contribution to the history of dentistry," *Journal of the American Dental Association* 28 (July): 1098–1107.

Asbell, Milton B., 1942. "The practice of dentistry among the ancient Hebrews," *The Hebrew Medical Journal* 1: 1–9 (text in English and Hebrew).

Asbell, Milton B., 1948. "Specimens of the dental art in ancient Phoenicia (fifth–fourth century BC)," *Bulletin of the History of Medicine* 22 (6): 812–821.

Ash, Major M. Jr. and Sigurd P. Ranfjord, 1982. *An Introduction to Functional Occlusion*. Philadelphia, PA: W. B. Saunders Co.

Athenaeus of Naucratis, 1927. *The Deipnosophists*, with an English translation by Charles Burton Gulick. London: W. Heinemann, Ltd.

Atilla, Gul, 1993. "A rare find in Anatolia: a tooth implant (mid-sixth century BC)," *Journal of Oral Implantology* 19 (1): 54–57.

Atteni, Luca, 2013. "The Pantanacci votive deposit: new anatomical discoveries," *Etruscan News* 15 (Winter): 1, 6.

Avivi-Arber, L. and G. A. Zarb, 1996. "Clinical effectiveness of implant-supported single-tooth replacement: the Toronto study," *International Journal of Oral and Maxillifacial Implants* 11 (3): 311–321.

Babbi, A., 2002. "Appliques e pendenti nuragici dalla Raccolta Comunale di Tarquinia." In O. Paoletti and L. Tamagno Perna, eds, *Etruria e Sardegna centro-settentrionale tra l'età del Bronzo Finale e l'arcaismo. Atti del XXI Convegno di Studi Etruschi ed Italici. Sassari-Alghero-Oristano-Torralba, 13–17 ottobre 1998*, 433–452. Pisa and Rome: Istituti Editoriali Poligrafici Internazionali.

Bachmann, H. G., 1995. "Gold analysis: from fire assay to spectroscopy—a review." In Giulio Morteani and Jeremy P. Northover, eds, *Prehistoric Gold in Europe. Mines Metallurgy and Manufacture*, 303–315. Dordrecht: Kluwer Academic. NATO ASI Series, Series E, Applied Sciences Volume 280.

Badre, Leila, 1986. "Machoire (No. 349)." In Eric Gubel, ed., *Les Pheniciens et Le Monde Méditerranéen* (exhibition catalogue), 266. Brussels: C. Coessens.

Badre, Leila, 2004. "93. Menschlicher Unterkiefer mit Golddrahthaterungen von gelockerten Zähnen." In Badisches Landesmuseum Karlsruhe (ed.), *Hannibal ad Portas—Macht und Reichtum Karthagos*, 292–293 (exhibition catalogue entry). Stuttgart: Konrad Theiss Verlag.

Baggieri, Gaspare, (ed.) 1996–1999. *L'Antica anatomia nell'arte dei donaria (Ancient Anatomy in the Art of Votive Offerings)*. Second edition of *"Speranza e Sofferenza" nei votive anatomici dell'antichità*. Rome: MelAMi. Reprint of exhibition catalogue.

Baggieri, Gaspare, 1998. "Appuntamento dal dentista etrusco," *Archeologia Viva* XVII, 70 (July–August): 66–69.

Baggieri, Gaspare, 1999. "Appointment with an Etruscan dentist," trans. and ed. Jane K. Whitehead, *Etruscan Studies* 6: 33–42.

Baggieri, Gaspare, 2001. "Le Protesi Dentarie Etrusche in Lega Aurea. Archeometallurgicia della Biocompatibilità," *Studi Etruschi* 64: 321–329.

Baggieri, Gaspare, 2005. *Odontoiatria dell'antichità in reperti osteo-dentari e archeologici*. Rome: MelAMi.

Baggieri, Gaspare and Luciana Allegrezza, 1994. "La protesi dentaria di Falerii Veteres," *Archeologia (Roma)* N.s. III (4/5): 4–5.

Baggieri, Gaspare and M. A. De Lucia, 1993. "Cenni di Odontoiatria Etrusca." In Luigi Capasso, ed., *Le Origini della Chirurgia Italiana*, 15–17. S. Atto Teramo: Officine Grafiche Edigrafital, for the Ministero dei Beni Culturali e Ambientali, Rome.

Baglione, Maria Paola, 1989. "Considerazioni sul 'ruolo' femminile nell'arcaismo e nel tardo arcaicmo." In A. Rallo, ed., *Le Donne in Etruria*, 107–119. Rome: "L'Erma" di Bretschneider (Studia Archeologica 52).

Baglioni, S., 1952. "Contributi alla conoscenza dell'arte dentaria àntica II," *Atti e Memorie dell'Accademia di Storia dell'Arte Sanitaria* (series 2) 18 (2): 14–74.

Bagnasco Gianni, G., 2013. "Tarquinia, sacred areas and sanctuaries on the Civita Plateau and on the coast: 'monumental complex,' Ara della Regina, Gravisca." In J. M. Turfa, ed., *The Etruscan World*, 594–612. London: Routledge.

Bailey, D. R. Shackleton, 1993. *Martial. Epigrams* (3 volumes). Cambridge, MA: Harvard University Press.

Baker, Patricia, 2004. "Roman medical instruments: archaeological interpretations of their possible 'non-functional' uses," *Social History of Medicine* 17: 3–21.

Ballér, P., 1992. "Medical thinking of the educated class in the Roman Empire: letters and writings of Plutarch, Fronto and Aelius Aristides." In A. Krug, ed., *From Epidaurus to Salerno (Ravello Symposium, 1990)*, 19–24. PACT 34.

Bannon, A. W., M. W. Decker, M. W. Holladay, P. Curzon, D. Donnelly-Roberts, P. S. Puttfarcken, R. S. Bitner, A. Diaz, A. H. Dickenson, R. D. Porsolt, M. Williams, and S. P. Arneric 1998. "Broad-spectrum, non-opioid analgesic activity by selective modulation of neuronal nicotinic acetylcholine receptors," *Science* 279: 77–81.

Bardinet, Thierry, 1990. "La Prothese Dentaire Au Temps des Pharaons: Mythe ou Realité?" *L'Information Dentaire* 29 (July 19): 2553–2555.

Bargellini, Sante, 1909. *Etruria meridionale*. Bergamo: Istituto italiano d'arte grafiche.

Barocchi, Paola and Daniela Gallo (eds), 1985. *L'Accademia etrusca*. Electa: Regione Toscana.

Bartels, Else M., Judith Swaddling, and Adrian P. Harrison, 2006. "An ancient Greek pain remedy for athletes," *Pain Practice* 6 (3): 212–218.

Bartoloni, Gilda, 1989. "Marriage, Sale and Gift. A proposito di alcuni corredi femminili dale necropolis populoniesi della prima età del ferro." In A. Rallo, ed., *Le Donne in Etruria*, 35–54. Rome: "L'Erma" di Bretschneider (Studia Archeologica 52).

Bartoloni, Gilda, 1991. "Populonia: characteristic features of a port community in Italy during the First Iron Age." In E. Herring, R. Whitehouse, and J. Wilkins, eds, *Papers of the Fourth Conference of Italian Archaeology [1990], Part 2. Archaeology of Power*, 101–115. London: Accordia Research Center.

Bartoloni, Gilda, 2006. "Madri di principi." In *Italo-Tusco-Romana: Festchrift für Luciana Aigner-Foresti zum 70. Geburtstag am 30. Juli 2006*, 13–22. Vienna: Holzhausen.

Bartoloni, Gilda, A. Berardinetti, and L. Drago, 2000. "Le communità della bassa valle tiberina e il Mediterraneo orientale prima della colonizzazzione greca." In F. Krinzinger, ed., *Die Ägäis und das westliche Mittelmeer. Beziehungen und Wechselwirkungen 8. bis 5. Jh.v.Chr. (Akten des Symposions Wien, 24. bis 27. März 1999)*, 525–533. Vienna: Österreichische Akademie der Wissenschaften.

Bartoloni, Gilda and Cristiano Grottanelli, 1989. "I carri a due ruote nelle tombe femminili del Lazio e dell'Etruria." In A. Rallo, ed., *Le Donne in Etruria*, 55–73. Rome: "L'Erma" di Bretschneider (Studia Archeologica 52).

Barton, Tamsyn, 1994. *Power and Knowledge: Astrology, Physiognomics, and Medicine in the Roman Empire*. Ann Arbor, MI: University of Michigan Press.

Baumann, Hellmut, 1993. *The Greek Plant World in Myth, Art and Literature*. Portland, OR: Timber Press.

Baumhammers, Andrejs, 1971. *Temporary and Semipermanent Splinting: An Atlas of Clinical Procedures*. Springfield, IL: Charles C. Thomas.

Bazzi, F., 1968. "La odontoiatria nell'opera di uno dei pionieri dell'arte dentaria," *Atti del XXI Congresso internazionale di storia della medicina, Siena, Italia, 22–28 settembre 1968*, 1: 855–867.

Beavis, Ian C., 1988. *Insects and Other Invertebrates in Classical Antiquity*. Exeter, UK: Exeter University Press.

Becker, Marshall Joseph, 1983. "Children's burials in Puglia from the Iron Age to the second century AD: cultural continuities," *Studi di Antichità* (Lecce) 4: 261–284.

Becker, Marshall Joseph, 1985. "Metric and non-metric data from a series of skulls from Mozia, Sicily and a related site," *Anthropologia Contemporanea* 8 (3): 211–228.

Becker, Marshall Joseph, 1988. "The contents of funerary vessels as clues to mortuary customs: identifying the *Os exceptum*." In Jette Christiansen and Torben Melander, eds, *Proceedings of the 3rd Symposium on Ancient Greek and Related Pottery (Copenhagen 1987)*, 25–32. Copenhagen: Nationalmuseet.

Becker, Marshall Joseph, 1990. "Etruscan social classes in the VI century BC: evidence from recently excavated cremations and inhumations in the area of Tarquinia." In Huberta Heres and Max Kunze, eds, *Die Welt der Etrusker: internationales Kolloquium, October 1988*, 23–35. Berlin: Akademie-Verlag.

Becker, Marshall Joseph, 1992a. "An Etruscan gold dental appliance in the collections of the Danish National Museum: evidence for the history of dentistry," *Tandlaegebladet: Danish Dental Journal* 96 (15): 695–700.

Becker, Marshall Joseph, 1992b. "Painful ostentation: decorative dental drilling among the classic period Maya of Central America before the coming of Columbus." Paper delivered at the session Pre-Columbian Science. Annual Meetings of the American Association for the Advancement of Science, Chicago, January 1992.

Becker, Marshall Joseph, 1992c. "Cultural uniformity during the Italian Iron Age: Sardinian Nuraghi as regional markers." In Robert H. Tykot and Tamsey K. Andrews, eds, *Sardinia in the Mediterranean: A Footprint in the Sea*, 204–209. Sheffield, UK: Sheffield Academic Press, Monographs in Mediterranean Archaeology 3.

Becker, Marshall Joseph, 1993a. "Human skeletons from Tarquinia: a preliminary analysis of the 1989 Cimitero site excavations with implications for the evolution of Etruscan social classes," *Studi Etruschi* 58: 211–248.

Becker, Marshall Joseph, 1993b. "Human sacrifice in Iron Age Italy: evidence from the 'Tombe Principesche,' numbers 926 and 928 at Pontecagnano (Salerno)," *Old World Archaeology Newsletter* 16 (2): 23–30.

Becker, Marshall Joseph, 1994a. "An analysis of the cremated human remains from Tomb XVII of the 1896 excavations at Satricum, Italy. Appendix 3.3." In Demetrius Waarsenburg, *The Northwest Necropolis at Satricum: An Iron Age cemetery in Latium Vetus*, 147–148. Doctoral Dissertation, Faculty of Letters, University of Amsterdam.

Becker, Marshall Joseph, 1994b. "Etruscan gold dental appliances: origins and functions as indicated by an example from Orvieto in the Danish National Museum," *Dental Anthropology Newsletter* 8(3): 2–8.

Becker, Marshall Joseph, 1994c. "Spurious 'examples' of ancient dental implants or appliances," *Dental Anthropology Newsletter* 9 (1): 5–10.

Becker, Marshall Joseph, 1994d. "Etruscan gold dental appliances: origins and functions as indicated by an example from Valsiarosa, Italy," *Journal of Paleopathology* 6 (2): 69–92.

Becker, Marshall Joseph, 1995a. "Female vanity among the Etruscans: the Copenhagen gold dental appliance." In Arthur C. Aufderheide, ed., *Actas del I Congreso Internacional de Estudios sobre Momias, 1992*, Volume II: 651–658. Santa Cruz de Tenerife: Museo Arqueologico y Etnologico de Tenerife.

Becker, Marshall Joseph, 1995b. "Human skeletal remains from the pre-colonial Greek Emporium of Pithecusa on Ischia (NA): culture contact in Italy from the early VIII to the II century BC." In Neil Christie, ed., *Settlement and Economy in Italy 1500 BC to AD 1500*, 273–281. Leicester, UK: Oxbow Monograph 41.

Becker, Marshall Joseph, 1995c. "Tooth evulsion among the ancient Etruscans: recycling in Antiquity," *Dental Anthropology Newsletter* 9 (3): 8–9.

Becker, Marshall Joseph, 1996. "An unusual Etruscan gold dental appliance from Poggio Gaiella, Italy. Fourth in a series," *Dental Anthropology Newsletter* 10 (3): 10–16.

Becker, Marshall Joseph, 1997. "Early dental appliances in the Eastern Mediterranean," *Berytus* 42 (1995–1996): 71–102.

Becker, Marshall Joseph, 1998a. "Etruscan gold dental appliances: evidence for cultural processes." In Antonio Guerci, ed., *Health and Diseases: Historical Routes, Volume 2 of the Proceedings of the 1st International Conference on Anthropology and History of Health and Disease*, 8–19. Genoa: Erga edizioni.

Becker, Marshall Joseph, 1998b. "The cremations in the Calabrese urn from Cerveteri and from other cinerary containers in the Museo Gregoriano Etrusco, Vatican Museums," *Bollettino—Monumenti, Musei e Gallerie Pontificie* XVIII: 57–73.

Becker, Marshall Joseph, 1999a. "Etruscan gold dental appliances: three newly 'discovered' examples in America," *American Journal of Archaeology* 103: 103–111.

Becker, Marshall Joseph, 1999b. "The Valsiarosa gold dental appliance: Etruscan origins for dental prostheses," *Etruscan Studies* 6: 43–73.

Becker, Marshall Joseph, 1999c. "Ancient 'dental implants': a recently proposed example from France evaluated with other claims," *International Journal of Oral and Maxillofacial Implants* 14: 19–29.

Becker, Marshall Joseph, 1999d. *Excavations in Residential Areas of Tikal: Groups with Shrines. Tikal Report 21*. Philadelphia, PA: The University Museum, University of Pennsylvania. University Museum Monograph 104.

Becker, Marshall Joseph, 1999e. "Calculating stature from in situ measurements of skeletons and from long bone lengths: an historical perspective leading to a test of Formicola's hypothesis at 5th century BCE Satricum, Lazio, Italy," *Rivista di Antropologia* (Rome) 77: 225–247.

Becker, Marshall Joseph, 2000a. "Reconstructing the lives of South Etruscan women." In Alison E. Rautman, ed., *Reading the Body: Representations and Remains in the Archaeological Record*, 55–67. Philadelphia, PA: University of Pennsylvania Press.

Becker, Marshall Joseph, 2000b. "Human skeletal remains recovered in the area of the Church of the Virgin Mary, Prague Castle, Czech Republic." In Jan Frolík, Jana Maříková-Kubkova, Eliška Růžičková and Antonín Zeman, *Nejstarší Sakrální Architektura Pražského Hradu*, 289–354. Prague: Peres (*Castrum Pragense*, Volume 3).

Becker, Marshall Joseph, 2000c. "Late roman skeletons from tombs of the fifth century CE at Metaponto (Basilicata) Italy," *Archaeological News* 23: 57–68.

Becker, Marshall Joseph, 2001. "Houselots at Tikal, Guatemala: it's what's out back that counts." In A. Ciudad Ruiz, M. J. Iglesias Ponce de León, and M. Carmen Martínez Martínez, eds, *Reconstruyendo la Ciudad Maya: El Urbanismo en las Sociedades Antiguas*, 427–460. Madrid: Publicaciones de la Sociedad Española de Estudias Mayas, No. 6.

Becker, Marshall Joseph, 2002a. "Etruscan female tooth evulsion: gold dental appliances as ornaments." In Gillian Carr and Patricia Baker, eds, *Practices, Practitioners and Patients: New Approaches to Medical Archaeology and Anthropology*, 236–257. Oxford: Oxbow Books.

Becker, Marshall Joseph, 2002b. "Etruscan tombs at Tarquinia: Heterarchy as indicated by human skeletal remains." In N. Negroni Catacchio, ed., *Paesaggi d'Acque—Ricerche a Scavi. Preistoria e Protostoria in Etruria: Atti del Quinto Encontro di Studi (12–14 May 2000)*, Volume II, 687–708. Milano: Onlus, for the Centro Studi di Preistoria e Archeologia.

Becker, Marshall Joseph, 2003. "Etruscan gold dental appliances: evidence for early 'parting' of gold in Italy through the study of ancient pontics." In Georges Tsoucaris and Janusz Lipkowski, eds, *Molecular and Structural Archaeology: Cosmetic and Therapeutic Chemicals*, 11–27. Dordrecht: Kluwer Academic (NATO Science Series, 117).

Becker, Marshall Joseph, 2004. "Etruscan skeletons of the Hellenistic period from the Casacce necropolis at Blera (Viterbo, Italy) excavated in 1982. Appendice II." In Gabriella Barbieri and Autori varie, (LAZIO) II. Blera (Viterbo). Località Casacce. *Necropoli rupestre di età ellenistica*, 175–189. *Notizie degli Scavi* (Serie IX) XIII–XIV (2002–2003): 89–190.

Becker, Marshall Joseph, 2005a. "Etruscan women at Tarquinia: skeletal evidence for tomb use," *Analecta Romana Instituti Danici* 31: 21–36.

Becker, Marshall Joseph, 2005b. "Cremations in five hut urns in the Museo Gregoriano Etrusco: implications for Iron Age cultural diversity." In Alessandro Mandolesi, *Materiale protostorico: Etruria et Latium Vetus*, 485–495. Cataloghi/Museo gregoriano etrusco, 9. Roma: "L'ERMA" di Bretschneider.

Becker, Marshall Joseph, 2006. "Etruscan women at Tarquinia: skeletal evidence for tomb use." (Abstracted from Becker 2005f, *Analecta Romana*). In Carol C. Mattusch, Alice A. Donohue, and Amy Brauer, eds, *Common Ground: Archaeology, Art, Science, and Humanities. Proceedings of the XVIth International Congress of Classical Archaeology*, 292–294. Boston, MA, August 23–26, 2003. Oxford: Oxbow Books.

Becker, Marshall Joseph, 2007. "Childhood among the Etruscans: mortuary programs at Tarquinia as indicators of the transition to adult status." In Ada Cohen and Jeremy B. Rutter, eds, *Constructions of Childhood in Ancient Greece and Italy*, 281–292. Hesperia, Supplement 41.

Becker, Marshall Joseph, 2008. "Grillz," *Anthropology News* 49 (5): 3.

Becker, Marshall Joseph, 2009. "Etruscan origins of pharmaceutical vessel shapes: four apothecary jars from Early Chiusi, Toscana, Italy." In Stefano Bruni, ed., *Etruria e Italia Preromana. Studi in onore di Giovannangelo Camporeale*, Volume I, 69–72. Rome: Fabrizio Serra Editore.

Becker, Marshall Joseph, 2011. "Etruscan infants: children's cemeteries at Tarquinia, Italy, as indicators of an age of transition." In Mike Lally and Alison Moore, eds, *(Re) Thinking the Little Ancestor: New Perspectives on the Archaeology of Infancy and Childhood*. BAR International Series 2271. Oxford: Archaeopress.

Becker, Marshall Joseph, 2012. "Coming of age in Etruria: Etruscan children's cemeteries at Tarquinia, Italy." *International Journal of Anthropology* 27 (1–2): 63–86.

Becker, Marshall Joseph, 2014. "Dentistry in ancient Rome: direct evidence based on the teeth from excavations at the Temple of Castor and Pollux in the Roman Forum," *International Journal of Anthropology* 29.4: 209–220.

Becker, Marshall Joseph, 2016, in press. "Spytihněv I (*c*.875–915), Duke of Bohemia: an osteobiographic perspective on social status and stature in the emerging Czech state." In Haagen D. Klaus, Mark N. Cohen, and Amanda Harvey, eds, *Bones of Complexity: Archaeological and Osteological Indicators of Prehistoric Heterarchy and Hierarchy*. Gainsville, FL: University Press of Florida.

Becker, Marshall Joseph, in press. "Human skeletal remains of the medieval period from the Farfa Abbey, Italy."

Becker, Marshall Joseph, n.d. a. "Two dental appliances in the Liverpool Museum and two in the Villa Giulia Museum, Rome." Field notes, May–June 1988.

Becker, Marshall Joseph, n.d. b. "The 'skull of Pliny' in the Museo Storico Nazionale dell'Arte Sanitaria, Rome." Field notes, 3 January 1991. Copy on file, West Chester University of Pennsylvania.

Becker, Marshall Joseph, n.d. c. "Deciduous molar retention among the Carthaginian colonists of Marsala, Sicily." Ms in process. Copy on file at West Chester University of Pennsylvania.

Becker, Marshall Joseph, n.d. d. "The *Os resectum*: evidence for the identification of one aspect of Roman funerary ritual from archaeological, anthropological, and epigraphical evidence." Ms on file, West Chester University of Pennsylvania.

Becker, Marshall Joseph, n.d. e. "Human skeletal remains of the fourteenth century from Burials along the Via S. Gerolamo, North of the apse of the deconsecrated Church of San Lorenzo, Cremona, Italy." Ms on file, Becker Archives, West Chester University of Pennsylvania.

Becker, Marshall Joseph, n.d. f. "The dental appliances used by President George Washington and by His Wife Martha." Paper on file, Becker archives, West Chester University of Pennsylvania.

Becker, Marshall Joseph and Alessia Donadio, 1992. "A summary of the analysis of cremated human skeletal remains from the Greek colony of Pithekoussai at Lacco Ameno, Ischia, Italy," *Old World Archaeology Newsletter* 16 (1): 15–23.

Becker, Marshall Joseph and Loretana Salvadei, 1992. "Analysis of the human skeletal remains from the Cemetery of Osteria dell'Osa." In Anna Maria Bietti Sestieri, ed., *Osteria dell'Osa*, 53–191. Rome: Quasar.

Becker, Marshall Joseph, MacIntosh Turfa, and B. Algee-Hewitt, 2009. *Human Remains from Etruscan and Italic Tomb Groups in the University of Pennsylvania Museum* (Biblioteca di Studi Etruschi 48). Pisa/Rome: Fabrizio Serra.

Bellagarda, Giorgio, 1965. "Antiche techniche nell'estrazione dei denti," *Minerva medica* 56: 892–900.

Belzoni, Giovanni B., 1820. *Narrative of the Operations and Recent Discoveries within the Pyramids, Temples, Tombs and Excavations in Egypt and Nubia.* London: John Murray.

Benedictine Monks (compilers), 1989. *The Book of Saints.* Sixth edition. Wilton, CT: Morehouse Publishing Company.

Benelli, Enrico, 2002. "Le formule onomastiche della *Tabula Cortonensis* e il valore del metronimico." In *La Tabula Cortonensis e il suo contest storico-archeologico. Atti del Incontro di studio 22 giugno 2001*, 93–100. (*Quaderni di Archeologia Etrusco-Italica* 28) Rome: Consiglio Nazionale delle Ricerche.

Benelli, Enrico, 2016. "Female slaves and slave-owners in ancient Etruria." In S. L. Budin and J. M. Turfa, eds, *Women in Antiquity: Real Women Across the Ancient World.* London: Routledge, 877–882.

Benner, Elisabeth, 1979. *Antique Medical Instruments.* Sotheby Parke Bernet: University of California Press.

Bennett, Storer, 1885. "Paper at the meetings of the Odontological Society of Great Britain on 'The Herbst Metho'," *Journal of the British Dental Association* 6: 28–31.

Bennike, Pia, 1985. *Paleopathology of Danish Skeletons: A Comparative Study of Demography, Disease and Injury.* Copenhagen: Akademisk Forlag.

Bennike, Pia and Lise Fredebo, 1986. "Dental treatment in the Stone Age," *Bulletin of the History of Dentistry* 34 (2): 81–87 (reprinted from *Tandlaegebladet, The Danish Dental Journal*, 1985, 89, number 12).

Bert, M., 1987. "Les implants lames," *Actualites Odonto-Stomatologiques* 159: 507–520.

Bertolino, V., 1955. "Nuovi studi sulla protesi dentaria fenicia," *Minerva Stomatologica* 4 (1): 30–32.

Bietti Sestieri, Anna Maria, 1992a. *The Iron Age Community of Osteria dell'Osa: A Study of Socio-Political Development in Central Tyrrhenian Italy.* Cambridge: Cambridge University Press.

Bietti Sestieri, Anna Maria, (ed.), 1992b. *La Necropoli Laziale di Osteria dell'Osa.* Rome: Quasar.

Biggs, Robert D., 1969. "Medicine in ancient Mesopotamia," *History of Science* 8: 94–105.

Billson, Charles James (ed.), 1895. *County Folk-Lore: Printed Extracts, No. 3. Leicestershire and Rutland. Issued by the Folk-Lore Society, Publication 37.* London: D. Nutt.

Bliquez, Lawrence, 1983. "Classical prosthetics," *Archaeology* 36: 25–29.

Bliquez, Lawrence, 1985. "Two lists of Greek surgical instruments and the state of surgery in Byzantine Times." In John Scarborough, ed., *Symposium on Byzantine Medicine*, 187–204. Dumbarton Oaks Papers, No. 38. Dumbarton Oaks Research Library and Collection. Washington, DC.

Bliquez, Lawrence, 1986. "Review of *Die Arzthäuser in Pompeii* (1984), by H. Eschebach," *Bulletin of the History of Medicine* 60: 116–117.

Bliquez, Lawrence, 1988. Review of *Eine Serie von Fälschungen römischer medizinischer Instrumentarien* by E. Künzl (1986), *Newsletter: Society for Ancient Medicine and Pharmacy* 16: 64–65.

Bliquez, Lawrence, 1994. *Roman Surgical Instruments and Other Minor Objects in the National Archaeological Museum of Naples.* Mainz: Philipp Von Zabern.

Bliquez, Lawrence, 1996. "Prosthetics in Classical Antiquity: Greek, Etruscan, and Roman prosthetics." In W. Haase, ed., *Aufstieg und Niedergang der römischen Welt. Teil II: Principat.* 37(3): 2640–2676. Berlin: De Gruyter.

Bliquez, Lawrence, 2015. *The Tools of Asclepius: Surgical Instruments in Greek and Roman Times.* Leiden: Brill. (A revision of J. S. Milne's (1907) Classic Study.)

Blumenbach, Johann-Friedrich, 1780. "Von den Zähnen der alten Aegyptier und von den Mumien," *Göttingisches Magazin der Wissenschaften und Litteratur* 1: 109–139.

Boardman, Sir John, 1980. *The Greeks Overseas: Their Early Colonies and Trade.* New and enlarged edition. London: Thames and Hudson.

Bobbio, Amedeo, 1958. "Excurso Histórico da Prótese Dental Fenícia, Etrusca e Romana," *Revista da Associacão Paulista dos Cirurgiões Dentistas* 12 (6): 360–374.

Böttiger, Carl, 1797. *Griechische Vasengemälde. Mit archäologischen und artistischen Erläuterungen der Originalkupfer. Ersten Bandes, Erster Heft.* Weimar: Industriecomptoir. (IV Nachrichten über die griechischen Vasen aus Briefen von Tischbein und Meyer (January 3, 1796: Naples).

Boissier, R., 1927. *L'evolution de l'Art Dentaire de l'antiquité à nos jours.* Paris: La Semaine dentaire.

Boissier, R., 1936. "L'art dentaire dans l'antiquité." In Maxime Laignel-Lavastine, ed., *Histoire Général de la Mèdicine*, Volume 1 of 3, 609–616. Paris: Albin Michel.

Bonet, V., 1995. "Les animaux occidentaux dans la pharmacopée de Pline." In *Homme et animal dans l'antiquité romaine*, 163–172. Actes of the Colloquium at Nantes, *Caesarodunum*, special number.

Bonfante, Larissa, 1981. "Etruscan couples and their aristocratic society," *Women in Antiquity. Women's Studies* 8 (1981) 157–187.

Bonfante, Larissa, 1984. "The women of Etruria." In John Peradotto and J. P. Sullivan, eds, *Women in the Ancient World: The Arethusa Papers*, 229–239. Albany, NY: State University of New York Press.

Bonfante, Larissa, 1986. "Daily life and afterlife." In Larissa Bonfante, ed., *Etruscan Life and Afterlife*, 232–278. Detroit, MI: Wayne State University Press.

Bonfante, Larissa, 1994. "Excursus: Etruscan women." In E. Fantham, H. P. Foley, N. B. Kampen, S. B. Pomeroy, and H. A. Shapiro, *Women in the Classical World*, 243–259. Oxford: Oxford University Press.

Bonfante, Larissa, 1995. "Etruscan sexuality and funerary art." In Natalie Boymel Kampen (with Bettina Bergman, Ada Cohen, and Eva Steh), eds, *Sexuality in Ancient Art: Near East, Egypt, Greece, and Italy*, 155–169. New York: Cambridge University Press.

Bonfante, Larissa, 1997. "Nursing mothers in Classical art." In A. O. Koloski Ostrow and C. L. Lyons (eds), *Naked Truths: Women, Sexuality, and Gender in Classical Art and Archaeology*, 174–196. London and New York: Routledge.

Bonfante, Larissa, 2003 (1875). *Etruscan Dress.* Updated edition. Baltimore, MD: Johns Hopkins.

Bonfante, Larissa, 2013. "Mothers and children." In J. M. Turfa, ed., *The Etruscan World*, 426–446. London: Routledge.

Bonfante, Larissa and Giuliano Bonfante, 2002. *The Etruscan Language: An Introduction.* Manchester: Manchester University Press.

Bonner, Campbell, 1950. *Studies in Magical Amulets, Chiefly Graeco-Egyptian.* Ann Arbor, MI: University of Michigan Press.

Borgonini Tarli, Silvana and Elena Repetto, 1985. "Antropologia dentaria nella Preistoria." In *Storia dell Odontoiatria*, 11–33. Milano: Ars Medica Antigua Editrice.

Boyer, Peter J., 2001. "Man of faith: can Jesse Jackson save himself?" *The New Yorker* October 22: 50–65.

Bradley, David, 1993. "Frog venom cocktail yields a one-handed painkiller," *Science* 261: 1117.

Bradley, Keith, 1998. "The Roman family at dinner." In Inge Nielsen and Hanne Sigismund Nielsen, eds, *Meals in a Social Context*, 36–55. Aarhus: Aarhus University Press.

Brånemark, P.-I., U. Breine, R. Adell, B. O. Hansson, J. Lindstöm, and A. Ohlsson, 1969. "Intra-osseous anchorage of dental prostheses," *Scandinavian Journal of Plastic and Reconstructive Surgery* 3: 81–100.

Brånemark, P.-I., B. O. Hansson, R. Adell, U. Breine, J. Lindstöm, O. Hallén, and A. Ohman, 1977. "Osseointergrated implants in the treatment of the edentulous jaw: experience from a 10-year period," *Scandinavian Journal of Plastic and Reconstructive Surgery Supplementum* 16, Stockholm: Almqvist and Wiksell.

Braun, August Emil, 1841 (1840). *Il laberinto di Porsenna, comparato coi sepolcri di Poggio-Gajella, ultimamente dissotterrati nell Agro Clusino.* Rome: A. Monaldi.

Braun, August Emil, 1855. "Scavi di Palestrina [letter to Pietro Cicerchia Rossi, from Braun]," *Bullettino dell'Instituto di Corrispondenza Archeologica* XI, XII: XLV–XLVIII.

Brendel, Otto J. 1995. *Etruscan Art.* New Haven, CT: Yale University Press (1995 edition with E. H. Richardson and F. R. Serra Ridgway; original edition 1978).

Briggs, L. Cabot, 1955. "The Stone Age races of Northwest Africa," *Bulletin of the American School of Prehistoric Research* 18: 1–98. Cambridge, MA: Harvard University, Peabody Museum.

Briggs, L. Cabot and M.-L. Margolis, 1951. "Remarques sur la coutume d'avulsion dentaire chez les peuples préhistoriques de l'Africa du Nord et du Sahara." In *Association Française pour l'Avancement des Sciences: Congrés de Tunis (9–16 Mai)* 1: 115–122.

Briquel, Dominique, 2013. "Etruscan origins and the ancient authors." In J. M. Turfa, ed., *The Etruscan World*, 36–55 [885–902]. London: Routledge.

Brothwell, Don R., 1963. *Digging up Bones: The Excavation, Treatment and Study of Human Skeletal Remains.* London: Trustees of the British Museum.

Brothwell, Don R., 1988. "Foodstuffs, cooking, and drugs." In Michel Grant and Rachel Kitzinger, eds, *Civilization of the Ancient Mediterranean*, Volume II, 247–264. New York: Charles Scribner.

Brothwell, D. R. and H. G. Carr, 1962. "The dental health of the Etruscans," *British Dental Journal* 113 (4): 207–210.

Brown, Lawrence Parmly, 1933. "Teeth in Museum of Alexandria," *International Dentistry* VI (23): 584.

Brown, Lawrence Parmly, 1934. "The antiquities of dental prosthesis (part I: to the close of the fifteenth century; part II: sixteenth and seventeenth centuries; part III: sections I and II)," *Dental Cosmos* 76: 828–836, 957–966, 1078–1084, 1155–1165.

Brown, Lawrence Parmly, 1936. "Appellations of the dental practitioner," *Dental Cosmos* 78: 246–258, 378–389, 481–495.

Brun, Robert, 1923. "Quelques italiens d'Avignon au XIVe siècle, II. Nadino da Prato, médecin de la cour pontificale," *Mélanges d'Archéologie et d'Histoire École Française de Rome* 40: 219–236.

Brunner, T. F., 1973. "Marijuana in ancient Greece and Rome? The literary evidence," *Bulletin of the History of Medicine* 47: 344–355.

Buccellato, A., P. Catalano, S. Musco, con la collaborazione di: C. Caldarini, G. Colonnelli, G. Fornaciari, M. Grandi, S. Minozzi, W. Pantano, C. Torri, and F. Zabotti, 2008. "Alcuni aspetti rituali evidenziati nel corso dello scavo della necropoli Collatina (Roma)." In John Scheid, ed., *Pour une archéologie du rite. Nouvelles perspectives de l'archéologie funéraire*, 59–88. Rome: Collection De L'École Française De Rome.

Buchner, Giorgio, 1979. "Early orientalizing: aspects of the Euboean connection [after 'Contributions à l'étude de la société et de la colonisation eubéennes' Naples 1975]." In David Ridgway and Francesca R. Ridgway, eds, *Italy Before the Romans: The Iron Age, Orientalizing and Etruscan Periods*, 129–144. New York: Academic Press.

Buchner, Giorgio and David Ridgway, 1993. *Pithekoussai I*, in 3 parts. *Monumenti Antichi* (Accademia Nazionale dei Lincei) Serie Monografica Volume IV (LV della Serie Generale). Rome: Giorgio Bretschneider.

Budge, E. A. W., 1913. *Syrian Anatomy, Pathology and Therapeutics*. London: Humphrey Milford.

Buerki, Robert A., 1988. "Caleb Taylor, Philadelphia druggist, 1812–1820: a preliminary analysis," *Pharmacy in History* 30: 81–88.

Caccioli, David A., "Kantharos or flower? Etruscan urn figures as indicators of romanization [abstract]," *American Journal of Archaeology* 105: 256.

Caelius Aurelianus, 1950. *On Acute Diseases and On Chronic Diseases*, trans. and ed. I. E. Drabkin. Chicago, IL: University of Chicago Press.

Cali, Giuseppe, 1901. *L'odontoiatria attraverso i secoli*. Naples: Tipografia dell'Unione.

Camporealef, Giovannangelo, ed., 2001. *Gli Etruschi fuori Etruria*. Verona: Arsenale.

Camporeale, Giovannangleo, 2013. "Foreign artists in Etruria." In J. M. Turfa, ed., *The Etruscan World*, 885–902. London: Routledge.

Cannizzaro, M., 1901. *Il cranio di Plinio*. London: Private edition.

Capasso, Luigi, 1985. "Dental pathology and alimentary habits reconstruction of Etruscan population [sic]," *Studi Etruschi* 53: 177–191.

Capasso, Luigi, 1986. "Etruria: Le Meraviglie dei Dentisti." In *La Medicina nell'Antichità = Archeo Dossier* (Novara) 13: 52–55.

Capasso, Luigi, ed., 1993. *Le Origini della Chirurgia Italiana*. S. Atto Teramo: Officine Grafiche Edigrafital, for the Ministero di Bene Culturale e Ambientale, Rome.

Capasso, Luigi, 2001. *I Fuggiaschi di Ercolano: Paleobiologia delle vittime dell'eruzione vesuviana del 79 d.C.* Rome; L'Erma di Bretschneider.

Capasso, Luigi and Gabriella Di Tota, 1993. "Etruscan teeth and odontology," *Dental Anthropology Newsletter* 8 (1): 4–7.

Carabelli, Georg, 1831. *Systematisches Handbuch der Zahnheilkunde*. Vienna: A. Doll & Baumüller & Seidel (Volume 1: 1831; Volume 2, with the subtitle "Anatomie des Mundes," was published in 1842). These volumes were reprinted in Leipzig by Zentralantiquariat der DDR, 1983.

Carroll, Diane Lee, 1970. "Drawn wire and the identification of forgeries in ancient jewelry," *American Journal of Archaeology* 74: 401.

Carroll, Diane Lee, 1972. "Wire drawing in antiquity," *American Journal of Archaeology* 76 (3): 321–323.

Casotti, Luigi, 1927. "Storia della protesi dentaria," *La Cultura Stomatologica* Anno IV (XII): 624–644.

Casotti, Luigi, 1933. "Impronte e portaimpronte," *La Stomatologia* 31: 36–58.

Casotti, Luigi, 1935. "Evoluzione della protesi dentaria." In *La Stomatologia in Italia* (Anno I–Fasc. VI Dicembre 1935–XIV), 28–48. Published in *Acta Medica Italica*.

Casotti, Luigi, 1947. "L'Odontotecnica degli Etruschi," *Rivista Italiana di Stomatologia* 2 (8): 661–678.

Casotti, Luigi, 1953. "Fenici, Ebrei ed arte dentaria," *Minerva Stomatologica* 2 (5): 237–238.

Casotti, Luigi, 1956. "Ouro e prótese junto aos Egípcios," trans. Amedeo Bobbio, *Revista da Associacão Paulista dos Cirurgiões Dentistas* 10 (3): 174–175.

Casotti, Luigi, 1957. "Vetulonia Etrusca e Stomatologia," *Rivista Italiana di Stomatologia* 12 (1): 97–112.

Casotti, Luigi, 1958. "Vetulonia: Etruscan dentistry," *Dental Abstracts* 3: 535–536.

Castorina, Alessandra, 1998. "Copia grande di antichi sepolcri. Sugli scavi delle necropoli in Italia meridionale tra Settecento e inizio Ottocento," *Rivista dell'Istituto Nazionale d'Archeologia e Storia dell'Arte* (series III, XIX–XX) 1996–1997: 305–344.

Catalano, Paola, Simona Minozzi, Stefano Musco, Gino Fornaciari (con la collaborazione di C. Caldarini, G. Colonnelli, G. Fornaciari, M. Grandi, S. Minozzi, W. Pantano, C. Torri, and F. Zabotti), 2007. "Le prime evidenze di odontotecnica nella Roma Imperiale: una protesi dentaria in oro rinvenuta in una tomba monumentale," (poster) *XVII Congresso dell'Associazione Antropologica Italiana, 26–29 Settembre 2007*, Cagliari.

Cataldi, Maria, 1993. *Tarquinia*. Rome: Quasar (for Regione Lazio Assessorato alla Cultura).

Cavenago, V., 1933. "Scienza ed arte dentaria nell'antichità mediterranea," *La Stomatologia* 31: 58–87.

Cederna, A. 1951 "Carsoli," *Notizie degli Scavi* 218–221.

Celsus, Aulus Cornelius, 1938. *De medicina* (8 books), trans. W. G. Spencer. Volume 3 (Loeb Classical Library No. 336). London: William Heinemann.

Cesaro, Roberto and F. W. von Hase, 1973. "Non-destructive radioisotope XRF analysis of early Etruscan gold objects," *Kerntechnik* 15 (12): 565–571.

Chandler, N. P., 1989. "Operative dentistry in the second century BCE," *Paleopathology Newsletter* 68: 11–12.

Chandler, N. P. and D. M. Fyfe, 1997. "Root canals of buried teeth: radiographic change due to crystal growth," *International Journal of Osteoarchaeology* 7 (1): 11–17.

Channing, Johannis (ed.), 1778. *Albucasis de Chirurgia. Arabice et Latine*. Oxford: Clarendon.

Chemant (see Dubois de Chemant).

Chohayeb, A., 1991. "The dental heritage of ancient Egypt," *Bulletin of the History of Dentistry* 39: 65–69.

Chu, Hsi-T'ao, 1958. "The use of amalgam as filling material in dentistry in ancient China," *Chinese Medical Journal* 76: 553–555.

Ciarallo, A., 1993. "L'uso delle piante nella pratiche mediche di epoca romana." In Luigi Capasso, ed., *Le Origini della Chirurgia Italiana*, 49–53. S. Atto Teramo: Officine Grafiche Edigrafital, for the Ministero di Bene Culturale e Ambientale, Rome.

Ciasca, Raffaele, 1927. *L'arte dei medici e speziali*. Biblioteca Toscana, Volume IV. Florence: Leo S. Olschki.

Cicero, 1928. *De Re Publica; De Legibus*, trans. Clinton W. Keyes. London: William Heinemann.

Cigrand, Bernard J., 1892. *The Rise, Fall and Revival of Dental Prosthesis*. Chicago, IL: Severinghaus.

Cigrand, Bernard J., 1893. *The Rise, Fall and Revival of Dental Prosthesis*. Second, revised and enlarged edition. Chicago, IL: Periodical Publishing House.

Clawson, M. Don, 1933. "A Phoenician dental appliance of the 5th century BC," *Transactions of the American Dental Society of Europe* [for the year] 1933," 142–160.

Clawson, M. Don, 1934. "Phoenician dental art," *Berytus* 1: 23–31.

Cohen, R. A., 1959. "Methods and materials used for artificial teeth, [abridged]," *Proceedings of the Royal Society of Medicine* 52: 775–786.

Cohen, R. A., 1962. "Notes on the identification, description and dating of ivory dentures," *British Dental Journal* 115: 259–263.

Colonna, Giovanni, 1974. "Preistoria e Protostoria di Roma e del Lazio." In Bruno d'Agostino, Paolo Enrico Arias, and Giovanni Colonna, eds, *Popoli e Civiltà dell'Italia Antica*, Volume 2, 275–346. Rome: Biblioteca di Storia Patria.

Colonna, Giovanni, 1977. "Un aspetto oscuro del Lazio antico: Le Tombe del VI–V secolo a. C.," *La Parola del Passato* 174: 131–165.

Colonna, Giovanni, 1988. "La produzione artigianale." In A. Momigliano and A. Schiavone, eds, *Storia di Roma*, Volume I: 291–316. Turin: Einaudi.

Colonna, G. 1993. "Ceramisti e donne padrone di bottega nell'Etruria arcaica." In G. Meiser, ed., *Indogermanica et Italica. Festschrift fur Helmut Rix zum 65. Geburtstag*, 61–68. Innsbruck: Institut fur Sprachwissenschaft.

Colyer, Sir Frank, 1952. *Old Instruments Used for Extracting Teeth*. London: Staples Press.

Connell, Brian, 2012. "Dental disease." In Brian Connell, Amy Gray Jones, Rebecca Redfern, and Don Walker, *A Bioarchaeological Study of Medieval Burials at the Site of St. Mary Spital*, 40–60. (MOLA Monograph 60.) London: Museum of London Archaeology.

Connor, Walter Robert, 1968. *Theopompus and Fifth-Century Athens*. Washington, DC: Center for Hellenic Studies.

Conrad, Lawrence, Michael Neve, Roy Porter, Vivian Nutton, and Andrew Wear, 1995. *The Western Medical Tradition: 800 BC–1800 AD*. Cambridge: Cambridge University Press.

Cook, D. C., 1981. "Koniag Eskimo tooth ablation: was Hrdlicka right after all?" *Current Anthropology* 22: 159–163.

Cornell, Tim and Kathryn Lomas (eds), 1995. *Gender and Ethnicity in Ancient Italy* (Specialist Studies on Italy 6). Accordia Research Institute: University of London.

Corruccini, Robert S. and Elsa Pacciani, 1989. "'Orthodontistry' and dental occlusion in Etruscans," *Angle Orthodontist* 59 (1): 61–64.

Corruccini, Robert S. and Elsa Pacciani, 1991. "Ortodonzia e Occlusione Dentale negli Etrusci," *Studi Etruschi* 57: 189–194.

Cowell, M., 1977. "Energy dispersive X-ray fluorescence analysis of ancient gold alloys." In *PACT: revue du Groupe européen d'études pour les techniques physiques, chimiques et mathématiques appliquées à l'archéologie*. PACT I, 76–85. Strasbourg: Conseil de l'Europe, Assemblée parlementaire.

Cozza, A. and A. Pasqui, 1981. *Carta Archeologica D'Italia (1881–1897): Materiali per Agro Falisco. Forma Italiae, Serie II, Documenti 2*. Florence: Leo S. Olschki for Unione Accademica Nazionale.

Craddock, Paul T., 2000a. "Historical survey of gold refining: 1. Surface treatments and refining worldwide, and in Europe Prior to AD 1500." In Andrew Ramage and Paul

Craddock, eds, *King Croesus' Gold: Excavations at Sardis and the History of Gold Refining*, 27–53. Cambridge: Archaeological Exploration of Sardis (with the British Museum). Archaeological Exploration of Sardis Monograph Series, 11.

Craddock, Paul T., 2000b. "Replication experiments and the chemistry of gold refining." In Andrew Ramage and Paul Craddock, eds, *King Croesus' Gold: Excavations at Sardis and the History of Gold Refining*, 175–183. Cambridge: Archaeological Exploration of Sardis (with the British Museum). Archaeological Exploration of Sardis Monograph Series, 11.

Craddock, Paul T., 2000c. "Early history of the amalgamation process, the platinum group element inclusions, assaying in antiquity." In Andrew Ramage and Paul Craddock, eds, *King Croesus' Gold: Excavations at Sardis and the History of Gold Refining*, 233–250. Cambridge: Archaeological Exploration of Sardis (with the British Museum). Archaeological Exploration of Sardis Monograph Series, 11.

Craddock, Paul T., 2009. *Scientific Investigation of Copies, Fakes and Forgeries.* Amsterdam: Butterworth-Heinemann (Elsevier).

Crawfurd, Raymond, 1914. "Martial and medicine," *Proceedings of the Royal Society of Medicine. Section: History of Medicine* (December 3, 1913, London) 7: 15–29.

Cristofani, Mauro, 1983. "Introduzione." In Mauro Cristofani and Marina Martelli, eds, *L'oro degli Etruschi*, 8–16. Novara: Istituto Geografico De Agostini.

Cristofani, Mauro, 1994. "Un etrusco a Egina," *Studi Etruschi* 59 (1993): 159–162.

Cristofani, Mauro and Marina Martelli (eds), 1983. *L'Oro degli Etruschi*. Novara: Istituto Geografico De Agostini.

Crubézy, E., L. G. Pascal Murail and J.-P. Bernadou, 1998. "False teeth of the Roman world," *Nature* 391: 29.

Cucina, A., R. Macchiarelli, L. Bondioli, J. F. Jarrige, and A. Coppa, 2001. "Human molar drillings in the 8th millennium BC Neolithics [sic] from Mehrgarh, Pakistan: First cases of dental care?" American Association of Physical Anthropology, Meeting Abstracts. March.

Cuozzo, Mariassunta, 2013. "Etruscans in Campania." In J. M. Turfa, ed., *The Etruscan World*, 301–318. London: Routledge.

Cüppers, Heinz, 1981. *Kranken- und Gesundheitspflege in Trier und dem Trierer Land von der Antike bis zur Neuzeit.* Trier: Selbstverlag Rheinisches Landesmuseum.

Czarnetzki, Alfred, and S. Ehrhardt, 1990. "Re-dating the Chinese amalgam-filling of teeth in Europe," *International Journal of Anthropology* 5: 325–332.

Czarnetzki, Alfred, and Kurt W. Alt, 1991. "Eine Frontzahnbrüke aus Flusspferdzahn— Deutschlands älteste Prothese?" *Zahnärztztliche Mitteilungen* 81: 216–219.

Dall'Osso, C., 1907. "Gli Etruschi e l'odontojatria," *Rivista Italiana di Odontojatria* 4 (1): 62–66.

Dalton, Van Broadus, 1946. *Genesis of Dental Education in the United States.* Columbus, OH: Spahr and Glenn.

Darenburg, C. and E. Saglio, 1918. *Dictionnaire des antiquités grecques et romaines d'aprés les textes et les monuments*, Volume III/2: p. 1679. Paris: Hachette.

Dasti, Luigi, 1877. Letter to W. Helbig (see under Helbig 1877).

Dasti, Luigi, 1878. *Notizie Storiche archeologiche di Tarquinia e Corneto.* Rome: Tipografia dell'Opinione.

D'Atri, Valeria and Piero Alfredo Gianfrotta, 1986. "Un Relitto con Dolia a Ladispoli," *Bollettino D'Arte Supplemento* 203–208.

Davide, D., 1972. "Survey of the skeletal and mummy remains of ancient Egyptians available in research collections," *Journal of Human Evolution* 1: 155–159.

Davies, Glenys, 1977. "Burial in Italy up to Augustus." In Richard Reece, ed., *Burial in the Roman World*, 13–19. London: Council for British Archaeology.

Davies, Malcomb and Jeyayaney Kathirithamby, 1986. *Greek Insects*. London: Duckworth.

Davies, Roy W., 1970. "The Roman medical service," *Saalburg-Jahrbuch* 27: 84–104.

Davies, Roy W., 1972. "Some more military medici," *Epigraphische Studien, Sammelband* 9: 1–11.

Dawson, Warren R., 1923. "Egyptian medicine under the copts in the early centuries of the Christian era," *Proceedings of the Royal Society of Medicine, Section of History of Medicine (London)* 17: 50–57.

Dawson, Warren R., 1935. "Studies in the Egyptian medical texts: V," *Journal of Egyptian Archaeology* 21: 37–40.

Dawson, Warren R., 1938. "Review of *The Papyrus Ebers: The Greatest Egyptian Medical Document*, trans. B. Ebbell (1937)," *Journal of Egyptian Archaeology* 24: 250–251.

Dawson, Warren R., 1953. "Egypt's place in medical history." In Edgar Ashworth Underwood, ed., *Science, Medicine, and History*, Volume I: 47–60. London: Oxford University Press.

Dawson, Warren R. and P. H. K. Gray, 1968. *Catalogue of Egyptian Antiquities in the British Museum I. Mummies and Human Remains*. London: Trustees of the British Museum.

de Angelis, Francesco, 2013. "The reception of Etruscan culture: Dempster and Buonarotti." In J. M. Turfa, ed., *The Etruscan World*, 1130–1135. London: Routledge.

de Chauliac, Guy, 1363 (manuscript). *La Grande Chirugie* de M. Guy de Chauliac, medicin tres-fameux de l'Université de Montpellier, composé l'an de grâce 1363. Restituée par M. Laurens Ioubert. Tournon: Claude Michel, 1598.

Dechaume, Michel and Pierre Huard, 1977. *Histoire Illustrée de l'Art Dentaire. Stomatologie et Odontologie*. Paris: Editions Roger Dacosta. (Italian translation, 1988: *Storia Illustrata dell'Arte Dentaria. Odontoiatria e Stomatologia*. Saronno, Varese: Ciba-Geigy edizione.

Dechaume, Michel and Pierre Huard, 1988. *Storia Illustrata dell'Arte Dentaria. Odontoiatria e Stomatologia*. Saronno, Varese, Italy: Ciba-Geigy edizione. Translated from *Histoire Illustrée de l'Art Dentaire* (1984). Editions Roger Dacoste.

De Forest, Mary (ed.), 1993. *Woman's Power, Man's Game: Essays on Classical Antiquity in Honor of Joy M. King*. Wauconda, IL: Bolchazy-Carducci.

de Gérauldy, Claude Jaquier, 1737. *L'art de Conserver les dents: Ouvrage utile & necessaire*. Paris: P. G. Le Mercier.

Della Seta, Alessandro, 1918. "Satricum [pages 233–320]," and "Praeneste [page 444]." In *Museo di Villa Giulia* (catalogue). Rome: Danesi editore.

Della Seta, Alessandro, 1928. *Italia Antica dalla caverna preistorica al Palazzo imperiale*. Bergamo: Istituto italiano d'arte grafiche.

Delpino, F. 2002. "Brocchette a collo oblique dall'area etrusca." In O. Paoletti and L. Tamagno Perna, eds, *Etruria e Sardegna centro-settentrionale tra l'età del Bronzo Finale e l'arcaismo. Atti del XXI Convegno di Studi Etruschi ed Italici. Sassari-Alghero-Oristano-Torralba, 13–17 ottobre 1998*, 363–385. Pisa and Rome: Istituti Editoriali Poligrafici Internazionali.

De Lucia Brolli, Maria Anna, 1991. *Civita Castellana. Il Museo Archeologico dell'Agro Falisco*. Rome: Quasar.

De Lucia Brolli, Maria Anna, and Jacopo Tabolli, 2013. "The Faliscans and the Etruscans." In J. M. Turfa, ed., *The Etruscan World*, 259–280. London: Routledge, 259–280.

de Marinis, S., 1961. *La tipologia del banchetto nell'arte etrusca arcaica*. Rome: "L'Erma" di Bretschneider.

Demetriou, Denise, 2012. *Negotiating Identity in the Ancient Mediterranean: The Archaic and Classical Multiethnic Emporia*. Cambridge: Cambridge University Press.

Demortier, Guy, 1986. "LARN experience in nondestructive analysis of gold artifacts," *Nuclear Instruments and Methods in Physics Research* B 14: 152–155.

Demortier, Guy, 1988. "The soldering of gold in antiquity," *Materials Research Society Symposium, Proceedings* 123: 193–198.

Demortier, Guy, 1995. "IBA applications to ancient metallic items." In M. A. Respaldiza and J. Gómez Camacho, eds, *Applications of Ion Beam Analysis Techniques to Arts and Archaeometry*, 91–114. Seville: Universidad de Sevilla.

Demortier, Guy, 2000. "Essential of PIXE and RBS for archaeological purposes." In Guy Demortier and A. Adriaens, eds, *Ion Beam Study of Art and Archaeological Objects: A Contribution by Members of the COST G1 Action*, 125–136. Luxembourg: Office for Official Publications of the European Communities.

Demortier, G., F. Fernandez-Gomez, M. A. Ontalba Salamanca, and P. Coquay, 1998. "PIXE in an external microbeam arrangement for the study of finely decorated tartesic gold jewellery items," *Nuclear Instruments and Methods in Physics Research* B 158: 275–280.

Demortier, Guy, Yvon Morciaux, and Daphné Dozot, 1999. "PIXE, XRF and GRT for the global investigation of ancient gold artefacts," *Nuclear Instruments and Methods in Physics Research* B 150: 640–644.

Dempster, Thomas (1579?–1625), 1726. *De Etruria regali libri septum*, Volume II (of 2), ed. Thomas Coke. Florentiae: apud J. C. Tartinium. Collections of Bryn Mawr College.

Deneffe, Victor, 1899. *La Prothése dentaire dans l'Antiquité*, ed. H. Caals). Paris: J.-B. Bailliere & fils.

Denker, A. and K. H. Maier, 1999. "Looking deep into the object." In G. Demortier and A. Adriaens, eds, *Ion Beam Study of Art and Archaeological Objects: A Contribution by Members of the COST G1 Action*, 81–83. Luxembourg: Office for Official Publications of the European Communities.

Dennis, George, 1888–1889. "The new Etruscan Museum at the Villa Papa Giulio at Rome," *Journal of the British and American Society (Rome)* 1: 150–168.

De Puma, Richard Daniel, 1987. "Etruscan gold jewelry techniques," *Field Museum of Natural History Bulletin* 58 (9): 7–15.

De Puma, Richard Daniel, 2013. *Etruscan Art in the Metropolitan Museum of Art*. New York: Metropolitan Museum of Art.

d'Errico, F., G. Villa, and G. Fornaciari, 1986. "Dental esthetics of an Italian Renaissance noblewoman, Isabella d'Aragona: a case of chronic mercury intoxication," *Ossa* 13: 207–228.

De Santis, A. 1995. "Contatti fra Etruria e Lazio Antico alla Fine dell'VIII sec. a.C.: La Tomba del Guerriero di Osteria dell'Osa." In N. Christie, ed., *Settlment and Economy in Italy 1500 BC to AD 1500* (Papers of the Fifth Conference of Italian Archaeology, 1992), 41: 365–375. Oxford: Oxbow Monograph.

De Simone, Carlo, 1995. *Tirreni a Lemnos: Evidenza Linguistica e Tradizioni Storiche*. Florence: Leo S. Olschki. Biblioteca di "Studi Etruschi" 23.

De Vecchis, Beniamino, 1925. *Trattato di Odontoiatria e Protesi Dentaria*. Napoli: Cultura Stomatologica.

De Vecchis, Beniamino, 1929. *Dentisti, Artisti, Pazienti nella Storia, nelle lettere, nella vita pratica*. Torino: Cultura Stomatologica.

De Vecchis, Beniamino, 1939. "La scoperta di un nuovo apparecchio protesico dell'Epoca Romana," *La Stomatologia Italiana* 1: 84–85.

DeVoto, G., 1980. "Analisi comparativa delle oreficerie di Preneste (tomba Barberini e Bernardini) e delle Fibula Prenestina (Museo Pigorina Roma). Appendice a M. Guarducci, La cosidetta Fibula Prenestina," *Lincei—Memorie Scienze morali*, Serie VIII, Volume XXIV (4): 546–548.

D'Hancarville, Pierre François (Pierre François Hughes), 1766–1777. *Collection of Etruscan, Greek, and Roman Antiquities from the Cabinet of the Honourable William Hamilton* (4 volumes). Naples: F. Morelli.

Dieck, Wilhelm, 1911. *Dresden, Hygiene-Ausstellung, 1911. Illustrierter Spezial-Katalog der Sondergruppe Zahnerkrankungen—nebst Anhang: Notwendigkeit und Wert der Zahnpflege.* Dresden: Wissenschaftliche Sondergruppe "Zahnerkrankungen."

Dieck, Wilhelm, 1934. "Das Zahnärzliche Institut der Universität Berlin im Rahmen der Entwicklung der Zahnheilkunde als Universitäts-Lehrfach," *Deutsche Zahn-Mund-Kieferheilkunde* 1: VII–XXIV.

Diodorus Siculus: See *Diodorus of Sicily, Library of History*, Volume 3, with an English translation by C. H. Oldfather, 1939. Cambridge MA: Harvard University Press (Loeb Classical Library).

Ditch, L. E. and J. C. Rose, 1972. "A multivariate dental sexing technique," *American Journal of Physical Anthropology* 37: 61–64.

Donais, Mary Kate and David George, 2012. "Using handheld XRF to aid in phasing, locus comparisons, and material homogeneity assessment at an archaeological excavation." In A. N. Shugar and J. L. Mass, eds, *Handheld XRF for Art and Archaeology: Studies in Archaeological Sciences* 3, 349–377. Leuven: Leuven University Press.

Donaldson, J. A., 2013. "The use of gold in dentistry: an historical overview, part II," *Gold Bulletin* 13 (4): 160–165.

Drabkin, I. E., 1944. "On medical education in Greece and Rome," *Bulletin of the History of Medicine* 15: 333–352.

Dubois de Chemant, Nicholas, 1788. *Dissertation sur les avantages des nouvelles dents et rateliers artificiels, incorruptibles et sans odeur, inventés par M. De Chemant, suivie d'une réfutation des assertions avancées par M. Dubois Foucou, le 18 Mai 1788.* London and Paris: L'Auteur and Gattey.

Dubois de Chemant, Nicholas, 1797. *A Dissertation on Artificial Teeth in General: Exposing the Defects and Injurious Consequences of All Teeth Made of Animal Substances.* London: J. Barker.

Düll, Rudolf (ed. and commentator), 1976. *Das Zwölf Tafelgesetz.* Munich: Tusculum Bücherei. (Reissue of 1944 edition).

Dunn, Carlo G., 1894. *L'Arte Dentaria fra gli Etruschi.* Florence: G. Barbèra.

Dussau, A., 1987. "The tooth 'worm' in Mesopotamia and ancient Egypt," *Le Chirurgien-dentiste de France* 57 (403): 28–33.

Duval, Jacques René, 1808. *Recherches historiques sur l'art du dentiste chez les anciens.* Paris: Croullebois (etc.).

Dvorsky-Rohner, Dorothy, 1995. "Greek domestic architecture: an ethnographic model for the interpretation of space," *Archaeological News* 20: 1–10.

Dysert, Anna, 2007. "Capturing medical tradition: Caelius Aurelianus' on acute diseases," *Hirundo: The McGill Journal of Classical Studies* 5: 161–173.

Ebbell, B. (translator), 1937. *The Papyrus Ebers: The Greatest Egyptian Medical Document.* Copenhagen: Levin and Munksgaard.

Echt, R. and W.-R. Thiele, 1987. "Etruskischer Goldschmuck mit gelöteter und gesinterter Granulation," *Archäologisches Korrespondenzblatt* 17: 213–222.

Echt, R. and W.-R. Thiele, 1994. "Sintering, welding, brazing and soldering as bonding techniques in Etruscan and Celtic goldsmithing." In Giulio Morteani and Jeremy P. Northover, eds, *Prehistoric Gold in Europe: Mines Metallurgy and Manufacture*, 435–451. Dordrecht: Kluwer Academic. NATO ASI Series, Series E, Applied Sciences Volume 280.

Edlund, Ingrid E. M., 1981. "A tomb group from Bisenzio in the Barrett collection, Buffalo, New York," *American Journal of Archaeology* 85: 81–83.

Eggebrecht, Arne (ed.), 1994. *Pelizaeus-Museum Hildesheim. Die ägyptische Sammlung.* Mainz am Rein: Verlag Philipp Von Zabern.

Einhorn, Art, 1973. Letter. *Current Anthropology* 14 (5): 521.

Ellis, William, 1979. *Journal of William Ellis.* Tokyo: Tuttle.

Emboden, William, 1980. *Narcotic Plants.* Revised edition. New York: Collier/Macmillan.

Emery, G. T., 1963. "Dental pathology and archaeology," *Antiquity* 37: 274–281.

Emmons, W. H., 1974. *Gold Deposits of the World.* New York: Arno Press.

Emptoz, François, 1987. "La Prothèse Dentaire dans la Civilisation Étrusque." In *Archéologie et Médecine: VII Recontre Internacionales d'Archéologie et d'Histoire (Antibes 1986)*, 545–560. Editions APDCA: Juan-les-Pins.

Enachesco, T., S. Pop, and V. Georgesco, 1962. "Le dimorphisme sexuel chez le nouveau-né, dimensions et proportions." In *VIe Congrés International des Sciences Anthropologiques et Ethnologiques (Paris 1960). Volume I: Rapport général et Anthropologie*, 157–162. Paris: Musée de L'Homme (Palais de Chaillot).

Engelmayer, Harry, 1964. "Zähne und Zahnkrankheiten in biblisch-talmudischer Sicht," *Deutsche zahnärztliche Zeitschrift* 19: 289–295.

Enwonwu. C. O., 1974. "Socio-economic factors in caries prevalence and frequency in Nigerians," *Caries Research* 8: 155–171.

Eogan, George, 1997. "'Hair-rings' and European Late Bronze Age society," *Antiquity* 71: 308–320.

Eriksson, K., 1988. "Dental care among the ancient Etruscans," *Hippokrates* 5: 14–22.

Errico (see d'Errico).

Eschebach, Hans, 1984. *Die Arzthäuser in Pompeii.* Feldmeilen, Switzerland: Raggi-Verlag (*Antike Welt*, Volume 15).

ET = Etruskische Texte (2 editions): regional corpus of known Etruscan inscriptions.

Euler (Professor Dr., Dir. Zahnärztlichen Universitätsinstitutes), 1928. Report to Junker, quoted in Junker 1929: 256–257.

Falchi, Isidoro, 1885. "V. Colonna [Necropoli di Vetulonia in Colonna]," *Notizie degli Scavi* 1885: 98–114 and "IV. Colonna [Necropoli di Vetulonia]," *Notizie degli Scavi* 1885: 398–417.

Falchi, Isidoro, 1891. *Vetulonia e la sua necropoli antichissima.* Florence: Edizione Anastatica (Reprinted 1965, Rome: "L'Erma" di Bretschneider).

Falchi, Isidoro, 1908. "Scavi a Vetulonia," *Notizie degli Scavi* V: 419–437.

Fantham, Elaine, Helene Peet Foley, Natalie Boymel Kampen, Sarah B. Pomeroy, and H. Alan Shapiro, 1994. *Women in the Classical World: Image and Text.* New York: Oxford University Press.

Farrar, John Nutting, 1888. *Treatise on the Irregularities of the Teeth and Their Correction*, Volume I. New York: The De Vinne Press.

Farrar, John Nutting, 1905. "Highest orthodontia. (facial beauty; etc.)," *Independent Practitioner* (which became the *International Dental Journal*), 2nd series, 10: 295–299.

Fauchard, Pierre, 1728. *Le Chirurgien Dentiste ou Traité des Dents* (2 volumes). Paris: Jean Mariette.

Fauchard, Pierre, 1746. *Le Chirurgien Dentiste ou Traité des Dents.* Second edition. Paris: Pierre-Jean Mariette.

Fauchard, Pierre, 1946. *The Surgeon Dentist or Treatise on the Teeth.* Translation of Fauchard's second edition, by Lilian Lindsay. London: Butterworth.

Faulkner, William, 1962/1999. *The Reivers: A Reminiscence.* New York: Vintage Books (Random House, 1999 edition).

Fayer, Carla, 1994. *La familia romana. Aspetti giuridici e antiquari.* I Problemi e Ricerche di Storia Antica, 16. Rome: "L'Erma"di Bretschneider.

Febres-Cordero, Foción, 1966. *Orígines de la odontología.* Caracas: Editorial Arte.

Fenelli, Maria, 1992. "I votivi anatomici in Italia, valore e limite delle testimonianze archeologiche." In A, Krug, ed., *From Epidaurus to Salerno* (Ravello Symposium 1990), PACT 34, 127–138.

Ferguson, Gregory S., Manoj K. Chaudhury, George B. Sigal, and George M. Whitesides, 1991. "Contact adhesion of thin gold films on elastomeric supports: cold welding under ambient conditions," *Science* 253: 776–778.

Feyerskov, O., P. Guldager Bilde, M. Bizzarro, J. Connelly, J. Thomsen, and B. Nyvad, 2012. "Dental caries in Rome year 50–100 AD," *Caries Research* 46 (5): 467–473.

Filderman, Jacques, 1931. "Notice sur une Prothèse fixe, datant d'avant J.-C.," *La Revue Odontologique* 52: 335–343.

Fischer, Klaus-Dietrich, 1987. "'Universorum ferramentorum nomina.' Frühmittelalterliche Listen chirurgischer Instrumente und ihr griechisches Vorbild," *Mittellateinisches Jahrbuch* 22: 28–44.

Fontan, Elisabeth, 2004. "92. Zahnersatz." In Badisches Landesmuseum Karlsruhe (ed.), *Hannibal ad Portas—Macht und Reichtum Karthagos*: 293 (exhibition catalogue entry). Stuttgart: Konrad Theiss Verlag.

Foreshaw, Roger J., 2010. "Were the dentists in ancient Egypt operative dental surgeons or were they pharmacists?" In Jenefer Cockitt and Rosalie David, eds, *Pharmacy and Medicine in Ancient Egypt: Proceedings of the Conferences Held in Cairo (2007) and Manchester (2008)*, 72–77. BAR IS 2141. Oxford: Archaeopress.

Formigli, Edilberto, 1979. "Modi di fabbricazione di filo metallico nell'oreficeria etrusca," *Studi Etruschi* 47: 281–292.

Formigli, Edilberto, 1983. "Appendice tecnica." In Mauro Cristofani and Marina Martelli, eds, *L'oro degli Etruschi*, 321–333. Novara: Istituto Geografico De Agostini.

Formigli, E., 1985. *Tecniche dell'oreficeria Etrusca e Romana: originali e falsificazioni.* Florence: Sansoni.

Formigli, E. (ed.), 1995. *Preziosi in oro: avorio, osso e corno : arte e tecniche degli artigiani etruschi: Atti del seminario di studi ed esperimenti, Murlo, 26 settembre-3 ottobre.* Siena: Nuova immagine; Sistema museale, Provincia di Siena.

Formigli, E. and Gerhard Nestler, 1994. *Granulazione etrusca: un'antica tecnica orafa.* Siena: Nuova imagine.

Fornaciari, G. and F. Mallegni. 1997. "I resti paleoantropologici." In M. Bonghi Jovino and C. Chiaramonte Treré, eds, *Tarquinia. Testimonianze archeologiche e ricostruzione storica*, 100–102. Rome: L'Erma di Bretschneider.

Fornaciari, G., M. G. Bogi, and E. Balducci, 1985–1986. "Dental pathology of the skeletal remains of Pontecagnano, Salerno, Italy, VII–IV centuries BC," *Ossa* 12: 9–31.

Foss, Pedar, 1994a. "Kitchens and dining rooms at Pompeii: the spatial and social relationship of cooking to eating in the Roman household." Ph.D. thesis, University of Michigan. Online: http://quemdixerechaos.com/pompeii/#a9 (consulted November 2014).

Foss, Pedar, 1994b. "Age, gender, and status divisions at mealtime in the Roman house," from Ph.D. thesis. Online: http://quemdixerechaos.com/pompeii/#a10 (consulted November 2014).

Foss, Pedar, 1995. "Social roles of cooking and dining in Roman houses." Online: www. UMICH.EDU/~pfoss/hgender.HTML (consulted November 2014).

Foster, E. W., 1879. "Celsus [especially 'Celsus concerning the teeth']," *Dental Cosmos* 21: 184–192, 235–241, 297–304.

Frassetto, Fabio, 1906. "Crani rinvenuti in tombe etrusche," *Atti della Società Romana di Antropologia* 12: 155–182.

Frazer, J. G., 1910. *Totemism and Exogamy*. London: Macmillan.

Frost, Honor (ed.), 1981. *The Punic Ship: Final Excavation Report*, Supplement to *Notizie degli Scavi*, series 8, 30.

Fujita, H., 1998. "The significance of ritual tooth ablation in Jomon peoples [Abstract, Poster Session C]", *Anthropological Science (Japan)* 106 (2): 173.

Funatsu, T., M. Inoue, R. Sasa, S. Kondo, and E. Wakatsuki, 1997. "Sexual dimorphism in the tooth-crown diameters of Japanese deciduous teeth. [Abstract A-10]," *Anthropological Science (Japan)* 106 (2): 155.

Gàbrici, Ettore, 1910. "Necropoli di età ellenistica a Teano dei Sidicini," *Monumenti Antichi* 20: cols. 5–152.

Galen, 1821–1833. *Claudii Galeni Opera Omnia* (20 volumes), ed. C. G. Kühn. Leipzig. Reprinted in 1964–1965 at Hildesheim: Georg Olms.

Galeotti, L., 1986–1988. "Considerazioni sul carro a due ruote nell'Etruria e nel *Latium vetus*," *Archeologia Classica* 38–40: 94–104.

Gambier, D. and F. Houet, 1991a. *France Upper Paleolithic*. Volume 6 (December) of *Hominid Remains: An Up-date*, ed. Rosine Orban. Supplement to *Anthropologie et Prehistoire*. Bruxelles: Laboratory of Anthropology and Human Genetics.

Gambier, D. and M. Lenoir, 1991b. "Les vestiges humains du Paléolithique supérieur en Gironde," *Bulletin de la Société d'Anthropologie du Sud-Ouest* 26 (1): 1–31.

Gardner, Robert, 1963. *Dead Birds* (Film: Dani People of the New Guinea Highlands). Harvard-Peabody Expedition to New Guinea.

Garn, S. M., A. B. Lewis, and R. S. Kerewsky, 1967. "Sex differences in tooth shape," *Journal of Dental Research* 46 (6): 1470.

Gasperini, Lidio, 1989. "La dignità della donna nel mondo etrusco e il suo lontano reflesso nell'onomastica personale romana." In A. Rallo, ed., *Le Donne in Etruria*, 181–190. Rome: "L'Erma" di Bretschneider (Studia Archeologica 52).

Gastaldi, Patrizia (ed.), 1998. *Studi su Chiusi Arcaica. Annali di Archeologia e Storia Ántica* (Nuova Serie N. 5). Naples: Istituto Universitario Orientale.

Gaultier, F., 2013. "Etruscan jewelry." In J. M. Turfa, ed., *The Etruscan World*, 914–927. London: Routledge.

Gautier, P., 1974. "Le Typikon du Christ Sauveur Pantocrator," *Revue des Etudes Byzantines* 32: 1–145.

Gauval, V. B., 1958. "Notes sur l'histoire de l'art dentaire dans la Bible et le Talmud," *Revue d'Histoire de la Médecine hébraïque* 11 (40): 63–70.

Geist-Jacobi, George Pierce, 1896. *Geschichte der Zahnheilkunde vom Jahre 3700 v. Chr bis zur Gegenwart*. Tübingen: Franz Pietzcker.

Geist-Jacobi, George Pierce, 1899. *Mittelalter und Neuzeit*. Berlin: Berlin Verlagsanstalt.

Gerlett, John, 1939. "Votive offerings," *Ciba Symposia* 1 (4): 122–125.

Ghalioungui, Paul, 1971. "Did a dental profession exist in ancient Egypt?" *Medical History* 15 (1): 92–94.

Ghalioungui, Paul, 1973. *The House of Life: Per Ankh. Magic and Medical Science in Ancient Egypt*. Second edition. Amsterdam: B. M. Israël.

Ghalioungui, Paul. 1987. *The* Ebers papyrus. *A New English Translation, Commentaries and Glossary*. Cairo: Academy of Scientific Research and Technology.

Ghalioungui, Paul and Zeinab El-Dawakhly, 1965. *Health and Healing in Ancient Egypt*. Cairo: Dar al-Maareb (Egyptian Organization for Authorship and Translation).

Ghinst, Irenée Jos. van der, 1930. "Les Étrusques, connaissaient-ils la pyorrée et la méthode prosthetique de traitement?" In *Atti VIII Congresso internazionale di storia della medicina*, (Rome, 22–27 September 1930), 406–407. Rome: Istituto poligrafico dello stato.

Giardino, Claudio, 2010 (1998). *I metalli nel mondo antico. Introduzione all'archeometallurgia*. Second edition. Bari: Laterza.

Giardino, Claudio. 2013. "Villanovan and Etruscan mining and metallurgy." In J. M. Turfa, ed., *The Etruscan World*, 721–737. London: Routledge.

Ginestet, Félix, 1927. "Prothèse de Contention Chez Les Phéniciens," *Revue de Stomatologie* 29 (1): 12–17.

Ginge, Birgitte, 1996. *Excavations at Satricum (Borgo Le Ferriere) 1907–1910: Northwest Necropolis, Southwest Sanctuary and Acropolis. Scrinium X*. Amsterdam: Thesis Publishers.

Ginge, Birgitte, Marshall Joseph Becker, and Pia Guldager, 1989. "Of Roman extraction," *Archaeology* 42 (4): 34–37.

Gleba, Margarita, 2008. *Textile Production in Pre-Roman Italy* (Ancient Textiles 4). Oxford: Oxbow Books.

Gleba, Margarita, 2012. "Italy: Iron Age." In M. Gleba and U. Mannering, eds, *Textiles and Textile Production in Europe From Prehistory to* AD *400*, 212–241. Oxford: Oxbow Books.

Gnade, Marajka, 1986. "De noordwest nekropool (pp. 120–121)" and De zuid-west nekropool (pp. 138–140)." In *Nieuw licht op een Oude Stad: Italiaanse en Nederlandse opgravingen in Satricum* (exhibition catalogue). Den Haag: Drukkerij Trio den Haag.

Godon, Charles Edouard, 1901. L'évolution de l'art dentaire: *L'Ecole Dentaire*, Paris: J.-B. Baillière et Fils.

Goose, D. H., 1963. "Dental measurement: an assessment of its value in anthropological research." In Don R. Brothwell, ed., *Dental Anthropology*, 125–148. New York: Pergamon Press.

Gorelick, Leonard and A. John Gwinnett, 1987a. *A History of Drills and Drilling*. New York State Dental Journal 53 (1): 35–39.

Gorelick, Leonard and A. John Gwinnett, 1987b. "Life and death of the tooth worm theory: or when I believe it, I will see it," *New York State Dental Journal* 53 (7): 21–25.

Gourevitch, Danielle, 2007. "Un livre récent d'histoire de l'odontoiatrie dans le monde étrusco-romain: lecture critique," *Actes de la Société française d'histoire de l'art dentaire* 12: 5–9. (Review article based on Baggieri 2005).

Grawinkel, Carl Julius, 1906. "Zähne und Zahnbehandlung der alten Aegypter, Hebräer, Inder, Babyloner, Assyrer, Griechen und Römer" (Ph.D. Dissertation, University Erlangen). Berlin: Berlinische Verlagsanstalt.

Gray, Peter Hugh Ker, 1966. *A Radiographic Skeletal Survey of Ancient Egyptian Mummies. Fourth European Symposium on Calcified Tissues.* Exerpta Medica International Congress Series, No. 120.

Gray, Peter Hugh Ker, 1967. "Radiography of ancient Egyptian mummies," *Radiography and Photography* 43 (2): 34–44.

Greif, Samuel, 1918. *Dentistry in the Bible and Talmud: A Valuable Contribution to the Early History of Dentistry.* New York: Who's Who Dental Publishing Company.

Griffenhagen, George B., 1992. "The *Materia Medica* of Christopher Columbus," *Pharmacy in History* 34: 131–145.

Grimm, Jacob, 1847. "Über Marcellus Burdigalensis," *Abhandlungen der Königlichen Akademie der Wissenschaffen zu Berlin,* 1847: 429–460.

Grimm, Jacob, 1855. "Über die Marcellischen Formeln," *Abhandlungen der Königlichen Akademie der Wissenschaffen zu Berlin,* 1855: 50–68.

Grmek, Mirko D. and Danielle Gourevitch, 1998. *Les maladies dans l'art antique.* Paris: Fayard.

Groenen, Marc, 1987. *Les représentations de mains négatives dans les grottes de Gargas et de Tibiran: Approche méthodologique.* Brussels: Faculté de philosophie et lettres/ Université libre de Bruxelles.

Guerini, Vincenzo, 1894a. "L'Art Dentaire chez les anciens peuples Italiens," *Revue Internationale D'Odontologie* (July): 393–396.

Guerini, Vincenzo, 1894b. "L'arte dentaria presso gli antichi popoli italiani," *Giornale Corrispondenze per Dentisti* 13: 185–188. (11th Congresso Internazionale di Medicina ed Igiene, 1894). Naples: Tipo-Litografiio Richter & Cie.

Guerini, Vincenzo, 1904. "Dental art among the Romans and Etruscans," *Dental Cosmos* 46: 278–280.

Guerini, Vincenzo, 1909. *A History of Dentistry from the Most Ancient Times Until the End of the Eighteenth Century.* Philadelphia, PA: Lea and Febiger.

Guerra, M. F., 2008. "An overview on the ancient goldsmith's skill and the circulation of gold in the past: the role of X-Ray based techniques," *X-Ray Spectrometry* 37: 317–327.

Guillemeau, Jacques, 1598. *Les oeuvres de chirurgie.* Paris: Nicolas de Louvain.

Guldager, Pia, 1990. "En tandklinik og skønhedssalon i Rom," *Tandlaegebladet (Danish Dental Journal)* 94 (10): 422–426.

Guldager, Pia and Karen Slej, 1986. "Il Tempio di Castore e Polluce," *Archeologia Viva* 5 (4): 24–37.

Gunter, Ann C., 2009. *Greek Art and the Orient.* Cambridge: Cambridge University Press.

Gurdon, Lady Eveline Camilla (ed. and collector), 1893. *County Folk-Lore: Printed Extracts,* No. 2. Suffolk. London: D. Nutt (Kraus Reprints, bound in Volume 37).

Gwinnett, A. John and Leonard Gorelick, 1979. "Inlayed teeth of ancient Mayans: a typological study using the SEM," *Scanning Electron Microscopy* 2: 575–580.

Haack, Marie-Laurence, 2013. "Modern approaches to Etruscan culture." In J. M. Turfa, ed., *The Etruscan World,* 1136–1145. London: Routledge.

Hallscheid, Sabin, 1986. *Die zahnmedizinische Karikatur.* Köln: Arbeiten der Forschungsstelle des Instituts für Geschichte der Medizin der Universität zu Köln.

Hamarneh, Sami Khalaf, and Glenn Sonnendecker, 1963. *A Pharmaceutical View of Abulcasis al-Zahrāwī in Moorish Spain.* Leiden: Brill.

Hamdî (Hamdy), Osman and Theodore Reinach, 1892. *Une nécropole Royale à Sidon: fouilles de Hamdy Bey.* Paris: Ernest Leroux (re-issued in 1987). Istanbul: Archaeology and Art Publications).

Hamilton, Sir William, 1791. *Collection of Engravings from Ancient Vases mostly of Pure Greek Workmanship Discovered in Sepulchres in the Kingdom of the Two Sicilies but Chiefly in the Neighbourhood of Naples MDCCLXXXIX and MDCCLXXX. Now in the Possession of Sir William Hamilton.* Volume 1. Naples: William Tischbein.

Handler, Jerome S., 1994. "Determining African birth from skeletal remains: a note on tooth mutilation," *Historical Archaeology* 28: 113–119.

Harrington, Spencer P. M., 1995. "Children of the African burial ground," *Archaeology* 48 (5): 14–15.

Harris, Chapin Aaron, 1839. *The Dental Art: A Practical Treatise on Dental Surgery.* Baltimore, MD: Armstrong and Berry (Facsimile reprint. The Classics of Dentistry Library, Birmingham, Alabama, 1979).

Harris, Chapin Aaron and Joseph Fox, 1855. *Diseases of the Human Teeth: Their Natural History and Structure, with the Mode of Applying Artificial Teeth.* Philadelphia, PA: Lindsay.

Harris, Edward F., 1997. "A strategy for comparing odontometrics among groups," *Dental Anthropology* 12 (1): 1–6.

Harris, James E. and Paul V. Ponitz, 1980. "Dental health in ancient Egypt." In Aidan and Eve Cockburn, eds, *Mummies, Disease, and Ancient Cultures*, 45–51. Cambridge: Cambridge University Press.

Harris, James E., Zaki Iskander, and Shafik Farid, 1975. "Restorative dentistry in ancient Egypt: an archaeological fact!" *Journal of the Michigan Dental Association* 57: 401–404.

Harrison, A. P. and E. M. Bartels, 2006. "A modern appraisal of ancient Etruscan herbal practices," *American Journal of Pharmacology and Toxicology* 1(1): 21–24.

Harrison, A. P. and J. M. Turfa, 2010. "Were natural forms of treatment for Fasciola hepatica available to the Etruscans?" *International Journal of Medical Sciences* 7(5): 282–291.

Harrison, Adrian P., Steen H. Hansen, and Else M. Bartels, 2012. "Transdermal opioid patches for pain treatment in ancient Greece," *Pain Practice* 12 (8): 620–625.

Hartland, Edwin Sidney (ed.), 1892. "Taken from, Gloucestershire notes and queries, 1881: Vol. 1: 43." County Folk-Lore, Printed Extracts No. 1. Gloucestershire: D. Nutt, for the Folk-Lore Society.

Hartmann, Axel, 1970. *Prähistorische Goldfunde aus Europa; spektralanalytische Untersuchen und deren Auswertung.* Volume 3 of the series, *Studien zu den Anfängen der Metallurgie*, ed. K. Bittel, A. Hartmann, H. Otto, E. Sangmeister, H. Schickler, and M. Schröder. Berlin: Gebrüder Mann Verlag.

Hartmann, Axel, 1982. *Prähistorische Goldfunde aus Europa; spektralanalytische Untersuchen und deren Auswertung II.* Volume 5 of the series, *Studien zu den Anfängen der Metallurgie*, ed. K. Bittel, A. Hartmann, H. Otto, E. Sangmeister, H. Schickler, and M. Schröder. Berlin: Gebrüder Mann Verlag.

Haynes, Sybille, 2000. *Etruscan Civilization: A Cultural History.* Los Angeles, CA: The J. Paul Getty Museum.

Heck, Steven D., J. Chester Siok, Karen J. Krapacho, Paul R. Kelbaugh, Peter F. Thadeio, Melissa J. Welch, Robert D. Williams, Alan H. Ganong, Mary E. Kelly, Anthony J. Lanzetti, William R. Gray, Douglas Phillips, Thomas N. Parks, Hunter Jackson, Michael K. Ahlijanian, Nicholas A. Saccomano, and Robert A. Volkmann. 1994. "Functional consequences of posttranslational isomerization of Ser[46] in a calcium channel toxin," *Science* 266: 1065–1068.

Helbig, Wolfgang, 1877. "I. Scavi (a. Scavio di Corneto). [Letter: Dasti to Helbig]," *Bullettino dell'Instituto di Corrispondenza Archeologica* 4: 56–64.

Helbig, Wolfgang, 1886. "Scavi di Capodimonte," *Mittheilungen des Kaiserlichen Deutschen Archaeologischen Institutes, Roemische Abteilung [= Römische Mitteilungen]* I: 18–36.

Helbig, Wolfgang, 1969. *Führer durch die öffentlichen Sammlungen klassicher Altertümer in Rom*, Volume III (fourth edition, ed. Hermione Speier). Tubingen: Ernst Wasmuth.

Hencken, Hugh, 1968. *Tarquinia and Etruscan Origins*. London: Thames and Hudson.

Henderson, J. 2002. *Aristophanes. Frogs, Assembleywomen, Wealth*. (Loeb Classical Library) Cambridge, MA: Harvard University Press.

Henry, P. J., W. R. Laney, T. Jemt, D. Harris, P. H. Krogh, G. Polizzi, G. A. Zarb, and I. Herrmann, 1996. "Osseointegrated implants for single-tooth replacement: a prospective 5-year multicenter study," *International Journal of Oral and Maxillofacial Implants* 11 (4): 450–455.

Henzen, G., 1855. "Scavi di Palestrina," *Monumenti Annali e Bulletini Pubblicati dall'Instituto di Corrispondenza Archeologica* I: 74–87 (Fas. I/ Gotha: Hugo Scheube).

Herbst, Wilhelm, 1885. *Das Füllen der Zahne mit Gold, &c., nach Deutscher Methode*. Berlin: C. Ash & Sons.

Heurgon, Jacques, 1964. *Daily Life of the Etruscans*. Translated from the French by James Kirkup (original French edition 1961). New York: The Macmillan Company.

Heyne, R., 1924. "Zähne und Zahnärztliches in der schönen Literatur der Römer." Doctoral dissertation, Leipzig.

Hideji, H., 1986. "Rules of residence in the Jomon Period, based on the analysis of tooth extraction." In R. J. Pearson, ed., *Windows on the Japanese Past: Studies in Archaeology and Prehistory*, 293–310. Ann Arbor, MI: University of Michigan Center for Japanese Studies.

Hillert, Andres, 1990. *Antike Arztedarstellungen*. Frankfurt am Main: Peter Lang (Marburger Schriften zur Medizingeschichte, Bd. 25).

Hillier, Bill and Julienne Hanson, 1989. *The Social Logic of Space*. Cambridge: Cambridge University Press.

Hippocrates, 1923/1931. *Hippocrates: Ancient Medicine*. Volumes 1, 2, and 4, trans. W. H. S. Jones. London: William Heinemann. Reprinted 1995.

Hippocrates, 1928. *Hippocrates: Ancient Medicine*. Volume 3, trans. E. T. Withington. London: William Heinemann.

Hirt, Margerite, 1986. "Le statut social du médecin à Rome et dans les provinces occidentales sous le Haut-Empire." In *Archéologie et Médecin: VIIIémes Recontres Internationales d'Archéologie et d'Histoire d'Antibes*, 95–107. Juan-les-Pins: Association pour la Promotion et la Diffusion des Connaissance Archéologiques, 1987.

Hobbs, Christopher, 1992. "Garlic: the pungent panacea," *Pharmacy in History* 34: 152–157.

Hockley, A. 1858. "Mr. Hockley on mechanical dentistry," *Quarterly Journal of Dental Science* I (April 1857–January 1858): 393–403.

Hoffmann-Axthelm, Walter, 1970. "The history of tooth replacement," *Dental Science and Research* 8 (9): 81–87.

Hoffmann-Axthelm, Walter, 1973. *Die Geschichte der Zahnheilkunde*. Berlin: Buch- und Zeitschriften Verlag; Die Quintessenz.

Hoffmann-Axthelm, Walter, 1981. *A History of Dentistry*, trans. H. M. Koehler. Chicago, IL: Quintessence Publishing Company.

Hoffmann-Axthelm, Walter, 1985. *Die Geschichte der Zahnheilkunde*. Second edition. Berlin: Quintessenz Verlags-GmbH.

Hooton, E. A., 1917. "Oral surgery in Egypt during the Old Empire," *African Studies* 1: 29–32.

Horstmanshoff, H. F. J., 1990. "The ancient physician: craftsman or scientist," *Journal of the History of Medicine* 45: 176–197.

Hostetler, K. L. 2004–2007. "Serpent iconography," *Etruscan Studies* 10: 203–209.

Hrdlicka, Ales, 1940. "Ritual ablation of front teeth in Siberia and America," *Smithsonian Miscellaneous Collections* 99 (3): 1–37.

Humphrey, John W., John P. Oleson, and Andrew N. Sherwood, 1998. *Greek and Roman Technology: A Sourcebook. Annotated Translations of Greek and Latin Texts and Documents.* London: Routledge.

Hung-Kuan-Chih, 1954. "Some problems in classified materia medica and explanatory materia medica," *Chinese Journal of Medical History* 3: 100 ff. (cited in Czarnetzki and Ehrhardt 1990).

Hunt, L. B., 1975. "Bartholomaeus Anglicus on gold: the modern views of a medieval encyclopaedist," *The Gold Bulletin* (Marshalltown, South Africa: International Gold Corporation) 8: 22–27.

Huntsman, Theresa and Marshall Joseph Becker, 2013. "An analysis of the cremated human remains in a terracotta cinerary urn of the third-second century BCE from Chiusi, now in the Metropolitan Museum of Art in New York," *Etruscan Studies* 16 (2): 153–164.

Iaia, Cristiano, 2007. "Elements of female jewellery in Iron Age Latium and southern Etruria: Identity and cultural communication in a boundary zone," in *Scripta praehistorica in honorem Biba Teržan*, 519–531. Ljubljana: Nardoni musej Slovenije.

Irish, Joel D., 2006. "Who were the ancient Egyptians? Dental affinities among the Neolithic through postdynastic peoples," *American Journal of Physical Anthropology* 129 (4): 529–543.

Iskander, Zaky and James E. Harris, 1977. "A skull with a silver bridge to replace a central incisor," *Annales du Service des Antiquités de l'Egypte* 62: 85–90.

Iskander, Zaky, James E. Harris, and Shafik Farid, 1978. "Further evidence of dental prosthesis in Ancient Egypt," *Annales du Service des Antiquités de l'Egypte* 63: 103–113.

Jackson, J. W., 1915. "Dental mutilations in Neolithic human remains," *Journal of Anatomy and Physiology* 49: 72–79.

Jackson, Ralph P. J., 1986. "A set of Roman medical instruments from Italy," *Britannia* 17: 119–167.

Jackson, Ralph P. J., 1987. "A set of surgical instruments from Roman Italy," *Archéologie et Médécine* 413–428.

Jackson, Ralph P. J., 1988. *Doctors and Diseases in the Roman Empire.* London: British Museum Publications.

Jackson, Ralph P. J., 1990. "Roman doctors and their instruments: recent research into ancient practice," *Journal of Roman Archaeology* 3: 5–27.

Jackson, Ralph P. J., 1993. "Roman medicine; the practitioners and their practices," *Aufstieg und Niedergang der römischen Welt* 37 (1): 79–101.

Jacob, Irene and Walter Jacob (eds), 1993. *The Healing Past: Pharmaceuticals in the Biblical and Rabbinic World.* Leiden: E. J. Brill.

Jacquart, Danielle, 1992. "Les traductions médicales de Gérard dr Crémone." In Pierluigi Pizzamiglio, ed., *Gerardo da Cremona*, 57–70. Annali della Biblioteca Statale e Libreria Civica di Cremona, XLI (1990).

Jamieson, L. M., 2006. "Traditional tooth gauging education tool for use in remote Ugandan community," *Health Education Research* 21 (4): 477–487.

Jannot, Jean-René, 2009. "The lotus, poppy and other plants in Etruscan funerary contexts." In J. Swaddling and P. Perkins, eds, *Etruscan by Definitio: Papers in Honour of Sybille Haynes, MBE.* British Museum Research Publication Number 173: 81–86.

Jashemski, Wilhelmina Feemster, 1999. *A Pompeian Herbal: Ancient and Modern Medicinal Plants*. Austin, TX: University of Texas Press.

Jashemski, Wilhelmina Feemster, ed., 2002. *Natural History of Pompeii*. Oxford: Oxford University Press.

Jason, David, 1998. "In his element," *Entertainment Centre. British Airways High Life* (March): 18.

Jenkins, Ian and Kim Sloan, 1996. *Vases and Volcanoes: Sir William Hamilton and His Collection*. London: British Museum Press.

Johnstone, Mary A., 1932a. "The Etruscan collection in the free public museums of Liverpool," *Annals of Archaeology and Anthropology, Liverpool* 19: 121–137, plates XCIII–XCIV.

Johnstone, Mary A., 1932b. "The Etruscan collection in the Public Museum of Liverpool," *Studi Etruschi* 6: 443–452.

Jonckheere, Frans, 1958. *Les médecins de l'Égypte pharaonique: Essai de Prosopographie. La Médecine Egyptienne*, No. 3. Brussels: Fondacion Egyptienne Reine Elisabeth.

Jones, Alfred, 1884. "Dentistry amongst the ancient Greeks and Romans," *Journal of the British Dental Association* 5: 407–413.

Jones, W. H. S., 1946. *Philosophy and Medicine in Ancient Greece*. Baltimore, MD: Johns Hopkins Press.

Jones, W. H. S., 1953. "Ancient documents and contemporary life, with special reference to the Hippocratic Corpus, Celsus and Pliny." In E. Ashworth Underwood, ed., *Science, Medicine and History: Essays on the Evolution of Scientific Thought and Medical Practice Written in Honour of Charles Singer*, 100–110. London: Oxford University Press.

Jonson, Ben, 1607. *Volpone; or, The foxe*. (A play first acted in 1605). London: Printed for T. Thorppe.

Joshel, Sandra R., 1992. *Work, Identity and Legal Status at Rome: A Study of the Occupational Inscription*. Norman, OK: University of Oklahoma Press.

Junker, Hermann, 1914. "Vorbericht über die 3. Grabung bei den Pyramiden von Gizeh, Jänner-April 1914," *Anzeiger Wiener Akademie Wissenschaften, Phil.-hist. Klasse* 51: 140–183.

Junker, Hermann, 1927. "Die Stele des Hofarztes Irj. Das Spezialistentum in der Ägyptische Medizin," *Zeitschrift für Ägyptische Sprache und Altertumskunde (Leipzig)* 63: 53–70.

Junker, Hermann, 1929. *Gîza I. Band I: Die Mastabas der IV. Dynastie auf dem Westfriedhof. Bericht über die von der Akademie der Wissenschaften . . . Grabungen auf dem Friedhof des Alten Reiches bei den Pyramiden von Gîza*, 256–257. Vienna: Hölder-Pichler-Tempsky.

Junker, Hermann, 1934. *Gîza II. Band II. Die Mastabas der beginnenden V. Dynastie auf dem Westfriedhof. [Denkschriften der Östereichische] Akademie der Wissenschaften in Wien, Philosophisch-historische Klasse. Denkschriften* 69. Vienna, Leipzig: Hölder-Pichler-Tempsky.

Kajava, Mika, 1994. *Roman Female Praenomina: Studies in the Nomenclature of Roman Women. Acta Instituti Romani Finlandiae*, XIV. Rome.

Kanaseki, Takeo, 1962. "The custom of teeth extraction [ablation] in ancient China." In *VIe Congrés International des Sciences Anthropologiques et Ethnologiques (Paris 1960). Volume I: Rapport général et Anthropologie*, 201–205. Paris: Musée de L'Homme (Palais de Chaillot).

Kaplony, Peter, n.d. *Die Inschriften der Ägyptischen Frühzeit*. Printed in German Dissertations in Classical Literature and Philology, Volume 177, No. 5 (set 2).

Kazhdan, A., 1984. "The image of the medical doctor in Byzantine literature of the tenth to twelfth centuries." In John Scarborough, ed., *Symposium on Byzantine Medicine*, 43–51. Dumbarton Oaks Papers, No. 38. Dumbarton Oaks Research Library and Collection: Washington, DC.

Keil, Baldur, 1977/1978. "Eine Prothese aus einem fränkischen Grab von Griesheim, Kreis Darmstadt-Dieburg," *Fundberichte aus Hessen* 17/18: 195–211.

Keith, A., 1931. *New Discoveries Relating to the Antiquity of Man*. London: Williams & Norgate.

Kenney, E. J. (ed.), 1980. *Latin Literature: The Cambridge History of Classical Literature*, II. Cambridge, England: Cambridge University Press.

Kennedy, K. A. r., V. N. Misra, and C. B. Burrow, 1980. "Dental mutilations in prehistoric India," *Current Anthropology* 22: 285–286.

Ker, Walter Charles Allen (trans.), 1968, 1978. *Epigrams/Martial* (2 volumes; reissued from the 1927 translations, see under Martial 1927). Loeb Classical Library 94–95. Cambridge, MA: Harvard University Press.

Kerr, J. G., 1894. "Dentistry in China," *Scientific American* 71: 198 (abstracted from the *Dental Register*).

Kerr, N. W., 1986. "A method of assessing periodontal status in archaeologically derived skeletal material," *Journal of Paleopathology* 2 (2): 67–78.

Kieser, Julius A., 1990. *Human Adult Odontometrics: The Study of Variation in Adult Tooth Size*. Cambridge: Cambridge University Press.

Kikwilu, E. N. and J. F. R. Hiza, 1997. "Tooth bud extraction and rubbing of herbs by TH in Tanzania: prevalence, and sociological and environmental factors influencing the practices," *International Journal of Paediatric Dentistry* 7: 19–24.

King, Helen, 1988. "The early anodynes: pain in the ancient world." In R. D. Mann, ed., *The History of the Management of Pain*, 51–62. Park Ridge, NJ: Parthenon.

Koch, Charles R. E. (ed.), 1909. *History of Dental Surgery*, Volume 1. Fort Wayne, IN: The National Art Publishing Company (1910).

Kocsis, A., S. Olàh and S. Cencetti, 1994. "Abnormal dental characteristics in an Etruscan specimen (6th century BC). Case Report." In Jacopo Moggi-Cecchi, ed., *Aspects of Dental Biology: Palaeontology, Anthropology and Evolution*, 373–378. Florence: International Institute for the Study of Man.

Koenen, Constantin, 1904. "Beschreibung von Novaesium" (Chapter 3 of "*Novaesium*"), *Bonner Jahrbücher (Jahrbücher des Vereins von Altertumsfreunden in Rheinlande)*, 111/112: 97–242.

Kondo, S., K. Nakajima, E. Wakatsuki, and T. Funatsu, 1997. "Sexual dimorphism in the crown component of the mandibular molars [Abstract A-9]," *Anthropological Science [Japan]* 106 (2): 155.

Koritzer, R. T., 1968. "Apparent tooth preparation in a Middle Mississippian Indian culture," *Journal of Dental Research* 47: 839.

Kornemann, K., 1989. "Literaturstudien über die problematische Existenz eines Zahnärztstandes im Alten Reich Ägyptens." Medical Dissertation: Berlin.

Kreil, Günther, 1994. "Conversion of L- to D-amino acids: a posttranslational reaction," *Science* 266: 996–997.

Kron, Geoffrey. 2013. "Fleshing out the demography of Etruria." In J. M. Turfa, ed., *The Etruscan World*, 56–75. London: Routledge.

Krumbacher, Karl, 1897. *Geschichte der byzantinischen litteratur von Justinian zum ende des Oströmischen Reiches (527–1453)* (2 volumes). Munich: C. H. Beck.

Künzl, Ernst, 1982. "Medizinische Instrumente aus Sepulkralfunden der römischen Kaizerzeit," *Bonner Jahrbücher* 182: 1–131.

Künzl, Ernst, 1986. "Eine Serie von Fälschungen römischer medizinischer Instrumentarien," *Archäologisches Korrespondenzblatt* 16: 333–339.

Künzl, Ernst, 1993. "Ein invorsichhtiger Arzt? Römisches Bronzebesteck mit chirurgischen Werkzeugen, aus dem Rhein gebaggert bei Mainz." In *Jehre Kultur und Geschichte in Nassau: dargestellt an Objekten der Sammlung Nassauuischer Altertümer des Museums Wiesbaden*, 99–103. Wiesbaden: Verlag des ereins für Nassauische Altertumskunde und Geschichtsforschung.

Künzl, Ernst and Thomas Weber, 1991. "Das spätantike Grab eines Zahnarztes zu Gadara in der Dekapolis," *Damaszener Mitteilungen* 5: 81–118.

Lamacki, W. F., 2014. "The tragic story of William Taggart," *CDS Review* 107 (4): 95–99.

Lambrechts, Roger, 1970. *Les inscriptions avec le mot 'tular' et le bornage étrusque.* Florence: L. S. Olschki.

Lancaster, Susannah, 2001. "Flashing a smile: dental inlaying among the Late Classic Maya." Paper presented at the Annual Meetings of the Society for American Archaeology, New Orleans (April 19).

Lanciani, Rodolfo Amedeo, 1892. *Pagan and Christian Rome.* New York: Benjamin Blom (Reissued in 1967).

Lanciani, Rodolfo Amedeo, 1893. *Ein unvorsichtiger Arzt? Römisches Bronzebesteck mit chirurgischen Werkzeugen, aus dem Rhein gebaggert bei Mainz. 200 000 Jahre Kultur und Geschichte in Nassau.* Wiesbaden: Verein für Nassauische Altertumskunde und Geschichtsforschung.

Laviosa, Clelia, Luigi Capasso, and Gaspare Baggieri, 1993. "Catalogo della Mostra." In Luigi Capasso, ed., *Le Origini della Chirurgia Italiana*, 97–132. S. Atto Teramo: Officine Grafiche Edigrafital, for the Ministero dei Beni Culturali e Ambientali, Rome.

Lazer, Estelle, 2009. *Resurrecting Pompeii.* London: Routledge.

Leake, Chauncy D., Sanford V. Larkey, and Henry F. Lutz, 1953. "The management of fractures according to the Hearst Medical Papyrus." In A. Ashworth Underwood, ed., *Science, Medicine and History*, 61–74. London: Oxford University Press.

Leca, Ange Pierre, 1971. *La Médicine Egyptienne au temps des Pharaons.* Paris: Dacosta.

Leca, Ange Pierre, 1976. *Les Momies.* Paris: Hachette.

Lechtmann, Heather and Arthur Steinberg, 1970. "Bronze joining: a study in ancient technology." In Suzannah Doehringer, David Gordon Mitten and Arthur Steinberg, eds, *Art and Technology: A Symposium on Classical Bronzes*, 5–35. Cambridge, MA: MIT Press.

Leek, Frank Filce, 1966. "Observations on the dental pathology seen in ancient Egyptian skulls," *Journal of Egyptian Archaeology* 52: 59–64.

Leek, Frank Filce, 1967a. "Reputed early Egyptian dental operation, an appraisal." In D. R. Brothwell and A. T. Sandison, eds, *Diseases in Antiquity*, 702–705. Springfield, IL: Charles C. Thomas.

Leek, Frank Filce, 1967b. "The practice of dentistry in ancient Egypt," *Journal of Egyptian Archaeology* 53: 51–58.

Leek, Frank Filce, 1972. "Did a dental profession exist in ancient Egypt during the 3rd Millenium BC?" *History of Medicine* 16: 404–406.

Leek, Frank Filce, 1979. "The dental history of the Manchester mummies." In A. Rosalie David, ed., *The Manchester Museum Mummy Project: Multidisciplinary Research on Ancient Egyptia Mummified Remains*, 65–77. Manchester: Manchester University Press.

Leek, Frank Filce, 1981. "Reévaluation des Arguments en Faveur de l'Existence d'une Profession Dentaire au Troisiéme Millenaire avant J.-C. en Egypte," *Bulletin et Mémoires de la Société d'Anthropologie de Paris* 8 (Series XIII): 377–380.

Lefkowitz, Mary R. and Maureen B. Fant, 2005. *Women's Life in Greece and Rome: A Sourcebook in Translation*. Third edition. Baltimore, MD: Johns Hopkins.

Lefoulon, Joachim Pierre, 1844. *A New Treatise on the Theory and Practice of Dental Surgery.* Translated from the French by Thomas E. Bond, Jr. Baltimore, MD: Woods and Crane for The American Society of Dental Surgeons.

Lehrberger, G., 1995. "The gold deposits of Europe: an overview of the possible metal sources for prehistoric gold objects." In Giulio Morteani and Jeremy P. Northover, eds, *Prehistoric Gold in Europe. Mines Metallurgy and Manufacture*, 115–144. Dordrecht: Kluwer Academic. NATO ASI Series, Series E, Applied Scences Volume 280.

Leighton, Robert, 2004. *Tarquinia: An Etruscan City*. London: Duckworth.

Lembke, Katja, 2001. *Phönizische anthropoide Sarkophage*. Mainz am Rhein: Philipp von Zabern.

Lentini, R., 1995. "Dentifrici e igiene orale nel mondo romano," *Medicina nei Secoli* 7 (2): 351–366.

Leopold, Henricus M. R., 1923. *Uit de Leerschool der spade I*. Zutphen: W. J. Thieme & Cie.

Levi, Donata, 1985a. "Collezionismo etrusco tra musei accademici e raccolte private (1724–1750)." In Paola Barocchi and Daniela Gallo, eds, *L'Accademia etrusca*, 109–120. Electa: Regione Toscana.

Levi, Donata, 1985b. "68. Maffei, Scipione, Museum Veronense." In D. Levi "Collezionismo etrusca tra musei, accademici e raccolte private (1725–1750)," 120–121. In Paola Barocchi and Daniela Gallo, eds, *L'Accademia etrusca*, 109–121. (Catalogue of a show held in Cortona, 1985). Florence and Milan: Electa.

Levi, Doro, 1931. "Carta archeologica di Vetulonia," *Studi Etruschi* 5: 13–40.

Li, Shizhen, 2003 [1596]. Compendium of Materia Medica (Ben cao Gang mu), in 6 volumes (English version). Beijing, China: Foreign Languages Press.

Lilley, J. D. 2002. "Seianti Hanunia Tlesnasa: some observations on the dental features." In J. Swaddling and J. Prag, eds, *Seianti Hanunia Tlesnasa: The Story of an Etruscan Noblewoman*, 23–26. London: British Museum Occasional Paper Number 100.

Linderer, Joseph, 1848. *Handbuch der Zahnheilkunde* (second and enlarged edition, from the 1837 version). Volume II. Berlin: Schlesingerische Buch- und Musikhandlung. (Volume I by C. J. Linderer and Joseph Linderer issued in 1842).

Linderer, Joseph, 1851. *Die Zahnheilkunde nach ihrem neusten Standpunkte; ein Lehrbuch für Zahnärtzte und Aerzte.* Erlangen: J. J. Palm und E. Enke.

Linderer, Joseph and C. J. Linderer, 1842. *Handbuch der Zahnheilkunde*. Volume I. Berlin: Schlesingerische Buch- und Musikhandlung.

Lindsay, Lilian, 1953. "Dental anatomy from Aristotle to Leeuwenhoek." In E. Ashworth Underwood, ed., *Science, Medicine and History*, 123–128. London: Oxford University Press.

Liston, M. A. (2012) "Reading the bones: interpreting the skeletal evidence for women's lives in ancient Greece." In S. L. James and S. Dillon, eds, *A Companion to Women in the Ancient World*, 125–140. Blackwells' Companions to the Ancient World, Malden, MA: Wiley- Blackwell.

Llagostera Cuenca, Esteban, 1978. *Radiological Examination of the Egyptian Mummies of the Archaeological Museum of Madrid.* Madrid: Raycar S.A.

Lloyd-Morgan, Glenys and S. P. Girardon, 1988. "The Etruscan collection." In M. Gibson and S. M. Wright, eds, *Joseph Mayer of Liverpool, 1803–1886*, 77–85 (Society of Antiquaries, Occasional Papers N.S. XI, London, 1988.)

Loraux, Nicole, 1993. *The Children of Athena: Athenian Ideas about Citizenship and the Division Between the Sexes*, trans. Froma I. Zeitlin. Princeton, NJ: Princeton University Press.

Lo Schiavo, F. 2002. "Osservazioni sul problema dei rapporti fra Sardegna ed Etruria in età nuragica—II." In O. Paoletti and L. Tamagno Perna, eds, *Etruria e Sardegna centrosettentrionale tra l'età del Bronzo Finale e l'arcaismo. Atti del XXI Convegno di Studi Etruschi ed Italici. Sassari-Alghero-Oristano-Torralba, 13–17 ottobre 1998*, 51–70. Pisa and Rome: Istituti Editoriali Poligrafici Internazionali.

Lucas, A., 1937. "Notes on myrrh and stacte," *Journal of Egyptian Archaeology* 24: 27–33.

Lucian, 1961a. "'A professor of public speaking' (rhetorum praeceptor)." In *Lucian, Volume 4*, trans. A. M. Harmon, 133–171. London: William Heinemann (from the 1925 edition).

Lucian, 1961b. *The Dialogues of the Dead, Lucian, Volume 7*, trans. M. D. Macleod. London: William Heinemann.

Lufkin, Arthur Ward, 1948. *A History of Dentistry.* Second edition. Philadelphia, PA: Lea & Febiger.

Lukacs, John R. and B. E. Hemphill, 1990. "Traumatic injuries of prehistoric teeth: new evidence from Baluchistan and Punjab Provinces, Pakistan," *Anthropologischer Anzeiger* 48 (4): 351–363.

Macchiarelli, Roberto, L. Salvadei, and L. Bondioli, 1995. "Odontometric variation and biological relationships among the Italic (Latins, Samnites, Paeligni, Picenes) and Imperial Roman populations." In Jacopo Moggi-Cecchi, ed., *Aspects of Dental Biology: Palaeontology, Anthropology and Evolution*, 419–436. Florence: International Institute for the Study of Man.

McKechnie, Paul, 1989. *Outsiders in the Greek Cities in the Fourth Century BC.* London and New York: Routledge.

Macnamara, Ellen, 1973. *Everyday Life of the Etruscans.* New York: Dorset Press (1987 reprint).

Mallegni, Francesco, M. Brogi, and E. Balducci, 1980. "Paleodontologia dei reperti umani di Pontecagnano (Salerno), VII–IV sec. a.C.," *Archivio per l'Antropologia e la Etnologia* 114: 63–93.

Mallegni, Francesco, Stefano Bruni, Mario Piombino Mascali, Fulvio Bartoli, and Emiliano Carnieri, 2005. "Paleobiologia del marinaio romano di Pisa San Rossore," *Archeologia Maritima Mediterranea* 1 (2004): 77–88.

Mancinelli Scotti, F. 1917. *Storia topografica di Roma, Narce, Falerii: epoca della pietra italica, etrusca, romana.* Rome: Officina Poligrafica Romana.

Manconi, Dorica and Nicholas Whitehead, 1994. "Imperial incorporation: the advent of Rome (the city)." In Caroline Malone and Simon Stoddart, eds, *Territory, Time and State: The Archaeological Development of the Gubbio Basin*, 178–187. Cambridge: Cambridge University Press.

Manniche, Lise, 1989. *An Ancient Egyptian Herbal.* London: British Museum, and Austin TX: University of Texas Press.

Manzi, Giorgio, Elena Santandrea, and Pietro Passarello, 1997. "Dental size and shape in the Roman Imperial Age: two examples from the area of Rome," *American Journal of Physical Anthropology* 102: 469–479.

Marcellus Empiricus, 1889. *De Medicamentis*, ed. Georg Helmreich. Leipzig: B. G. Teubner.

Marcellus Empiricus, 1968. *Marcellus Über Heilmittel* (in 2 volumes), ed. Max Niedermann. *Corpus Medicorum Latinorum* V. Second edition, revised by Eduard Liechtenhan. Berlin: Akademie-Verlag.

Marcellus of Side, 1851. *Poetae bucolici et didactici. Theocritus, Bion, Moschus. Recognovit et praefatione critica instruxit C. Fr. Ameis; Nicander, Oppianus, Marcellus Sideta de piscibus, Poeta de herbis, recognovit F.S. Lehrs; Phile de animalibus, elephant, plantis, etc. . . .* Paris: Didot: 165–167, repeated at end of book with critical apparatus (pp. cxxiii–cxxv).

Marcellus of Side, 1888. *Marcelli Sidetae medici fragmenta*, ed. O. Schneider. Leipzig: Teubner.

Marin (see under Terribile Wiel Marin).

Marinis (see de Marinis).

Martelli, Andrea and Luca Nasorri, 1998. "La Tomba dell'Iscrizione nella Necropoli di Poggio Rienzo." In Patrizia Gastaldi, ed., *Studi su Chiusi Arcaica*, 81–101. Annali di Archeologia e Storia Ántica (Nuova Serie N. 5). Naples: Istituto Universitario Orientale.

Martial, 1897. *The Epigrams of Martial*, trans. various authors. London: George Bell and Sons.

Martial, 1927. *Martial: Epigrams*, trans. Walter C. A. Ker (in 2 volumes). London: William Heinemann.

Martinelli, Nicholas and S. Charles Spinella, 1981. *Dental Laboratory Technology*. Third edition. St. Louis, IL: C. V. Mosby Company.

Marvitz, Leif, 1982. "Tandlaegekunst." In *Etruskernes Verden: Livet og døden hos et oldtidsfolk i Italien*, 49 (catalogue). Copenhagen: The Authors and The National Museum of Denmark.

Marz, Ilona, 2010. "Zahnschiene aus Gold: Ein Grabfund aus römischer Zeit." In *Der Zweite Blick: Besondere Objekte aus den historischen Sammlungen der Charité*, eds Beate Kunst, Thomas Schnalke and Gottfried Bogusch, 41–49. Berlin: Walter de Gruyter.

Mas, Julio, 1984. "Excavaciones en el Yacimiento Submarino de 'San Ferreol' (Costa de Cartagena)." In *VI Congresso Internazionale de Arqueologia Submarina Cartagena 1982)*, 189–224. Madrid: Ministerio de Cultura.

Masali, Luca, 1985. "La cura dei denti presso i popoli mesopotamici." In G. Vogel and G. Gambacorta, eds, *Storia della odontoiatria*, 47–50. Milan: Ars Medica Antiqua.

Masali, Luca and Alberto Peluso, 1985. "L'odontoiatria nell'antico Egitto." In G. Vogel and G. Gambacorta, eds, *Storia della odontoiatria*, 51–66. Milan: Ars Medica Antiqua Editrice.

Masali, Melchiorre, 1980. "Physical anthropology of the Egyptians." In Ilse Schwidetsky, Bruno Chiarelli, Olga Necrasov, eds, *Physical Anthropology of European Populations*, 369–376. Berlin: De Gruyter.

Matrone, J., 1909. *Précis historique sur les fouilles exécutées par M.r l'ingenieur J. Matrone près de l'anciènne bourgade de la marine de Pompéi: Boscotrecase (prés de Naples)*. Naples: Tipografia Gennaro Avallone (copy at the British School at Rome).

Maugham, W. Somerset, 1934. "Honolulu." In *East and West: The Collected Short Stories of W. Somerset Maugham*, 125–147. Garden City, NY: Garden City Publishing Co.

Maxwell-Hyslop, K. B., 1956. "Urartian bronzes in Etruscan tombs," *Iraq* 18: 150–167.

May, Meredith, 2005. "The gold standard of style: no longer just for tough guys, glittering grills go mainstream," San Francisco Chronicle/SF Gate, May 1, 2005. Online: www.sfgate.com/bayarea/article/BAY-AREA-The-gold-standard-of-style-No-longer-2637779.php (consulted December 30, 2014).

Mayer, Joseph, 1852. *Egyptian Museum: No. VIII, Colquitt-Street, Liverpool.* 1852 (April 15). (Booklet/guide to Mayer's museum in Colquitt Street, Liverpool. Archival copy in the World Museum Liverpool is annotated with inventory numbers by Charles T. Gatty.)

Mayor, Adrienne, 2010. *The Poison King.* Princeton, NJ: Princeton University Press.

Mays, Simon, 1998. *The Archaeology of Human Bones.* London: Routledge.

Meeks, N. D., 2000. "Scanning electron microscopy of the refractory remains and the gold." In Andrew Ramage and Paul Craddock, eds, *King Croesus' Gold: Excavations at Sardis and the History of Gold Refining*, 99–156. Cambridge: Archaeological Exploration of Sardis (with the British Museum). Archaeological Exploration of Sardis Monograph Series, 11.

Meiser, G., ed., 2014. *Etruskische Texte. Editio minor.* Second edition, 2 vols. Hamburg: Baar.

Mello, E., P. Parrini, and Edilberto Formigli, 1982. "Etruscan filigree: welding techniques of two gold bracelets from Vetulonia," *American Journal of Archaeology* 87: 548–551.

Menconi, A. and Gino Fornaciari, 1985. "L'odontoiatria etrusca." In G. Vogel and G. Gambacorta, eds, *Storia della odontoiatria*, 89–97. Milan: Ars Medica Antiqua Editrice.

Mengarelli, R., 1898. "X. Conca. Nuove scoperte nella tenuta di Conca nel territorio dell'antica Satricum," *Notizie degli Scavi* 1896: 166–171.

Merbs, C. F., 1968. "Anterior tooth loss in Arctic populations," *Southwestern Journal of Anthropology* 24: 20–32.

Mérie, Gyulen and Janos Nemeskéri, 1959. "Bericht über eine ein bei einer Mumie verwandete Nasenprothese [Budapest]," *Zeitschrift für ägypische Sprache und Altertumskunde* 84: 76–78.

Michaelides, Demetrius, 1984. "A Roman surgeon's tomb from Nea Paphos," *Report of the Department of Antiquities, Cyprus* 315–332.

Micheloni, Placido, 1976. *Storia dell'odontoiatria. I. Dalla preistoria al tempo di Roma.* Rome: Tipografia Editrice Italia (Volume I of 3: Vols. II and III are titled *Il mondo dei denti e la sua storia*).

Miller, Judith. 2008. "Dental health and disease in ancient Egypt." In Rosalie David, ed., *Egyptian Mummies and Modern Science*, 52–70. Cambridge: Cambridge University Press.

Miller, Stephen G., 1981. "Excavations at Nemea 1980," *Hesperia* 50: 45–67.

Milne, John Stewart, 1907. *Surgical Instruments in Greek and Roman Times.* Oxford: Clarendon Press.

Milner, G. R. and C. S. Larsen, 1991. "Teeth as artifacts of human behavior: intentional mutilation and accidental modification." In Marc A. Kelley and Clark Spencer Larsen, eds, *Advances in Dental Anthropology*, 357–378. New York: Wiley-Liss.

Mingoli, A., 1953. "Invenzione dei denti porcellanacei di Giuseppangelo Fonzi," *Clinica Odontoiatrica* 8: 7–15.

Minozzi, Simona, Gino Fornaciari, Stefano Musco, and Paola Catalano, 2007. "A gold dental prosthesis of Roman Imperial Age," *The American Journal of Medicine* 120 (5): e1–e2. Online with color photos: www. paleopatologia.it/articoli/stampa2. php?recordID=69 (consulted July 18, 2013).

Minozzi, Simona, Paola Catalano, Carla Caldarini, and Gino Fornaciari, 2012. "Paleopathology of human remains from the Roman Imperial Age," *Pathobiology* 79: 268–283.

Minto, Antonio, 1943. *Populonia.* Florence: Istituto di Studi Etruschi/Rinascimento del Libro.

M'Manus, Charles, 1905. "On the history of dentistry from the earliest times," *International Dental Journal* 26: 826–832.

Modi, Jamshedji Jivanji, 1931. "Dentistry in ancient India," *The Indian Dental Journal* 6 (1): 1–15 (copy bound with Sudhoff reprints, The Library of the Dental School of the University of Pennsylvania: D617.673/.SU22).

Moisan, M., 1990. "Les plantes narcotiques dans le Corpus hippocratique." In Paul Potter, Gilles Maloney, and Jacques Desautels, eds, *La maladie et les maladies dans la Collection hippocratique*, 381–391. Actes du VIe Colloque international hippocratique (September 1987). Quebec: Les Editions du Sphinx.

Møller-Christensen, V., 1958. *Bogen om Aebelholt Kloster*. Copenhagen: Dansk Videnskabs Forlag.

Møller-Christensen, V., 1961. *Bone Changes in Leprosy*. Copenhagen: Munksgaard.

Møller-Christensen, V., 1969. "Tandpleje i middelalderen [Dental treatment in the Middle Ages]," *Nordisk Medicinhistorisk Aarsbok, Supplement II*.

Møller-Christensen, V., S. N. Bakke, R. S. Melsom, and A. E. Waaler, 1952. "Changes in the anterior nasal spine and the alveolar process of the maxilla in leprosy," *International Journal of Leprosy* 20 (3): 335–340.

Molleson, Theya, 1992. "Mortality patterns in the Romano-British cemetery at Poundbury Camp, Dorchester." In Steven Bassett, ed., *Death in Towns. Urban responses to the dying and the dead*, 43–55. Leicester and New York: Leicester University Press.

Molleson, Theya, and Margaret Cox, with H. A. Waldron and D. K. Wittaker 1993. *The Spitalfields Project. Volume 2: The Anthropology: The Middling Sort*. CBA Research Report 86. London: Council for British Archaeology.

Molnar, Stephen, 1971. "Human tooth wear, tooth function and cultural variability," *American Journal of Physical Anthropology* 34: 175–189.

Moltesen, Mette, 1987. *Wolfgang Helbig: Brygger Jacobsen's Agent i Rom 1887–1914*. Copenhagen: Ny Carlsberg Glyptotek.

Moltesen, Mette and Cornelia Weber-Lehmann, 1991. *Catalogue of the Copies of Etruscan Tomb Paintings in the Ny Carlsberg Glyptotek*. Ny Carlsberg Glyptotek: Copenhagen.

Moltesen, Mette and Marjatta Nielsen (eds), 1996. *Etruria and Central Italy 450–30* BC (catalogue). Copenhagen: Ny Carlsberg Glyptotek.

Monardes, Nicholas, 1967 [1577]. *Joyfull News Out of the Newe Founde Worlde*, trans. John Frampton. New York: AMS Press Edition.

Monier, Stéphane and Thibault Monier, with Danielle Gourevitch, 2008. "L'Art dentaire chez les Étrusques," *Actualites Odonto-Stomatologiques* 243: 279–293.

Moorehead, Terence F., 1983. "Chirurgia, medicina, dentifricium," *British Dental Journal* 154 (10): 340–342.

Morimoto, Iwataro, 1998. "Attrition on incisors of Asuka and Muromachi Japanese females, probably due to their oral work in spinning ramie into yarn," *Paleopathology Newsletter* 103: 6–7 (summary of a 1995 paper in *Japanese in Anthropological Science* 103 (5): 447–465).

Morris, A. G., 1993. "Human remains from the early Iron Age sites of Nanda and KwaGandaganda, Mngeni Valley, Natal, South Africa," *Natal Museum Journal of Humanities* 5: 83–98.

Morris, A. G., 1998. "Dental mutilation in southern African history and prehistory with special reference to the 'Cape Flats Smile'," *South African Dental Journal* 53: 179–183.

Morteani, Giulio, 1995. "Mineral economics, mineralogy, geochemistry and structure of gold deposits: an overview." In Giulio Morteani and Jeremy P. Northover, eds,

Prehistoric Gold in Europe. Mines Metallurgy and Manufacture, 97–113. Dordrecht: Kluwer Academic. NATO ASI Series, Series E, Applied Scences Volume 280.

Morteani, Giulio and Jeremy P. Northover (eds), 1994. *Prehistoric Gold in Europe: Mines Metallurgy and Manufacture.* Dordrecht: Kluwer Academic. NATO ASI Series, Series E, Applied Scences Volume 280.

Mouton, Claude, 1746. *Essay d'odontotechnie, ou dissertation sur les dents artificielles. Où l'on démontre que leur usage.* Paris: A. Boudet.

Müller, Karl (ed.), 1841–1872. *Fragmenta Historicum Graecorum . . . Apollodori Bibliotheca . . .* (5 volumes). Paris: A. F. Didot. (Scriptorum graecorum bibliotheca, Volume 11a–e.)

Mummery, John R., 1870. "On the relations amongst the ancient inhabitants," *Transactions of the Orthodontic Society of Great Britain* 2: 22.

Muratori, G., 1968. "Giovanni Arcolano, pioniere della odontoiatria—e della chirurgia della bocca. Sua opera e dei principali artefici del 400–500," *Atti del XXI Congresso internazionale di storia della medicina, Siena, Italia, 22–28 settembre 1968* I: 869–873.

Murray, Oswyn (ed.), 1990. *Sympotica: Symposion on the Symposion* (the 1984 conference). Oxford: Oxford University Press.

Musílek, Ladislav, Tomáš Čechák, and Tomáš Trojek, 2012. "X-ray fluorescence in investigations of cultural relics and archaeological finds," *Applied Radiation and Isotopes* 70: 1193–1202.

Musitelli, Sergio, 1995. "Pagine di Odontoiatria e di Odontologia nel Mondo Antico," *Medicina nei Secoli: Arte e Scienza* 8 (2): 207–235.

Musitelli, Sergio, 1996. "An outline of odontoiatry and odontology in the ancient world," *Medicina nei Secoli* 8 (2): 207–235.

Myers, Charles W. and John W. Daly, 1993. "Tropical poison frogs," *Science* 262: 1193.

Naso, Alessandro, 2011. "Protesi dentarie auree in Etruria e nel Lazio." In Simona Rafanelli and Paola Spaziani, eds, *Etruschi: Il privilegio della bellezza.* Sansepolcro Italy: Aboca, 146–154.

Nataf, Daniele, 1988. "Magie, Medicine et Art Dentaire dans l'Egypte pharaonique [Part 1]," *Revue Odonto Stomatologie* 17: 323–332.

Nataf, Daniele, 1989. "Magie, Medicine et Art Dentaire dans l'Egypte pharaonique [Part 2]," *Revue Odonto Stomatologie* 18: 31–41.

Nati, Danilo, 2012. *La collezione Bruschi Falgari. Materiali del Museo Archeologico Nazionale di Tarquinia*, 20 (Archeologia 168), Rome: G. Bretschneider.

Neiburger, E. J., 1992. *The Dentists' Handbook.* Waukegan, IL: Andent.

Neiburger, E. J., 2000. "Dentistry in ancient Mesopotamia," *Journal of the Massachusetts Dental Society* 49 (2): 16–19.

Neiburger, E. J., M. Cohen, J. Lieberman, and M. Lieberman, 1998. "The dentition of Abraham's people: why Abraham left Mesopotamia," *The New York State Dental Journal* 64 (9): 25–29.

Nepos, Cornelius, 1904. *Corneli Nepotis Vitae*, ed. Eric Otto Winstedt. Oxonii: E. Typographes Clarendoniano. Scriptorum classicorum biblioteca Oxoniensis.

Nestler, Gerhard and Edilberto Formigli, 1994/2001. *Granulazione etrusca. Un'antica arte orafa.* Siena: nuova imagine. (Reprinted 2001.)

Newmyer, Stephen, 1993. "Asaph the Jew and Greco-Roman pharmaceutics." In Irene Jacob and Walter Jacob, eds, *The Healing Past. Pharmaceuticals in the Biblical and Rabbinic World*, 107–120. Leiden: E. J. Brill.

Nickol, Thomas, 1991. "'To have and have not': remarks on extraction in 'eight books on medicine' of Celsus," *Bulletin of the History of Dentistry* 39 (1): 21–24.

Nicolini, G., 1992. "Gold wire techniques of Europe and the Mediterranean around 300 BC." In Giulio Morteani and Jeremy P. Northover, eds, *Prehistoric Gold in Europe: Mines Metallurgy and Manufacture*, 453–470. Dordrecht: Kluwer Academic. NATO ASI Series, Series E, Applied Sciences Volume 280.

Nielsen, Inge, 1992. "The Metellan Temple." In Inge Nielsen and Birte Poulsen, eds, *The Temple of Castor and Pollux I*, 87–117. Rome: De Luca for the Soprintendenza Archeologica di Roma.

Nielsen, Inge and Jan Zahle, 1987. "The Temple of Castor and Pollux on the Forum Romanum. Preliminary Report on the Scandinavian Excavations 1983–1985," *Acta Archeologica* 56 (1985): 1–30.

Nielsen, Marjatta, 1975. "The lid sculptuires of Volaterran cinerary urns." In P. Bruun, ed., *Studies in the Romanization of Etruria (Acta Instituti Romani Finlandiae 5)*, 263–404. Rome: Bardi.

Nielsen, Marjatta, 1985. "Women in late Etruscan society." In K. Jexlev, ed., *Fromhed og verdslighed i middelalder og renaissance. Festskrift til Thelma Jexlev*, 192–202. Odense: Odense Universitetsvorlag.

Nielsen, Marjatta, 1986 "Late Etruscan cinerary urns from Volterra at the J. Paul Getty Museum: a lid figure altered from male to female, and an ancestor to satirist Persius," *Getty Museum Journal* 14: 43–58.

Nielsen, Marjatta, 1988–1989. "Women and family in a changing society: a quantitative approach to late Etruscan burials, *Analecta Romana Instituti Danici* 17–18: 53–98.

Nielsen, Marjatta, 1989. "La donna e la famiglia nella tarda società etrusca." In A. Rallo, ed., *Le Donne in Etruria*, 121–145. Rome: "L'Erma" di Bretschneider (Studia Archeologica 52).

Nielsen, Marjatta, 1990. "Sacerdotesse e associazioni cultuali femminili in Etruria: testimonianze epigrafiche e iconografiche," *Analecta Romana Instituti Danici* 19: 45–67.

Nielsen, Marjatta, 1992. "Portrait of a marriage: the old Etruscan couple from Volterra." In *Ancient Portraiture: Image and Message. Acta Hyperborea: Danish Studies in Classical Archaeology* 4: 89–141. Copenhagen: Museum Tusculanum Press, University of Copenhagen.

Nielsen, Marjatta, 1996. "Burial customs in Etruria [pages 20–27] and sarcophagi and cinerary urns." In Mette Moltesen and Marjatta Nielsen, eds, *Etruria and Central Italy 450–30 BC.* (Catalogue), 43–128. Copenhagen: Ny Carlsberg Glyptotek.

Nielsen, Marjatta, 1998. "Etruscan women: a cross-cultural perspective." In Lena Larsson Lovén and Agneta Strömberg, eds, *Aspects of Women in Antiquity (Proceedings of the First Nordic Symposium on Women's Lives in Antiquity (1997)*, 69–84. Jonsered: Paul Åströms Förlag.

Nielsen, Marjatta, 2007. "Late Etruscan sarcophagi as expressions of status for women and men in public roles and personal status." In Lena Larsson Lovén and Agneta Strömberg, eds, *Men and Women in Antiquity: Proceedings of the Third Nordic Symposium on Gender and Women's History in Antiquity (Copenhagen 3–5 October 2003)* 57–72. Sävedalen: Paul Åströms Förlag.

Nobel, Gabriel, 1909. *Zü geschichte der zahnheilkunde im Talmud*. Leipzig: Druck von W. Drugulin.

Norman, C. R., 2009. "Warriors and weavers: sex and gender in Daunian stelae." In K. Lomas and E. Herring, eds, *Gender Identities in Italy in the First Millennium BC*, 37–54. Oxford: BAR IS, vol. 1983.

Norman, Camilla R., 2011a. "The tribal tattooing of Daunian women,"*European Journal of Archaeology* 14:1–2, 133–157.

Norman, Camilla R., 2011b. "Weaving, gift and wedding: a local identity for the Daunian stelae." In M. Gleba and H, Horsnæs, eds, *Communicating Identity in Italic Iron Age Communities*, 33–49. Oxford: Oxbow Books.

Norman, Camilla R. 2012. "The Iron Age stelae of Daunia (Italy)." Dissertation. The University of Sydney.

Norman, Camillla R., 2016. "Daunian women: costume and actions commemorated in stone." In S. L. Budin and J. M. Turfa, eds, *Women in Antiquity: Real Women Across the Ancient World*. London: Routledge, 865–876.

Northcote, James Spencer, 1878. *Epitaphs of the Catacombs, Or, Christian Inscriptions in Rome During the First Four Centuries*. London: Longmans, Green, and Co.

Nunn, John F., 1996. *Ancient Egyptian Medicine*. Norman, OK: University of Oklahoma Press.

Nutting, J. and J. L. Nuttall, 1977. "The maleability of gold," *Gold Bulletin* 10: 2–8.

Nutton, Vivian, 2004. *Ancient Medicine*. London: Routledge.

O'Brien, William J. (ed.), 1989. *Dental Materials: Properties and Selection*. Chicago, IL: Quintessence Publishing Company.

Oefele, Felix Freiherr von, 1902. *Materialien zur Bearbeitung babylonischer Medizin*. Berlin: W. Peiser.

Oefele, Felix Freiherr von, 1917. "Babylonian titles of medical textbooks," *Journal of the American Oriental Society* 37: 250.

Økland, Jorunn, 1995. "'*In Publicum Procurrendi*': women in the public space of Roman Greece." In Lena Larsson Lovén and Agneta Strömberg, eds, *Aspects of Women in Antiquity: Proceedings of the First Nordic Symposium on Women's Lives in Antiquity (Göteborg 12–15 June 1997)*, 127–141. Jonsered: Paul Åströms Förlag.

Önnerfors, A., 1993. "Magische Formeln im Dienste römischer Medizin." In *Aufstieg und Niedergang der Römischen Welt* 37 (1): 157–226.

Ontalba Salamanca, M. A., G. Demortier, F. Fernndez Gomez, P. Coquay, J. L. Ruvulcaba-Sil, and M. A. Respaldiza, 1998. "PIXE and SEM studies of Tartesic gold artefacts," *Nuclear Instruments and Methods in Physics Research* B 136–138: 851–857.

Oranje, P., N. Noriskin, and T. W. B. Osborn, 1935. "The effect of diet upon dental caries in the South African Bantu," *South African Journal of Medical Sciences* 1: 57–62.

Origo, Iris, 1963. *The Merchant of Prato: Francesco di Marco Datini*. Harmondsworth, UK: Penguin Books.

Oyamada, J., Y. Kitagawa, Y. Manabe, and Rokutanda, A., 2000. "People of the Samurai class kept their antemortem lost teeth," *Dental Anthropology* 14: 7–14.

Pacciani, Elsa and Robert S. Corruccini, 1986. "Studio Epidemiologico comparativo sull'occlusione dentale," *Antropologia Contemporanea* 9: 57–64.

Pacciani, Elsa and Fiorenza Sonego, 1998. "La tomba dell'Iscrizione era una tomba di famiglia?" In Patrizia Gastaldi, ed., *Studi su Chiusi Arcaica*, 103–105. (*Annali di Archeologia e Storia Ántica*, Nuova Serie N. 5). Naples: Istituto Universitario Orientale.

Packard, Francis R., 1921. *Life and Times of Ambroise Paré (1510–1590)*. New York: P. B. Hoeber.

Pagano, Mario, 1996. "La nuova pianeta della città e di alcuni edifici pubblici di ercolano," *Cronache ercolanesi* 26: 229–262.

Pagano, Mario, 1997. *I Diari di scavo di Pompeii, Ercolano e Stabiae di Francesco e Pietro La Vega (1764–1810)*. (Soprintendenza Archeologica di Pompeii Monografie 13.) Rome: L'Erma di Bretschneider.

Pannozzo, Enrica, 1986. "Esplorazione archeologiche e collezionismo: dal ritrovamento fortuito allo scavo sistematico, dalla raccolta privata al museo pubblico." In Giovanella Morghen, ed., *Bibliotheca Etrusca. Fonti letterarie e figurative tra XVIII e XIX secolo nella Biblioteca dell'Istituto Nazionale di Archeologia e Storia dell'Arte*, 21–59. Rome: Istituto Poligrafico e Zecca dello Stato.

Papabasileiou, G. A., 1903. "Anaskaphai en Euboia," *Praktika tis en Athinais Archaiologikis Etaireias tou Etous* 1902: 61–72 (*en Eretria*: 63–65).

Paré, Ambroise, 1564. *Dix Livres de la chirurgie avec le magasin des instruments necessaires à icelle*. Paris: Jean Le Roger.

Paré, Ambroise, 1585. *Les oeuvres d'Ambroise Paré* (in 28 volumes). Fourth edition. Paris: G. Buon.

Parrini, Paolo, Edilberto Formigli, and Emilio Mello, 1982. "Etruscan granulation: analysis of orientalizing jewelry from Marsiliana d'Albenga," *American Journal of Archaeology* 86: 118–121.

Paton, W. R., 1956. *The Greek Anthology*. Volume IV (5 volumes). Cambridge, MA: Harvard University Press.

Paul of Aegina, 1844–1847. *The Seven Books of Paulus Aegineta* (3 volumes), trans. F. Adams. London: Sydenham Society.

Paul of Aegina, 1924. *Paulus Aegineta* (part 2, Books V–VII), ed. I.L. Heiberg. *Corpus Medicorum Graecorum* IX, 2. Leipzig: B. G. Teubner.

Pedani Dioscuridis Anazarbi, 1958. *Materia Medica*, ed. Max Wellman (5 *libri* in 3 volumes). Berlin: Weidmann.

Pedersen, P. O., 1978. "The dentition of King Christian the Third," *Ossa* 6: 229–242.

Pelagatti, Paola, 1985. "Il museo di Villa Giulia e gli altri musei dell'Etruria Meridionale nell'ultimo triennio," *Studi Etruschi* 51: 511–534.

Penso, Giuseppe, 1984. *Le Médicine Romaine*. Paris: Editions R. Dacosta.

Penso, Giuseppe, 1985. *La Medicina Romana* (translation of Penso 1984). Italy: Ciba-Geigy.

Peréz-Pérez, A., C. Lalueza, M. Hernández, and D. Turbón, 1992. "Análisis del patrón de estriación dentaria: variabilidad intrapoblacional en la serie medieval de La Olmeda (Palencia)." In *Nuevas perspectivas en Antropología. VII Congresso Español de Antropología Biológica*, 731–740. Granada: Universidad de Granada, Imprenta Provincial.

Perine, George H., 1883. "A history of dentistry from the earliest period to the present time," *New England Journal of Dentistry* 2 (6): 161–166, 199–205, 269–273, 343–345.

Perkins, Philip, 1999. *Etruscan Settlement, Society and Material Culture in Central Coastal Etruria*. BAR International Series, Number 788. Oxford: John and Erika Hedges.

Petrie, W. M. Flinders, 1914. *Amulets*. London: Constable.

Pfaff, Philipp, 1756. *Abhandlung von den Zähnen des menschlichen Körpers und deren Krankheiten*. Berlin: Haude and Spencer.

Pfeiffer, K., 1978. "Was there dentistry in highly cultured old Mesopotamia?" *Zahnärztlicher Gesundheitsdienst (Bundesverbandes der Zahnärtzte)* 15 (2): 8–10.

Pfeiffer, S., J. C. Dudar, and S. Austin, 1989. "Prospect Hill: skeletal remains from a 19th-century Methodist cemetery, Newmarket, Ontario [Canada]," *Northeast Historical Archaeology* 18: 29–48. Online: http://digitalcommons.buffalostate.edu/neha/vol18/iss1/4 (consulted March 22, 2016).

Philbrook, B. F., 1897. "Cast fillings," *Transactions of the Iowa State Dental Society*, 1897: 277–279. (Paper read before the Iowa State Dental Society, Thirty-fourth Annual Meeting, Des Moines, Iowa.) Cedar Rapids, Iowa: T.S. Metcalf.

Piergili, B., 1906–1907. "Gold crown del VI secolo av. G. C.," *La Stomatologia* 5: 319.

Pietrusewsky, Michael and Michele T. Douglas, 1992. "Tooth ablation in old Hawaii," *The Journal of the Polynesian Society* 102 (3): 255–272.

Piette, Michel, Guy Demortier, and Fraz Bodart, 1986. "PIXE analysis of solders on ancient gold artifacts with a nuclear microprobe." In A. D. Romig, Jr. and W. F. Chambers, eds, *Microbeam Analysis*, 333–336. San Francisco, CA: San Francisco Press.

Pinch, Geraldine, 1995. *Magic in Ancient Egypt*. Austin, TX: University of Texas Press.

Pindborg, J. Jørgen and L. Marvitz, 1960. *Tandlaegen i kunsten; en ikonografi. København: Munksgaard: The Dentist in Art*. Translated from the Danish by Gillian Hartz. Chicago, IL: Quadrangle Books.

Pingel, V., 1995. "Technical aspects of prehistoric gold objects on the basis of mineralogical analysis." In Giulio Morteani and Jeremy P. Northover, eds, *Prehistoric Gold in Europe: Mines Metallurgy and Manufacture*, 385–398. Dordrecht: Kluwer Academic. NATO ASI Series, Series E, Applied Scences Volume 280.

Pinto-Cisternas, Juan, Jacopo Moggi-Cecchi, and Elsa Pacciani, 1995. "The lateral incisor trait." In Jacopo Moggi-Cecchi, ed., *Aspects of Dental Biology: Palaeontology, Anthropology and Evolution*, 333–339. Florence: International Institute for the Study of Man.

Piperno, Arrigo, 1910. "Un pó di Stomatologia del passato (1500–1800)," [Estratto dalla] *Stomatologia* 8: 3–32. Milano: Casa Edit. L. F. Cogliati.

Pirzio Biroli Stefanelli, Lucia, 1992. *L'Oro dei Romani: Gioielli di Età Imperiale*. "L'Erma" di Bretschneider: Roma.

Pittau, Massimo, 1997. "La lingua etrusca: Grammatica e lessico," *GLOSSA* 4. Nuoro, Sardinia: Insula.

Pizzamiglio, Pierluigi (ed.), 1992. "Gerardo da Cremona," *Annali della Biblioteca Statale e Libreria Civica di Cremona* 41 (1990).

Platschick, Carlo, 1904–1905. "La via percorsa dall'odontoiatria (Section I of "Primo Trattato Italiano di Odontotecnica")," *La Stomatologia* 3: 237–256.

Pleket, H. W., 1995. "The social status of physicians in the Graeco-Roman world." In Ph. van der Eijk, H. F. J. Horstmanshoff, and P. H. Schrijvers, eds, *Ancient Medicine in its Socio-Cultural Context*, Volume I, 27–34. (Papers of the Leiden Congress, 1992.) Amsterdam: Rodopi (*Clio Medica* 27).

Pliny, 1870–1898. *C. Plini Secundi naturalis historiae libri XXXVII*. Volume 1 (1870) ed. Ludwig von Jan; Volumes 2–6 (1875–1898) ed. Karl Friedrich T. Mayhoff. Leipzig: B. G. Teubner.

Pliny, 1962. *Natural History*. Volume X: Books 36–37, ed. D. E. Eichholz. London: William Heinemann.

Pliny, 1963. *Natural History*. Volume VIII: Books 28–32, ed. W. H. S. Jones. London: William Heinemann.

Podestà, G., 1947. "Le satire Lucianeschi di Teodore Prodromo," *Aevum* 21: 17–22.

Pollux, 1900. *Pollucis Onomasticon*, ed. Eric Bethe. Part I (containing Books I–V) of Volume IX, from *Lexicographi Graeci*. Leipzig: B. G. Teubner. Online: http://babel. hathitrust.org/cgi/pt?id=inu.32000001852062;view=1up;seq=5 (consulted June 6, 2014).

Polscher, Walter, 1908. "Altitalische Zahnersatzkunst—moderne Brückenarbeit," *Deutsche Zahnärztliche Wochenschrift* 11: 5–8.

Ponting, Matthew J. and Pablo Fernandez-Reyes, 2015. "Report on the analysis by scanning electron microscope with energy-dispersive spectrometry (SEM-EDS) of two Etruscan gold denture fittings." Manuscript report, University of Liverpool.

Porter, Roy and Mikulas Teich (eds), 1995. *Drugs and Narcotics in History*. Cambridge: Cambridge University Press.

Pot, Tjeerd, 1985. "Two Etruscan gold dental appliances, found in 19th century excavations at Satricum and Praeneste," *Mededelingen van het Nederlands Instituut te Rome* 47 (New Series 11): 35–39.

Potter, Tim, 1978. *The Changing Landscape of South Etruria.* London: Paul Elsk.

Poulsen, Birthe, 1992. "The written sources." In Inge Nielsen and Birte Poulsen, eds, *The Temple of Castor and Pollux I*, 54–60. Rome: De Luca for the Soprintendenza Archeologica di Roma.

Poulsen, Frederik, 1927. *Aus einer alten Etruskerstadt.* Copenhagen: Bianco Lunos Bogtrykkeri.

Powell, Marvin, 1993. "Drugs and pharmaceuticals in ancient Mesopotamia." In Irene Jacobs and Walter Jacobs, eds, *The Healing Past: Pharmaceuticals in the Biblical and Rabbinic World*, 46–67. Leiden: E. J. Brill.

Powers, Rosemary, 1988. "Operative dentistry in the second century BCE," *Paleopathology Newsletter* 63: 13–14.

Preuss, Julius, 1971. *Biblisch-talmudische Medizin.* New York: KTAV Publishing House (from the 1911 edition).

Proskaur, Curt, 1979. "A pictorial history of dentistry. Part I: prehistoric, Egyptian, Assyrian. Part II: Etruscan, Roman, and Greek," *TIC* 38 (2): 8–10, (3): 13–14. (*TIC* was a dental journal published by Ticonium Corporation of Albany NY, now discontinued.)

Prossinger, Hermann, 1998. "The reconstruction of missing tooth dimensions as a prerequisite for sex determination." In Kurt W. Alt, Friedrich W, Rösing, and Maria Teschler-Nicola, eds, *Dental Anthropology: Fundamentals, Limits, and Prospects*, 501–518. Vienna: Springer.

Puccioni, Nello, 1904. "Dello deformazioni e mutilazioni artificiali etniche più in uso," *Archivio per L'Antropologia e la Etnologia* 34: 355–402.

Puech, Pierre-François F., 1987. "Examen microsopique d'une momie egyptienne," *Nouvelles Archives du Musée d'Histoire Naturelle de Lyon*, Fascicule 25: 58–60.

Puech, Pierre-François F., 1995. "Dentistry in ancient Egypt: Junkers' teeth," *Dental Anthropology Newsletter* 10 (1): 5–7.

Puech, Pierre-François, C. Serratrice, and F. F. Leek, 1983. "Tooth wear as observed in ancient Egyptian skulls," *Journal of Human Evolution* 12: 617–629.

Puech, Pierre-François, Francois Cianfarani, and Stella Puech, 1990. "Les Dents, des singes à Mozart," *L'Information Dentaire* 72 (22): 2003–2008.

Pulak, C. 1998. "The Uluburun shipwreck: an overview," *International Journal of Nautical Archaeology* 27: 188–224.

Pulak, C. 2001. "The cargo of the Uluburun ship and evidence for trade with the Aegean and Beyond." In L. Bonfante and V. Karageorghis, eds, *Italy and Cyprus in Antiquity: 1500–450 BC*, 13–60. Nicosia: Severis Foundation.

Purland, T. Jr., 1831. *Practical Directions for Preserving the Teeth.* London: S. Highley.

Purland, T. Jr., 1857–1858. "Dental memoranda," *Quarterly Journal of Dental Science* I: 63–65, 201–204, 342–346, 460–463; II (1858): 121–123, 242–243, 353–355, 490–493.

Quenouille, Jean-Jacques, 1975. "La Bouche et les dents dans l'Antiquité égyptienne." Doctoral Thesis (Dental Surgery) presented at the University Claude-Bernard, Lyon (No. 437), France.

Quenouille, Jean-Jacques, 1977. "Les papyrus médicaux," *Information Dentaire* 23: 29–43.

Quintarelli, L., 1946. "L'odontoiatria nella storia," *Clinica Odontoiatrica* 2 (March): 34–36, 54–56, 102–104.

Rafanelli, Simona and Paola Spaziani, eds, 2011. *Etruschi: Il privilegio della bellezza.* Sansepolcro, Italy: Aboca. (2011 exhibition, Centro Studi Aboca Museum.)

Rallo, Antonia, 1989a. "Classi sociali e mano d'opera femminile." In A. Rallo, ed., *Le Donne in Etruria*, 147–156. Rome: "L'Erma" di Bretschneider (Studia Archeologica 52).

Rallo, Antonia, 1989b. "La cosmesi." In A. Rallo, ed., *Le Donne in Etruria*, 173–179. Rome: "L'Erma" di Bretschneider (Studia Archeologica 52).

Ramage, Andrew and Paul Craddock (eds), 2000a. *King Croesus' Gold: Excavations at Sardis and the History of Gold Refining*. Cambridge, MA: Harvard University Press for the Archaeological Exploration of Sardis. Archaeological Exploration of Sardis Monograph Series, 11.

Ramage, Andrew and Paul Craddock, 2000b. "Prologue." In Andrew Ramage and Paul Craddock, eds, *King Croesus' Gold: Excavations at Sardis and the History of Gold Refining*, 10–13. Cambridge: Archaeological Exploration of Sardis (with the British Museum). Archaeological Exploration of Sardis Monograph Series, 11.

Ramage, Nancy H., 1989. "A list of Sir William Hamilton's property," *The Burlington Magazine* 131 (1039): 704–706.

Ramage, Nancy H., 1990 "Sir William Hamilton as collector, exporter, and dealer: the acquisition and dispersal of his collections," *American Journal of Archaeology* 94: 469–480.

Ramos Calvo, P. M., 1986. "Dentistry in antiquity: Egypt, Hippocrates, Galen and Celsus. [In Spanish]," *Revista española de Estomatologia* 34: 427–437.

Rastrelli, Anna, 1998. "La necropoli di Poggio Gaiella." In Patrizia Gastaldi, ed., *Studi su Chiusi Arcaica*, 57–79. (Annali di Archeologia e Storia Ántica, Nuova Serie No. 5). Naples: Istituto Universitario Orientale.

Rath, Gernot, 1958. "Notizie storiche sulle protesi dentarie," *Symposium Ciba [Milano]* 6 (1): 9–18. Copy at Consiglio Nazionale di Ricerca, Roma.

Rathje, Annette, 1989. "Alcune considerazioni sulle lastre da Poggio Civitate con figure femminili." In A. Rallo, ed., *Le Donne in Etruria*, 75–84. Rome: "L'Erma" di Bretschneider (Studia Archeologica 52).

Rathje, Annette. 2007. "Etruscan women and power." In Lena Larsson Lovén and Agneta Strömberg, eds, *Public Roles and Personal Status: Men and Women in Antiquity. Proceedings of the Third Nordic Symposium on Gender and Women's History in Antiquity (Copenhagen 3–5 October 2003)*, 19–34. Sävedalen: Paul Åströms Förlag.

Rathje, A. 2013. "The banquet through Etruscan history." In J. M. Turfa, ed., *The Etruscan World*, 823–830. London: Routledge.

Raub, Ch. J., 1995. "The metallurgy of gold and silver in prehistoric times." In Giulio Morteani and Jeremy P. Northover, eds, *Prehistoric Gold in Europe: Mines Metallurgy and Manufacture*, 243–259. Dordrecht: Kluwer Academic. NATO ASI Series, Series E, Applied Sciences Volume 280.

Rawson, Beryl, 1991. "Adult–child relationships in Roman society." In Beryl Rawson, ed., *Marriage, Divorce and Children in Ancient Rome*, 7–30. Oxford: Clarendon Press.

Recke, Matthias, 2013. "Science as art: Etruscan anatomical votives." In J. M. Turfa, ed., *The Etruscan World*, 1068–1085. London: Routledge.

Recke, Matthias and Waltrud Wamser-Krasznai, (2008). *Kultische Anatomie. Etruskische Körperteil-Votive aus der Antikensammlung der Justus-Liebig-universität Giessen (Stiftung Ludwig Stieda)*. Ingolstadt: Deutsches Medizinhistorisches Museum.

Reid, Nicholas and Klaus Wagensonner, 2014. "My tooth aches so much," *Cuneiform Digital Library Bulletin* 2014: 3. Online: http://cdli.uda.edu/pubs/cdlb/2014/cdlb2014_003.html (consulted July 31, 2014).

Reinach, Salomon, 1892 (see under O. Hamdî).

Reinach, Salomon, 1918. *"Medicus."* In Charles Daremburg and M. Edmond Saglio, eds, *Dictionnaire des Antiquités Grecques et Romaines*, Volume 3, part 2 (L–M): 1669–1700. Paris: Librairie Hachette.

Renan, Ernest, 1864. *Mission de Phénicie e le Campagne de Sidon*. Paris: Imprimerie impériale.

Rendeli, Mario, 1993. *Città aperte*. Rome: Gruppo Editoriale Internazionale.

Renzi, Martina, Ignacio Montero-Ruiz and Michael Bode, 2009. "Non-ferrous metallurgy from the Phoenician site of La Fonteta (Alicante, Spain): a study of provenance," *Journal of Archaeological Science* 36: 2584–2596.

Rey, R., 1993. *Histoire de la douleur*. Paris: La Découverte.

Reynolds, David West, 1997. "The lost architecture of ancient Rome: insights from the Severan Plan and the regionary catalogues," *Expedition* 39 (2): 15–24.

Richardson, L. Jr., 1992. *A New Topographical Dictionary of Ancient Rome*. Baltimore, MD: Johns Hopkins Press.

Richter, G. M. A., 1966. *The Furniture of the Greeks, Etruscans and Romans*. London: Phaidon.

Riddle, John M., 1985. *Dioscorides on Pharmacy and Medicine*. Austin, TX: University of Texas Press. History of Science Series, 3.

Riddle, John M., 1987. "Folk tradition and folk medicine: recognition of drugs in classical antiquity." In John Scarborough, ed., *Folklore and Folk Medicine*, 33–61. Madison, WI: American Institute of the History of Pharmacy.

Riddle, John M., 1992. *Quid pro quo: Studies in the History of Drugs*. Aldershot, UK: Variorum.

Riddle, John M., 1993. "High medicine and low medicine in the Roman empire." In *Aufstieg und Niedergang der Römischen Welt* 37 (1): 102–120.

Ridgway, David, 1992. *The First Western Greeks*. Cambridge: Cambridge University Press.

Ridgway, David, 1997. "Nestor's Cup and the Etruscans," *Oxford Journal of Archaeology* 16, 3: 325–344.

Ridgway, David, 2000. "The first Western Greeks revisited," in D. Ridgway, F. R. Serra Ridgway, M. Pearce, E. Herring, R. D. Whitehouse, and J. B. Wilkins, eds, *Ancient Italy in its Mediterranean Setting: Studies in honour of Ellen Macnamara*, 179–191. London: Accordia Research Institute, University of London.

Riethe, P. and A. Czarnetzki, 1983. "Amalgam- und Goldfolienfüllung Anno Domini 1601," *Deutsche Zahnärztliche Zeitschrift* 38: 610–616.

Riis, Poul Jorgen, 1941. *Tyrrhenika: An Archaeological Study of the Etruscan Sculpture in the Archaic and Classical Periods*. Copenhagen: Einar Munksgaard.

Ring, Malvin E., 1985. *Dentistry: An Illustrated History*. New York: Harry N. Abrams.

Ring, Malvin E., 1986. "Dentistry in ancient Rome," *Compendium* 7: 715–716, 718.

Risdon, D. L., 1938. "A study of the cranial and other human remains from Palestine excavated at Tell Duweir (Lachish) by the Wellcome-Marston Archaeological research expedition," *Biometrika* 31: 99–166.

Ritner, Robert K., 1993. *The Mechanics of Ancient Egyptian Magical Practice*. Studies in Ancient Oriental Civilization, Volume 54. Chicago, IL: The Oriental Institute of the University of Chicago Press.

Rix, H., ed., 1991. *Etruskische Texte. Editio minor*. First edition, 2 vols. Tübingen: Gunther Narr.

Rivault, A. A., 1953. "La contention en prothèse partielle fixe," *Minerva Stomatologica* 2 (1): 1–3.

Rizzo, M. Antonella, 1985. "Appendice I. Dati sulla risistenazione dei corredi e sulle nuove esposizione." In P. Pelagatti, ed., "Il museo di Villa Giulia e gli altri musei dell'Etruria Meridionale nell'ultimo triennio," *Studi Etruschi* 51: [511–534] 518–527.

Robb, John, 1994a. "Burial and social reproduction in the Peninsular Italian Neolithic," *Journal of Mediterranean Archaeology* 7: 29–75.

Robb, John, 1994b. "Anthropology and paleopathology of Neolithic human remains from Catignano (Pescara, Italy)," *Rivista di Antropologia* (Roma) 72: 197–224.

Robb, John, 1997a. "Violence and gender in early Italy." In Ann Olga Kosloski-Ostrow and Claire L. Lyons, eds, *Troubled Times: Osteological and Archaeological Evidence of Violence*, 43–65. New York: Routledge.

Robb, John, 1997b. "Intentional tooth removal in Neolithic Italian women," *Antiquity* 71: 659–669.

Roberts, Charlotte, 1986. "Leprogenic odontodysplasia." In E. Cruwys and R. Foley, eds, *Teeth and Anthropology*, 137–147. BAR International Series 291. Oxford: BAR.

Robetti, I., 1983. "Le nomenclature dentali," *Minerva Stomatologia* 32: 476.

Rodkinson, Michael L., 1896. *New Edition of the Babylonian Talmud: English Translation.* Revised and corrected by Isaac M. Wise. Volume I: *Tract Sabbath*. New York: New Amsterdam Book Company.

Rohner (see Dvorsky-Rohner).

Roldan, B., J. A. Sánchez, and B. Perea, 1992. "A human molar of the Roman period set in a silver ring [Abstract of a poster presentation from the 1992 Paleopathology Meeting, Barcelona]." In *Papers on Paleopathology* (distributed by the Paleopathology Association), 345. (Proceedings of the Ninth European Meeting of the Paleopathology Association. Abstracts from The Museu D'Arquelogia de Catalunya, Barcelona 1995.)

Rolleston, J. D., 1914. "Medical aspects of the Greek anthology," *Proceedings of the Royal Society of Medicine, London, Part II: Section of the History of Medicine* 7: 3–13, 30–56.

Romero, J., 1970. "Dental mutilation, trephination, and cranial deformation." In T. Dale Stewart, ed., *Handbook of Middle American Indians*, Volume 9: 50–67. Austin, TX: University of Texas Press.

Rosenthal, F., 1960. "Bibliographical notes on medieval Muslim dentistry," *Bulletin of the History of Medicine* 34 (1): 52–60.

Rösing, F. W., 1980. "Sexing immature human skeletons," *Journal of Human Evolution* 12: 149–155.

Rösing, F. W., G. Paul, and S. Schnutenhaus, 1995. "Sexing skeletons by tooth size." In Ralf J. Radlanski and Herbert Renz, eds, *Proceedings of the 10th International Symposium on Dental Morphology*, 373–376. Berlin: "M" Marketing Services C. and M. Brünner GbR.f

Rovira, Salvador and Martina Renzi, 2013. "Plata Tartésica: una revisión de la tecnología extractiva a la luz de nuevos hallazgos." In Juan M. Campos and Jaime Alver, eds, *Tarteso. El emporio del metal*, 473–488. Córdoba: Almuzara.

Rowland, Ingrid, 2001. "Etruscan secrets," *New York Review of Books* 48 (11): 12, 14–17.

Rowland, Ingrid, 2013. "Annius of Viterbo." In J. M. Turfa, ed., *The Etruscan World*, 1117–1129. London: Routledge.

Ruffer, Marc Armand, 1913. "Studies in palaeopathology in Egypt," *Journal of Pathology and Bacteriology* 18: 149–162.

Ruffer, Marc Armand, 1920. "Study of abnormalities and pathology of ancient Egyptian teeth," *American Journal of Physical Anthropology* 3: 335–382.

Ruffer, Marc Armand, 1921. *Studies in the Paleopathology of Egypt*. Chicago, IL: University of Chicago Press.

Russo, Andrea, 1992. "I preparatori di farmaci nella società romana," *PACT: From Epidaurus to Salerno 34*: 263–274.

Ryff, Walther Hermann, 1545. *Die gross Chirurgei, oder, volkommene Wundartzenei chirurgischen Handtwirckung eigentlicher Bericht, und Inhalt alles so der Wundartznei angehörig : mit künstlicher Fürmalung, klarer Beschreibung, und Anzeyg vilfaltiger Nutzbarkeyt und Gebrauchs, aller hierzu dienlicher und gebreuchlicher Instrument oder Ferrament.* . . . Franckfurt [am Meyn]: Chr. Eg. University of Pennsylvania Rare Books, Folio RD30.R94 1545.

Sabbah, Guy, and Philippe Mudry (eds), (1995). *La médecine de Celse. Aspects historiques, scientifiques et littéraires.* Publications de l'Université de Saint-Étienne, Centre Jean-Palerne. Mémoires XIII.

Sallou, F., 1975. "Archéologie dentaire: le spécimen de Junker," *Revue d'Odonto-Stomatologie* 4 (6): 521–531.

Salvadei, Loredana, 2002. *Valori metrici corone denti permanenti* [sic]. (Data from the adults at the Iron Age Cemetery at Osteria dell'Osa, Rome, Italy.) Ms on file, Becker archives, West Chester, PA: West Chester University,

Sanchez Canton, Francesco Javier, 1972. *Museo del Prado: Catálogo de las pinturas.* Madrid: Museo del Prado.

Sannibale, Maurizio, 2006. "Tra cielo e terra. Considerazioni su alcuni aspetti della religione etrusca a Vulci," *Studi Etruschi* 72 (2006/2009), 117–147.

Sannibale Maurizio, 2008a. "Gli ori della Tomba Regolini-Galassi: tra tecnologia e simbolo. Nuove proposte di lettura nel quadro del fenomeno Orientalizzante in Etruria", *Mélanges de l'École Française de Rome—Antiquité (MEFRA)* 120 (2): 337–367.

Sannibale, Maurizio, 2008b. "Iconografie e simboli orientali nelle corti dei principi etruschi," *Byrsa* 7.1 (2): 85–123.

Sannibale, Maurizio, 2013. "Orientalizing Etruria." In J. M. Turfa, ed., *The Etruscan World*, 99–133. London: Routledge.

Sannibale, Maurizio, 2015. "Giovanni Pinza a cento anni dai 'Materiali per l'Etnologia Antica Toscano-Laziale,'" *Rendiconti della Pontifica Accademia Romana di Archeologia* 87 (2014–2015): 189–291.

Santi, Fabrizio, 2002. "La famiglia Bruschi-Falgari e la sua collezione di antichità etrusche," *Bollettino della Società Tarquiniese d'Arte e Storia* 31: 159–188.

Saunders, J. B. de C. M., 1963. *The Transitions from Ancient Egyptian to Greek Medicine.* Lawrence, KS: University of Kansas Press.

Scarborough, John, 1969. *Roman Medicine.* Ithaca, NY: Cornell University Press.

Scarborough, John, 1979. "Nicander's toxicology, II: spiders, scorpions, insects and myriapods," *Pharmacy in History* 21: 3–34, 73–92.

Scarborough, John, 1985. "Introduction." In John Scarborough, ed., *Symposium on Byzantine Medicine*, ix–xvi. Dumbarton Oaks Papers, No. 38. Dumbarton Oaks Research Library and Collection: Washington, DC.

Scarborough, John, 1986. "Pharmacy in Pliny's *Natural History*: some observations on substances and sources." In Roger French and Frank Greenaway, eds, *Science in the Early Roman Empire: Pliny the Elder, His Sources and Influence*, 59–85. London: Croom Helm.

Scarborough, John, 1987. "Adaptations of folk medicines in the formal materia medica of classical antiquity." In John Scarborough, ed., *Folklore and Folk Medicine*, 21–32. Madison, WI: American Institute of the History of Pharmacy.

Scarborough, John, 1988. "Medical uses of insects [review]." In Gregory J. Higby and John Scarborough, eds, "In the literature," *Pharmacy in History* 30: 200–201.

Scarborough, John, 1990. "Review of *Antike Arztedarstellungen*, by A. Hillert," *Society for Ancient Medicine and Pharmacy: Newsletter* 18: 32–33.

Scarborough, John, 1996. "Drugs and medicines in the Roman world," *Expedition* 38 (2): 38–51.

Scarborough, John, 2000. "The life and times of Alexander Tralles," *Expedition* 39 (2): 51–60.

Scarborough, John, 2006. "More on Dioscorides' Etruscan herbs," *Etruscan News* 6 (Summer): 1, 9.

Scarborough, John and Vivian Nutton, 1982. "The preface of Dioscorides' *Materia Medica*: introduction, translation, commentary," *Transactions and Studies of the College of Physicians of Philadelphia* 4: 187–227.

Scatozza Höricht, Lucia Amalia, 1986. *I Vetri Romani di Ercolano*. Rome: "L'Erma" di Bretschneider.

Scharizer, E., 1961. "Kunstglieder im Altertum," *Monatsschrift für Unfallheiligkunde und Versicherungsmedizin* 64: 468–470.

Scheffer, Charlotte. 2007. "Women in Etruscan tomb-painting, in public roles and personal status." In Lena Larsson Lovén and Agneta Strömberg, eds, *Men and Women in Antiquity. Proceedings of the Third Nordic Symposium on Gender and Women's History in Antiquity (Copenhagen 3–5 October 2003)*, 35–53. Sävedalen: Paul Åströms Förlag.

Schneider, Wolfgang, 1985. *Paracelsus. Neues von seiner Tartarus—Vorlesung (1527/28)*. (Braunschweiger Veröffentlichungen zur Geschichte der Pharmazie und der Naturwissenschaften, Band 29.) Stuutgart: Deutscher Apotheker Verlag.

Schnitman, P. A. and L. B. Shulman (eds), 1979. *Dental Implants: Benefits and Risk (an NIH-Harvard Consensus Development Conference)*. Washington, DC: U.S. Department of Health and Human Services.

Schonack, Wilhelm, 1912. *Die Rezeptsammlung des Scribonius Largus*. Jena: Gustav Fischer.

Schöne, Hermann, 1903. "Zwei Listen Chirurgischer Instrumente," *Hermes* 38: 280–284.

Schortman, Edward M., 1989. "Interregional interaction in prehistory: the need for a new perspective," *American Antiquity* 54: 52–65.

Schwartz, Jeffrey H., Jaymie Brauer, and Penny Gordon-Larsen, 1995. "Brief communication: Tigaran (Point Hope, Alaska) tooth drilling," *American Journal of Physical Anthropology* 97: 77–82.

Schwartz, J. H., F. D. Houghton, L. Bondioli, and R. Macchiarelli, 2015. "Bones, teeth, and estimating age of perinates: Carthaginian infant sacrifice revisited," *Antiquity* 86: 738–745.

Schwartzberg, Lauren, 2014. "The ancient history of grills," *Vice Magazine* December 15. Online: www.vice.com/read/the-ancient-history-of-grills-456 (consulted December 15, 2014).

Schweitzer, G., 1936. *Dieck-Sammlung* (catalogue of the Dieck collection recently purchased by the University of Berlin). March.

Sclafani, Marina, 2010. "Deckel etruskischer Aschenkisten mit Ehepaardarstellungen hellenistischer Zeit." In A. Kieburg and A. Rieger, eds, *Neue Forschungen zu den Etruskern. (Beiträge der Tagung vom 07. bis 09. November 2008 am Archäologischen Institut der Universität Bonn)*, 123–130. (BAR IS 2163.) Oxford: Archaeopress.

Scott, G. Richard and Christy G. Turner II, 1997. *The Anthropology of Modern Human Teeth*. Cambridge Studies in Biological Anthropology 18. Cambridge: Cambridge University Press.

Scribonius Largus, 1983. *Compositiones* [*medicamentorum*], ed. Sergio Sconocchia. Leipzig: B. G. Teubner.

Seguin, Guillaume, Emmanuel d'Incau, Pascal Murail, and Bruno Maureille, 2014. "The earliest dental prosthesis in Celtic Gaul? The case of an Iron Age burial at Le Chêne, France," *Antiquity* 88: 488–500. Online: http://antiquity.ac.uk/ant/088/ant0880488.htm (consulted November 16, 2016).

Seta (see Della Seta).

Sforzini, Clementina, 1985. "Appendice II. Nota bibliografica sulla storia del Museo di Villa Giulia." In P. Pelagatti, ed., "Il museo di Villa Giulia e gli altri musei dell'Etruria Meridionale nell'ultimo triennio," *Studi Etruschi* 51: [511–534] 528–534.

Sgarbi, Vittorio (ed.), 1984. *Tutti i musei d'Italia.* Rozzano: Editoriale Domus.

Shapiro, Arthur K. and Elaine Shapiro, 1997. *The Powerful Placebo: From Ancient Priest to Modern Physician.* Baltimore, MD: Johns Hopkins University Press.

Shaw, R., 1931. "Artificial deformation of teeth: a preliminary report," *South African Journal of Science* 50: 116–121.

Shennan, S. J. (ed.), 1989. *Archaeological Approaches to Cultural Identity.* New York: Routledge.

Sherwin-White, Susan M., 1978. *Ancient Cos: An Historical Study from the Dorian Settlement into the Imperial period.* Göttingen: Vandenhoeck und Ruprecht.

Sigerist, Henry Ernest, 1955. *A History of Medicine,* Volume I. New York: Oxford University Press.

Simms, Ronda, 1995. "Mourning and community at the Athenian Adonia," *The Classical Journal* 93 (2): 121–141.

Simon, C., 1990. "Les restes humains de l'église du Grand-Saconnex, Genève," *Genava* 38: 67–75.

Sineo, Luca, 1996. "Using DNA to study the Etruscans: data from two sites." Paper presented at a conference on DNA Studies in Archaeological Research, organized by A. B. Chiarelli at The University of Rome (June 21).

Singer, R., 1952. "Artificial deformation of teeth," *South African Journal of Science* 50: 116–122.

Sissman, Isaac, 1968. "History of dentistry in Pennsylvania," *Pennsylvania Dental Journal* 35 (3): 5–121.

Small, Jocelyn P., 1971. "The banquet frieze from Poggio Civitate," *Studi Etruschi* 39: 25–61.

Ŝmelhaus, Stanislaus, 1938. "Untersuchungen über altezahnärztliche Instrumente, sowie über Art und Weise der Zahnextraktion." *Zeitschrift für Stomatologie* 36 (heft 23): 1353–1369; (heft 24): 1408–1425.

Ŝmelhaus, Stanislaus, 1939. "Untersuchungen über altezahnärztliche Instrumente, sowie über Art und Weise der Zahnextraktion," *Zeitschrift für Stomatologie* 37 (heft 1): 32–43; (heft 2): 97–106.

Smetánka, Zdeněk, 1988. *Stopa Magického Jednání na Pohřebišti za Jízdárnou Pražského Hradyu: Předběžná zpráva [A Trace of a Magical Procedure in the Early Mediaeval Cemetery Behind the Riding School of the Preague Castle: A Preliminary Report].* Sborník Kruhu přátel Muzea hlavního města Prahy 1: 47–55.

Smith, C. J., 1999. "Medea and Italy: barter and exchange in the archaic Mediterranean." In Gocha R. Tsetskhladze, ed., *Ancient Greeks West and East,* 179–206. Leiden: Brill.

Smith, F. B., 1894. "Method of manipulating gold as practised fifty years ago," *International Dental Journal* 15: 627–628.

Smith, Maurice, 1958. *A Short History of Dentistry*. London: Allan Wingate.

Snow, Dean R., 2013. "Sexual dimorphism in Early Upper Paleolithic cave art," *American Antiquity* 78 (4): 746–761.

Sogliano, A., 1901. "Il borgo marinaro presso il Sarno," *Notizie degli Scavi* 1901: 423–440.

Soranus of Ephesus [Soranus Ephesius], 1927. *Gynaeciorum*, ed. Ioannes Ilberg. *Corpus Medicorum Graecorum*, Volume 4. Leipzig: B. G. Teubner.

Spallicci, A., 1934. *I medici e la medicina in Marziale*. Milano: La Siringa.

Spink, M. S. and G. L. Lewis, 1973. *Albucasis on Surgery and Instruments* (English translation and commentary by Spink and Lewis). Berkeley, CA: University of California Press.

Spivey, Nigel, 1991. "The power of women in Etruscan society," *Accordia Research Papers* 2: 55–67.

Spivey, Nigel, 1995. "Review of *La civiltà di Chiusi e del duo territorio. Atti del XVII Convegno di Studi Etruschi ed Italici (various authors)*," *American Journal of Archaeology* 99: 364–365.

Spivey, Nigel, 1996. "Etruscomania and Etruscosense," *American Journal of Archaeology* 100: 170–173.

St. Hoyme, L. E. and R. T. Koritzer, 1971. "Commentary on prehistoric dentistry," *Dental Radiography and Photography* 44: 65.

Stannard, Jerry, 1974. "Squill in ancient and medieval *Materia Medica*, with special reference to its employment for dropsy," *Bulletin of the New York Academy of Medicine*. Second series, 50: 684–713.

Steinbeck, John, 1947. *The Wayward Bus*. New York: Bantam Books.

Steingräber, S., ed., 1986. *Etruscan Painting: Catalogue Raisonné of Etruscan Wall Painting*. New York: Harcourt Brace Jovanovich/ Johnson Reprints; English edition eds David and Francesca R. Ridgway.

Stermer Beyer-Olsen, Eva Margrete, and Verner Alexandersen, 1994. "Sex assessment of medieval Norwegian skeletons based on permanent tooth crown size," *International Journal of Osteoarchaeology* 5: 274–281.

Stern, W. B., 1994. "On non-destructive analysis of gold objects." In Giulio Morteani and Jeremy P. Northover, eds, *Prehistoric Gold in Europe. Mines Metallurgy and Manufacture*, 317–328. Dordrecht: Kluwer Academic. NATO ASI Series, Series E, Applied Scences Volume 280.

Sternberg, Esther M., 1998. "Unexpected effects: a review of Shapiro and Shapiro [*The Powerful Placebo*, 1997]," *Science* 280: 1901–1902.

Sterpellone, Luciano and Mahmoud Salem Elsheikh, 1990. *La Medicina Araba. L'Arte medica nei Califfati d'Oriente e d'Occidente*. N. p.: Ciba Edizione. (1995 Edition = Origgio [Varese]: Ciba.)

Stocker, Joannes, Adrianus Toll, and Jacques Le Maire, 1657. *Praxis aurea: ad corporis humani morbos omnes, ... Lugduni Batavorum*. Lyon: Adrianus Toll, Maire (from the 1634 second eidtion, by Johann Stockar).

Stoddart, R. W. 2002. "Remains from the sarcophagus of Seianti Hanunia Tlesnasa: pathological evidence and its implications." In J. Swaddling and J. Prag, eds, *Seianti Hanunia Tlesnasa: The Story of an Etruscan Noblewoman*, 29–38. London: British Museum Occasional Paper Number 100.

Stol, M., 1985. "Felix von Oefele and Babylonian medicine," *Janus* 22: 7–16.

Stopponi, Simonetta, 2013. "Orvieto, Campo della Fiera—*Fanum Voltumnae*." In J. M. Turfa, ed., *The Etruscan World*, 632–654. London: Routledge.

Straub, M., 1974. "Johannes Stocker: '*Ad dolorem dentium*'." Medical Dental Dissertation, Tübingen (110 pages).

Strauss, Evelyn, 1992. "New nonopioid painkiller shows promise in animal tests," *Science* 279: 32–33.

Strøm, Ingrid, 1990. "Relations between Etruria and Campania around 700 BC." In Jean-Paul Descoeudres, ed., *Greek Colonists and Native Populations: Proceedings of the First Australian Congress (1989)*, 87–97. Oxford: Clarendon Press.

Strömgren, Hedvig Lidforss, 1919. *Tandläkekonsten Hos Romarna*. Copenhagen: Henrik Koppels.

Strong, D. E. and J. B. Ward-Perkins, 1962. "The Temples of Castor in the Forum Romanum," *Papers of the British School at Rome* 30 (17): 1–30.

Strouhal, Eugen and Rutger Perizonius, 1993. "From Saqqara," *Paleopathology Newsletter* 84 (December): 7.

Sudhoff, Karl, 1908. "Zahnzangen aus der Antike," *Archiv für Geschichte der Medizin* 2 (1): 55–69. Leipzig: Barth.

Sudhoff, Karl, 1917. "Der Stelzfuss aus Capua," *Mitteilungen zur Geschichte der Medizin und der Naturwissenschaften* 16: 291–293.

Sudhoff, Karl, 1921. *Geschichte der Zahnheilkunde, Ein Leitfoden.* First edition. Leipzig: J. A. Barth.

Sudhoff, Karl, 1922. *Geschichte der Medizin.* Berlin: S. Karger.

Sudhoff, Karl, 1926. *Geschichte der Zahnheilkunde.* Second edition. Leipzig: J. A. Barth.

Sutter, Rita, 1996. "Dental museum opens wide," *Maryland in Baltimore (Magazine of the University of Maryland in Baltimore)* Fall: 16–19.

Suzuki, Hisashi, 1982. "Skulls of the Minatogawa Man." In Hisashi Suzuki and Kazuro Hanihara, eds, *The Minatogawa Man*, 7–49. Tokyo: University of Tokyo Press.

Swaddling, J., A. Oddy, and N. Meeks, 1991. "Etruscan and other early gold wire from Italy," *Jewellery Studies* 5: 7–21.

Swaddling, J. and J. Prag (eds) 2002. *Seianti Hanunia Tlesnas: The Story of an Etruscan Noblewoman.* London: British Museum Occasional Paper Number 100.

Szegedy-Maszak, Andrew, 1988. "Sun and stone: images of ancient, heroic times," *Archaeology* 41 (4): 20–31.

Tabanelli, Mario N., 1962. "La odontoiatria." In Mario N. Tabanelli, *La Medicina nel Mondo degli Etruschi*, 92–96. Florence: Leo S. Olschki.

Tabourian, Karekin G., 1932. *Mouth Hygiene.* Beirut: Author, 149 pp. Cited by Clawson (1933: 160 n. 10) as "First treatise on mouth hygiene in Armenia."

Tacuinus [*Tacvini*], (translator), 1532. *Aegritvdinum et Morborum ferme omnium Corporis humani, cum cures eorundem, by Bvhahylyha Byngezla.* Argent: Apud Ioannem Schottum librarium [bound with Abenguefit 1533, q.v.].

Tacuinus [*Tacvini*], 1533. "Domvs Sextadecima, Tacuinorum omniu continens canones introductorios." In *Sex Rervm non naturalium* 7–118. Careno: Sexti (see Abenguefit 1533 for location and details).

Taggart, William Henry, 1907. "A new and accurate method of making gold inlays," *Transactions of the New York Odontological Society*, 1907–1908: 2–14; 14–20 (includes discussion). (Paper presented to the New York Odontological Society in New York City.) Philadelphia: Press of the "Dental Cosmos"—The S. S. White Dental Mfg. Co.

Tallat von Vochenberg, Johannes, 1530. *Artzney: Buchlein der kreutter, wider* [sic] *allerlei kranckeyten und gebrechen der tzeen.* Leipzig: Michael Blum.

Tayles, N., 1996. "Tooth ablation in prehistoric Southeast Asia," *International Journal of Osteoarchaeology* 6 (4): 333–345.

Terribile Weil Marin, V. and Cleto Corrain, 1986. "Su di un esemplare di protesi dentaria totale dei primi dell'800," *Archivio per l'Antropologia e la Etnologia* 106: 227–230.

Terribile Weil Marin, V. and E. M. Cappelletti, 1995. "The embalming process of St. Gregorio Barbarigo [1697]," *Paleopathology Newsletter* 100: 5–7.

Terzioğlu, Arslan and Ilter Uzel, 1986. "Etruskische Goldbandprothese in Westanatolien entdeckt," *Apotheker Journal* 8.12 (December 15): 34–36.

Terzioğlu, Arslan and Ilter Uzel, 1987. "Die Goldbandprothese in etruskischer Technik. Ein neuer Fund aus Westanatolien," *Phillip Journal* 2: 109–112.

Teschler-Nicola, M., 1992. "Sexualdimorphismus der Zahnkronendurchmesser. Ein Beitrag zur Geschlechtsdiagnose subadulter Individuen anhand des frübronzezeitlichen Gräberfeldes von Franzhausen I, Niederösterreich," *Anthropologischer Anzeiger* 50: 51–65.

Teschler-Nicola, M. and Hermann Prossinger, 1998. "Sex determination using tooth dimensions." In Kurt W. Alt, Friedrich W, Rösing, and Maria Teschler-Nicola, eds, *Dental Anthropology: Fundamentals, Limits, and Prospects*, 501–518. Vienna: Springer Verlag.

Teschler-Nicola, M., Michaela Kneissel, Franz Brandstätter, and Hermann Prossinger, 1998. "A recently discovered Etruscan dental bridgework." In Kurt W. Alt, Friedrich W, Rösing, and Maria Teschler-Nicola, eds, *Dental Anthropology: Fundamentals, Limits, and Prospects*, 57–68. Vienna: Springer.

Teschler-Nicola, Maria, M. Berner, K. Kneissel, P. Roschger, and J. Haller, 1994a. "Very early dental bridgework. [Poster abstract]," *Homo* 45 Supplement: 132.

Teschler-Nicola, Maria, M. Berner, K. Kneissel, P. Roschger, F. Brandstätter, K. Wiltschke-Schrotta, and J. Haller, 1994b. "A very early dental bridgework [Poster: data from handouts]," Tenth European Meeting of the Paleopathology Association. Göttingen, Germany, August 29–September 3. Abstracted in *Papers on Paleopathology* (Göttingen Meeting Report, pp. 27–28).

Theophrastus, 1916. *Enquiry into Plants*, Volume 2, trans. Sir Arthur Hort. London: William Heinemann (Loeb Classical Library).

Theophrastus, 1988. *Recherches sur les Plantes* (3 volumes), trans. Suzanne Amigues Paris: Société d'Editions "Les Belles Lettres."

Thierfelder, C., 1987. "Zahnersatz im alten Berlin," *Medizin Aktuell* 13: 585.

Thoma, Kurt H., 1917. "Oral diseases of ancient nations and tribes," *Journal of the Allied Dental Societies* 12: 327–334.

Thompson, C.-J.-S., 1921. "La dentisterie historique au musée d'histoire médicale "Wellcome" à Londres," *La Semaine Dentaire* 3, 36 (September 4): 580–586.

Thompson, R. C. (ed.), 1923. *Assyrian Medical Texts from the Originals in the British Museum*. London: H. Milford and Oxford.

Tingay, Graham I. F. and John Badcock, 1989. *These Were the Romans*. Second edition. Chester Springs, PA: Dufour.

Torino, Marielva, Angelo Menconi, and Gino Fornaciari, 1996. "Le Protesi dentarie etrusche: errori di interpretazione." In Lanmarco Laquidara, ed., *Quaderni internazionali di Storia della Medicina e della Sanità. Numero speciale: Atti del 1 Congresso Nazionale della Società Italiana di Storia dell'Odontostomatologia*, Anno V (1): 119–125. Milan: Società Italiana di Storia dell'Odontostomatologia.

Torino, Marielva, Angelo Menconi, and Gino Fornaciari, 1997. "Le protesi dentarie auree nei gruppi umani a cultura Etrusca: nuove acquisizioni." In *Atti del XIX Convegno di Studi Etruschi ed Italici (Volterra, 15–19 ottobre 1995): Aspetti della cultura di*

Volterra etrusca fra l'età del ferro e l'età ellenistica e Contributi della ricerca antropologica alla conoscenza del popolo etrusco, 535–544. Florence: Olschki 1997.

Torrey, Charles C., 1920. "A Phoenician Necropolis at Sidon," *Annual of the American School of Oriental Research in Jerusalem* I (1919–1920): 1–27.

Touwaide, Alain, 1998. "Bibliographie historique de la botanique Textes Médicaux Antiques," *Lettre d'informations (Centre Jean-Palerne)* 31: 2–65.

Treggiari, Susan M., 1978. "Rome: urban labour." In *Seventh International Economic History Conference, Edinburgh 1978*, 162–165. Tonbridge, UK: Lewis Reprints, Ltd.

Treggiari, Susan M., 1979. "Lower class women in the Roman economy," *Florilegium* I: 65–86.

Treggiari, Susan M., 1981. "Urban labour in Rome: *Mercennarii* and *Tabernarii*." In Peter Garnsey, ed., *Non-Slave Labour in the Greco-Roman World*, 48–64. Cambridge: Cambridge Philological Society, Supplementary Volume no. 6.

Trillou, J.-A., 1976. "La prothèse dentaire égyptienne: mythe où réalite'?" *Le Chirurgien-Dentiste de France* (March 24): 59–60.

Trogmayer, Otto, 1960–1962. "I magyar temető Békésen," *Mora Ferenc Muzeum Evkonyve [Ertesitóje]* X–XII: 9–38.

Turfa, Jean MacIntosh, 1994. "Anatomical votives and Italian medical traditions." In Richard Daniel De Puma and Jocelyn Penny Small, eds, *Murlo and the Etruscans: Art and Society in Ancient Etruria*, 224–240. Madison, WI: University of Wisconsin Press.

Turfa, Jean MacIntosh, 2004. "[Weigeschenke: Altitalien und Imperium Romanum. 1. Italien.] B. Anatomical votives." In *Thesaurus Cultus et Rituum Antiquorum (ThesCRA) I. Processions—Sacrifices—Libations—Fumigations—Dedications*, 359–368. Los Angeles, CA: Getty Publications (and LIMC).

Turfa, Jean MacIntosh, 2005. *Catalogue of the Etruscan Gallery of the University of Pennsylvania Museum of Archaeology and Anthropology*. Philadelphia, PA: University Museum Press.

Turfa, Jean MacIntosh, 2006. "Etruscan religion at the watershed: before and after the fourth century BC." In P. Harvey and C. Schultz, eds, *Religion in Republican Italy* (Papers of Conference, New Haven, February 2003), 62–89. *Yale Classical Studies* 33. Cambridge: Cambridge University Press.

Turfa, Jean MacIntosh, 2009. "From the tombs of Bisenzio." In Stefano Bruni, ed., *Etruria e Italia Preromana. Studi in onore di Giovannangelo Camporeale*, Volume II, 525–533. Rome: Fabrizio Serra Editore.

Turfa, Jean MacIntosh, 2012a. "Buried in the height of fashion," *Expedition* 54(2): 7–9.

Turfa, Jean MacIntosh, 2012b. *Divining the Etruscan World: The Brontoscopic Calendar and Religious Practice*. Cambridge: Cambridge University Press.

Turfa, Jean MacIntosh, in press. *Catalogue of the Etruscan and Italic Collection in the World Museum Liverpool*, ed. Georgina Muskett.

Turfa, Jean MacIntosh, 2016. "The *Obesus Etruscus*: can the trope be true?" In S. Bell and A. Carpino, eds, *A Companion to the Etruscans*, 321–335. Oxford: Wiley-Blackwell.

Turfa, Jean MacIntosh and M. J. Becker, 2013. "Health and medicine in Etruria." In J. M. Turfa, ed., *The Etruscan World*, 855–881. London: Routledge.

Turner, Christy G., 1995. "Dental transfigurement and its potential for explaining the evolution of post-archaic Indian culture in the American Southwest," *Dental Anthropology* 14 (1): 1–6.

Ubelaker, Douglas H., 1996. "Skeletons testify: anthropology in forensic science," *Yearbook of Physical Anthropology* 39: 229–244.

Underwood, E. Ashworth (ed.), 1953. *Science, Medicine and History: Essays on the Evolution of Scientific Thought and Medical Practice* (2 volumes). London: Oxford University Press.

Ungar, Peter S., Frederick E. Grine, Mark F. Teaford, and Alejandro Pérez-Pérez, 2001. "A review of interproximal wear grooves on fossil hominin teeth with new evidence from Olduvai Gorge," *Archives of Oral Biology* 46: 285–292.

United Press International, 1997. "Bulgarian scientist gets Roman teeth," *UPI News Release* January 13.

United States Customs Laboratory, 1998. *Gold Fineness in Articles of Jewelry. United States Customs Laboratory Methods, USCL Manual 71-04.*

Vallois, H. V., 1971. "Le crâne-trophée capsien de Faïd Souar II, Algérie (Fouilles La place, 1954)," *L'Anthropologie* 75 (3–6): 191–220.

van der Ghinst, J. (see Ghinst).

van der Meer, L. Bouke, 1987. *The Bronze Liver of Piacenza: Analysis of a Polytheistic Structure.* Amsterdam: J. C. Gieben.

Van Marter, James Gilbert, 1885a. "Some evidences of prehistoric dentistry in Italy," *Independent Practitioner* 6: 1–5 (preceeded by plates).

Van Marter, James Gilbert, 1885b. "Prehistoric dentistry," *Archives of Dentistry* 2: 87–89 (brief summary of 1885a).

Van Marter, James Gilbert, 1885c. "Dell'odontojatria nei tempi antichi" [unsigned], *Giornale di Corrispondenza per Dentisti* 14: 227–231.

Van Marter, James Gilbert, 1886. "Further evidences of prehistoric dentistry," *Independent Practitioner* 7: 57–61, and plate.

Van Marter, James Gilbert, 1889. "Prehistoric dentistry: bridge work," *Dental Register* 43: 261.

Vargiu, R. and M. J. Becker, 2005. "Appendice: studio antropologico dei resti scheletrici umani." In M. Cataldi, "Sulle 'tombe a buca' di Tarquinia," 395–409. In *Dinamiche di sviluppo delle città nell'Etruria Meridionale. Veio, Caere, Tarquinia, Vulci. Atti del XXIII Convegno di Studi Etruschi ed Italici (1–6 ottobre 2001)*, 409–411. Pisa-Rome: Istituti Editoriali e Poligrafici Internazionali.

Vaûte, A., 1995. "Some experiences with the analysis of gold objects." In Giulio Morteani and Jeremy P. Northover, eds, *Prehistoric Gold in Europe: Mines Metallurgy and Manufacture*, 329–339. Dordrecht: Kluwer Academic. NATO ASI Series, Series E, Applied Scences Volume 280.

Verderame, Lorenzo, 1997. *A Bibliography of Ancient Mesopotamian Medicine.* Rome: University of Rome "La Sapienza."

Verger-Pratoucy, Jean-Claude, 1966. "Les rétentions dentaires préhistoriques," *Bulletin du Groupement International pour la Recherche Scientifique en Stomatologie et Odontologie* (Bruxelles) 4 (October): 457–469.

Verger-Pratoucy, Jean-Claude, 1968. "Recherches sur les mutilations dentaires pre-historiques." Thèse Doctorat en Médicine No. 179. Faculté Médicine et Pharmacie, Université de Bordeaux.

Verger-Pratoucy, Jean-Claude, 1975. "Histoire des Extractions Dentaires: Mise au Point Concernant la Période Préhistorique," *Actualités Odontostomatologiques* 111: 421–428.

Verger-Pratoucy, Jean-Claude, 1985. "Odontologie." In *La Prospection Archeologique de la Vallee du Nil, Facicle 15: Necropole de Missiminia*, 121–132. Paris: Editions du CNRS.

Verger-Pratoucy, Jean-Claude, 1995. "Un héros de la guerre d'indépendance américaine, premier odontologiste 'medico-légal'," *Information Dentaire* 5 (February 2): 355–358.

Vidal, François, 1983. "La pharmacologie bucco-dentaire au temps d'Auguste," *Le Chirurgien Dentiste de France* 194 (March 10): 21–30.

Vidal, François, 1984. "Caelius Aurelianus et la douleur dentaire '*de dolore dentium*'," *L'Information Dentaire* 28 (12/7): 2875–2888.

Villamil, Edgard (ed.), 1994. "Sonrisa etrusca. Ágina Rápida," *La Prensa [Honduras]* May 29.

Villard, Laurence, 1992. "Les vases dans la Collection Hippocratique: vocabulaire et usage," *Bulletin de Correspondance Hellénique* 116: 73–96.

Villard, Laurence and Francine Blondé, 1992. "Sur quelques vases présents dans la Collection Hippocratique: Confrontation des Données littéraires et archéologiques," *Bulletin de Correspondance Hellénique* 116: 97–117.

Vincenti, Valentina, 2009. *La Tomba Bruschi di Tarquinia*. Rome: Giorgio Bretschneider.

Vogel, G. and G. Gambacorta (eds), 1985. *Storia della odontoiatria*. Milan: Ars Medica Antiqua.

von Brunn, W., 1926. "Der Stelzfuss von Capua und die antiken Prothesen," *Archiv für Geschichte der Medizin* 18: 351–360 (Tafel XIII).

von Deines, H., H. Grapow, and W. Westendorf, 1958a. *Ubersetsung der medizinischen Texte*. Volume IV, 1 of *Grundriss der Medizin der alten Agypter*. Berlin: Akademie-Verlag.

von Deines, H., H. Grapow, and W. Westendorf, 1958b. *Ubersetsung der medizinischen Texte Erläuterungen*. Volume IV, 2 of *Grundriss der Medizin der alten Agypter*. Berlin: Akademie-Verlag.

von Hase, Friedrich-Wilhelm, 1976. "Palestrina (Praeneste), entry on gold from Bernadini Tomb." In G. Colonna, G. Bartoloni, E. Colonna di Paulo, and F. Melis, eds, *Civiltà del Lazio primitivo* (exhibition catalogue, Palazzo delle Esposizioni, Roma), 226–233. Rome: Multigrafica.

Waarsenburg, Demetrius J., 1991a. "*Auro dentes iuncti*: an inquiry into the study of the Etruscan dental prosthesis." In Marijka Gnade, ed., *Stips Votiva*, 241–247. Amsterdam: Allard Pierson Museum, University of Amsterdam.

Waarsenburg, Demetrius J., 1991b. "De Schedel van Plinius Maior," *Hermenevs (Tijdschrift voor antieke cultuur)* 63 (1): 39–43.

Waarsenburg, Demetrius J., 1994. "The northwest Necropolis of Satricum: an Iron Age cemetery in Latium Vetus." Doctoral Dissertation, Faculty of Letters, University of Amsterdam.

Waarsenburg, Demetrius J., 1995. *The Northwest Necropolis of Satricum: An Iron Age Cemetery in Latium Vetus*. (Scrinium VIII, Satricum III.) Amsterdam: Thesis Publishers.

Wade, A. D., J. Hurnanen, B. Lawson, D. Tampieri, and A. J. Nelson. 2012. "Early dental intervention in the Redpath Ptolemaic Theban male," *International Journal of Paleopathology* 2 (2012): 217–222.

Waite, W. H., 1885a. "Association intelligence, Western counties' branch [Letter; discussion]," *Journal of the British Dental Association [now British Dental Journal]* 6: 316–317; 499–512, and 2 figures.

Waite, W. H., 1885b. "Pre-historic dentistry, specimens exhibited," *The Dental Record* 5: 442–443.

Wallace, Rex E., 2008. *ZIKH RASNA. A Manual of the Etruscan Language and Inscriptions*. Ann Arbor, MI and New York: Beech Stave Press.

Wallace-Hadrill, Andrew, 1990. "The social spread of Roman luxury: sampling Pompeii and Herculaneum," *Papers of the British School at Rome* 58: 145–192.

Ward, G., 1962. "The origins of dental prosthesis: an outline," *British Dental Journal* 112 (1): 10–11.

Warmington, E. H. (ed. and trans.), 1938. *Remains of Old Latin. Volume III: Lucilius. The Twelve Tables*. Cambridge, MA: Harvard University Press (reprinted 1967).

Waters, Harold Orlan, 1998. "Letter to the editor," *The New Yorker* 74 (35): 7.

Weege, Fritz, 1913. "Das Museum der Villa Papa Giulio." In Wolfgang Helbig and W. Amelung, eds, *Führer durch die öffentlichen Sammlungen klassicher Altertümer in Rom*. Third edition. Volume II: 312–381. Leipzig: B. G. Teubner.

Weinberger, Bernhard Wolf, 1940. "Did dentistry evolve from the barbers, blacksmiths or from medicine?" *Bulletin of the History of Medicine* 8: 970, 976, 978–979.

Weinberger, Bernhard Wolf, 1941. "The Etruscan cast 'gold' crowns illustrated by Guerini," *Journal of the American Dental Association* 28: 1853–1854.

Weinberger, Bernhard Wolf, 1946. "Further evidence that dentistry was practiced in ancient Egypt, Phoenicia, and Greece," *Bulletin of the History of Medicine* 20: 188–195.

Weinberger, Bernhard Wolf, 1947. "The dental art in ancient Egypt," *Journal of the American Dental Association* 34 (3): 170–184.

Weinberger, Bernhard Wolf, 1948. *An Introduction to the History of Dentistry*. Volume 1. Saint Louis: C. V. Mosby (special edition by Gryphon Editions in Birmingham, Alabama, 1981).

Weisgerber, G. and E. Pernicka, 1995. "Ore mining in prehistoric Europe: an overview." In Giulio Morteani and Jeremy P. Northover, eds, *Prehistoric Gold in Europe: Mines Metallurgy and Manufacture*, 159–182. Dordrecht: Kluwer Academic. NATO ASI Series, Series E, Applied Scences Volume 280.

Weiss, Morris M., 1989. "Etruscan medicine," *Journal of Paleopathology* 2: 129–164.

West, Margaret, Andrew T. Ellis, Philip J. Potts, Christina Strelic, Christine Vanhoof, Dariusz Wegrzynek, and Peter Wobrauschek, 2012. "Atomic spectrometry update: X-ray fluorescence spectrometry," *Journal of Analytical Atomic Spectrometry* 27: 1603–1644.

Wharton, Edith, 1938. *The Buccaneers*. New York: D. Appleton-Century (see Book 2, Section 10).

White, Tim D., David Degusta, Gary D. Richards, and Steven G. Baker, 1997. "Brief communication: prehistoric dentistry in the American Southwest: a drilled canine from Sky Aerie in Colorado," *American Journal of Physical Anthropology* 103: 409–414.

Whitehouse, Ruth, 1992. "Tools the manmaker: the cultural construction of gender in Italian prehistory," *Journal of the Accordia Research Center* 3: 41–54.

Whittaker, D. K., 1993. "Oral health." In T. Molleson and M. Cox, eds, *The Spitalfields Project. Volume 2: The Anthropology. The Middling Sort*, 49–65. London: Council for British Archaeology.

Wilkinson, Richard H. 1994. *Symbol and Magic in Ancient Egypt*. London: Thames and Hudson.

Willis, M. S., L. E. Harris and P. J. Hergenrader, 2008. "On traditional dental extraction: case reports from Dinka and Nuer en route to restoration," *British Dental Journal* 204: 121–124.

Witcher, Rob, 2000. "Two regions, one hinterland: the Tiber Valley project." Paper presented in the session "Comparative survey archaeology," organized by Peter Attema and Rob Witcher. European Conference of Archaeology 2000. Lisbon.

Woodforde, John, 1967. *The Strange Story of False Teeth*. London: Routledge and K. Paul (1970 edition New York: Universe Books).

Zarb, G. A. and A. Schmitt, 1990. "The longitudinal clinical effectiveness of osseointegrated dental implants: the Toronto Study. Part III: problems and complications encountered," *Journal of Prosthetic Dentistry* 64 (2): 185–194.

Zarb, G. A. and A. Schmitt, 1992. "Osseointegration and the edentulous predicament: the 10-year-old Toronto study," *British Dental Journal* 172 (4): 135.

Zias, Joe E., 1993. "*Cannabis sativa* (hashish) as an effective medicine: the anthropological evidence [abstract]," *American Journal of Physical Anthropology*, Supplement 16: 215.

Zias, Joseph and Karen Numeroff, 1986a. "Case reports on paleopathology: no. 7," *Paleopathology Newsletter* 53 (March): 10–11.

Zias, Joseph and Karen Numeroff, 1986b. "Ancient dentistry in the Eastern Mediterranean: a brief review," *Israel Exploration Journal* 36: 65–67.

Zias, Joseph and Karen Numeroff, 1987. "Operative dentistry in the second century BCE," *Journal of the American Dental Association* 114: 665–666.

Zias, J. and Rosemary Powers, 1989. "Operative dentistry in the second century BCE (discussion ed. Eve Cockburn)," *Paleopathology Newsletter* 65: 11.

Index

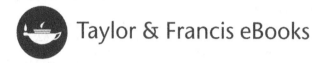

Milton Keynes UK
Ingram Content Group UK Ltd.
UKHW021843071024
449327UK00021B/1535

9 780367 595326